SECOND EDITION

DIFFERENTIAL DIAGNOSIS IN PEDIATRIC RADIOLOGY

SECOND EDITION

DIFFERENTIAL DIAGNOSIS IN PEDIATRIC RADIOLOGY

LEONARD E. SWISCHUK, M.D.

Professor of Radiology and Pediatrics
Director of Pediatric Radiology
Department of Radiology
University of Texas Medical Branch
Children's Hospital
Galveston, Texas

SUSAN D. JOHN, M.D.

Associate Professor of Radiology and Pediatrics
Department of Radiology
University of Texas Medical Branch
Children's Hospital
Galveston, Texas

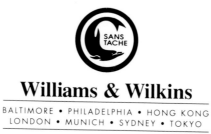

Williams & Wilkins

BALTIMORE • PHILADELPHIA • HONG KONG
LONDON • MUNICH • SYDNEY • TOKYO

A WAVERLY COMPANY

Editor: Charles W. Mitchell
Managing Editor: Marjorie Kidd Keating
Production Coordinator: Anne Stewart Seitz
Copy Editor: Carol Zimmerman
Designer: Norman W. Och
Illustration Planner: Wayne Hubbel

Copyright © 1995
Williams & Wilkins
428 East Preston Street
Baltimore, Maryland 21202, USA

Accurate indications, adverse reactions, and dosage schedules for drugs are provided in this book, but it is possible that they may change. The reader is urged to review the package information data of the manufacturers of the medications mentioned.

Printed in the United States of America

Chapter reprints are available from the Publisher.
First Edition 1984

Library of Congress Cataloging in Publication Data

Swischuk, Leonard E., 1937–
 Differential diagnosis in pediatric radiology / Leonard E.
Swischuk, Susan D. John.—2nd ed.
  p.   cm.
 Includes bibliographical references and index.
 ISBN 0-683-08046-6
  1. Pediatric radiology. 2. Children—Diseases—Diagnosis.
 3. Diagnosis, Differential. I. John, Susan D. II. Title.
  [D NLM: 1. Radiography—in infancy & childhood. 2. Diagnosis,
 Differential—in infancy & childhood. WN 240 S978d 1995]
RJ50.R3S89 1995
618.92′007572—dc20
DNLM/DLC
for Library of Congress   94-22469 CIP

DEDICATION

To my Wife and Best Friend,

JANIE

Leonard E. Swischuk, M.D.

To my Husband and Children,

DARRELL, DAVID AND DANIEL

Susan D. John M.D.

PREFACE

Since the publication of the First Edition of Differential Diagnosis in Pediatric Radiology, diagnostic imaging has undergone a veritable explosion in the number of available imaging modalities. Before embarking upon the second edition, we had to confront the problem of how far we wished to venture into the differential diagnoses of the findings seen with these new modalities. As we considered the day-to-day practice of pediatric diagnosis at our institution, it became clear that plain radiographs continue to provide crucial information in the early stages of diagnosing disease in children, and proper interpretation is pivotal in directing further diagnostic work-ups that can be both complex and expensive. In addition, because radiologists in training are now spending a larger percentage of their time learning to perform and interpret these more complex imaging studies, plain film interpretation skills are often given a lower priority. This is especially true in those areas where more sophisticated imaging has come to play a dominant role after plain films (e.g., brain, spinal cord, mediastinum). We therefore decided to keep plain radiograph diagnosis as the central focus of this text, with the addition of ultrasound, computerized tomography, or magnetic resonance imaging in specific areas where they are crucial to the diagnosis. Only in the chapter on the abdomen, where ultrasound has become a common screening examination for many abdominal problems, did we provide differential diagnoses for the various findings encountered. Our goal for this edition was to update the text, illustrations, and tables of differential diagnoses to include newly described entities and, when applicable, to discuss the role of the plain radiograph amidst the wide variety of available imaging techniques that can now be used to diagnose pathology in children.

We would like to thank our secretaries, Carmen Floeck and Thelma Sanchez, and our photographers, John Ellis and Lora Hofer, for their perseverance and assistance in preparing this book. The production of a book is dependent on the help of many individuals and with a radiology publication, manuscript and illustration preparation must be of the first order. We are extremely fortunate to have these people work with us.

Leonard E. Swischuk, M.D.
Susan D. John, M.D.

CONTENTS

CHAPTER 2—FACE, SINUSES, MASTOIDS, AND NECK

CHAPTER 3—ABDOMEN

CHAPTER 4—BONES AND SOFT TISSUES

CHAPTER 5—HEAD

CHAPTER 6—THE SPINE

Aeration Disturbances

BILATERAL OVERAERATION

Generally, bilateral overaeration of the lungs results from overly deep inspiratory efforts or expiratory obstruction (emphysema) of the lungs (Table 1.1). In terms of an overly deep inspiratory effort, the problem often simply is that of an overexuberant normal breath, accentuated by a voluntary Valsalva maneuver. What happens is that the technician tells the child to take a deep breath and "hold it," and in response, the patient performs a Valsalva maneuver. In infants, the same phenomenon occurs just before a cry. Fortunately, such artifactual overaeration usually is more pronounced on one view of the chest than the other, and in this way, one can determine that overaeration is not fixed. This is important because, if overaeration is fixed, further evaluation of the problem is required.

Another cause of bilateral, nonobstructive overinflation of the lungs is air hunger, a phenomenon present in patients who are oxygen deficient. In such patients, as long as pulmonary compliance is relatively normal, overbreathing to adequately oxygenate the blood leads to overdistended lungs. This most commonly occurs in patients with cyanotic heart disease. Another form of "air hunger" occurs in the acidotic infant, and actually, this situation is more common than that which occurs with hypoxemia. Acidotic patients, in an attempt to blow off excessive carbon dioxide, "overbreathe" and overinflate their lungs (Fig. 1.1). The finding, of course, is nonspecific and can occur with any number of metabolic disturbances leading to acidosis, but in the pediatric patient (especially the infant), it most commonly is due

to diarrhea and severe dehydration (9). These patients also tend to demonstrate transient microcardia (10) and decreased pulmonary blood flow due to the low blood volume induced by the severe degree of fluid loss. Such decreased blood flow causes the pulmonary blood vessels to be smaller than normal, the lungs to be oligemic, and hyperlucency to be even more pronounced (9).

Table 1.1
Bilateral Overaeration

Nonobstructive overation	
Overexuberant inspiration Air hunger-dehydration-acidosis	} Very common
Air hunger-cyanotic heart disease	} Moderately common
Obstructive emphysema (peripheral)	
Viral lower respiratory tract infection (bronchitis, bronchiolitis)	} Very common
Asthma Cystic fibrosis	} Common
Immunologic deficiency Thermal bronchiolitis Cutis laxa Antitrypsin deficiency Multiple peripheral F.B. Graft-vs.-host bronchiolitis	} Rare
Obstructive emphysema (central)	
Vascular ring	} Moderately common
Mediastinal mass or cyst Enlarged lymph nodes Laryngotracheal foreign body	} Uncommon
Endotracheal mass	} Rare

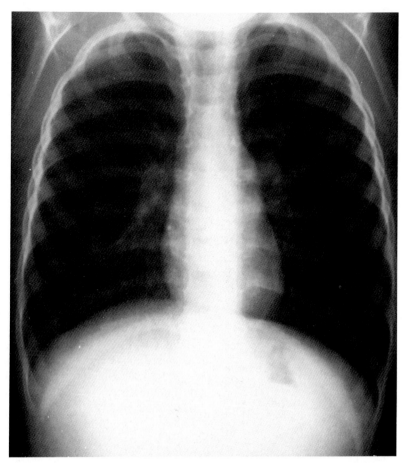

Figure 1.1. Overaeration due to dehydration. Note the overdistended but clear lungs. Also note that the heart is smaller than normal (dehydration causes microcardia).

When airway obstruction is the cause of overaeration, increased lung size and radiolucency are more fixed, and the obstruction can be central (trachea or upper airway) or peripheral (bronchial). Central obstruction is far less common, but when it occurs the obstruction usually is located from somewhere just below the glottis to the carina. Obstructions above this level tend to cause underaeration more than overaeration (i.e., inspiratory obstruction predominates). With peripheral obstruction, air trapping is diffuse and the lungs become larger and radiolucent. Clinically, these patients often demonstrate expiratory wheezing.

Central obstruction usually is caused by extratracheal compressive lesions, for endotracheal lesions such as inflammatory granulomas, tumors, foreign bodies, tracheal stenoses (congenital or acquired), and ectopic endotracheal thyroid tissue are relatively rare. Extratracheal lesions causing airway compression include entities such as abnormal blood vessels, mediastinal cysts or tumors (primary and secondary), and enlarged lymph nodes (inflammatory or tumorous).

In terms of vascular abnormalities, congenital anomalies rather than acquired aneurysms or other dilations are the usual problem. Most often, one is dealing with a true vascular ring, and the main radiographic clue to its presence is a right-side aortic arch (Fig. 1.2). The reason for this is that in the two most common vascular rings (double aortic arch and right side aorta with aberrant left subclavian artery and ligamentum arteriosum or ductus arteriosus), a right aortic arch is present. With double aortic arch, the two arches encircle the trachea and esophagus, while with aberrant left subclavian artery, the right aortic arch, in combination with the aberrant left subclavian artery traveling behind the esophagus and the ligamentum arteriosum or ductus arteriosus extending from the left subclavian artery to the pulmonary artery, constitute the ring (Fig. 1.2). **Thus, if the aortic arch is on the left, a vascular ring causing airway obstruction is a very remote possibility.**

A right aortic arch produces one or more of the following findings: deviation of the trachea to the left, ipsilateral indentation and compression of the trachea, and a right paratracheal mass or lump. This latter finding, of course, represents the aortic knob which, with right aortic arch, usually is somewhat higher in position than it would be if it were normal and on the left. In addition, there is absence of the aortic knob on the left, and on lateral view, when a vascular ring exists, anterior tracheal deviation also may occur. Unfortunately, not all of these findings are clearly present in all patients.

After these observations are made, confirmation of the presence of a vascular ring is best accomplished with a barium esophagram, where the vessels comprising the ring produce opposing indentations on the esophagus. Occasionally, these indentations lie directly across from one another, but more often, they are offset, producing a reverse-S configuration (Fig. 1.2*B*). Posterior indentation of the esophagus also is present, but since such indentation can be seen with other asymptomatic arterial anomalies, it is the reverse-S configuration that is most important

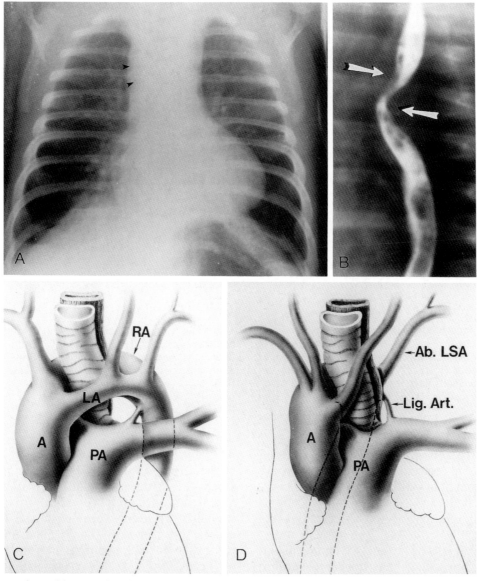

Figure 1.2. Overaeration with vascular ring. A. Frontal view demonstrating marked overaeration of both lungs. **B.** Barium swallow demonstrating characteristic reverse-S indentation of the esophagus *(arrows)*. In other cases, the indentations lie directly across from each other. **C. Double aortic arch.** Note the two arches of the aorta; the right *(RA)* usually is larger and higher than the left *(LA)*. Both unite behind the esophagus and the resultant encircling ring is obvious. Aorta *(A)*, pulmonary artery *(PA)*. **D. Right aortic arch with aberrant left subclavian artery and ligamentum arteriosum or ductus arteriosus.** The ring in this anomaly is completed by the ligamentum arteriosum *(Lig. Art.)* or patent ductus arteriosus, which connects the aberrant left subclavian *(Ab. LSA)* artery (passing behind the esophagus) with the left pulmonary artery (passing in front of the trachea). Aorta *(A)*, pulmonary artery *(PA)*.

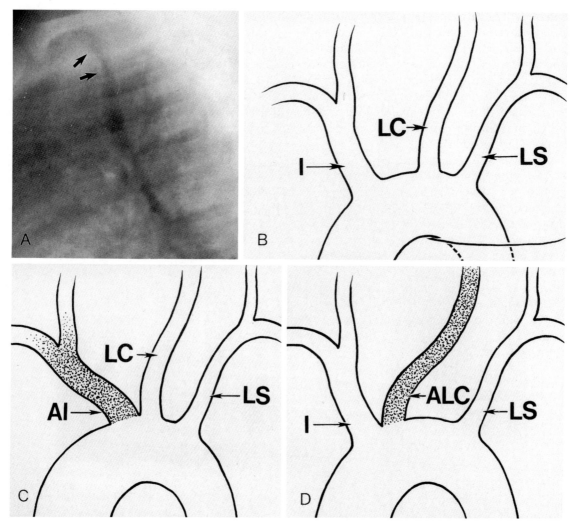

Figure 1.3. Anomalous innominate or left common carotid artery. A. Note the characteristic anterior indentation and posterior displacement of the trachea *(arrows)* that can be produced by either one of these anomalies. The anomalous innominate artery is much more common, but in both conditions the indentation most often is asymptomatic. **B. Normal arrangement of vessels.** Note normal separation of the three great arteries; the innominate *(I)*, left common carotid *(LC)*, and left subclavian *(LS)* arteries. **C. Anomalous innominate** *(AI)* artery. The innominate artery arises too far to the left. **D. Anomalous left common carotid** *(ALC)* artery. The left carotid artery arises too far to the right.

to note. Classically, aortography was used for the definitive diagnosis of vascular rings, however, magnetic resonance imaging (MRI) has become an excellent method for demonstrating both the anomalous vessels and their relationship to the narrowed trachea (2) (see Fig. 1.37).

In other patients with obstructing vascular anomalies, anterior compression of the trachea is encountered on lateral chest films. Although controversy exists regarding the cause of this compression, in most cases it is most likely due to a slightly anomalous origin of either the innominate or left common carotid artery (Fig. 1.3). The former is much more common, but even then, most of these cases produce

no symptoms (10). Occasionally, severe obstruction of the airway results (1), but the finding of anterior tracheal indentation should be treated with caution, and significance attached only if other causes of airway obstruction have been excluded. Although bronchoscopy can identify the tracheal narrowing, demonstration of the anomaly is best accomplished with MRI (13). MRI shows the relationship of the mediastinal vessels to the narrowed trachea without exposure to ionizing radiation or intravascular contrast material (4). Although surgical intervention often is not required, severe cases are treated by surgically tacking the anomalous artery to the posterior surface of the sternum. This procedure frequently is less than completely corrective since the original compression of the trachea usually results in some degree of focal tracheomalacia. It is this associated problem that can cause lingering airway obstruction even after the vessel is lifted off the trachea. Fortunately, in most cases, by the age of 4 or 5 years, the child outgrows the problem and the indentation and symptoms disappear. Anterior tracheal indentation is not seen in older children (1).

Mediastinal cysts, tumors, or enlarged lymph nodes causing compression of the airway usually are identified by the unilateral or bilateral mediastinal widening that they produce. In addition, compression and deformity of the tracheal air column are seen, but overall, the plain film findings are nonspecific. Barium esophagrams also usually are nonspecific, and eventually one must employ procedures such as MRI, computerized tomography (CT), aortography, or I^{131} isotope studies (thyroid masses) for final delineation. Bronchography seldom is necessary in the investigation of these lesions.

Obstructive emphysema secondary to widespread peripheral bronchial or bronchiolar obstruction classically occurs in viral lower respiratory tract infection (including infantile bronchiolitis), asthma, and cystic fibrosis (3, 6) (Fig. 1.4). With viral lower respiratory tract infection, one of the main problems is

bronchitis associated with bronchospasm. Bronchial inflammation leads to mucosal edema, hypersensitive bronchi with exaggerated expiratory constriction and air-trapping, and obstructive emphysema. The entire problem is seen in its worst form with acute infantile bronchiolitis. Indeed, in the most severe cases, the lungs hardly change in size between inspiration and expiration; the thoracic cage is grossly overdistended and the diaphragmatic leaflets are flattened or even slightly inverted. Parahilar, peribronchial infiltrates along with segmental and lobar atelectasis also commonly occur. To a lesser extent, similar peripheral bronchial obstruction with parahilar, peribronchial infiltration occurs with viral lower respiratory tract infections throughout childhood, but it is the infant with bronchiolitis (0 to 2 years of age with peak incidence around 6 months) who demonstrates overaeration most profoundly.

Findings similar to those seen with viral bronchiolitis also can be seen in infants with cystic fibrosis, and actually, it is not uncommon for these infants to present with a bronchiolitis-like picture on a number of occasions before the proper diagnosis is established. Asthma, chronic aspiration, certain immunologic deficiency problems, and graft-vs.-host disease (5) also produce generalized overaeration and parahilar, peribronchial infiltrates.

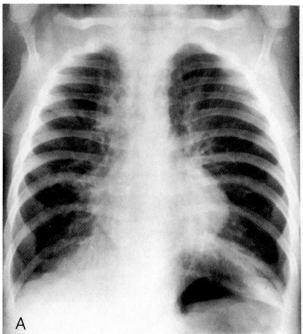 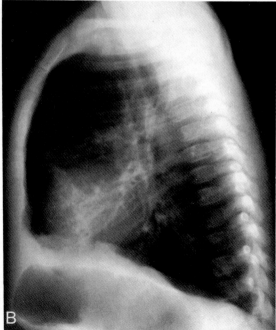

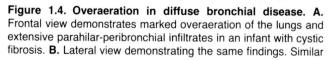

Figure 1.4. Overaeration in diffuse bronchial disease. A. Frontal view demonstrates marked overaeration of the lungs and extensive parahilar-peribronchial infiltrates in an infant with cystic fibrosis. **B.** Lateral view demonstrating the same findings. Similar findings can be seen in patients with viral lower respiratory tract infection and asthma. In bronchiolitis, often there is less parahilar-peribronchial infiltration.

Generalized overaeration due to bronchial or bronchiolar constriction, generally unassociated with pulmonary infiltrates, is seen with α_1-antitrypsin deficiency (12), congenital cutis laxa (8), and thermal bronchiolar damage secondary to smoke or hot air inhalation. Occasionally, multiple foreign body fragments can be inhaled into numerous bronchi (11), resulting in diffuse bilateral air-trapping. All of these conditions are rather rare, however.

Finally, a word regarding **intercostal bulging and cervical herniation of the lungs,** as seen with obstructive emphysema, is in order. It is true that such bulging of the lungs through the various soft tissue spaces of the thoracic cage occurs with obstructive emphysema, but it also can be seen in a normal infant performing a Valsalva maneuver, just before starting to cry. In addition, although **flattening of the diaphragmatic leaflets is a common feature of obstructive emphysema, to a degree, it also can be seen in nonobstructive overaeration. Most often, this also occurs in the normal patient performing a voluntary Valsalva maneuver.** Consequently, before one accepts flattening of the diaphragmatic leaflets as a definite finding, one should be sure that it is present on both views. Only then can one be certain that it is due to fixed airway obstruction.

REFERENCES

1. Berdon WD, Baker DH, Bordiuk J, Mellins R: Innominate artery compression of trachea in infants with stridor and apnea. *Radiology* 92:272–278, 1969.
2. Bisset GS, Strife JL, Kirks DR, Bailey WW: Vascular rings: MR imaging. *AJR* 149:251–256. 1987.
3. Eggleston PA, Ward BH, Pierson WE, Bierman CW: Radiographic abnormalities in acute asthma in children. *Pediatrics* 54:442–449, 1974.
4. Fletcher BD, Cohn RC: Tracheal compression and the innominate artery: MR evaluation in infants. *Radiology* 170:103, 1989.
5. Johnson FL, Stokes DC, Gruggiero M, Dalla-Pozza L, Callihan TR: Chronic obstructive disease after bone marrow transplantation. *J Pediatr* 105:370–376, 1984.
6. Kirkpatrick JA, Wagner ML: Roentgen manifestations of bronchiolitic inflammatory disease. *Pediatr Clin North Am* 10:633–642, 1963.
7. Koch DA: Roentgenologic considerations of capillary bronchiolitis. *AJR* 82:433–436, 1959.
8. Merton DF, Rooney R: Progressive pulmonary emphysema associated with congenital generalized elastolysis (cutis laxa). *Radiology* 113:691–692, 1974.
9. Nathan MH: Diagnosis of dehydration, acidosis, and gastroenteritis in infants from chest radiography. *Radiology* 83:297–305, 1964.
10. Swischuk LE: Microcardia: an uncommon diagnostic problem. *Am J Roentgenol Radium Ther Nucl Med* 103:115–118, 1968.
11. Swischuk LE: Acute respiratory distress with cyanosis. *Pediatr Emerg Care* 3:209–210, 1987.
12. Talamo RC, Levison H, Lynch MJ, Hercz A, Hyslop NE Jr, Bain HW: Symptomatic pulmonary emphysema in childhood associated with hereditary α_1-antitrypsin and elastase inhibitor deficiency. *J Pediatr* 79:20–26, 1971.
13. Vogl TJ, Wilimzig C, Hofmann U, Dresel S, Lissner J: MRI in tracheal stenosis by innominate artery in children. *Pediatr Radiol* 21:89–93, 1991.

BILATERAL UNDERAERATION

The most common cause of bilateral underaeration is a poor inspiratory effort, and while many times this occurs because the infant is too sick, weak, or depressed to initiate good respiratory activity, more often it is due to faulty radiographic technique (Table 1.2). However, underaeration also can be due to diaphragmatic elevation secondary to large abdominal masses or fluid collections, diaphragmatic paralysis, and central obstruction of the airway (1, 2). Any number of intraluminal or extraluminal airway lesions can cause such obstruction (Fig. 1.5), but actually these lesions more commonly result in overaeration due to expiratory air trapping. Underaeration, usually chronic, also occurs with muscular or neurologic disease.

In those cases where impaired air entry is the cause of underaeration, paradoxical inspiratory phase widening of the superior mediastinum and cardiac silhouette occurs (2). Under normal circumstances, of course, during inspiration, both the superior mediastinum and cardiac silhouette become smaller, but with inspiratory obstruction, negative intrathoracic pressures increase and paradoxical enlargement of the heart and mediastinum occurs. It is not always easy to appreciate these changes, but to avoid missing them, one should keep this phenomenon in mind.

REFERENCES

1. Blazer S, Naveh Y, Friedman A: Foreign body in the airway: a review of 200 cases. *Am J Dis Child* 134:68–71, 1980.
2. Capitanio MA, Kirkpatrick JA: Obstructions of the upper airway in children as reflected on the chest radiograph. *Radiology* 107:159–161, 1973.

Table 1.2
Bilateral Underaeration

Poor inspiration	}	Very common
Abdominal distension (mass, fluid, etc.)	}	Common
Primary muscle disease Neurologic disease Diaphragmatic paralysis	}	Moderately common
Inspiratory airway obstruction	}	Uncommon

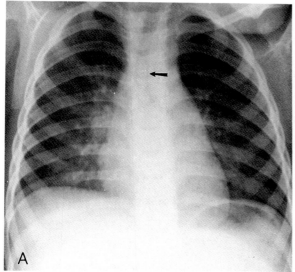
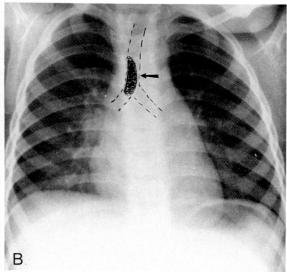

Figure 1.5. Underaeration with tracheal foreign body. A. This is an inspiratory film (note distended trachea), but the lungs are underaerated. The reason is that there is a peanut, just vaguely visible *(arrow)* in the trachea. **B.** Peanut and trachea outlined. (Courtesy of C. J. Fagan, M.D.)

UNEQUAL LUNG AERATION, SIZE, AND VASCULARITY (WHICH SIDE IS ABNORMAL?)

To one degree or another, lung size, aeration, and vascularity (pulmonary blood flow) are interrelated, but the relationships are not always the same. In other words, in some cases, a lung may be enlarged, hyperlucent, and undervascularized, while in others, it may be large, hyperlucent, but normally vascularized. Each set of circumstances represents a different pathophysiologic disturbance, and information about which is present usually can be derived from plain chest films. A problem arises, however, when one is uncertain as to which side is abnormal. This is a frequent dilemma, but if one applies four simple rules to one's analysis of the initial inspiratory film and the subsequent inspiratory-expiratory film sequence, one almost always will be able to decide which lung is abnormal (Table 1.3). However, before embarking on this discussion, it might be emphasized that certain artifactual physical factors such as

Table 1.3
Unequal Lung Size, Aeration, and Blood Flow (Which Side Is Abnormal?)

Inspiratory film
  Side with normal or ↑ vascularity usually is normal
  Side with ↓ vascularity usually is abnormal
  Small, *completely* opaque side is abnormal

Inspiratory-expiratory films
  Side which changes size less, or not at all, is abnormal

thick, overlying soft tissues, absence of soft tissue, poor tube centering, grid cutoffs, and patient rotation, must be entirely eliminated as causes of "apparently" unequal aeration (Fig. 1.6). This seems straightforward, but it is important.

RULE 1: IF VASCULARITY IS DECREASED, THE LUNG IS ABNORMAL

This rule holds whether the lung is large or small. Decreased pulmonary blood flow in these lungs can be due to pulmonary artery obstruction, hypoplasia, absence, or spasm (Fig. 1.7). Spasm usually is a reflex phenomenon (secondary to local hypoxia and subsequent acidosis) that occurs when a lung ceases to ventilate normally (i.e., infection, atelectasis, obstruction). It is as if the pulmonary artery "knew" that there was little use in sending blood to the nonventilating lung, and although the phenomenon is nonspecific, it can occur rather quickly after ventilation is impaired. With pulmonary artery hypoplasia or absence (agenesis), it is not difficult to see why pulmonary blood flow is diminished and, similarly, with pulmonary artery obstruction, the problem is straightforward (i.e., intravascular embolus or extrinsic compression by an adjacent mediastinal cyst or tumor). When the problem is obstructive emphysema, in addition to reflex arterial spasm, the overdistended lung also exerts a direct squeezing effect on the blood vessels. When these factors act together they can markedly reduce pulmonary blood flow (Fig. 1.7A).

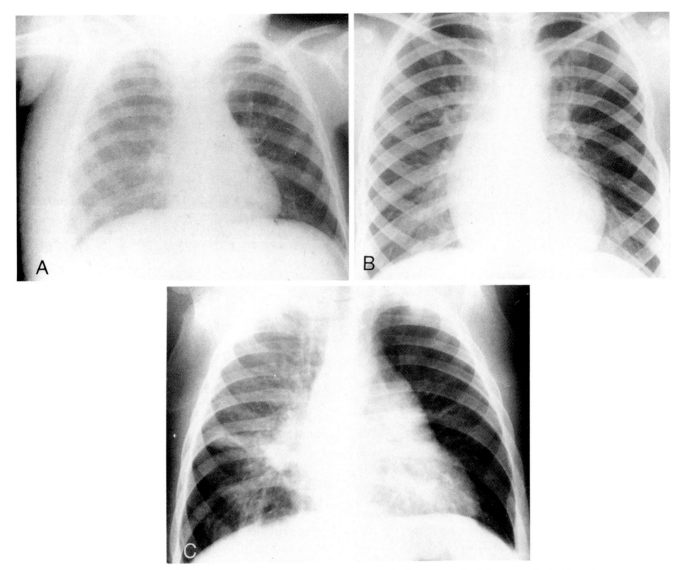

Figure 1.6. "Apparent" unequal aeration. A. The left lung appears more radiolucent than the right, but the vascularity is equal. Opacity over right lung is due to edematous soft tissues secondary to a burn. **B.** The left lung is slightly more radiolucent than the right. This is due to absence of the left pectoralis muscle. Note associated underdevelopment of the upper five ribs on the left. **C.** Rotation to the left causes the left lung to appear more radiolucent. The mediastinal edge also appears sharper. This patient had a viral lower respiratory tract infection with parahilar-peribronchial infiltrates and some linear atelectasis on the right. Actually, lung aeration is equal, but appears unequal because of rotation.

RULE 2: IF PULMONARY VASCULARITY IS NORMAL OR INCREASED, THE LUNG PROBABLY IS NORMAL

This is the corollary of rule 1. In other words, if a lung demonstrating decreased pulmonary vascularity is abnormal, then one demonstrating normal or increased blood flow should be normal. This may seem an almost foolishly simplistic rule, but one will come to see its usefulness when dealing with a large, radiolucent, or hyperlucent lung on one side and a small, radiolucent lung on the other (Fig. 1.8). If the large lung, in such cases, is compensatorily overinflated, one may be tempted to call it abnormal because it is so large. However, one will reverse one's opinion once the pulmonary vasculature is assessed, for the vessels will seem to be normal or increased.

Evidence of such shift in blood flow may be more obvious in certain cases than in others, for usually the shift takes a little time to develop. As a consequence, the shift might be less pronounced with acute problems such as atelectasis due to foreign bodies, and very florid in chronic problems such as unilateral pulmonary artery and lung agenesis or

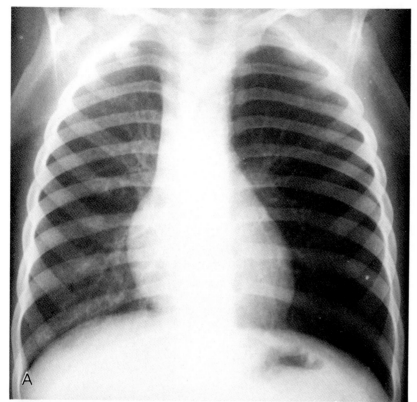

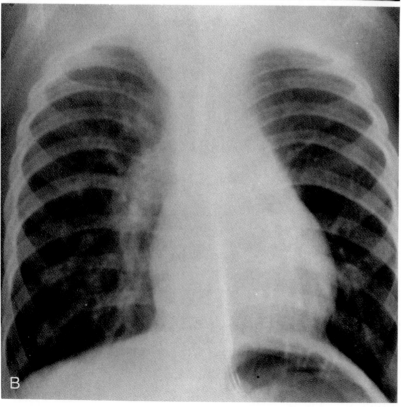

Figure 1.7. Hyperlucent lung with decreased vascularity. A. The left lung is hyperlucent, slightly larger than the right, and shows diminished vascularity. The problem is obstructive emphysema due to a foreign body in the left bronchus. **B.** This patient also demonstrates decreased vascularity on the left, but in addition, the left lung is small and radiolucent. The problem is congenital hypoplasia of the left lung. In both cases, decreased vascularity is the clue to the radiolucent lung being the abnormal one.

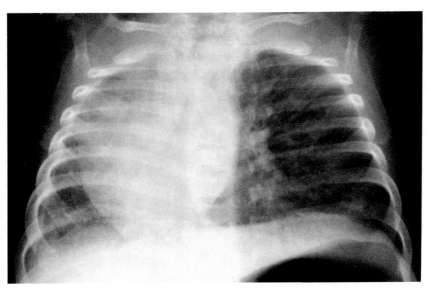

Figure 1.8. Hyperlucent lung with normal or increased vascularity. At first one might pick the more radiolucent and larger left lung as the abnormal one (i.e., obstructive emphysema). However, note that its vascularity is increased rather than decreased. For this reason, the left lung should not be abnormal and, indeed, the real problem is partial agenesis (upper lobe) of the right lung with compensatory overaeration of the left lung. More than normal volumes of blood are flowing through the left lung because the right lung cannot accept a normal flow of blood.

hypoplasia. Nonetheless, one often can be surprised to see how rapidly such blood shift can occur with an acute problem.

RULE 3: A SMALL, COMPLETELY OPAQUE HEMITHORAX IS THE ABNORMAL HEMITHORAX

The **key word** to the proper interpretation of cases demonstrating this finding is **complete.** In other words, the involved hemithorax must be completely opaque, and the best way to evaluate whether it is, is to inspect the costophrenic angle. If the angle is opaque, then the hemithorax is totally opaque, and if it is not, then the hemithorax is not completely opaque. This is an important distinction, because if a small hemithorax is deemed totally opaque, it is abnormal and the diagnosis should be either total atelectasis or agenesis of the lung (Fig. 1.9A). Atelectasis in such cases can be presumed resorptive (i.e., secondary to obstruction) and not compressive (i.e., compression by an overdistended contralateral lung), for no matter how large a pathologically obstructed, overdistended lung becomes, it does not compress the other lung to the point of total opacification (Fig. 1.9B). This rule, however, holds for the inspiratory film only, for if the film is made during expiration, the normal lung can be totally compressed. This phenomenon is difficult, if not impossible, to accomplish during inspiration.

As a side point, the same pathophysiology exists with large, opaque masses in the chest, because no matter how large they become, they seldom cause total compression and complete opacification of the contralateral lung.

RULE 4: WITH INSPIRATION-EXPIRATION, THE LUNG CHANGING SIZE LEAST, OR NOT AT ALL, IS THE ABNORMAL LUNG

The preceding three rules are applied to the inspiratory chest film, and the inspiratory-expiratory film sequence will either confirm the inspiratory film findings or solve the problem in those cases where uncertainty persists. On the inspiratory-expiratory film sequence the lung that changes size least, or not at all, is the abnormal lung. This is true of a lung that is hypoplastic, emphysematous because of obstruction, atelectatic, or agenetic. In essence, one is simply documenting the fact that the volume of air moving in and out of the lung is abnormal. The degree of abnormality, of course, determines the degree of change, but virtually always, discrepancy between the two sides exists (Figs. 1.10 and 1.11). The only exception occurs with mild unilateral, congenital hypoplasia of a lung, where the mildly hypoplastic lung functions in nearly normal or completely normal fashion.

In the vast majority of cases, with the four rules applied, one seldom needs fluoroscopy for the assess-

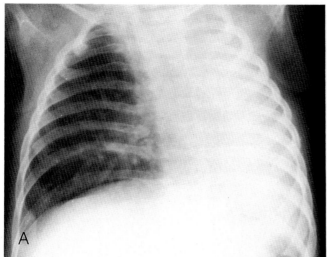

Figure 1.9. Small opaque hemithorax. A. Agenesis of the left lung. Note the small, totally opaque left hemithorax in this young infant. No air at all is present in the left lung. The right lung shows compensatory hyperinflection, and as might be expected, slightly engorged pulmonary vascularity. **B.** This patient has a similar opacified hemithorax except that there is a triangle of aerated lung *(arrow)* in the left costophrenic angle. Even though the left hemithorax is nearly totally opaque, this triangle of aerated lung should cause one to look at the other side more critically. In this case, the right lung is emphysematously overdistended because of congenital lobar emphysema, which is causing compression of the left lung. However, even though the right lung is markedly enlarged, it does not completely compress the left lung.

ment of unequal aeration. This is not to denounce the procedure, but merely to indicate that plain films usually suffice. However, if fluoroscopy is performed, one will note characteristic mediastinal shift and ipsilateral diaphragmatic immobilization.

LARGE OPAQUE HEMITHORAX

A large opaque hemithorax is due most often to large accumulations of fluid in the pleural space, and in children, pus (empyema) is most common (Table 1.4). Other types of fluid include serous, bloody, or chylous effusions, but after the newborn period, chyle accumulations are uncommon. In older infants and children, chylothorax most often occurs after thoracic surgery or chest trauma as a result of thoracic duct injuries. Bloody effusions usually occur in association with chest trauma, but occasionally bleeding can occur with rupture of a congenital aneurysm of the ductus arteriosus (usually in an infant) or with a blood dyscrasia. However, the latter two conditions are rare, and consequently, in the pediatric age group, **pleural fluid is pus until proven otherwise.**

Radiographically, it is impossible to differentiate one type of fluid from another, and the findings with any type of fluid depend primarily on the volume of fluid present. In advanced cases, contralateral shift of the mediastinum is seen. In addition, inversion of the ipsilateral diaphragmatic leaflet often occurs (especially on the left), and of course the lung on the same side is completely compressed and airless (Fig. 1.12). In less advanced cases, however, the lung is less compressed, the opaque hemithorax nearly normal or normal in size, and the findings often confusing. The reason for this is that residual aeration of the incompletely compressed lung is present and, to the inexperienced viewer, suggests that consolidation, rather than fluid in the pleural space, is the problem (see Fig. 1.18).

Table 1.4
Large Opaque Hemithorax

Pus (empyema)	}	Most common
Effusion with lymphoma, neuroblastoma	}	
Hemothorax		Common
Effusion with tuberculosis		
Fungal disease		
Chest tumor		
Pancreatitis	}	Uncommon
Abdominal tumors and infections		
Chylothorax		
Large mass or cyst (fluid filled)		
Diaphragmatic hernia (airless)	}	Rare
Fluid-filled lung (bronchial atresia, congenital lobar enphysema)		

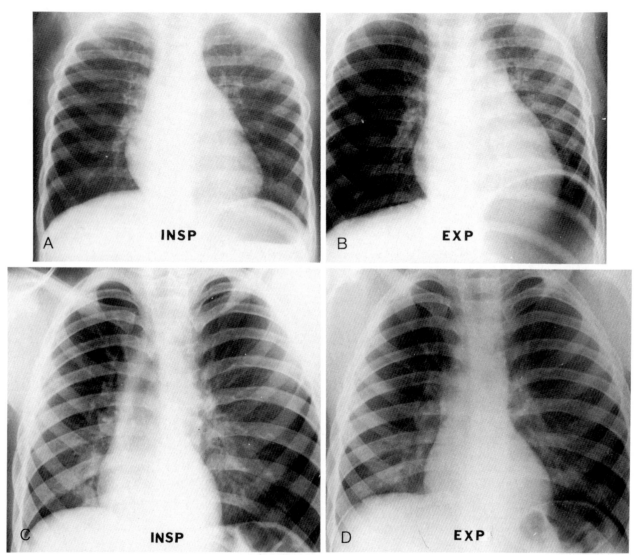

Figure 1.10. Value of inspiratory-expiratory film sequence.
A. On this inspiratory view, one would have considerable difficulty determining that an obstructing foreign body is present. **B.**
Expiratory view, however, clearly demonstrates air-trapping in
the right lung, consistent with a foreign body in the right main
bronchus. **C.** Inspiratory view in a patient with asthma demonstrates a large radiolucent left lung and a small radiolucent right
lung. One must look closely to note that the vascularity is diminished on the right, suggesting that the right lung is abnormal. **D.**
Expiratory film demonstrates that the left lung deflates normally
while the right lung changes very little in size. The right main
bronchus was obstructed by a mucous plug.

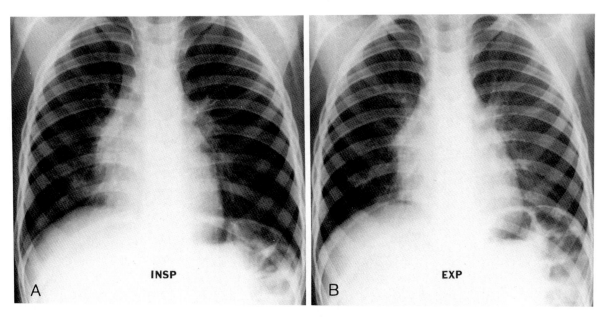

Figure 1.11. Inspiratory-expiratory sequence: lung that changes size least is the abnormal lung. A. On this **inspiratory view,** note that the left lung is much larger than the right. However, vascularity is about the same on both sides, making it difficult to determine which lung is abnormal. **B. Expiratory film** clearly shows that the left lung is the one that changes volume most markedly. The right lung, in fact, has not changed size at all and, on expiration, becomes the larger lung. This clearly indicates the presence of obstructive emphysema on the right which, in this patient with asthma, was due to an obstructing mucous plug.

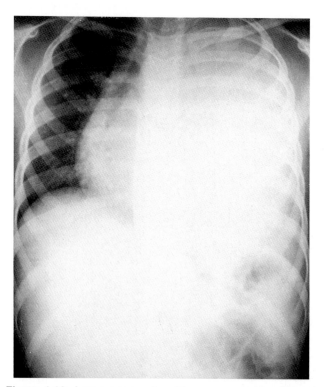

Figure 1.12. **Large opaque hemithorax: empyema.** There is no problem in deciding that the abnormality is on the left. The entire left hemithorax is opacified, the mediastinum is shifted to the right, and the left diaphragmatic leaflet and stomach are depressed. In addition, there is no air in the left lung. This patient had a pneumococcal empyema that was completely compressing the lung.

Empyemas can be seen with any number of bacterial infections, but most commonly occur with staphylococcal, hemophilus, and pneumococcal pneumonias. Staphylococcal pneumonia has a wide age range, while hemophilus pneumonia tends to occur in infants and young children (under 2 years of age). Pneumococcal pneumonias have an age range comparable to that of staphylococcal infections, except that they are slightly less common in the young infant. With massive serous pleural effusions, a number of underlying diseases can be present, but most commonly the cause is kidney disease such as the nephrotic syndrome, or an intrathoracic or abdominal tumor such as lymphoma or neuroblastoma. Other intrathoracic tumors (e.g., teratoma, pulmonary blastoma, mesothelioma) are far less common, but also can be associated with massive pleural effusions (Fig. 1.13). Quite rarely, large pleural effusions can occur with primary pulmonary tuberculosis, fungal disease, and even viral infections (1, 4). Pleural effusions with the collagen vascular diseases and acute glomerulonephritis, are common, but to have an effusion so massive that total opacification of the hemithorax results is rare. On the right, massive unilateral pleural effusions can occur with subphrenic or hepatic tumors or abscesses, and on the left, with subphrenic abscesses or pancreatic infections. Less frequently, pancreatitis produces the same findings on the right.

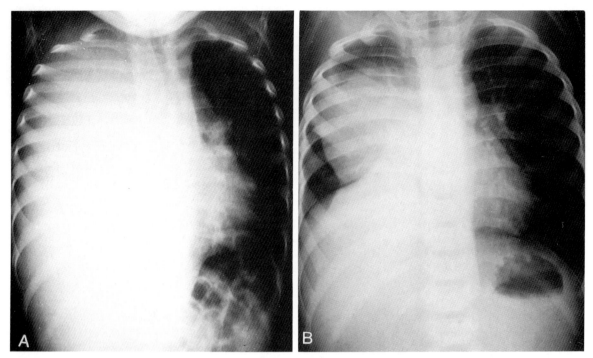

Figure 1.13. Large opaque hemithorax: large pleural effusion with underlying tumor. A. The findings are nonspecific and suggest a large fluid accumulation on the right. **B.** After thoracentesis, a large mass remains. This was a teratoma.

Figure 1.14. Large opaque hemithorax: large mass. A large lymphoma-infiltrated thymus gland is producing the opaque right hemithorax in this patient. The clue to the presence of a large mass rather than a large collection of pleural fluid is the triangle of aerated lung seen in the right costophrenic angle *(arrow)*.

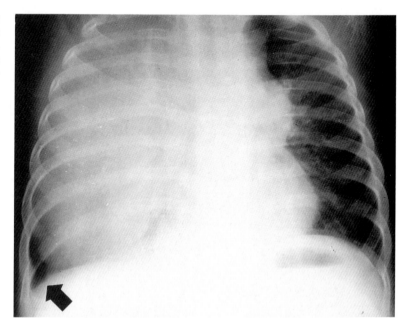

Other causes of a totally opaque hemithorax are unlikely to occur beyond the neonatal period, for they include the fluid-filled lung of congenital lobar emphysema or bronchial atresia (2, 3), the solid right lung syndrome (5), and the airless diaphragmatic hernia. Occasionally, one can encounter a patient with a large cyst or intrathoracic mass that causes near total opacification of a hemithorax, but in most of these cases, residual aeration of the ipsilateral lung is present, seen as a triangular radiolucency in the costophrenic angle (Fig. 1.14). It is most important to make this latter observation, for when the radiolucent triangle is seen, pleural fluid cannot be the cause of opacification. Ultrasound can quickly verify the presence or absence of pleural fluid (see Fig. 1.19) and also can be used to localize the best site for thoracentesis.

REFERENCES

1. Cho CT, Hiatt WO, Behbehani AM: Pneumonia and massive pleural effusion associated with adenovirus type 7. *Am J Dis Child* 126:92–94, 1973.
2. Fagan CJ, Swischuk LE: The opaque lung in lobar emphysema. *Am J Roentgenol Radium Ther Nucl Med* 114:300–304, 1972.
3. Griscom NT, Harris GBC, Wohl MEB, Vawter GF, Eraklis AJ: Fluid-filled lung due to airway obstruction in the newborn. *Pediatrics* 43:383–390, 1969.
4. Pinckney L, Parker BR: Primary coccidioidomycosis in children presenting with massive pleural effusion. *AJR* 130:247–249, 1978.
5. Swischuk LE, Hayden CK Jr, Richardson J: Neonatal opaque right lung. *Radiology* 141:671–673, 1981.

SMALL TO NORMAL OPAQUE (HAZY) HEMITHORAX

For the most part, a distinctly small and hazy or opaque hemithorax indicates volume loss, and almost always one is dealing with atelectasis or pulmonary agenesis (2, 3) (Table 1.5). Of course, the degree to which the lung is hazy or opaque depends on the amount of aerated lung present, and this also influences the degree of compensatory overaeration of the contralateral lung. With partial agenesis (one or two lobes only) or incomplete atelectasis, the hemithorax is hazy, while with complete atelectasis or total unilateral pulmonary agenesis, it is opaque (Fig. 1.15). Atelectasis, of course, is much more common, and leading the list of causes are conditions such as improper endotracheal tube positioning, mucous plugs (most often secondary to viral lower respiratory tract infection and/or asthma), and foreign bodies. When an otherwise healthy child is found to

have an opaque hemithorax that shows evidence of volume loss, a bronchial foreign body should be strongly suspected (6). Endobronchial granulomas and tumors are far less common, as are extrinsic, compressive lesions such as strategically located mediastinal cysts, masses, or abnormal vessels.

Regarding abnormal vessels, the one most commonly encountered (although still quite rare) is the aberrant left pulmonary artery, or "pulmonary sling" (1, 4, 5, 7). In this condition, the left pulmonary artery, as it arises anomalously from the right pulmonary artery, swings around the right side of the carina and compresses the right bronchus (see Fig. 1.38*B*). Most often, there is variable underaeration of the right lung, but occasionally, obstructive emphysema can result (1). This condition is discussed more fully under Focal Tracheobronchial Narrowings (p. 32).

As noted earlier, when atelectasis or agenesis is partial, the involved hemithorax is small and hazy rather than small and opaque (Fig. 1.15). Partial agenesis, for the most part, is a problem of the right lung, and usually the upper and middle lobes are the agenetic lobes. The anomaly commonly is associated with abnormalities such as accessory diaphragm, abnormal veins (scimitar syndrome), sequestration, and arteriovenous fistula (2, 3). This constellation of abnormalities also has been called the hypogenetic right lung syndrome (3). Overall, the condition is rather innocuous, but the findings in these children frequently are misinterpreted as pulmonary infection or atelectasis (Fig. 1.16). Indeed, many of these patients are subjected to procedures such as bronchoscopy, computerized tomography (CT), or pulmonary angiography, but all should be avoided.

There are a few instances where a hemithorax is opaque or hazy and yet relatively normal in size (Table 1.5). Most often, this occurs when fluid layers along the posterior chest wall in a patient who is examined in the supine position (Fig. 1.17). With the aerated lung located above the fluid, the end result is a hazy but relatively normal size hemithorax. Another condition in which a hemithorax is opaque and yet of relatively normal size is during the development of an empyema. In such cases, the volume of fluid is not large enough to completely compress the lung, but yet large enough to cause considerable opacification of the hemithorax (Fig. 1.18*A*). Because the lung is incompletely compressed, some parenchymal aeration and air bronchograms remain, and because of this, one often is led to believe that consolidation is the problem. However, total consolidation of an entire lung (all lobes) is rather uncommon (Fig. 1.18*B*). In problem cases, ultrasound should be uti-

Table 1.5
Small or Normal Size Opaque Hemithorax

Small opaque or hazy hemithorax		
Atelectasis	}	Common
Pulmonary agenesis	}	Rare
Normal size opaque or hazy hemithorax		
Pleural fluid on supine film	}	Common
Developing empyema	}	Moderately common
Total lung consolidation (all lobes on one side)	}	Rare

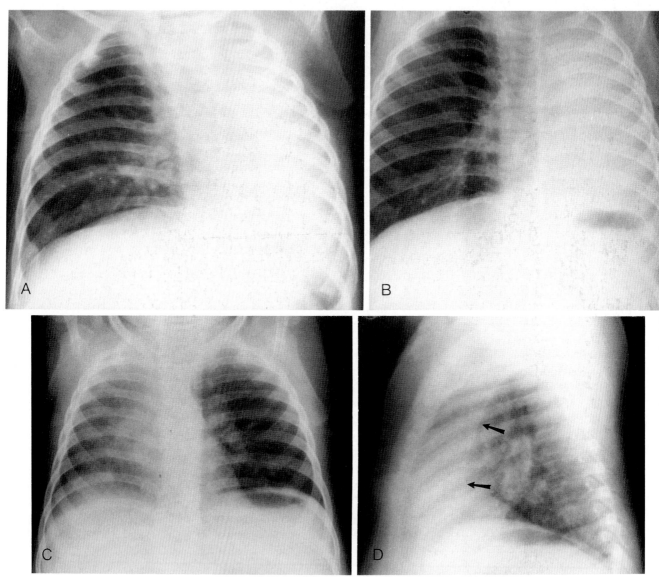

Figure 1.15. Small opaque or hazy hemithorax. A. Total agenesis of the left lung produces a small, opaque hemithorax on the left and an overdistended lung on the right. However, note that vascularity in the right lung is increased. **B.** Total atelectasis of the left lung produces a small opaque left hemithorax and an overdistended radiolucent right lung. **C.** Agenesis of the right upper and middle lobes produces a small, semiopaque, or hazy, right hemithorax. **D.** Lateral view demonstrating typical retrosternal opacity *(arrows)*, due to the aerated lower lobe abutting areolar soft tissue replacing the absent middle and upper lobes.

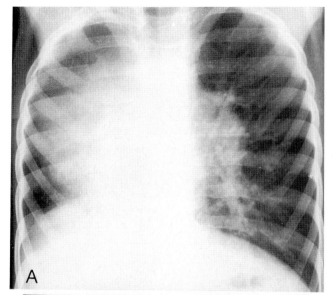

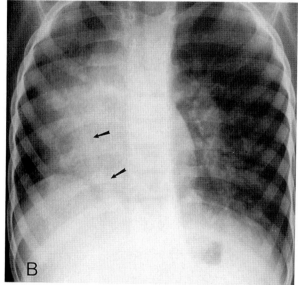

Figure 1.16. Small hazy (semiopaque) hemithorax mimicking pneumonia. A. A pneumonia might erroneously be suggested on the right. However, one should ask, "Why is there so much volume loss on the right?" and "Why are the pulmonary artery and its branches so prominent on the left?" These are unusual findings for an acute pneumonia, and suggest that the problem is on the right, chronic, and due either to atelectasis or agenesis. **B.** Another view (overpenetrated) in the same patient 3 years earlier demonstrates an abnormal vein characteristic of the scimitar syndrome. This is consistent with the diagnosis of a hypogenetic right lung with middle and upper lobe agenesis.

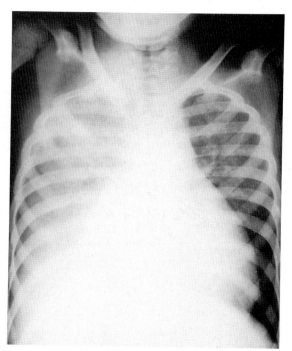

Figure 1.17. Opaque, normal size hemithorax. Posterior layering of pleural fluid in the supine position produces partial opacification of the right hemithorax. The lung size, however, remains normal, as fluid has layered along the posterior surface. The patient also has cardiomegaly.

2. Currarino G, Williams B: Causes of congenital unilateral pulmonary hypoplasia: a study of thirty-three cases. *Pediatr Radiol* 15:15–24, 1985.
3. Felson B: Pulmonary agenesis and related anomalies. *Semin Roentgenol* 7:17–30, 1972.
4. Jue KL, Raghib G, Amplatz K, Adams P Jr, Edwards JE: Anomalous origin of the left pulmonary artery from the right pulmonary artery. *AJR* 95:598–610, 1965.
5. Philip T, Sumerling MD, Fleming J, Grainger RG: Aberrant left pulmonary artery. *Clin Radiol* 23:153–159, 1972.
6. Seibert RW, Seibert JJ, Williamson SL: The opaque chest: when to suspect a bronchial foreign body. *Pediatr Radiol* 16:193–196, 1986.
7. Tesler UF, Balsara RH, Niguidula F: Aberrant left pulmonary artery (vascular sling): report of five cases. *Chest* 66:402–407, 1974.

LARGE RADIOLUCENT (HYPERLUCENT) HEMITHORAX

Most often, a large, hyperlucent hemithorax is caused by obstructive or compensatory emphysema of an entire lung (Table 1.6), and when emphysema is compensatory, almost always it is secondary to complete atelectasis or agenesis of the contralateral lung. Occasionally, it is due to contralateral pneumonectomy, but in childhood, this is a rare situation. In any of these cases, the large, hyperlucent lung is easy to identify, and with its normal or increased

lized to determine whether pleural fluid is present (Fig. 1.19).

REFERENCES

1. Capitanio MA, Ramos R, Kirkpatrick JA: Pulmonary sling: roentgen observations. *Am J Roentgenol Radium Ther Nucl Med* 112:28–34, 1971.

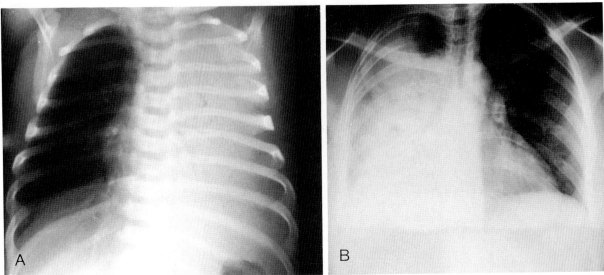

Figure 1.18. Opaque, normal size hemithorax. A. Developing empyema compresses the lung on the left. However, an air bronchogram still is present as the lung is not totally compressed. The air bronchogram is central, attesting to the developing empyema. **B.** Consolidating pneumonia of the right lung produces opacity of the entire right lung, except for the apex. Again the hemithorax is normal in size. Note, however, that air bronchograms extend more peripherally than in part **A,** and hence suggest consolidation.

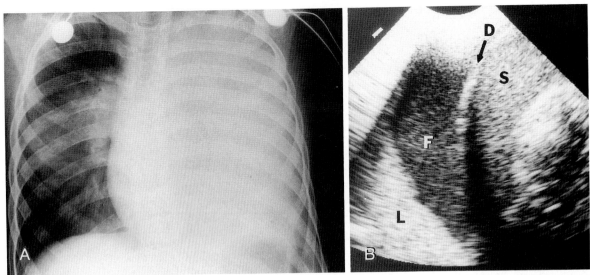

Figure 1.19. Opaque hemithorax: empyema. A. Note the opaque left hemithorax. Total consolidation of the left lung might erroneously be suggested; however, note that although a central air bronchogram is present, no air bronchograms are seen in the periphery as would be expected with a total lung consolidation. **B.** Ultrasonogram demonstrates a large collection of fluid *(F)* under the compressed left lung *(L),* overlying the diaphragm *(D).* Spleen *(S).*

vascularity, should be chosen as the normal lung (Fig. 1.20).

When classic obstructive emphysema (i.e., progressive enlargement of a lung) is the cause of a large, hyperlucent lung, the emphysematous lung is fixed in overdistension, and its vascularity usually is diminished (Fig. 1.21). The degree of diminution of vascularity depends on the degree and duration of overdistension and, thus, in early or mild cases, vascularity still may appear relatively normal. In such cases, inspiratory-expiratory film sequences are extremely helpful (Fig. 1.22).

Most commonly, obstructive emphysema is caused by an endobronchial foreign body, but next most common is a mucous plug. Such plugs usually are seen with viral lower respiratory tract infections and/or asthma. Endobronchial lesions such as inflammatory granulomas (i.e., tuberculosis) or endobronchial tumors are much less common causes of

obstructive emphysema, and so are extrinsic, compressive lesions such as mediastinal cysts, tumors, and abnormally dilated or located blood vessels.

Congenital lobar emphysema is another common cause of hyperlucency of one side of the chest. Usually the condition is discovered in infancy, but there are cases where the patient grows into childhood with little or no respiratory difficulty. In any case, it is the left upper lobe that is involved most often, and if emphysema is pronounced, the entire lung may falsely appear emphysematous. If one is fortunate enough to also see the triangular, compressed lower lobe just against the spine, the diagnosis of upper lobe obstructive emphysema is almost assured (Fig. 1.23A). Right upper and right middle lobe involvement are next most common, and opinion differs as to which is more common. In our experience, upper lobe involvement is slightly more common. Middle lobe emphysema can be difficult to assess because the secondary compressive atelectasis of the upper and lower lobes by the expanded middle lobe often is erroneously considered to be the primary abnormality (Fig. 1.24).

After obstructive emphysema is determined to be present, the need for further investigation depends on whether the problem is acute or chronic. If it is acute and present in a patient with asthma or a viral lower respiratory tract infection, a mucous plug is the most likely cause and little needs to be done. The patient should be encouraged to cough, but regardless, the plug usually eventually dislodges on its

Table 1.6
Large Hyperlucent (Radiolucent) Hemithorax

Obstructive emphysema Compensatory emphysema[a]	Common
Pneumothorax	Moderately common
Cystic disease of the lung Large pneumatocele Diaphragmatic hernia (stomach)	Relatively rare

[a]Changes size on inspiration-expiration.

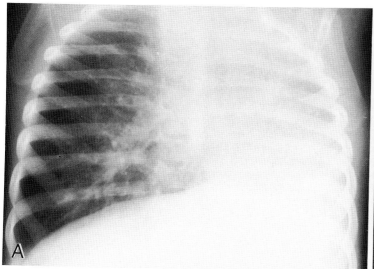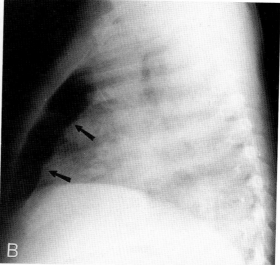

Figure 1.20. Large hyperlucent lung: compensatory emphysema. A. Note the large, hyperlucent right lung. Also note that the pulmonary vascularity is engorged, suggesting that the right lung must be the normal lung. The left lung is collapsed secondary to mucous plugging from a viral lower respiratory tract infection. **B.** Lateral view demonstrating anterior mediastinal herniation *(arrows)* of the compensatorily overinflated right lung, a common phenomenon with an overdistended lung.

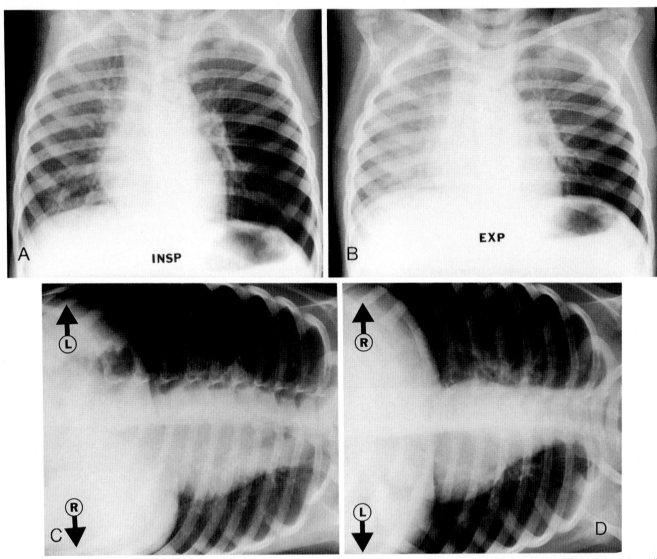

Figure 1.21. Large hyperlucent lung: obstructive emphysema. A. Inspiratory film in a patient with an obstructing foreign body on the left. The left lung, especially the left lower lobe, is large, hyperlucent, and undervascularized. **B.** Expiratory film confirms air-trapping in the left lung, mainly in the left lower lobe. **C.** Decubitus film with the right side down shows that the right lung collapses (becomes smaller and hazy). The left lung is radiolucent and remains overdistended. **D.** Decubitus film with the left side down. Note that the left lung has remained radiolucent (air cushion effect due to obstructive emphysema). The right lung is normally aerated. The findings confirm obstructive emphysema of the left lung; it should have collapsed.

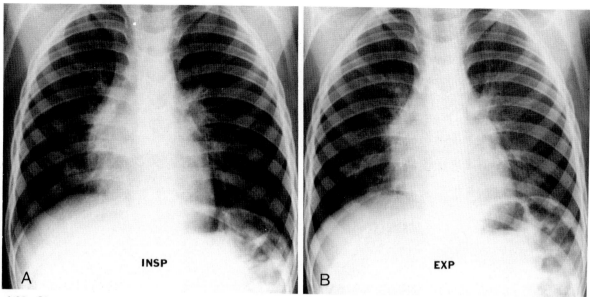

Figure 1.22. Obstructive emphysema: subtle findings. A. On the inspiratory view, obstructive emphysema on the right could easily be missed. The right lung may be slightly more radiolucent than the left. **B.** Expiratory film, clearly demonstrates the presence of obstructive emphysema on the right.

own. If, by clinical history, the presumptive diagnosis is a foreign body, however, bronchoscopy is the next step. There is seldom need for other radiographic studies, but if uncertainty prevails, fluoroscopy can be helpful. On fluoroscopy, obstructive emphysema results in decreased motion of the depressed, ipsilateral diaphragmatic leaflet and contralateral shift of the mediastinum on expiration. If fluoroscopy is unavailable one can obtain decubitus views (2). The principle behind decubitus views is that when an obstructed lung is in the dependent position (the "down" side in the decubitus position), it acts as an air cushion and does not deflate. Normally, the dependent lung deflates because of compression. The phenomenon can be enhanced by asking the patient to exhale while the film is being obtained.

Conditions producing findings similar to obstructive emphysema of a lung include cystic disease of the lung, large postinflammatory pneumatoceles, left-side diaphragmatic hernias with an air-filled stomach in the chest (1, 4), and pneumothorax (5). As far as cystic disease of the lungs is concerned, occasionally a large solitary cyst or postinflammatory pneumatocele can occupy a hemithorax, but more often the problem is multiple cysts in congenital cystic adenomatoid malformation (3). Although early in the neonatal period the cysts in this lesion are very small and fluid-filled, as the patient grows older, there is progressive replacement of the fluid with air (due to the air-drift phenomenon via the ducts of

Lambert and pores of Kohn) and improved visualization of the cysts. At first they appear small and bubbly, then larger and more thin-walled, and eventually, so large that they coalesce and virtually obliterate the septae between them. It is in these latter two stages that the findings are difficult to differentiate from those of an emphysematous lung or a large pneumothorax (Fig. 1.23B).

Diaphragmatic hernias on the left side containing an air-filled stomach are a rather uncommon cause of a large, unilateral hyperlucent hemithorax, but the findings can be puzzling (Fig. 1.23C). Such hernias can be secondary to blunt abdominal trauma (either acute or on a delayed basis), but most are delayed congenital herniations through the foramen of Bochdalek. Finally, massive pneumothoraces also can produce a large, hyperlucent hemithorax, but the findings usually are very straightforward (Fig. 1.23D). On the other hand, anterior pneumothoraces occurring in patients lying in the supine position can pose a more perplexing problem. Such pneumothoraces most commonly occur in the neonate but also occur in older children. In such cases, radiolucency of the hemithorax is due to air accumulating over the anterior surface of the lung, and also to compression of the lung by the pleural air. Together, these factors cause pulmonary blood flow to be diminished and the lung to become hyperlucent (Fig. 1.25). The degree of increased radiolucency depends on the volume of free air present.

Another clue to the presence of an anterior pneu-

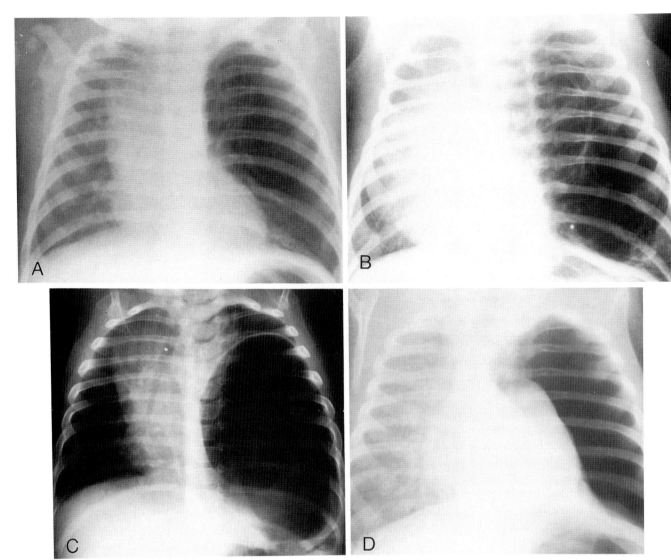

Figure 1.23. Large hyperlucent hemithorax: various causes. A. Congenital lobar emphysema. Note the overdistended left lung. Vascularity is diminished and the secondarily compressed lower lobe is just barely visible. **B. Congenital cystic adenomatoid malformation.** At this stage of the disease, the cysts become very large and the septae quite thin. The lung is hyperlu-cent and devascularized. **C. Delayed diaphragmatic hernia with gastric herniation.** Note the distended stomach in the left hemithorax. (Courtesy of Virgil Graves, M.D.) **D. Large tension pneumothorax on the left.** The pneumothorax was a complication of air-trapping due to a viral lower respiratory tract infection.

mothorax is that the ipsilateral mediastinal edge usually appears sharper than its mate on the other side (Fig. 1.25). This is not an absolutely pathognomonic finding, for similar sharpness can be seen with an emphysematous overdistended lung (see Fig. 1.23A) or a hypoplastic, underperfused lung (see Fig. 1.27). However, it still is a very useful sign of anterior pneumothorax. The reason the ipsilateral mediastinal edge is sharper with anterior pneumothorax is that free air rather than normal lung parenchyma abuts the mediastinal edge.

In all these entities, hyperlucency results because the ratio of air to blood in the lungs is altered in favor of air. In other words, with obstructive emphysema, the blood vessels are compressed and constricted, and with congenital hypoplasia, they are absent or small. As a result, less blood than normal is carried through the lungs. The lung then becomes hyperlucent and, at the same time, the presence of fewer, smaller, and less filled blood vessels results in less blurring (increased sharpness) of the ipsilateral mediastinal edge.

In the newborn and young infant, an anterior pneumothorax sometimes compresses the normal

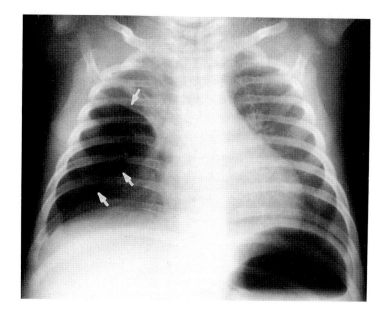

Figure 1.24. Congenital right middle lobe emphysema. Note typical overdistension of the right middle lobe with associated compressive atelectasis of both the right upper and right lower lobes *(arrows)*.

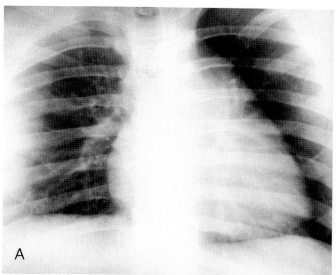

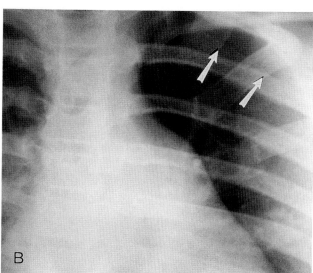

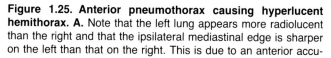

Figure 1.25. Anterior pneumothorax causing hyperlucent hemithorax. A. Note that the left lung appears more radiolucent than the right and that the ipsilateral mediastinal edge is sharper on the left than that on the right. This is due to an anterior accumulation of air (i.e., anterior pneumothorax). **B.** Film obtained a few moments later, in expiration, demonstrates typical findings of a pneumothorax *(arrows)*.

Figure 1.26. Bilateral anterior pneumothorax. Note the upward and medial compression of the lobes of the thymus gland, causing a mass-like appearance in the superior mediastinum *(arrows)*.

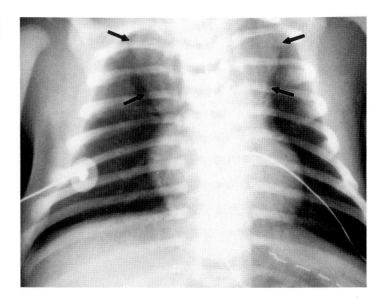

thymus gland, especially if the pneumothorax is under tension. The result is a convex distortion of the superior mediastinum that can resemble a mass (6). The mass-like appearance is even more prominent when the pneumothoraces are bilateral (Fig. 1.26).

REFERENCES

1. Brill PW, Gershwind ME, Krasna IH: Massive gastric enlargement with delayed presentation of congenital diaphragmatic hernia: report of three cases and review of the literature. *J Pediatr Surg* 12:667–674, 1977.
2. Capitanio MA, Kirkpatrick JA: The lateral decubitus film, an aid in determining air-trapping in children. *Radiology* 103:460–462, 1972.
3. Madewell JE, Stocker JT, Korsower JM: Cystic adenomatoid malformation of the lung: morphologic analysis. *AJR* 124:436–448, 1975.
4. Siegel MJ, Shackelford GD, McAlister WH: Left-sided congenital diaphragmatic hernia: delayed presentation. *AJR* 137:43–46, 1981.
5. Swischuk LE: Two lesser known but useful signs of neonatal pneumothorax. *AJR* 127:623–627, 1976.
6. O'Keeffe FN, Swischuk LE, Stansberry SD: Mediastinal pseudomass caused by compression of the thymus in neonates with anterior pneumothorax. *AJR* 156:145–148, 1991.

SMALL, RADIOLUCENT (HYPERLUCENT) HEMITHORAX

The commonest causes of a small, hyperlucent hemithorax are congenital pulmonary hypoplasia (with ipsilateral pulmonary artery hypoplasia or absence), and the Swyer-James syndrome (Table 1.7). Congenital hypoplasia of the lung may or may not be associated with congenital heart disease (3), but when it

Table 1.7
Small Hyperlucent Hemithorax

Pumonary artery and lung hypoplasia[a] Swyer-James lung[b]	Moderately common
Postradiation[b] Pulmonary vein atresia or stenosis[b] Pulmonary embolus[a]	Rare

[a] Changes size on inspiration-expiration.
[b] May show scarring or reticulation.

is, persistent truncus arteriosus and tetralogy of Fallot are most likely. With persistent truncus arteriosus, hypoplasia may occur on either side, but with tetralogy of Fallot, it usually occurs on the left. In the absence of congenital heart disease, left-side hypoplasia also is favored. If underdevelopment of the right lung occurs, usually it takes the form of right upper and/or middle lobe agenesis. The lower lobe is normal, but in combination with agenesis of the other lobes, a small and hazy, rather than radiolucent, hemithorax results (see Fig. 1.16).

With congenital hypoplasia of the lung, the patient is usually asymptomatic, and in our experience, such lungs are not prone to repeated pulmonary infections. Indeed, most of the time their discovery is totally incidental. Increased radiolucency of the lung results from decreased pulmonary blood flow (i.e., hypoplastic or absent pulmonary artery), and in some cases the findings are quite striking (Fig. 1.27). An important feature of these lungs is that they change size on inspiration-expiration, and even though the degree of change may not be as great as

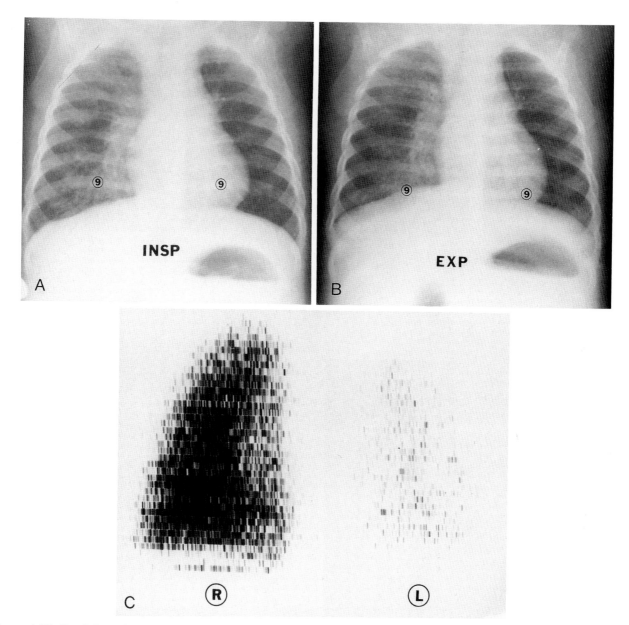

Figure 1.27. Small hyperlucent hemithorax: pulmonary hypoplasia. A. On this inspiratory view, note that the left lung is smaller but more radiolucent (undervascularized) than the right lung. This also is causing increased sharpness of the left mediastinal edge. The ninth ribs are marked. **B.** Expiratory film in the same infant demonstrates that both lungs change size during expiration, but the left does so a little less than the right. The ninth ribs are marked again. **C.** Isotope perfusion study demonstrates markedly decreased perfusion of the left lung.

in a totally normal lung, significant change does occur (Fig. 1.27). It is this feature, more than any other, that serves to distinguish the congenitally hypoplastic lung from the one acquired in the Swyer-James or MacLeod syndromes (2, 4–6, 10).

Classically, the Swyer-James lung results from a severe inflammatory episode that produces an obliterative bronchiolitis. This is especially likely to occur with viral infections (2, 5), but also can be seen with other pulmonary infections or with chronic foreign bodies. The end result is a small, hyperlucent lung that does not change much in size between inspiration and expiration. In addition, while many of these lungs are totally clear, others demonstrate parenchymal scarring or reticulation. For this reason, we have expanded the classic definition of the Swyer-James lung to include such variations. From the purist's standpoint, however, the lung should be free of infiltrates, small, hyperlucent, and demonstrative of obstructive emphysema.

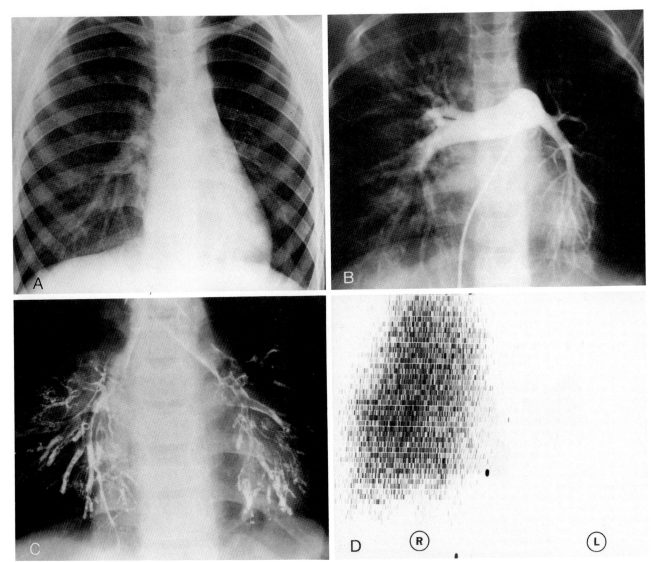

Figure 1.28. Small hyperlucent hemithorax: acquired hypoplasia (Swyer-James lung). A. Note the small, hyperlucent, and undervascularized left lung. The right lung shows slight compensatory overaeration and increased pulmonary blood flow. This patient, when an infant, had a normal chest film, but later acquired a severe infection of the left lung. **B.** Pulmonary arteriogram demonstrates characteristic decreased flow to the left lung and small, constricted pulmonary arteries. Those in the left lower lobe are crowded because of partial left lower lobe atelectasis, which is seen as opacity behind the left side of the heart on the chest film in part **A. C.** Bronchogram demonstrating moderate bronchiectatic changes on the left, especially in the left lower lobe, and less filling of the small peripheral bronchioles than on the normal right side. Also note that both the right and left major bronchi are about equal in size. If congenital hypoplasia were the problem, the left bronchus would be significantly smaller than the right (recall, however, that the normal left bronchus often is a little smaller than the right). Also note that the bronchi of the left lower lobe are crowded, confirming the presence of atelectasis. **D.** Perfusion isotope scan demonstrates virtually no isotope activity in the left lung.

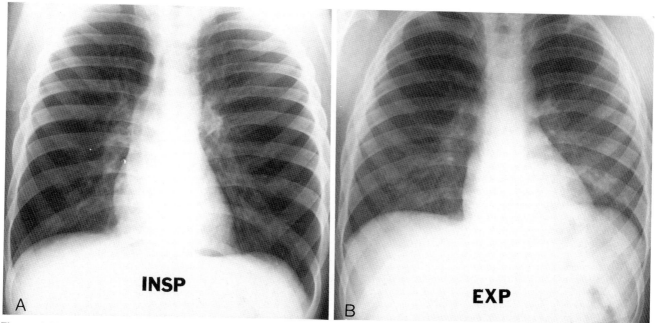

Figure 1.29. Small hyperlucent hemithorax: endobronchial obstruction. A. On this inspiratory view, note that the right lung is more radiolucent than the left. However, it is a little smaller than the left lung and the vascularity is slightly diminished. Be- cause of the decreased vascularity in the right lung, one should suspect the right lung to be abnormal. **B.** Expiratory view clearly demonstrates air trapping in the right lung due to an underlying foreign body.

When a small, hyperlucent lung is demonstrated to be congenital in origin, there is little reason to perform any other radiographic studies, because usually no specific therapy is indicated. Of course, isotope perfusion scans will be abnormal, and pulmonary arteriograms will show ipsilateral pulmonary artery hypoplasia or absence, but these findings are expected and are no different from those seen in the Swyer-James lung (Fig. 1.28). If, on the other hand, a patient is decreed to have a Swyer-James lung, then it must be determined whether the lung is a problem to the patient. This can take the form of repeated pulmonary infections or cyanosis resulting from desaturation due to intrapulmonary shunting. Classically, bronchography was used to evaluate Swyer-James lung and would reveal two types of bronchial disease. The first is that seen in the classic Swyer-James lung, where the obliterative bronchiolitis leads to nonfilling of the peripheral bronchioles and a normal bronchial tree proximal to this level. In other cases, however, widespread bronchiectasis in the more proximal bronchi occurs (Fig. 1.28). Bronchograms are now seldom performed, however, as high-resolution CT reveals similar changes and is more sensitive in detecting areas of air-trapping (7, 8).

After congenital or acquired pulmonary hypopla-sia, the next most common cause of a small hyperlucent hemithorax is bronchial obstruction. At first, this may appear to be a strange statement, for most often one thinks of atelectasis or obstructive emphysema as the two findings associated with this problem. However, at a certain stage of bronchial obstruction, the involved lung may appear smaller and more radiolucent than normal. The vascularity in such a lung usually is slightly decreased, an important observation that is frequently missed. Once one makes this observation, inspiratory-expiratory film sequences should be obtained. During inspiration and expiration, the smaller, abnormal, hyperlucent lung changes its size very little or not at all (Fig. 1.29). In these cases the abnormal air flow to and from the lung is such that, during inspiration, enough air gets into the lung to prevent the development of atelectasis, but during expiration, not enough is trapped to allow the lung to become progressively enlarged. The end result is a "balanced-obstructed" lung. Other rather rare causes of a unilateral, small hyperlucent hemithorax include post-irradiation lung, pulmonary embolus (very rare in children), and pulmonary vein atresia or stenosis (9).

A final variation of the small, hyperlucent lung is one that demonstrates some degree of reticularity. For the most part, if one encounters such a lung, the

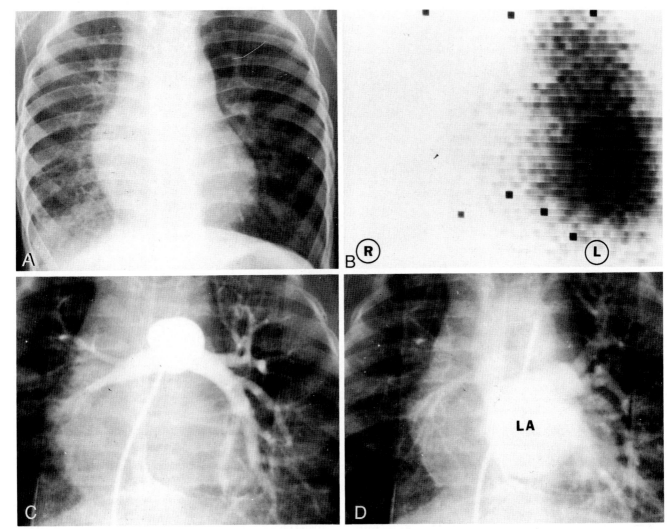

Figure 1.30. Small reticular lung: pulmonary vein atresia. A. Note that the right lung is smaller than the left and possesses a diffuse reticularity, especially in its lower half. For the most part, such reticulation should suggest unilateral pulmonary vein atresia or a variation of the Swyer-James lung. **B.** Isotope perfusion study demonstrates no isotope uptake in the right lung. **C.** Pulmonary arteriogram, early phase. Note markedly diminished blood flow to the right lung and characteristically small, con- stricted, and tapered pulmonary artery branches. **D.** Pulmonary arteriogram, later phase. The small vessels on the right are the pulmonary artery branches visualized in part **C.** They demon- strate extreme stasis of contrast material, and hence markedly impaired pulmonary blood flow. Also note that there are no drain- ing pulmonary veins on the right. On the left, veins are present and, in fact, are a little larger than normal. Left atrium *(LA).* A bronchogram in this patient was normal.

best possibilities are unilateral pulmonary atre- sia or stenosis (1), acquired hypoplasia with paren- chymal scarring (Swyer-James lung) and, occasion- ally, postirradiation lung. Cases of unilateral pulmonary vein atresia may be difficult to differenti- ate from the Swyer-James lung until pulmonary ar- teriograms are performed. In pulmonary vein atre- sia, draining pulmonary veins will not be visualized (Fig. 1.30). The reticulations present in patients with pulmonary vein atresia are due to chronic intersti- tial pulmonary edema and ensuing fibrosis, and probably also to compensatorily dilated lymphatics. In the Swyer-James lung and the postirradiation lung, reticularity is due to pulmonary fibrosis.

REFERENCES

1. Belcourt CL, Roy DL, Nanton MA, Finley JP, Gillis DA, Krause VW, Aterman K: Stenosis of individual pulmo- nary veins: radiologic findings. *Radiology* 161:109–112, 1986.
2. Cumming GR, MacPherson RI, Chernick V: Unilateral

hyperlucent lung syndrome in children. *J Pediatr* 78:250–260, 1971.

3. Currarino G, Williams B: Causes of congenital unilateral pulmonary hypoplasia: a study of thirty-three cases. *Pediatr Radiol* 15:15–24, 1985.
4. Kogutt MS, Swischuk LE, Goldblum R: Swyer-James syndrome (unilateral hyperlucent lung) in children. *Am J Dis Child* 125:614–618, 1973.
5. MacLeod WM: Abnormal transradiancy of one lung. *Thorax* 17:230–239, 1962.
6. MacPherson RI, Cumming GR, Chernick V: Unilateral hyperlucent lung: a complication of viral pneumonia. *J Can Assoc Radiol* 20:225–231, 1969.
7. Marti-Bonmati L, Perales RF, Catala F, Mata JM, Calonge E: CT findings in Swyer-James syndrome. *Radiology* 172:477–480, 1989.
8. Moore ADA, Godwin JD, Dietrich PA, Vershakelen JA, Henderson WR Jr: Swyer-James syndrome: CT findings in eight patients. *AJR* 158:1211–1215, 1992.
9. Swischuk LE, L'Heureux P: Unilateral pulmonary vein atresia or stenosis (diagnostic roentgenographic and clinical features). *AJR* 135:667–672, 1980.
10. Swyer P, James C: Case of unilateral pulmonary emphysema. *Thorax* 8:133–136, 1953.

Focal Aeration Disturbances

Focal aeration disturbances, either atelectatic or emphysematous, can result from any of the problems leading to similar aeration disturbances involving the entire lung. These conditions have been discussed in previous sections and do not require reiteration, except to note that the commonest cause of focal atelectasis is mucous plugging due to viral lower respiratory tract infection or asthma. The commonest cause of obstructive emphysema is a foreign body (1, 5). In addition, it might be noted that areas of atelectasis and obstructive emphysema frequently coexist in some patients. For the most part, this occurs with endobronchial lesions such as granulomas, tumors, or multiple foreign bodies, and unless one is aware of the phenomenon, the findings can be puzzling. This is especially true when the right middle lobe is involved (Fig. 1.31).

An unusual condition resulting in localized overinflation of a portion of the lung (usually a lobe) is the bronchial atresia-mucocele syndrome (2–4, 6). In the newborn, this condition manifests as a solid, fluid-filled lobe distal to the atretic portion of the bronchus. The early radiographic findings are those of a pulmonary mass, but later, as fluid clears, the lung becomes emphysematous (by way of the air-drift phenomenon through the pores of Kohn). Mucous impactions distal to the site of bronchial atresia appear as a nodule or small mass, and in combination, the findings are pathognomonic (Fig. 1.32).

REFERENCES

1. Eggleston PA, Ward BH, Pierson WE, Bierman CW: Radiographic abnormalities in acute asthma in children. *Pediatrics* 54:442–449, 1974.
2. Genereux GP: Bronchial atresia: a rare cause of unilateral lung hypertranslucency. *J Can Assoc Radiol* 22:71–82, 1971.
3. Oh KS, Dorst JP, White JJ, Haller JA Jr, Johnson BA, Byrne WD: Syndrome of bronchial atresia or stenosis with mucocele and focal hyperinflation of the lung. *Johns Hopkins Med J* 138:48–53, 1976.
4. Schuster SR, Harris GBC, Williams A, Kirkpatick J, Reid L: Bronchial atresia: a recognizable entity in the pediatric age group. *J Pediatr Surg* 13:682–689, 1978.
5. Shopfner CE: Aeration disturbances secondary to pulmonary infection. *Am J Roentgenol Radium Ther Nucl Med* 120:261–273, 1974.
6. Talner LB, Gmelich JT, Liebow AA, Greenspan RH: The syndrome of bronchial mucocele and regional hyperinflation of the lung. *Am J Roentgenol Radium Ther Nucl Med* 110:675–686, 1970.

TRACHEOBRONCHIAL AIR SHADOW ABNORMALITIES

The tracheal air shadow almost always is visible in infants and children, but in the young infant, since the trachea is mobile, the air column normally may become rather tortuous during expiration (Fig. 1.33). Characteristically, during expiration it buckles anteriorly and to the right (4), and in some cases, produces an almost right-angle configuration at the level of the thoracic inlet (Fig. 1.33). This should not be misinterpreted for deviation due to a mass, for when a mass or vascular ring displaces the trachea, acute bends are not present; rather, focal curving contours are seen (Fig. 1.34). It has been suggested that herniation of the thymus gland into the neck during expiration contributes to the normal tracheal deviation seen in Fig. 1.33 (10).

GENERALIZED TRACHEAL DIAMETER CHANGES

In infants, it has been stated that it should be considered abnormal if, during inspiration, the trachea is less than 3 mm in diameter (6). This is probably true, but the whole problem is rather rare, for there are very few, if any, causes of narrowing of the entire trachea on inspiration. Even cases of congenital tracheal stenosis usually are more focal than generalized. On expiration, however, the entire trachea may narrow to a diameter of less than 3 mm. In some of these cases, the trachea simply is hypercollapsible, and even though it is quite narrow during expiration, no particular symptoms arise and obstructive emphysema does not develop. On the other

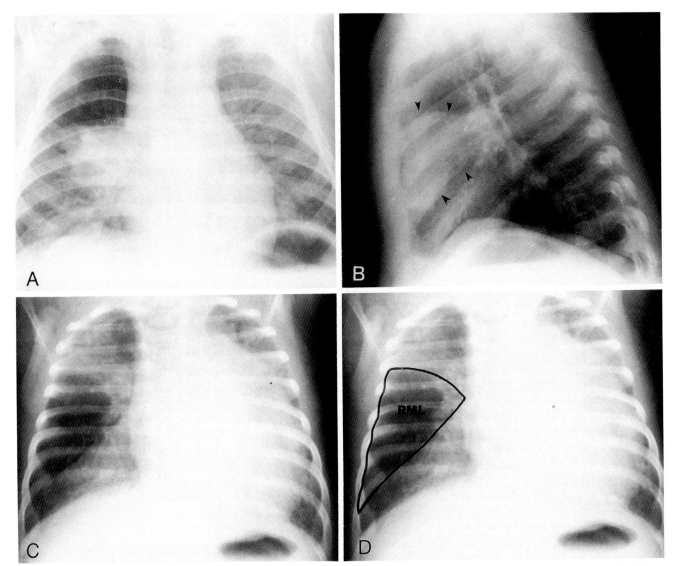

Figure 1.31. Focal aeration disturbances. A. Right middle lobe atelectasis and right upper lobe emphysema. Note what at first appears to be a large, dense, right hilum. Also note that the right upper lobe is hyperlucent due to obstructive emphysema. **B.** Lateral view demonstrates the opacity seen on frontal view to be a partially collapsed right middle lobe *(arrows)*. These findings were secondary to a large endobronchial granuloma due to atypical tuberculous infection. **C. Middle lobe emphysema.** Note the triangular radiolucency in the right midlung field. This is characteristic of an overdistended right middle lobe, and the opacities above and below are the partially collapsed right upper and lower lobes. **D.** Diagrammatic outlining of the emphysematous right middle lobe *(RML)*. This patient had congenital right middle lobe emphysema and also had a large ventricular septal defect (note cardiomegaly and vascular engorgement).

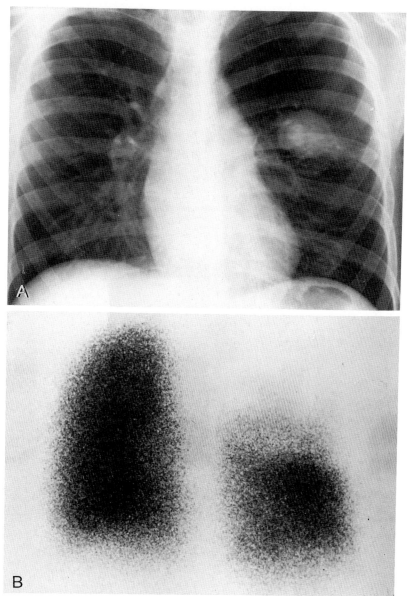

Figure 1.32. Bronchial atresia with mucocele: hyperinflation syndrome. A. Note the hyperinflated left upper lobe. The vascularity is diminished, and the lobe is larger than normal. Also note the large central nodule representing impacted mucus (i.e., mucocele). **B.** Isotope scan showing no uptake in left upper lobe.

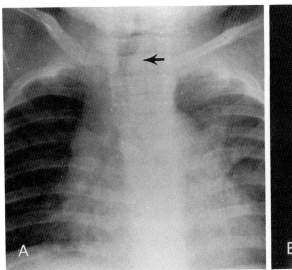
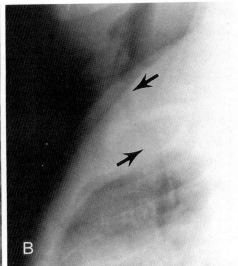

Figure 1.33. Normal tracheal buckling. A. Frontal view showing characteristic deviation of the trachea to the right on expiration. Note the almost right angle bend *(arrow)* at the level of the thoracic inlet. **B.** Lateral view demonstrating extreme tortuosity of the entire airway *(arrows)* causing a "pseudomass" configuration to develop behind the pharynx and upper trachea.

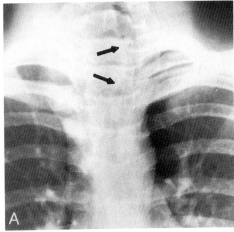
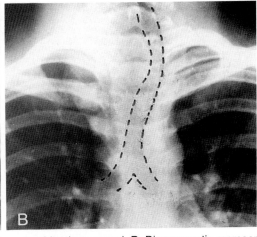

Figure 1.34. Pathologic tracheal deviation. A. Note minimal compression and marked deviation of the trachea to the left *(arrows)* by a thyroid adenoma. The superior mediastinum also is wider than normal. **B.** Diagrammatic representation of tracheal deviation seen in part **A.**

hand, the same phenomenon can occur in infants with bronchiolitis and/or reactive airway disease (Fig. 1.35A and B). The phenomenon often is explained on the basis of generalized tracheomalacia (1), but this condition is rare. Another rare cause of diffuse tracheal narrowing is intramural mucopolysaccharide deposition in the storage diseases (13).

A generalized increase in the diameter of the trachea and major bronchi is an uncommon problem, but does occur in tracheobronchomegaly (8, 11, 16). In this condition, elastic tissue deficiency allows the trachea and bronchi to distend to greater than normal diameters during inspiration (Fig. 1.35C and D),

and although the condition has been considered congenital, most likely it is the result of an acquired necrotizing bronchiolitis. Inspired air is blocked by the obliterated bronchioles, leading to chronic overdistension of the more proximal bronchi and trachea (11). However, the trachea may not dilate as much as the bronchi (Fig. 1.35).

FOCAL TRACHEOBRONCHIAL NARROWINGS

Focal, often eccentric, tracheobronchial narrowings can result from the compressive effects of

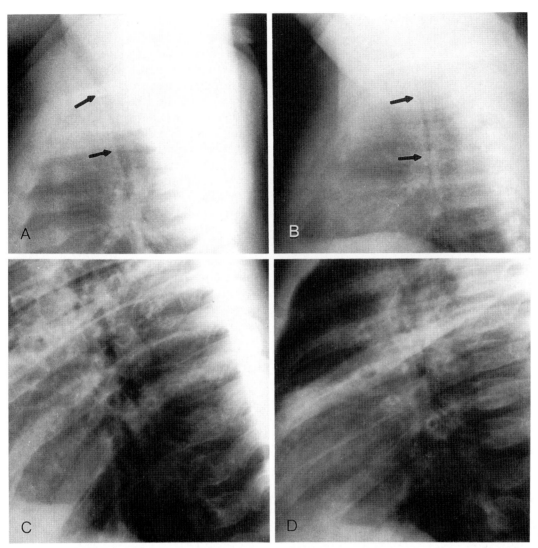

Figure 1.35. Hypercollapsible trachea. A. Inspiratory view demonstrating normal tracheal diameter *(arrows)*. **B.** Expiratory view demonstrates marked diminution of tracheal diameter *(arrows)*. This patient had wheezing that cleared with epinephrine. Eventually, the infant developed asthma. **C. Tracheobron-** **chomegaly.** Inspiratory view demonstrating large cystic structures scattered throughout the lung. These are overly dilated bronchi. **D.** Expiratory film. Characteristically, the bronchi collapse (i.e., note how much smaller the cystic areas appear).

abnormally located or dilated blood vessels and paratracheal cysts, masses, or inflammations. They also can result from encroachment upon the airway by endotracheal or endobronchial lesions. Circumferential narrowings are less common and usually are due to congenital or acquired stenoses, or focal areas of tracheomalacia. None of these lesions are particularly common, but with the widespread use of endotracheal tubes in the neonate, acquired tracheal stenosis is becoming more common. Usually these narrowings are located within 1 inch of the vocal cords. Narrowings in this area are discussed more completely in Chapter 2.

Focal tracheomalacia occurs with any lesion that causes compression of the trachea in utero. Consequently, it can be seen with compressive vascular anomalies or rings (1, 2, 7, 12, 14), paratracheal cysts or masses, or even the dilated proximal pouch of esophageal atresia (5). In these cases, there is inhibition of normal cartilage development and focal softening of the trachea (Fig. 1.36). In the older infant and child, focal tracheomalacia usually is the result of damage to the trachea during endotracheal intubation.

Not all vascular abnormalities cause tracheal compression to the point of the development of focal tracheomalacia. However, with true vascular rings (e.g., double aortic arch), anomalous innominate or

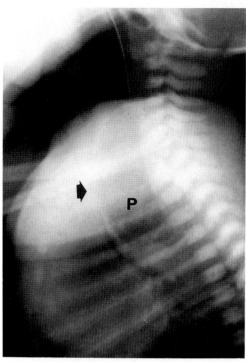

Figure 1.36. Focal tracheomalacia. In this infant with esophageal atresia, the air-filled proximal esophageal pouch *(P)* is producing a focal narrowing of the adjacent trachea *(arrow)*.

left common carotid artery, and anomalous left pulmonary artery (pulmonary sling), the problem is common. With vascular rings, a right-sided aortic arch usually is present, and this will produce compression of the trachea from the right side. Narrowing of the trachea may be seen on both frontal and lateral views, and also is vividly demonstrable with MRI (Fig. 1.37). Anomalous innominate or left common carotid artery abnormalities (see p. 4) characteristically produce anterior compression of the trachea (Fig. 1.38A). With the pulmonary sling (9, 15), the left pulmonary artery, as it arises from the right pulmonary artery, swings around the trachea and produces an indentation just above the carina on the right (Fig. 1.38B). On lateral view, since the aberrant left pulmonary artery travels between the esophagus and the trachea, a characteristic posterior indentation on the trachea is produced (Fig. 1.38C). A concomitant anterior indentation on the adjacent esophagus also can be seen when barium studies are performed. The pulmonary sling anomaly usually is symptomatic while the anomalous innominate or left common carotid abnormality, although producing apnea in some patients (2), tends to be asymptomatic (14). Double aortic arch and right aortic arch with aberrant left subclavian artery and encircling ductus arteriosus or ligamentum arter-

iosus (true vascular rings) usually are symptomatic. Congenital stenosis of the trachea or bronchi is rather uncommon but does occur (Fig. 1.39). These narrowings can occur anywhere along the tracheobronchial tree. Acquired stenoses are becoming more common with the widespread use of tracheostomies and long-term endotracheal intubation. These narrowings tend to occur in the subglottic portion of the trachea, or slightly lower when related to a tracheostomy tube. A peculiar form of congenital tracheal narrowing occurs with complete cartilaginous rings. In infants with this condition, the cartilaginous rings are solid and produce variable lengths of tracheal stenosis. The anomaly is associated with aberrant left pulmonary artery and hence the term "the ring-sling complex" (3) has been used. The typical findings consist of anterior indentation of the trachea and posterior indentation of the esophagus by the left pulmonary artery that travels between the trachea and esophagus, associated with an area of stenosis of the trachea (Fig. 1.38C).

Finally, an unusual but not uncommon, tracheal narrowing can occur with impacted esophageal foreign bodies (Fig. 1.40A). In these cases paraesophageal edema occurs rather rapidly, and although at first problems with dysphagia may be present, eventually respiratory obstructive symptoms predominate. These infants often self-adjust their diets, slowly switching to liquids and avoiding solids. Therefore, the presence of the impacted esophageal foreign body frequently is a surprise. Narrowing of the trachea may remain for a few days after the foreign body has been removed (Fig. 1.40B).

AIR BRONCHOGRAM

When air is seen in the bronchi, the term "air bronchogram" is used, and while such a phenomenon occurs in the trachea and major bronchi in normal individuals, when it is seen beyond the second branching of the bronchial tree, it becomes pathologic. In such cases, the pulmonary parenchyma loses its normal aeration and becomes hazy or opaque, either due to atelectasis or to the accumulation of some type of fluid in the alveoli (i.e., exudate, edema, or blood). The air in the small bronchi that are surrounded by the opacified alveoli becomes visible as an air bronchogram. Exudate (pus) is seen with consolidating pneumonias, edema fluid from any number of cardiac or noncardiac causes, and blood from traumatic injury, venous infarction, or bleeding disorders. Regardless of the cause, the findings are about the same (Fig. 1.41), but with compressive atelectasis, the air-filled bronchi in the

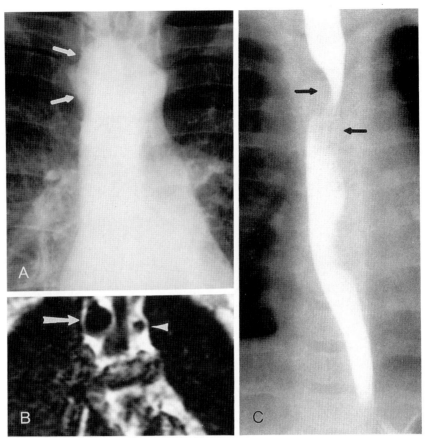

Figure 1.37. Focal tracheomalacia: double aorta. A. Note the prominent aortic arch on the right compressing and displacing the trachea to the left *(arrows)*. **B.** MRI demonstrates the larger and more superior right arch *(arrow)* and the small left arch *(ar-rowhead)*. **C.** Esophogram on another patient with a double aorta shows the impression made by the larger right arch above the smaller indentation by the left arch, creating the reverse S-sign *(arrows)*.

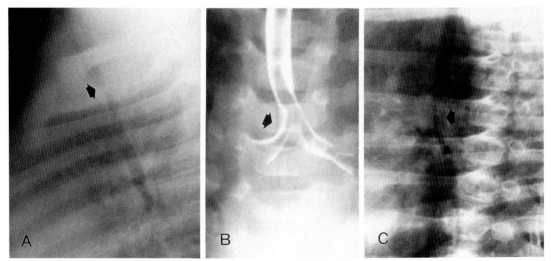

Figure 1.38. Focal tracheal narrowings with vascular anomalies. A. Anomalous innominate artery. Note characteristic anterior tracheal indentation *(arrow)* produced by an anomalous innominate artery. **B. Pulmonary sling.** Characteristic tracheal indentation on the right, just at the level of the carina *(arrow)*. **C.** Lateral view, same patient, demonstrating characteristic posterior indentation and compression of the trachea *(arrow)*. (Parts **B** and **C** courtesy of Joe Jackson, M.D., Corpus Christi, Texas.)

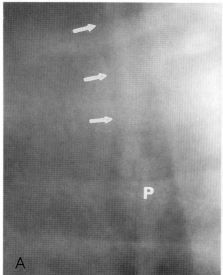 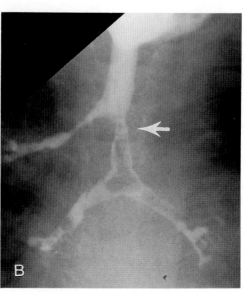

Figure 1.39. Focal tracheal narrowing: stenosis. A. Long segment tracheal stenosis *(arrows)* is present in this patient with the pulmonary ring-sling complex. The aberrant left pulmonary artery *(P)* as it travels between the trachea *(T)* and esophagus *(E)* produces corresponding indentations on both of these structures. **B.** Bronchogram in another patient with a short segment congenital tracheal stenosis *(arrow)*.

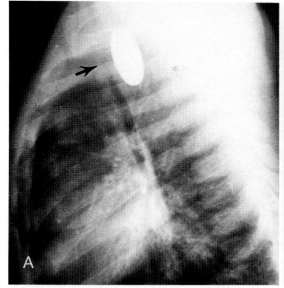 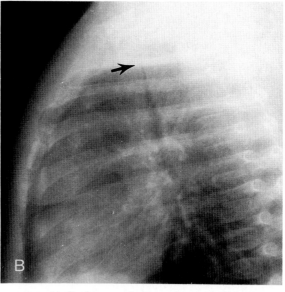

Figure 1.40. Focal tracheal narrowing: esophageal foreign body. A. Esophageal foreign body (a coin) causing paraesophageal inflammation and compression of the trachea *(arrow)*. **B.** Same patient. Narrowing *(arrow)* persists after the coin has been removed. Such narrowing can develop within 2 or 3 days after the foreign body becomes lodged and characteristically remains for a few days after its removal.

collapsed lobe are clustered close together. If bronchiectasis also is present, the bronchi become nodular and dilated (Fig. 1.41*B* and *C*).

Rarely, air bronchograms can be seen with extensive interstitial disease (i.e., see Fig. 1.78*B*), and in such cases, although the alveoli are relatively free of disease, the interstitium is so thickened by infiltrate, edema, or fibrosis that the alveoli are compressed to a near-airless state. Alveolar disease then is erroneously suggested because the radiograph cannot differentiate between alveoli that are packed full of fluid and those squeezed shut by extensive interstitial infiltrate (i.e., both are airless).

REFERENCES

1. Baxter JD, Dunbar JS: Tracheomalacia. *Ann Otol Rhinol Laryngol* 72:1013–1023, 1963.

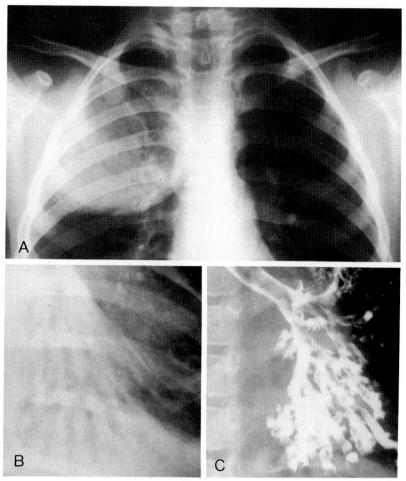

Figure 1.41. Air bronchogram. A. Consolidating pneumonia. Note the air bronchogram in the consolidated right upper lobe due to *Klebsiella* pneumonia. **B.** Air bronchogram with atelectasis and bronchiectasis. Note the dilated, tortuous air-filled bronchi in the left lower lobe. They are crowded because of atelectasis and dilated because of bronchiectasis. **C.** Bronchogram demonstrating the left lower lobe bronchiectatic changes.

2. Berdon WD, Baker DH, Bordiuk J, Mellins R: Innominate artery compression of trachea in infants with stridor and apnea. *Radiology* 92:272–278, 1969.
3. Berdon WE, Baker DH, Wung Jen-Tien, Chrispin A, Kozlowski K, de Silva M, Bales P, Alford B: Complete cartilage ring tracheal stenosis associated with anomalous pulmonary artery: the ring-sling complex. *Radiology* 152:57–64, 1984.
4. Chang L, Lee F, Gwinn J: Normal lateral deviation of the trachea in infants and children. *Am J Roentgenol Radium Ther Nucl Med* 109:247–251, 1970.
5. Cook RCM, Bush GH: Tracheal compression as a cause of respiratory symptoms after repair of oesophageal atresia. *Arch Dis Child* 53:246–248, 1978.
6. Donaldson SW, Thompsett AC Jr: Tracheal diameter in the normal newborn infant. *Am J Roentgenol Radium Ther Nucl Med* 67:785–787, 1952.
7. Fletcher BD, Cohn RC: Tracheal compression and the innominate artery: MR evaluation in infants. *Radiology* 170:103–107, 1989.
8. Hunter TB, Kuhns LR, Roloff MA, Holt JF: Tracheobronchiomegaly in an eighteen month old child. *AJR* 123:687–690, 1975.
9. Jue KL, Raghib G, Amplatz K, Adams P Jr, Edwards JE: Anomalous origin of the left pulmonary artery from the right pulmonary artery. *AJR* 95:598–610, 1965.
10. Mandell GA, Bellah RD, Boulden MEC, Sherman NH, Harcke HT, Padman RJ, McNicholas KW: Cervical trachea: dynamics in response to herniation of the normal thymus. *Radiology* 186:383–386, 1993.
11. Mitchell RE, Burgy RG: Congenital bronchiectasis due to deficiency of bronchial cartilage (Williams-Campbell syndrome). *J Pediatr* 87:230–232, 1975.
12. Möes CAF, Izukawa T, Trusler GA: Innominate artery compression of the trachea. *Arch Otolaryngol* 101:733–738, 1975.
13. Peters ME, Arya S, Langer LO, Gilbert EF, Calson R, Adkins W: Narrow trachea in mucopolysaccharidoses. *Pediatr Radiol* 15:225–228, 1985.
14. Swischuk LE: Anterior tracheal indentation in infancy and early childhood: normal or abnormal? *Am J Roentgenol Radium Ther Nucl Med* 112:12–17, 1971.
15. Tesler UF, Balsara RH, Niguidula F: Aberrant left pulmonary artery (vascular sling): report of five cases. *Chest* 66:402–407, 1974.
16. Williams HE, Landau LI, Phelan PD: Generalized bronchiectasis due to extensive deficiency of bronchial cartilage. *Arch Dis Child* 47:423–428, 1972.

Free and Loculated Air

Free air can accumulate in the pleural space (pneumothorax), mediastinum (pneumomediastinum), pericardial cavity (pneumopericardium), and in the heart itself (pneumocardium). The most common of these, of course, is pneumothorax.

PNEUMOTHORAX

Pneumothorax is more common in the neonate than in older children, and most commonly it occurs in infants receiving positive pressure ventilation. Spontaneous pneumothorax is less common in children than in adults, although a familial form has been described (13). Generally, when pneumothorax is present in a child, some underlying problem such as chest trauma, asthma (1), or ruptured pneumatocele is the cause. Chest trauma probably is most common, however (Table 1.8).

Table 1.8
Free and Loculated Air

Pneumothorax	
Chest trauma Neonatal pneumothorax	Common
Asthma Foreign body	Uncommon
Obstructive emphysema—other causes Esophageal perforation Spontaneous pneumothorax Ruptured lung cyst or pneumatocele	Rare
Mediastinal air	

A. Pneumomediastinum
   Asthma
   Trauma
   Iatrogenic
	Common

Foreign body Paroxysmal coughing Esophageal perforation	Rare
B. Air in mediastinal viscera (hiatus hernia, esophagus, colon interposition)	Common
Pneumopericardium	
Trauma Positive pressure ventilation	Uncommon
Gas-forming infection	Rare
Pneumocardium	
Penetrating trauma Iatrogenic	Uncommon

With pneumothorax, air can outline the lung circumferentially, or can accumulate along any of its surfaces. This is important to appreciate, for one can encounter subpulmonic, medial, and anterior air accumulations, and when any of these occur alone, they may be missed or misinterpreted. Classically, however, free air tends to produce a band of hyperlucency (vascular marking-free) between the chest wall and the underlying lung (Fig. 1.42A).

Medial pneumothorax, that is, a collection of air between the mediastinum and the inner lung edge, most commonly occurs in supine position and in the neonate (7, 11), but can be seen in older children (Fig. 1.42B). This type of pneumothorax must be differentiated from the normal radiolucent halo around the heart occasionally produced by juxtapositioning of the left cardiac border and the lower lobe pulmonary artery, and from pneumopericardium. When a medial pneumothorax is suspected, decubitus views can be helpful, because the air will shift (rise) to a more familiar location, that is, against the lateral chest wall. Expiratory views also can enhance visualization of the pneumothorax.

Anterior pneumothorax, that is, free air layered over the anterior surface of the lung in patients examined in the supine position, also poses a considerable diagnostic problem. Although first described in the neonate (11), this pattern also can occur in older children. When present, pneumothorax produces hyperlucency of the involved hemithorax (due to increased air in the pleural space and compression of the lung below it) and exaggerated sharpness of the ipsilateral mediastinal edge (see Fig. 1.25). This latter finding results from air abutting the mediastinum and is important to note because often no other findings of pneumothorax are present. In infants, when the pneumothorax is under some tension, the thymus gland can be compressed medially and superiorly, giving the false impression of a superior mediastinal mass (8) (Fig. 1.42C).

PNEUMOMEDIASTINUM

The commonest cause of pneumomediastinum in the pediatric age group is airway obstruction in patients with asthma (1, 6, 9), and although pneumomediastinum also can occur with obstructing foreign bodies and other focal or generalized airway obstructions, all of these situations are rather uncommon (Table 1.8). Next most commonly after asthma, pneumomediastinum can be seen with chest trauma and iatrogenically after endoscopy or during positive pressure ventilation. Paroxysms of coughing also occasionally can lead to pneumomediastinum

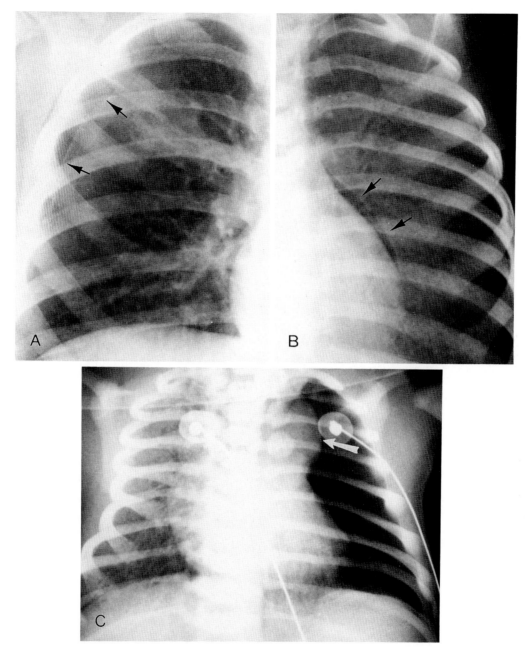

Figure 1.42. A. Typical pneumothorax. Note the free edge of the right lung *(arrow).* Some air also is present outside the chest wall because of penetrating chest trauma. **B. Medial pneumothorax.** Note the medial pneumothorax *(arrows)* in this patient whose lung was biopsied for verification of *Pneumocystis carinii* pneumonia (note hazy lungs). **C. Anterior pneumothorax.** In this supine infant, the pneumothorax lies anteriorly, causing increased radiolucency of the left hemithorax, increased sharpness of the left heart border, and upward and medial compression of the thymus gland *(arrow).*

but the situation does not arise very often. Pneumomediastinum secondary to spontaneous esophageal perforation also is rare.

Air in the mediastinum produces irregular gas collections within the soft tissues of the superior mediastinum, with the air frequently outlining the undersurface of the thymus gland. In other cases, the air may extend into the soft tissues of the neck or chest wall. This is termed "subcutaneous emphysema" (Fig. 1.43A) and, indeed, there may be more air in the extrathoracic soft tissues than in the mediastinum itself. Air in the mediastinum often is visualized better on lateral than on frontal views, and occasionally can track downward and produce simi-

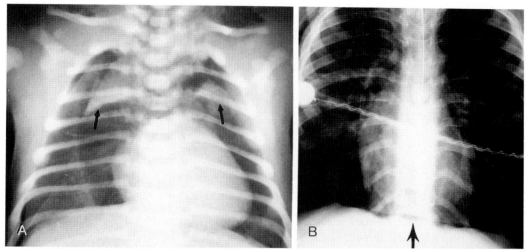

Figure 1.43. Pneumomediastinum. A. Characteristic central air collections surrounding the heart and elevating the lobes of the thymus gland *(arrows).* The free air has also dissected into the subcutaneous tissues of the neck. Bilateral pneumothoraces are also present. **B.** Continuous diaphragm sign *(arrow)* of pneumomediastinum in a patient with a lacerated trachea.

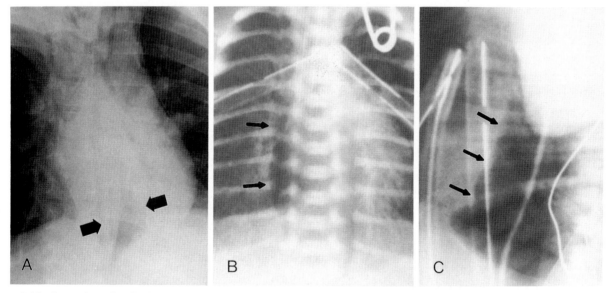

Figure 1.44. Central mediastinal air collections. A. Air in inferior pulmonary ligament *(arrows).* Note typical appearance of such air *(arrows)* in this location. This patient also has left lower lobe atelectasis, right upper lobe atelectasis, and air in the superior mediastinum, all of which resulted from massive aspiration of foreign material. **B.** Neonate with air in the retroesophageal space or ligament *(arrows).* **C.** Lateral view demonstrates the typical location of this air *(arrows).*

lar irregular collections of air in the lower mediastinum. In other cases, air can pass into the abdominal cavity to produce pneumoperitoneum. Pneumomediastinal air may also accumulate along the diaphragmatic leaflets (between the diaphragm and the parietal pleura) and mimic a subpulmonic pneumothorax. If such air crosses the superior surface of the diaphragm, it will outline the diaphragm in its entirety (5) constituting the continuous diaphragm sign (Fig. 1.43B). Finally, it might be noted that

pneumomediastinal air also can accumulate in the inferior pulmonary ligaments and, as such, produce a characteristic oblong or oval air collection behind the heart (Fig. 1.44A). Such air collections commonly occur with blunt chest trauma (2–4, 10) and with positive pressure-assisted ventilation. A similar air collection can occur in the retroesophageal space (ligament) and most commonly is seen in neonates receiving positive pressure ventilation (Fig. 1.44B and C). These latter air collections must be differentiated from the circular to oval collection of air in a hiatus hernia (Fig. 1.45*A*). Air in a dilated esophagus also can be seen with gastroesophageal reflux (Fig. 1.45*B* and *C*). This finding, termed "mega-aeroesophagus," is most common in the perinatal period and in children with cerebral palsy or mental retardation (12). A final cause of air in the mediastinum is that seen with colon interposition or the so-called "gastric tunnel" (Fig. 1.46). In these cases where the esophagus is absent or destroyed, an interposing piece of colon or stomach is placed in the anterior mediastinum, and swallowed air accumulates in these structures.

PNEUMOPERICARDIUM

Pneumopericardium generally is uncommon in the pediatric age group, but can be seen with chest trauma and positive pressure-assisted ventilation. The latter mechanism accounts for many pericardial air collections in the neonate, but in older children

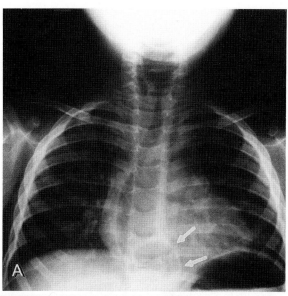

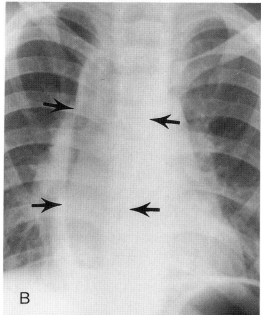

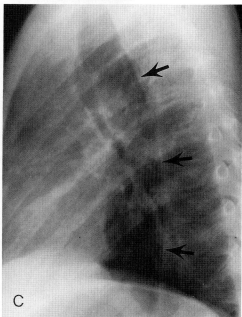

Figure 1.45. Air in the esophagus. A. Note typical appearance of air in the hiatus hernia *(arrows)*. There is also air in the esophagus, indicating the presence of gastroesophageal reflux. *B* and

C. Note the air-filled, dilated esophagus *(arrows)*. The presence of such mega-aeroesophagus is a reliable plain film sign of gastroesophageal reflux.

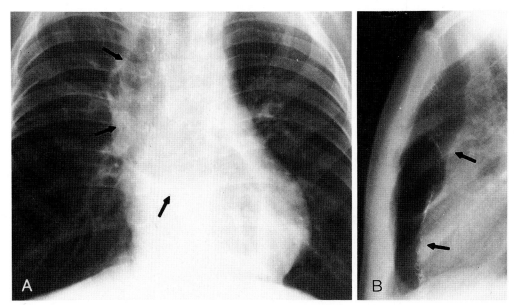

Figure 1.46. Retrosternal gastric tunnel. A. Note air outlining the retrosternally transferred stomach *(arrows).* **B.** Lateral view demonstrating similar findings *(arrows).*

the problem usually is trauma. With small-volume air collections, air may not surround the entire heart, but still, most often enough air is present to allow visualization of part or all of the pericardial sac (a thin white stripe) (Fig. 1.47*A*).

PNEUMOCARDIUM

Air within the heart is quite rare and almost always is secondary to penetrating trauma of the heart (Fig. 147*B*) or trauma to the large peripheral blood vessels resulting in air embolus of the heart. However, it also can be seen on an iatrogenic basis, secondary to positive pressure ventilation (usually in a neonate) or following accidental introduction of air into the vascular system during intravenous injections.

FREE AIR AND FLUID

Air, when combined with fluid in any of the foregoing compartments, results in air-fluid levels on upright or decubitus views. In the pleural space, such air-fluid levels can be seen with pyopneumothorax or hemopneumothorax (Fig. 1.48*A*). Air-fluid levels in the pleural space also occur with esophageal perforation, and air-fluid levels in the mediastinum can be seen with hiatus hernia, esophageal obstruction, and occasionally with hemo- or pyopneumopericardium. Air-fluid levels also can be seen in the inferior pul-

monary ligament. The fluid in these cases usually is blood due to chest trauma (Fig. 1.48*B*).

REFERENCES

1. Bierman CW: Pneumomediastinum and pneumothorax complicating asthma in children. *Am J Dis Child* 114:42–50, 1967.
2. Fagan AH, Rogers BM, Talbert JL: Traumatic mediastinal pneumatoceles. *Radiology* 120:11–18, 1976.
3. Felman AH, Rogers BM, Talbert JL: Traumatic paramediastinal air cyst: a case report. *Pediatr Radiol* 4:120–121, 1976.
4. Hyde I: Traumatic paramediastinal air cysts. *Br J Radiol* 44:380–383, 1971.
5. Levin B: Continuous diaphragm sign: newly recognized sign of pneumomediastinum. *Clin Radiol* 24:337–338, 1973.
6. McSweeney WJ, Stempel DA: Non-iatrogenic pneumomediastinum in infancy and childhood. *Pediatr Radiol* 1:139–144, 1973.
7. Moskowitz PS, Griscom NT: The medial pneumothorax. *Radiology* 120:143–147, 1976.
8. O'Keeffe FN, Swischuk LE, Stansberry SD: Mediastinal pseudomass caused by compression of the thymus in neonates with anterior pneumothorax. *AJR* 156:145–148, 1981.
9. Ozonoff M: Pneumomediastinum associated with asthma and pneumonia in children. *AJR* 95:112–117, 1965.
10. Ravin C, Smith GW, Lester PD, McLoud TC, Putman CE: Post-traumatic pneumatocele in the inferior pulmonary ligament. *Radiology* 121:39–41, 1976.
11. Swischuk LE: Two lesser known but useful signs of neonatal pneumothorax. *AJR* 127:623–627, 1976.
12. Swischuk LE, Hayden CK Jr, van Caillie B: Mega-aeroe-

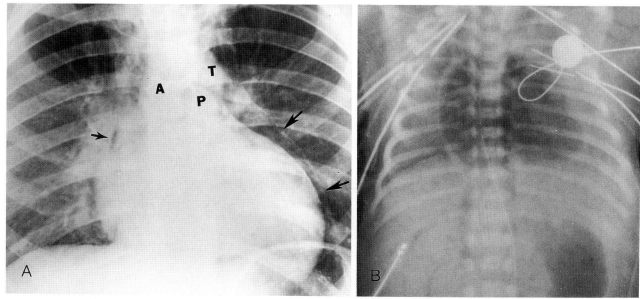

Figure 1.47. A. Pneumopericardium. Note air within the pericardial sac *(arrows)*, outlining the heart. Air also is present around the great vessels, and associated pneumomediastinum has outlined the thymus gland *(T)*. Aorta *(A)*. Pulmonary artery

(P). **B. Pneumocardium.** The heart is filled with air as a complication of positive pressure ventilation in this premature neonate. Also note intravascular air within the liver.

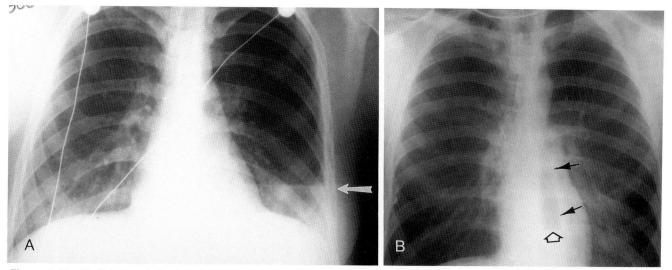

Figure 1.48. Air-fluid levels in the chest. A. Note the air-fluid level in the left lower hemithorax *(arrow)* in a patient with a hemopneumothorax secondary to a stab wound. **B.** Air-fluid level in a trauma-induced lung cyst in the inferior pulmonary ligament

(open arrow). (Reprinted with permission from Fagan, CJ, Swischuk LE: Traumatic lung and paramediastinal pneumatoceles. *Radiology* 120:11–18, 1976.)

sophagus in childhood: a sign of esophageal sphincter dysfunction. *Radiology* 141:73–76, 1981.
13. Wilson WG, Aylsworth AS: Familial spontaneous pneumothorax. *Pediatrics* 64:172–175, 1979.

Pleural Space and Fissure Thickening

THICKENING OF THE PLEURAL SPACE

Thickening of the pleural space can be generalized or localized, and when generalized, most often is due to some type of fluid collection. Fibrous pleural thickening is less common in children. Any type of fluid can accumulate in the pleural space, but pus (i.e., empyema) and serous effusions are the most common (Table 1.9). Empyema can accompany a variety of bacterial pneumonias, but most commonly is seen with staphylococal, *Hemophilus influenzae,* and *Streptococcus pneumoniae* infections (4, 8). Pleural fluid accumulations with *Mycoplasma pneumoniae* consolidations occur, but pleural fluid collections are rare with mycoplasma or viral bronchitis.

Serous pleural effusions commonly occur with renal diseases (e.g., acute glomerulonephritis, ne-

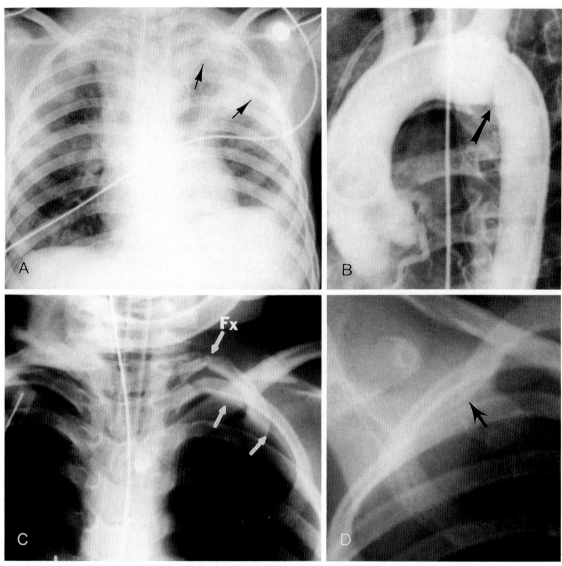

Figure 1.49. Pleural fluid over apex of the lung. A. Aortic rupture. Note the left apical pleural cap *(arrows)*. The superior mediastinum is widened and the esophageal tube is displaced to the right. **B.** Aortogram demonstrating an intimal flap due to an aortic injury *(arrow)*. **C.** Rib fracture. Note fluid over the apex of the left lung *(arrows)*. Also note the rib fracture *(Fx)*, and note that the mediastinum is not widened and that the tracheal and esophageal tubes are not displaced. A chest tube is present on the right for a pneumothorax. **D.** Normal apical soft tissues mimicking pleural thickening *(arrow)*.

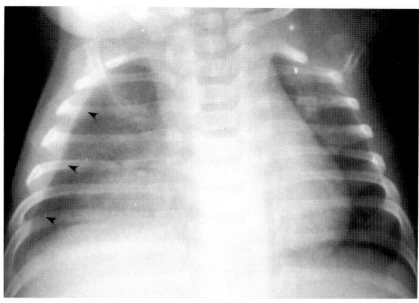

Figure 1.50. Pleural fluid. Note characteristic appearance of pleural fluid accumulating laterally *(arrows)*. One should recall that this fluid actually surrounds the lung, which is why the whole lung appears a little hazy.

Table 1.9
Pleural Space and Fissure Thickening

Pleural space thickening		
Fluid		
Empyema	}	
Serous effusion	}	Common
Blood		
Chyle	}	Uncommon
Pleural fibrosis	}	Common
Underlying rib lesions	}	Uncommon
Pleural tumor	}	Rare
Pleural fissure thickening		
Serous effusion		
Purulent effusion	}	
Blood	}	Common
Adjacent pulmonary edema		
Chyle	}	Rare
Focal subpleural thickening		
Underlying rib lesions	}	Common
Pleural tumor	}	Rare

nal diseases (e.g., acute glomerulonephritis, nephrotic syndrome, chronic renal failure), with tumors such as lymphoma and neuroblastoma, and with congestive heart failure. Blood in the pleural space most commonly occurs with chest cage and lung trauma, and less commonly with bleeding disorders, intravascular catheter erosions (1), aortic rup-

ture, and very infrequently with rupture of a ductus arteriosus aneurysm. With aortic rupture, fluid often accumulates over the left lung apex, because the point of rupture commonly is in that portion of the transverse arch which lies in communication with the left pleural space. Blood leaks over the top of the lung to produce the apical cap sign (7), a finding that should suggest aortic injury when seen with a widened mediastinum (Fig. 1.49A and B). Apical caps also can occur with an underlying upper rib fracture (Fig. 1.49C). Chylothorax is most common in newborn infants, and can occur spontaneously or secondary to superior vena cava thrombosis (5). Chylous effusions in patients beyond the neonatal period usually result from thoracic duct injury during chest trauma or thoracic surgery.

The most typical appearance of fluid in the pleural space is that which results when fluid accumulates over the lateral and apical portions of the lung (Fig. 1.50). Similar fluid accumulations can be seen on lateral view, occurring along either the anterior or posterior chest walls. Posteriorly, a costophrenic angle meniscus can be a clue to the presence of such fluid. If fluid accumulates over the diaphragmatic leaflets, a subpulmonic effusion results and an abnormality of diaphragmatic contour is seen (see Fig. 1.102A). Over the apex, pleural fluid accumulation must be differentiated from normal soft tissues that, to the uninitiated, may have an appearance virtually indistinguishable from fluid (Fig. 1.49D). This finding is common in children as well as adults and is due to normal subpleural fat and muscle (9).

Thickening of the pleural space due to fibrosis is less common in children, but must be differentiated from pleural fluid. This usually is accomplished with decubitus views which show that fibrous thickening does not change its configuration, whereas fluid shifts with changes in position. However, one must remember that in some cases of empyema or clotted blood, the fluid is so thick or so loculated that it also does not shift.

LOCALIZED THICKENINGS OF THE PLEURA

Localized thickening of the pleura almost always is related to old infection, trauma, or thoracic surgery involving the pleura or to some underlying lesion of the rib (Table 1.9). Focal rib abnormalities encountered include fractures with associated hematoma, osteomyelitis, and metastatic disease or leukemic lesions of the ribs (Fig. 1.51). When leukemic involvement of the ribs is extensive, the pleural thickening may be more diffuse than localized (6). Primary rib tumors and primary pleural tumors are quite rare. **Pleural fissure thickening,** when minimal, can be due to accumulation of fluid in the fissure or accumulation of fluid in the immediate subpleural space (Fig. 1.52). Actually, in the early stages of interstitial pulmonary edema, the latter

probably is more common and results from distension of the subpleural lymphatics. When the finding is due to actual pleural fluid, the fluid most often is serous (Table 1.9) and the degree of thickening depends on the amount of fluid present. In more severe cases, actual loculations of fluid can be seen (Fig. 1.52B) and sometimes such loculations can mimic a pulmonary mass. Thickening of the pleural fissure secondary to fibrosis is uncommon in the pediatric age group but occasionally can occur after infection or trauma.

Localized **thickening over the apex** of the lungs most often is due to normal soft tissues. Thereafter one should consider some type of fluid collection, and lastly an underlying rib lesion or pleural fibrosis. The causes of apical fluid collections are the same as for generalized fluid accumulations. However, one should be aware of the propensity for blood to accumulate over the apex with aortic rupture (see Fig. 1.49).

REFERENCES

1. Amodio JB, Abramsono SJ, Berdon WE, Solar C, Markowitz R, Kasznica J: Iatrogenic causes of large pleural fluid collections in the premature infant: ultrasonic and radiographic findings. *Pediatr Radiol* 17:104–108, 1987.
2. Bean WJ, Jordan RB, Gentry H, Nice CM: Fissure lines in the pediatric roentgenogram. *Am J Roentgenol Radium Ther Nucl Med* 106:109–113, 1969.

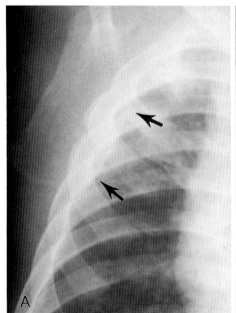
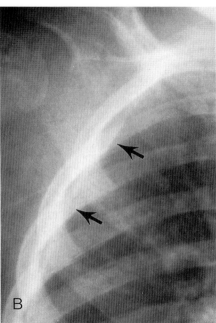
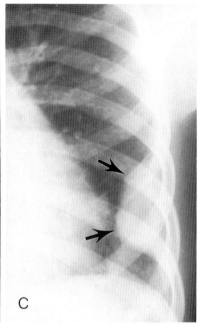

Figure 1.51. Localized pleural thickening. A. Note typical localized pleural thickening *(arrows)* and periosteal new bone deposition on adjacent ribs, due to chest tube placement for drainage of pleural fluid. **B.** Localized subpleural fluid collections *(arrows)* due to osteomyelitis of the rib, which became radiographically visible on later films. **C.** Pleural thickening secondary to leukemic involvement of the rib *(arrows).*

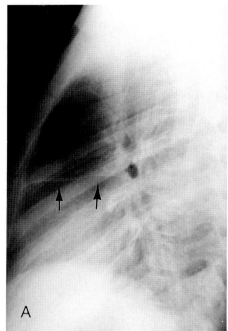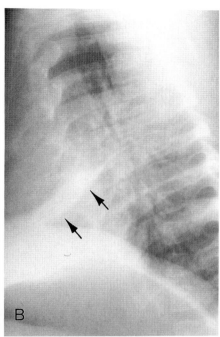

Figure 1.52. Pleural fissure thickening. A. Early fluid. Note that the minor fissure *(arrows)* in this patient with glomerulonephritis and pulmonary edema is slightly thickened. **B.** Loculated pleural effusion in the major fissure causes marked thickening of the fissure *(arrows).*

3. Fine NL, Smith LR, Sheedy PF: Frequency of pleural effusions in mycoplasma and viral pneumonias. *N Engl J Med* 283:791–793, 1970.
4. Highman JH: Staphylococcal pneumonia and empyema in childhood. *AJR* 106:103–108, 1969.
5. Kramer SS, Taylor GA, Garfinkel DJ, Simmons MA: Lethal chylothoraces due to superior vena caval thrombosis in infants. *AJR* 137:559–563, 1981.
6. Seigel MJ, Shackelford GD, McAlister WH: Pleural thickening: an unusual feature of childhood leukemia. *Radiology* 138:367–369, 1981.
7. Simeone JF, Minagi H, Putman CE: Traumatic disruption of the thoracic aorta: significance of the left apical extrapleural cap. *Radiology* 117:265–268, 1975.
8. Smith PL, Gerald B: Empyema in childhood followed roentgenographically: decortication seldom needed. *AJR* 106:114–117, 1969.
9. Vix V: Extrapleural costal fat. *Radiology* 112:563–565, 1974.

Calcifications in the Chest

A number of different calcifications can occur in the chest of a child, but almost always when calcification is seen, the disease process is chronic or healed. Most calcifications can be classified as flocculent, irregular, curvilinear, or punctate (Table 1.10).

FLOCCULENT AND IRREGULAR CALCIFICATIONS

Irregular calcifications commonly are seen in granulomatous pulmonary nodules or lymph nodes (Fig. 1.53*A* and *B*). Most commonly, the underlying infection is tuberculosis or fungal disease, but every so often similar calcifications can be seen in tumors undergoing necrosis, either spontaneously or after therapy (Fig. 1.53*C*). Flocculent calcification within a pulmonary nodule can be seen in postinflammatory granulomas, but is most characteristic of a hamartoma (see Fig. 1.64*B*). These lesions are rare, but the flocculent calcification belies the presence of cartilage, and therefore is a significant diagnostic feature of the lesion.

Irregular calcifications of various sizes also occur in old thrombi in the superior and inferior vena cavae (3, 6, 10) or portal vein, and while many are idiopathic (probably the result of dehydration, sepsis, or infection in infancy), others are the result of indwelling catheters or shunt tubes for hydrocephalus. The location of these calcified thrombi is what identifies them as such (Fig. 1.53*D*) and some may have a characteristic bullet shape. Other less common causes of irregular or flocculent calcification include calcific pericarditis, pleural calcification secondary to old infections, calcification in an old pulmonary he-

Table 1.10
Calcifications in the Chest

Flocculent or irregular	
Granulomas (nodules)	} Common
Old inflamed lymph nodes	
Old thrombi in IVC or SVC[a]	} Moderately common
Necrotic or treated tumor	
Calcific pericarditis	
Pleural calcifications	
Teratoma	
Old pulmonary hematoma	} Rare
Hamartoma	
Cardiac valve	
Myocardial infarction	
Linear and curvilinear	
Pleura	
Pericardium	} Uncommon
Vascular	
Calcification of cyst wall	} Rare
Punctate calcifications	
Old healed granulomatous disease	} Common
Calcification of ligamentum arteriosum	} Uncommon
Osteogenic sarcoma metastases	
Chickenpox pneumonia	
Pulmonary microlithiasis	} Rare
Hypercalcemia states	
Sarcoidosis	

[a] IVC, inferior vena cava; SVC, superior vena cava.

matoma or old pneumonia, calcified cardiac valves, calcification in a cartilaginous rib tumor, and, rarely, calcification of the myocardium after infarction.

LINEAR AND CURVILINEAR CALCIFICATIONS

These calcifications occur within the walls of blood vessels or cysts, or in serous membranes such as the pericardium and pleura. With these latter structures, calcification almost always is secondary to old inflammatory disease or trauma, and poses no real difficulty in identification. Vascular calcifications are relatively uncommon in the pediatric age group, but idiopathic calcification of the great vessels can occur in the young infant, and within the aorta of children with the candidiasis-endocrinopathy syndrome (7) and Singleton-Merten syndrome (5) (Fig. 1.54A). Calcifications in great vessel aneurysms, mycotic or otherwise, are uncommon (11), and so are calcifications in vascular grafts or in the patch used for cor-

rection of infundibular stenosis in tetralogy of Fallot (9). In the latter cases, aneurysmal dilation of the repaired infundibular region precedes the appearance of calcification, but when calcification occurs, it is rather characteristic (Fig. 1.54B). Calcification within the walls of bronchogenic cysts is rare (Fig. 1.54C), but calcification of acquired cysts such as echinococcal cysts is considerably more common. Overall, the frequency of parasitic cysts depends on the geographic location of one's practice.

Curvilinear lymph node calcifications resulting in "eggshell" calcifications are rare in children. However, occasionally in tuberculous or fungal infections lymph nodes can calcify in such a fashion (see Fig. 1.53B).

PUNCTATE CALCIFICATIONS

Punctate, parenchymal calcifications can be single or multiple, and most often result from tuberculous or histoplasma infections (Fig. 1.55A). Of course, they also can be seen with other fungal diseases, and their main differential diagnosis, especially when multiple, is that of normal blood vessels seen on end. Other causes of multiple punctate calcifications in the lung parenchyma include chickenpox pneumonia (usually in immunologically suppressed patients) and pulmonary microlithiasis (12). Both problems, however, are extremely rare in children. Calcification due to bone formation within metastatic nodules from osteogenic sarcoma can be punctate, but such nodules seldom are discovered before the presence of the primary tumor is known.

A peculiar, small, often punctate, calcification is that which occurs in the ligamentum arteriosum (2). This calcification is located between the aorta and pulmonary artery, and although frequently punctate, it also can be comma- or flame-shaped (Fig. 1.55B). The characteristic location of this calcification is what suggests its origin, and it is more commonly seen on CT of the chest than on plain chest radiographs (1).

MISCELLANEOUS CALCIFICATIONS

Diffuse calcification of the lungs is very uncommon, but metastatic calcification in the form of calcified masses or nodules has been reported in hypercalcemic states such as chronic renal failure or hypervitaminosis D and following cardiac surgery (4, 8). In such cases, calcium is deposited in the interstitium of the lungs, much the same as in other soft

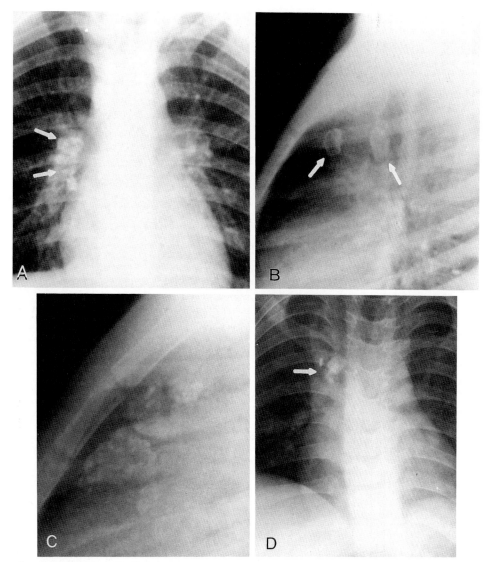

Figure 1.53. Irregular calcifications. A. Note typical irregular calcification of lymph nodes in the right hilar region *(arrows)* in this patient with old healed tuberculosis. **B.** Lateral view showing the calcified, shell-like periphery of the paratracheal and anterior mediastinal lymph nodes *(arrows)*. **C.** Old calcified posttreatment lymphoma lymph nodes in the mediastinum. **D.** Note the typically irregularly calcified thrombus in the superior vena cava *(arrow)*. Also note the tip of the adjacent shunt tube in this patient shunted for hydrocephalus.

tissues of the body. Formed calcifications representing bony structures, or even teeth, are characteristic of teratomas, but these tumors also can exhibit nonspecific, irregular calcifications.

REFERENCES

1. Bisceglia M, Donaldson JS: Calcification of the ligamentum arteriosum in children: a normal finding on CT. *AJR* 156:351, 1991.
2. Currarino G, Jackson JH Jr: Calcifications of ductus arteriosus and ligamentum Botalli. *Radiology* 94:139–142, 1970.
3. Kassner EG, Baumstark A, Kinkhabwala MN, Ablow RC, Haller JO: Calcified thrombus in the inferior vena cava in infants and children. *Pediatr Radiol* 4:167–171, 1976.
4. Mani TM, Lallemand D, Corone S, Mauriat P: Metastatic pulmonary calcifications after cardiac surgery in children. *Radiology* 174:463, 1990.
5. Singleton EB, Merten DF: An unusual syndrome of widened medullary cavities of the metacarpals and phalanges, aortic calcification and abnormal dentition. *Pediatr Radiol* 1:2–7, 1973.
6. Singleton EB, Rosenberg HS: Intraluminal calcification of the inferior vena cava. *AJR* 86:556–560, 1961.
7. Shikata A, Sugimoto T, Kosaka K, Tehara T, Kido SO, Matsuo H, Sawada T, Berdon WE, Herrod HG, Parvey L:

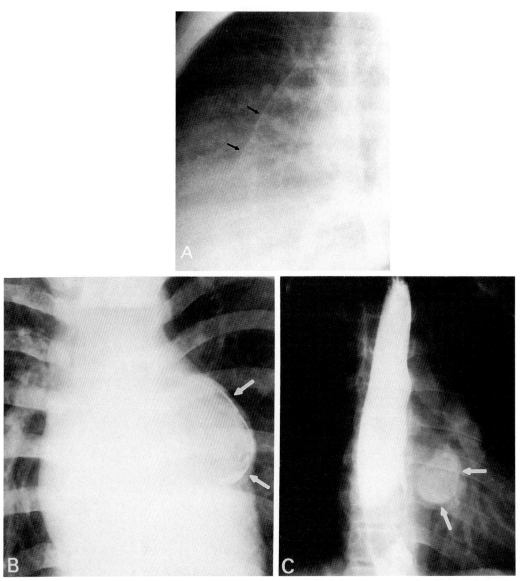

Figure 1.54. Curvilinear calcifications. A. Linear calcification in aorta in patient with Singleton-Merten syndrome. **B.** Typical calcification *(arrow)* in the dilated patch used for correction of tetralogy of Fallot. **C.** Unusual calcification in bronchogenic cyst *(arrows).*

Thoracic aortic calcification in 3 children with candidiasis-endocrinopathy syndrome. *Pediatr Radiol* 23:100–103, 1993.

8. Slovis TL, Chand N, Shanovos TO, Fleischmann LE, Brough AJ: Pulmonary calcifications in a child with renal failure. *Pediatr Radiol* 6:112–115, 1977.

9. Swischuk LE, Alexander A, Hayden CK Jr, Sapire DW: Postoperative lumps and bumps in congenital heart disease: their significance. *Perspect Radiol* 3:45–52, 1990.

10. Tseng CH, Chang GKJ, Lora F: Congenital calcified thrombosis of inferior vena cava, bilateral renal veins and left spermatic vein. *Pediatr Radiol* 6:176–177, 1977.

11. Viat P, Cattelain C, Gallez A: Acquired pulmonary artery aneurysm in an infant. *Pediatrics* 65:89–93, 1980.

12. Volle E, Kaufmann HJ: Pulmonary alveolar microlithiasis in pediatric patients: review of the world literature and two new observations. *Pediatr Radiol* 17:439–442, 1987.

Pulmonary Cavities

Larger cavities most often are the result of pneumatoceles or pulmonary abscesses (Table 1.11). An abscess usually is a complication of bacterial pneu-

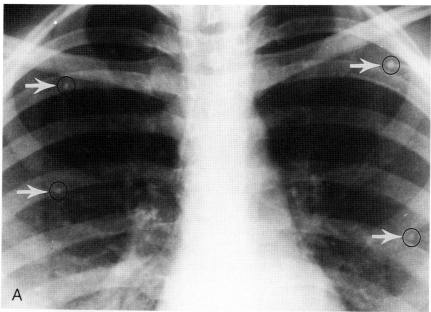

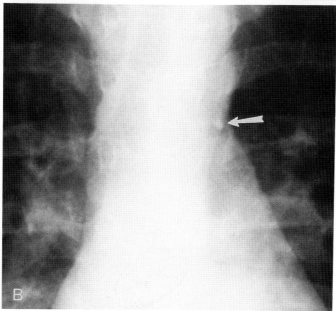

Figure 1.55. Punctate calcifications. A. Note numerous small punctate calcifications in this patient with healed histoplasmosis *(arrows).* These densities are located too far out in the periphery to be blood vessels. When central, however, they can be difficult to differentiate from blood vessels seen on end. Also, note calcifications in right hilar nodes. **B.** Small punctate calcification *(arrow)* in typical location of ligamentum arteriosum.

monia but also can be seen with infection secondary to chronic foreign bodies in the tracheobronchial tree. Air-fluid levels frequently are present in abscesses and their walls are variably thickened and hazy (Fig. 1.56A). Haziness is due to surrounding inflammation, and in most cases, serves to distinguish the abscess from a pneumatocele or the rare congenital pulmonary cyst (Fig. 1.56B). Unless these latter lesions become infected, their walls remain thin and discrete. An abscess has this appearance only after being treated.

The commonest cause of a pneumatocele is infection and, most commonly, the infection is staphylococcal pneumonia (3). However, pneumatoceles also can be seen with other acute bacterial pneumonias (1, 4, 9, 17) and even with tuberculosis (12). They

Table 1.11
Pulmonary Cavities

Pneumatocele-inflammatory[a] Pulmonary abscess[a]	}	Common
Pneumatocele-traumatic[a] Pneumatocele-hydrocarbon pneumonia[b] Echinococcal cyst[c]	}	Uncommon
Solitary cyst (congenital) Adenomatoid malformation[a] Cavitary tuberculosis Cavitating pneumonia Cavitating hematoma Cavitating infarct Lymphangioma of the lung	}	Rare

[a] Frequently multiple.
[b] May be multiple.
[c] Common in endemic areas.

also are common in the hyper-IgE syndrome where staphylococcal infections are common. In any given case the pneumatoceles can be single or multiple (Fig. 1.56D and E), and in some cases can become so large that a tension phenomenon is induced (Fig. 1.56D). Occasionally, pneumatoceles can rupture and produce a pneumothorax, but most often they slowly resolve and disappear with no trace that they ever were present. Other causes of pneumatoceles include hydrocarbon pneumonitis (2, 8) and histiocytosis-X (7). In all of these cases, pneumatoceles result from bronchial obstruction (i.e., by inflammatory exudate, endobronchial granulomas, extrinsic pressure from lymph nodes or peribronchial infiltrates), causing air-trapping and alveolar rupture distal to the point of obstruction.

Another form of lung pneumatocele is that which occurs with blunt, compressive chest trauma (5, 6, 14). Although it is not known exactly how such a pneumatocele develops, it is believed that compressive forces cause temporary occlusion of a bronchus, buildup of pressures beyond the point of occlusion, and then rupture of the temporarily overdistended alveoli. These pneumatoceles may be single or multiple (Fig. 1.56C), and similar air collections can occur in the inferior pulmonary ligament (see Fig. 1.44A). Traumatic pneumatoceles usually are clinically innocuous and most often gradually disappear within two to three weeks.

Cavitary primary tuberculosis is very rare in children (15) and, actually, most reported cases probably are cases of pneumatocele formation rather than cases of necrotic cavity development. Other rare cavitary lesions include cavitating posttraumatic pulmonary hematomas, cavitating infarcts, pulmonary

lymphangioma (13), and echinococcal cysts (10, 16). Echinococcal cysts, of course, are more common in certain geographic areas than others. Multiple large, thin-walled, cystic cavities also can be seen with congenital cystic adenomatoid malformation of the lung. This lesion is initially solid and fluid-filled in the neonate, but gradually the fluid in the cystic areas is replaced with air and, as air accumulates, the cysts become quite large (11). Indeed, they can fill the entire hemithorax, even to the point of mimicking a pneumothorax (see Fig. 1.23B). Small cavitary pulmonary nodules will be discussed in the section on pulmonary nodules (see p. 58).

REFERENCES

1. Asmar BI, Thirumoorthi MC, and Dajani AS: Pneumococcal pneumonia with pneumatocele formation. *Am J Dis Child* 132:1091–1093, 1978.
2. Baghassarian OM, Weiner S: Pneumatocele formation complicating hydrocarbon pneumonitis. *AJR* 95:104–111, 1965.
3. Boisset GF: Subpleural emphysema complicating staphylococcal and other pneumonias. *J Pediatr* 81:259–266, 1972.
4. Chitayat D, Diamant R, Lazenick R, Spirer Z: Hemophilus influenzae type B pneumonia with pneumatocele formation. *Clin Pediatr* 19:151–152, 1980.
5. Fagan CJ, Swischuk LE: Traumatic lung and paramediastinal pneumatoceles. *Radiology* 120:11–18, 1976.
6. Felman AH, Rodgers BM, Talbert JL: Traumatic paramediastinal air cyst. *Pediatr Radiol* 4:120–121, 1976.
7. Godwin JD, Webb WR, Savoca CJ, Gamsu G, Goodman PC: Multiple thin-walled cystic lesions of the lung. *AJR* 135:593–604, 1980.
8. Harris VJ, Brown R: Pneumatoceles as a complication of chemical pneumonia after hydrocarbon ingestion. *AJR* 125:513–537, 1975.
9. Johnson F: Cavitating lesions in a cold agglutinin positive pneumonia. *Pediatr Radiol* 6:181–182, 1977.
10. Katz R, Murphy S, Kosloske A: Pulmonary echinococcosis: a pediatric disease of the southwestern United States. *Pediatrics* 65:1003–1006, 1980.
11. Madewell JE, Stocker JT, Korsower JM: Cystic adenomatoid malformation of the lung: morphologic analysis. *AJR* 124:436–448, 1975.
12. Matsaniotis N, Kattamis CH, Economov-Mavrou, C, Kyriaakou M: Bullous emphysema in childhood tuberculosis. *J Pediatr* 71:703, 1967.
13. Milovic I, Oluic D: Lymphangioma of the lung associated with respiratory distress in a neonate. *Pediatr Radiol* 22:156, 1992.
14. Ravin C, Smith GW, Lester PD, McLoud TC, Putman CE: Post-traumatic pneumatocele in the inferior pulmonary ligament. *Radiology* 121:39–41, 1976.
15. Solomon A, Rabinowitz L: Primary cavitating tuberculosis in childhood. *Clin Radiol* 23:483–485, 1972.
16. Thumler J, Munoz A: Pulmonary and hepatic echinococcosis in children. *Pediatr Radiol* 7:164–171, 1978.
17. Warner JO, Gordon I: Pneumatoceles following haemophilus pneumonia. *Clin Radiol* 32:99–105, 1981.

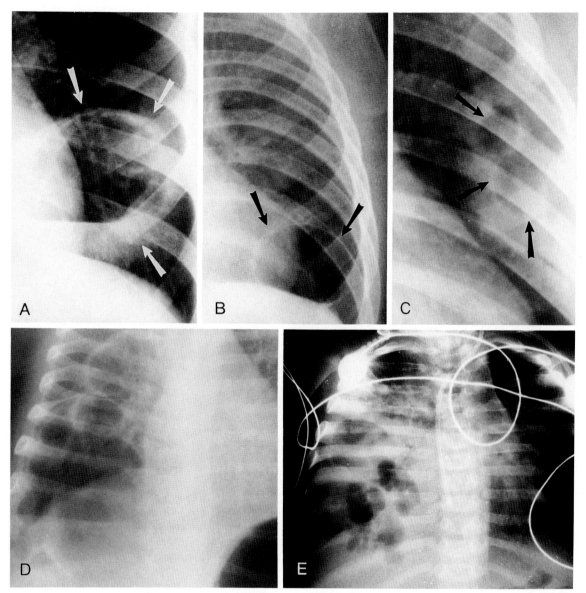

Figure 1.56. Cavities in the lungs. A. Abscess. Note the rather thick, fuzzy wall and an air-fluid level *(arrows)*. **B. Congenital lung cyst** with a thin wall *(arrows)* in the left lower lobe. A solitary pneumatocele would look the same. **C. Posttraumatic pneumatoceles** *(arrows)* with surrounding evidence of pulmonary contusion. **D. Multiple pneumatoceles** in the right lung secondary to staphylococcal pneumonia. **E. Pneumatoceles in tuberculosis.** These are uncommon and, ordinarily, this film would be more suggestive of staphylococcal infection.

Bubbly Lungs

A bubbly pattern in the lungs most commonly occurs in the neonate, especially the premature neonate. In such infants, a bubbly pattern can result from overdistension of the terminal bronchioles and alveolar ducts in hyaline membrane disease, pulmo- nary interstitial emphysema in children requiring positive pressure ventilation, or from the uneven pattern of alveolar aeration seen with the Wilson-Mikity and bronchopulmonary dysplasia syndromes (Fig. 1.57) (2, 3). The bubbles in all these conditions can be diffuse and bilateral or more focal. Unilateral focal bubbles can be seen with cystic adenomatoid malformation (Fig. 1.58) (1).

In older children, cylindrical or saccular bronchi-

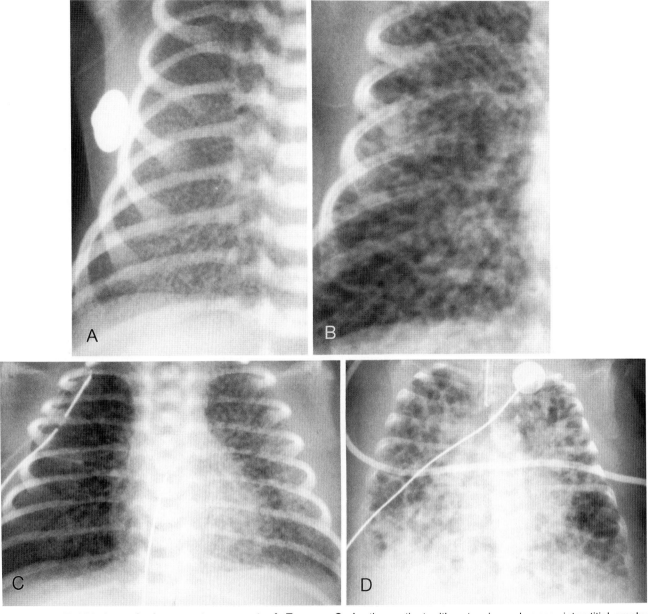

Figure 1.57. Bubbly lungs in the premature neonate. A. Type I bubbles of hyaline membrane disease. Note the small central bubbles that represent the distended terminal bronchioles. **B. Type II bubbles-pulmonary interstitial emphysema.** Note the serpiginous air collections that extend farther into the lung periphery representing air in the interstitial space and lymphatics.

C. Another patient with extensive pulmonary interstitial emphysema. **D. Type III bubbles-bronchopulmonary dysplasia.** Note the characteristic coarse bubbly pattern of advanced bronchopulmonary dysplasia. Unlike pulmonary interstitial emphysema bubbles, which remain fixed on inspiration and expiration, the bubbles in bronchopulmonary dysplasia collapse upon expiration.

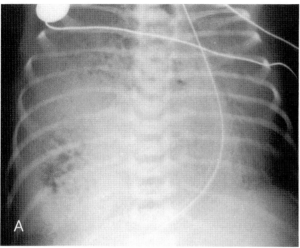

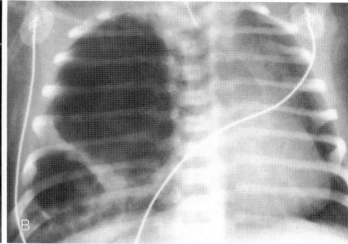

Figure 1.58. Cystic adenomatoid malformation. A. In this very young infant, the cysts remain largely fluid filled. Note the ap- pearance of multiple small air-filled spaces within the lesion. **B.** Another patient demonstrating large air-filled cysts.

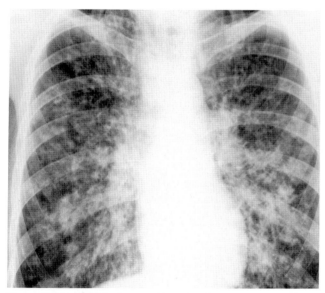

Figure 1.59. Bubbly lungs. Note the fine architecture of the bronchiectatic spaces (i.e., bubbles) in this patient with bronchi- ectasis from cystic fibrosis.

ectasis is a much more common cause of bubbly lungs (Fig. 1.59). Focal bronchiectasis often is seen with chronic foreign bodies or severe pulmonary in- fections that destroy bronchial walls.

REFERENCES

1. Madewell JE, Stocker JT, Korsower JM: Cystic adeno- matoid malformation of the lung: morphologic analysis. *AJR* 124:436–448, 1975.
2. Swischuk LE: Bubbles in hyaline membrane disease. *Radi- ology* 122:417–426, 1977.
3. Westcott JL, Cole SR: Interstitial pulmonary emphysema in children and adults: roentgenographic features. *Radiol- ogy* 111:367–378, 1974.

Large or Prominent Hilar Regions

Hilar prominence, or enlargement, can be bilat- eral or unilateral (Table 1.12) and, overall, the com- monest cause is lymph node enlargement. In some cases of hilar lymph node enlargement, the nodes are discretely outlined, while in others adjacent in- flammatory changes cause the edges of the nodes to be fuzzy and indistinct (Fig. 1.60*A*). These latter findings are the result of associated interstitial, peri- bronchial inflammation that classically occurs with viral lower respiratory tract infections (1, 3, 7). How- ever, these changes also can be seen with asthma, cystic fibrosis, chronic aspiration, fungal disease, and occasionally *Mycoplasma pneumoniae* infection. In the foregoing conditions adenopathy usually is bilat- eral, a configuration generally not seen with com- mon bacterial pneumonias.

When bilateral adenopathy is discrete, one's first consideration still should be viral lower respiratory tract infection, but, in addition, one should give seri- ous consideration to fungal infections, metastatic disease, the reticuloendothelioses TB, and the leuke- mia-lymphoma group of diseases. Much less com- monly (mainly because the diseases are rare in chil- dren), one also can encounter bilateral adenopathy with sarcoidosis (2) and Wegener's granulomatosis.

The second most common cause of bilateral hilar prominence is pulmonary artery dilation. When the pulmonary arteries are dilated bilaterally, the most

Table 1.12
Large or Prominent Hilar Regions

Bilateral
A. Adenopathy
  Viral infection
  Mycoplasma pneumoniae infection } Common

  Cystic fibrosis
  Fungal infection
  Chronic aspiration
  Tuberculosis } Moderately common

  Sarcoidosis
  Wegener's granulomatosis
  Reticuloendothelioses
  Metastases
  Leukemia-lymphoma } Rare

B. Pulmonary artery enlargement
  Pulmonary hypertension } Moderately common

  Absent pulmonary valve } Rare

Unilateral
A. Adenopathy
  Tuberculosis
  Mycoplasma pneumoniae infection
  Bacterial pneumonia
  Superior segment, lower lobe pneu-
    monia artifact } Common

  Fungal infections
  Metastases } Uncommon

B. Pulmonary artery enlargement
  Pulmonary stenosis with left pulmo-
    nary artery enlarged } Uncommon

  Absent pulmonary valve with unilat-
    eral absent pulmonary artery } Rare

common underlying problem is pulmonary hypertension, and its cause usually is an underlying left-to-right shunt or a cardiac admixture lesion (Fig. 1.60B). In either case, excessive volumes of blood flowing through the lungs in time induce muscular hypertrophy of the media of the peripheral pulmonary arterioles and, eventually, pulmonary hypertension. Pulmonary hypertension secondary to left-side obstructing lesions such as aortic stenosis, coarctation of the aorta, mitral stenosis, and myocardial disease is less common, especially in young infants. If left untreated, however, such left-sided lesions can eventually cause chronic pulmonary arteriolar changes and pulmonary hypertension. In addition, acquired rheumatic valvular disease is more prevalent in the older child. Idiopathic pulmonary hypertension is rare in the pediatric age group and so is hypertension due to pulmonary artery emboli.

A very rare cause of bilateral pulmonary artery enlargement leading to prominent hilar regions is congenital absence of the pulmonary valve (4, 6). This condition, often associated with tetralogy of Fallot, produces gross insufficiency of the absent pulmonary valve and, characteristically, massive enlargement of the main, right, and left pulmonary artery branches (Fig. 1.60C). The peripheral pulmonary vessels in these patients are very thin, and the zone of demarcation between the dilated proximal pulmonary artery and its peripheral branches often is so abrupt that hilar masses are suggested. In addition, in many of the cases associated with tetralogy of Fallot, the left pulmonary artery is absent and thus only the right hilum will appear enlarged.

The commonest cause of **unilateral hilar enlargement** in the pediatric age group is pulmonary infection (Fig. 1.61) and, most commonly, it will be primary tuberculosis (5, 8). In some of these cases adenopathy may be discrete, but in others it may be obscured by atelectasis or even obstructive emphysema (Fig. 1.61B and C). Bilateral adenopathy in primary pulmonary tuberculosis also occurs, but is far less common.

Other causes of unilateral hilar lymph node enlargement include fungal disease, *Mycoplasma pneumoniae* infection, and bacterial pneumonias. Unilateral hilar enlargement also can occur with metastatic disease, the leukemia-lymphoma group of diseases, and absence of the pulmonary valve with concomitant absence of the left pulmonary artery (i.e., right hilar enlargement is present). Indeed, any time one pulmonary artery is absent, the other tends to enlarge and produce a unilaterally prominent hilar region. Valvular pulmonary stenosis causes left hilar prominence due to poststenotic enlargement of the pulmonary artery, where the jet of blood passing through the stenotic valve is so directed that it causes dilation of the main pulmonary artery and left branch (Fig. 1.62).

Finally, before leaving the topic of unilateral hilar enlargement, one should make note of the artifactually prominent hilar region produced by a superior segment lower lobe pneumonia. On lateral view, of course, the hilar region is not enlarged, and the pneumonia is clearly located posteriorly in the superior segment of the corresponding lower lobe. On frontal view, however, because it is superimposed on the hilar region, the region itself appears enlarged (Fig. 1.63A and B). A similar problem occasionally can arise with anterior segment right upper lobe consolidation.

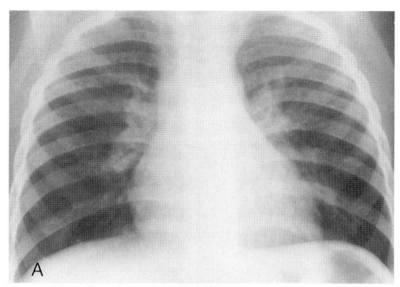

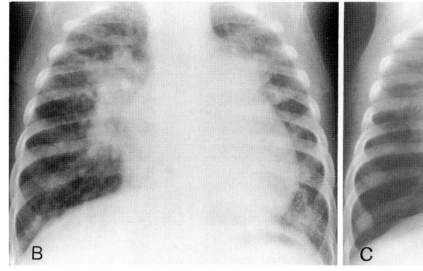

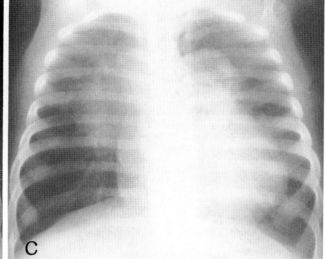

Figure 1.60. Bilateral hilar prominence. A. Adenopathy. Characteristic bilateral hilar adenopathy in a patient with viral lower respiratory tract infection. **B. Large pulmonary arteries** causing prominent bilateral hilar regions (the left is partially ob-scured by the heart) in patient with a large ventricular septal de-fect and pulmonary hypertension. **C. Large pulmonary arteries** causing large bilateral hilar regions in a patient with dilation sec-ondary to absence of the pulmonary valve.

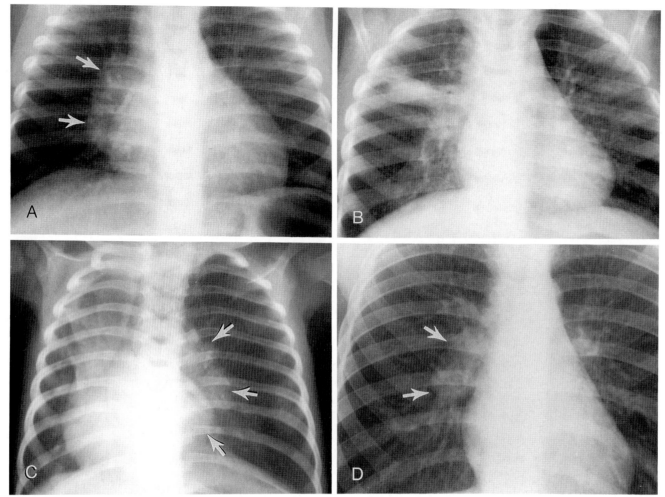

Figure 1.61. Unilateral hilar prominence. A. Note the right hilar mass *(arrows)* due to lymphadenopathy in this child with primary tuberculosis. **B.** Another patient with a prominent right hilum due to tuberculous lymphadenopathy. The opacity in the right upper lobe is atelectasis, which commonly accompanies the lymphadenopathy of primary tuberculosis. **C.** The left hilar adenopathy *(arrows)* could be overlooked because of the large obstructed left lung and associated mediastinal shift to the right. Again the problem was tuberculosis, in this case with bronchial obstruction. **D.** Right hilar adenopathy in a patient with histoplasmosis *(arrows)*.

REFERENCES

1. Conte P, Heitzman ER, Markarian B: Viral pneumonia roentgen-pathological correlations. *Radiology* 95:267–272, 1970.
2. Merten DF, Kirks DR, Grossman H: Pulmonary sarcoidosis in childhood. *AJR* 135:673–679, 1980.
3. Osborne, D: Radiologic appearance of viral disease of the lower respiratory tract in infants and children. *AJR* 13:29–33, 1978.
4. Osman MZ, Meng CCL, Girdany BR: Congenital absence of the pulmonary valve: report of eight cases with review of the literature. *Am J Roentgenol Radium Ther Nucl Med* 106:58–69, 1969.
5. Leung AN, Müeller NL, Pineda PR, FitzGerald JM: Primary tuberculosis in childhood: radiographic manifestations. *Radiology* 182:87–91, 1992.
6. Pernot C Hoeffel JC, Henry M, Stehlin H, Worms AM, Louis JP: Congenital absence of the pulmonary valve: radiological findings in infants. *Ann Radiol* 15:217–222, 1972.
7. Scanlon GA, Unger JD: The radiology of bacterial and viral pneumonias. *Radiol Clin North Am* 11:317–338, 1973.
8. Weber AL, Bird KT, Janower ML: Primary tuberculosis in childhood with particular emphasis on changes affecting the tracheobronchial tree. *AJR* 103:123–132, 1968.

Pulmonary Nodules

Pulmonary nodules can be solitary or multiple, calcified or uncalcified, and cavitary or solid (Table 1.13). The commonest cause of a solitary nodule in a

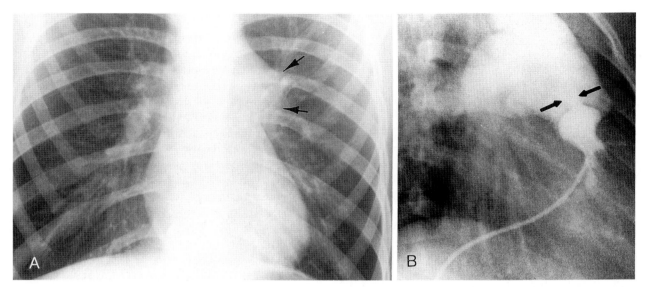

Figure 1.62. Pulmonary valve stenosis. A. Note the prominent left hilar region produced by a large pulmonary artery, due to pulmonary stenosis with poststenotic dilation of the main pulmo- nary artery and its left branch *(arrows)*. **B.** Angiogram shows the jet of blood *(arrows)* passing through the stenotic valve that is responsible for the dilation.

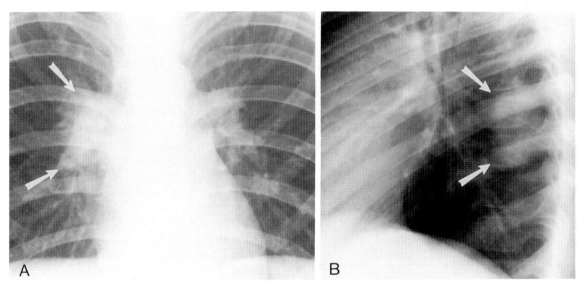

Figure 1.63. Superior segment pneumonia mimicking unilat- eral adenopathy. A. Note the dense, prominent hilar region on the right *(arrows)*. **B.** Lateral view shows that it is due to superim- position of a superior segment, lower lobe pneumonia *(arrows)*.

child is infection, usually healed primary tuberculo- sis. Tuberculous nodules may or may not contain cal- cification, and are more common than similar nod- ules caused by fungal infections (Fig. 1.64A). Residual nodules (healed granulomas) from other pulmonary infections are quite rare, including those seen with acute or healed atypical measles pneumo- nia (9, 10, 22, 23).

A relatively common cause of an apparent lung nodule is acute, consolidating pneumonia (see Fig. 1.65B), usually pneumococcal. The fact that the con- solidation is first seen as a pulmonary nodule is strictly fortuitous, for it just happens that in the early stages of consolidation the pneumonia can ap- pear nodular or spherical (16). A few hours later, its configuration changes and it becomes more ill-de- fined and typical. As a side point, it might be noted that these pneumonias also can appear as pulmonary or mediastinal masses. In all of these cases, the clue to proper diagnosis is the clinical history, for these children invariably have findings such as tachypnea, cough, high fever (103°F or over), or chest pain,

Table 1.13
Pulmonary Nodules

Solitary nodule		
Granuloma-tuberculosis[a]	}	Common
Granuloma-fungal[a]		
Consolidating pneumonia	}	Moderately common
Metastases[d]		
Small abscess[d]		
Small cyst		
Hamartoma[a]		
Nipple shadow		
Other primary neoplasia		
Sarcoidosis[b,d]		
Pulmonary varix or arterio-venous malformation		
Cutaneous nodules		
Mucous plugs (asthma)	}	Rare
Mucocele (bronchial atresia)		
Healed (posttraumatic) hematoma[b,d]		
Postinfarct		
Collagen vascular disease[d]		
Atypical measles[b]		
Old pneumonia[b]		
Primary tumor		
Multiple nodules		
Multiple nodules		
Granulomas[a] (TB, fungus)	}	Common
Metastases[d]	}	Moderately common
Laryngeal papillomatosis[d]		
Multiple abscesses[c]	}	Uncommon
Multiple emboli[d]		
Wegener's granulomatosis[c]		
Sarcoidosis[b,d]		
Mucous plugs		
Cutaneous lesions (artifact)		
Collagen vascular disease[d]	}	Rare
Lymphoma		
Multiple hamartomas[b]		
Other primary tumors		

[a] Commonly calcify.
[b] May calcify.
[c] Commonly cavitate.
[d] May cavitate.

clearly suggesting that a pulmonary infection is the problem.

All other causes of a solitary pulmonary nodule are rare, and one of the rarest is a pulmonary tumor. For the most part, one cannot tell one tumor from another except in those cases where typical flocculent cartilage calcifications are present. In such cases, a hamartoma should be the diagnosis (Fig. 1.64B). One of the most often reported, but still rare, primary pulmonary tumors is the pulmonary blastoma (8, 14). Other sporadically reported primary lung tumors include plasma cell granuloma (11), leiomyosarcoma (1), choristoma (21), congenital mesenchymoma (6), and squamous cell carcinoma (18). Solitary pulmonary metastases can occur, but usually more than one nodule is apparent when metastatic tumor is present. Occasionally, a small bronchogenic cyst can appear in the periphery of the lung and suggest a pulmonary nodule, but more often they are located in juxtaposition to the tracheobronchial tree (Fig. 1.65C). Rarely, these cysts can calcify (see Fig. 1.54C).

When a nodule is associated with trailing vascular feeders and drainers, one can suggest the diagnosis of pulmonary varix or arteriovenous malformation (Fig. 1.65A), and MRI or CT can delineate these vessels to better advantage. If a pulmonary nodule is associated with hyperinflation and hyperlucency of the lung around and distal to it, bronchial atresia with a mucocele should be the diagnosis (5, 13, 17). In these cases, bronchial atresia exists from birth, but as time goes by, mucous accumulates distal to the area of atresia and forms a mucocele (see Fig. 1.32). The lung distal to the obstruction receives air by the air-drift phenomenon (i.e., air from the adjacent normal lung passes to the obstructed lung through the pores of Kohn and ducts of Lambert) and then becomes distended. This leads to hyperlucency and oligemia of the involved lobe, and the plain film findings are virtually diagnostic. Similar nodular accumulations of mucus can occur on a transient basis in children with asthma, but they are not associated with regional hyperinflation (20).

Lesions on the skin that might project through the lungs as a pulmonary nodule, including nipple shadows, generally are uncommon in the pediatric age group. Of course, the simplest way to determine whether such a pseudonodule is present is: (a) to be aware of the typical location of a nipple shadow (i.e., lower third of the lung fields), and (b) to know whether the patient has any cutaneous lesions (e.g., neurofibromatosis). If one does not judge the nodule to be within the pulmonary parenchyma on both frontal and lateral views, one has to suspect it as being a skin lesion. Oblique views also often can be used to demonstrate that such a nodule is not in the chest. Other causes of a solitary pulmonary nodule include a small abscess, sarcoidosis, healed (posttraumatic) hematoma, healed pulmonary infarct, collagen vascular disease, and old healed pneumonia (Table 1.13).

The two most common causes of **multiple nodules** in the chest are inflammatory granulomas and pulmonary metastases (Table 1.13). Granulomas, however, are more common and, for the most part,

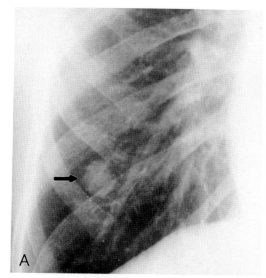
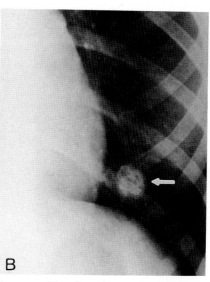
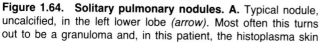

Figure 1.64. Solitary pulmonary nodules. A. Typical nodule, uncalcified, in the left lower lobe *(arrow).* Most often this turns out to be a granuloma and, in this patient, the histoplasma skin test was positive. Granulomas also frequently show central calcification. **B.** Hamartoma with typical flocculent calcification of cartilage *(arrow).*

include tuberculous and fungal infections (Fig. 1.66*B*). Fungal infections, however, are a more common cause of multiple granulomas. These granulomas usually are quite uniform in size and may show punctate calcifications (see Fig. 1.53*A*). Metastatic nodules often show greater variation in size (Fig. 1.66*C*). Another interesting cause of multiple pulmonary nodules is juvenile laryngeal papillomatosis (19). These patients are first seen with hoarseness due to a papilloma growing in or around the vocal cords. Once surgical intervention or tracheostomy is accomplished, seeding of the papilloma into the distal bronchial tree can occur, and then pulmonary nodules develop (Fig. 1.66*A*). Some of these nodules may cavitate. Other causes of multiple pulmonary nodules include: multiple pulmonary abscesses (3), multiple emboli, Wegener's granulomatosis (15), multiple hemangiomas of the lung (2), multiple hamartomas (4, 7), sarcoidosis, collagen vascular diseases, lymphoma, and mucous plugs in cystic fibrosis (Fig. 1.66*D*) or asthma (20).

Calcifications within pulmonary nodules are most commonly seen with granulomas, as discussed earlier in this section. Healed hematomas, old pulmonary infarcts, and old healed pneumonias can also appear as calcified pulmonary nodules. The flocculent calcifications of a pulmonary hamartoma are characteristic, but this is a rare lesion. Calcification within a nodule can be verified with conventional or computed tomography, but the latter modality is more sensitive (12). Metastatic pulmonary nodules, as a rule, do not calcify, but those due to osteogenic

sarcoma may show ossification. Such ossification cannot be distinguished from calcification, but on a practical basis, the fact that a primary osteosarcoma is present usually is well known before metastatic nodules develop.

CT also is useful for demonstrating cavities within nodules. Cavitating nodules most commonly occur with multiple pulmonary abscesses, septic emboli, Wegener's granulomatosis, and laryngeal papillomatosis (19). However, cavitation can also occur with metastatic disease (Fig. 1.66*C*), sarcoidosis, the collagen vascular diseases, and a variety of fungal infections.

REFERENCES

1. Beluffi G, Bertolotti P, Mietta A, Manara G, Luisetti M: Primary leiomyosarcoma of the lung in a girl. *Pediatr Radiol* 16:240–244, 1986.
2. Brill PW, Symchych P, Winchester P: Capillary hemangioma of the lung. *Radiology* 124:184, 1977.
3. Felman AH, Shulman ST: Staphylococcal osteomyelitis, sepsis and pulmonary disease. *Radiology* 117:649–655, 1975.
4. Futrell JW, McKillop DB, Izant RJ Jr: Angiomatous hamartoma in an infant. *Am J Dis Child* 128:96–99, 1974.
5. Genereux GP: Bronchial atresia: a rare cause of unilateral lung hypertranslucency. *J Can Assoc Radiol* 22:71–82, 1971.
6. Haller FO, Kauffman SL, Kassner EG: Congenital mesenchymal tumour of the lung. *Br J Radiol* 50:217–219, 1977.
7. Hull MT, Gonzalez-Crussi F, Grosfeld JL: Multiple pulmonary fibroleiomyomatous hamartomata in childhood. *J Pediatr Surg* 14:428–431, 1979.

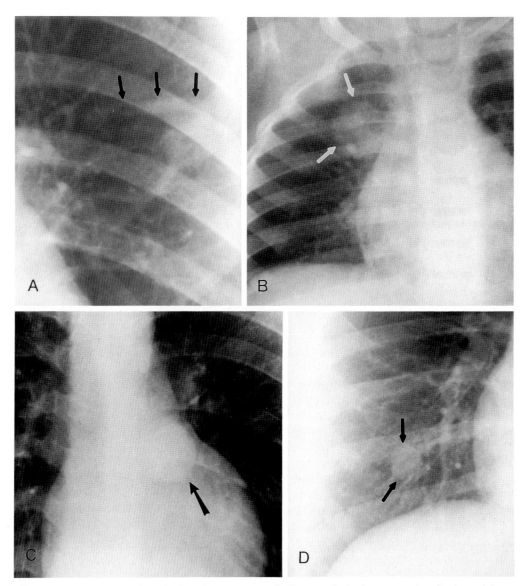

Figure 1.65. Solitary pulmonary nodules. A. Arteriovenous malformation. Note the irregular shaped nodule in the left upper lobe with an associated trailing vessel *(arrows).* **B. Nodular consolidating pneumonia *(arrows).*** The finding, at first, suggests a pulmonary nodule, but the patient had a high fever and clinical findings typical of pneumonia. Such nodular pneumonias are common in childhood and usually are due to pneumococcal infections. **C.** Small nodule due to a **bronchogenic cyst *(arrow).*** The typical location suggests the diagnosis. **D.** Solitary metastasis *(arrows)* in an adolescent with a history of a molar pregnancy.

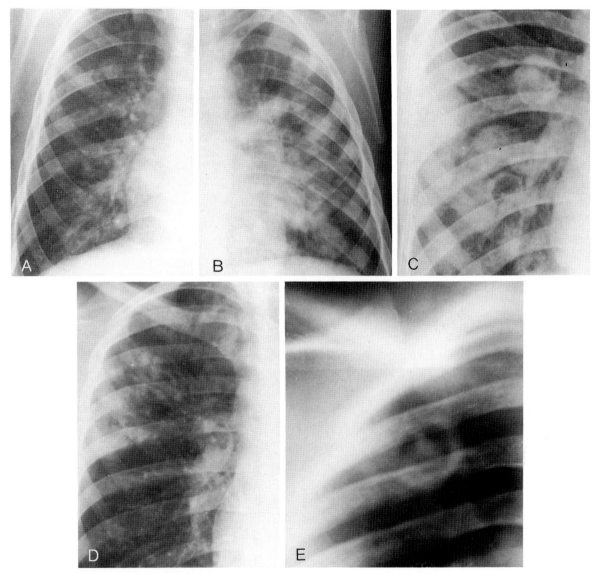

Figure 1.66. Multiple pulmonary nodules. A. Multiple, but somewhat indistinct, pulmonary nodules in juvenile papillomatosis. **B.** Numerous, ill-defined nodules due to granulomas in actinomycosis. **C.** Typical appearance of metastatic nodules, some of which have cavitated. They are smooth-edged and of variable size. **D.** Mucous plugs in cystic fibrosis. Note numerous mucous plugs presenting as nodules in the lung. They are especially prominent in the right upper lobe. **E.** Small cavitary nodule with central nidus, typical of aspergillosis. The small nidus often is termed the "fungus ball." This patient had immunologic deficiency.

8. Kovanlikaya A, Pirnar T, Olgun N: Pulmonary blastoma: a rare case of childhood malignancy. *Pediatr Radiol* 22:155, 1992.

9. Margolin FR, Gandy TK: Pneumonia of atypical measles. *Radiology* 131:653–655, 1979.

10. Mitnick, J, Becker, MH, Rothberg, M, Genieser, NB: Nodular residua of atypical measles pneumonia. *AJR* 134:257–260, 1980.

11. Monzon CM, Gilchrist GS, Burgert EO, O'Connell EJ, Telander RL, Hoffman AD, Li, Chin-Yang: Plasma cell granuloma of the lung in children. *Pediatrics* 70:268–274, 1982.

12. Muhm JR, Brown LR, Crowe JK, Sheedy PF II, Hattery RR, Stephens DH: Comparison of whole lung tomography and computed tomography for detecting pulmonary nodules. *AJR* 131:981–984, 1978.

13. Oh KS, Dorst JP, White JJ, Haller JA Jr, Johnson BA, Byrne WD: Syndrome of bronchial atresia or stenosis with mucocele and focal hyperinflation of the lung. *Johns Hopkins Med J* 138:48–53, 1976.

14. Ohtomo K, Araki T, Yashiro N, Lio M: Pulmonary blastoma in children: two case reports and review of the literature. *Radiology* 147:101–104, 1983.

15. Orlowski JP, Clough JD, Dyment PG: Wegener's granulomatosis in the pediatric age group. *Pediatrics* 61:83–90, 1978.

16. Rose RW, Ward BH: Spherical pneumonias in children simulating pulmonary and mediastinal masses. *Radiology* 106:179–182, 1973.

17. Schuster SR, Harris GBC, Williams A, Kirkpatrick J, Reid L: Bronchial atresia: a recognizable entity in the pediatric age group. *J Pediatr Surg* 13:682–689, 1978.

18. Shelley BE, Lorenzo RL: Primary squamous cell carcinoma of the lung in childhood. *Pediatr Radiol* 13:92–94, 1983.

19. Smith L, Gooding CA: Pulmonary involvement in laryngeal papillomatosis. *Pediatr Radiol* 2:161–166, 1974.

20. Swischuk LE: *Emergency Imaging of the Acutely Ill or Injured Child.* Williams & Wilkins: Baltimore, 1994:106.

21. Wat K, Toomey F, Wat BY, Reiber N: Pulmonary choristoma in a neonate. *AJR* 139:377–379, 1982.

22. Wood BP, Bernstein RM: Pulmonary nodular "pneumonia" during the acute atypical measles illness. *Ann Radiol* 21:193–198, 1978.

23. Young LW, Smith DI, Glasgow LA: Pneumonia of atypical measles, residual nodular lesions. *Am J Roentgenol Radium Ther Nucl Med* 110:439–448, 1970.

Infiltrates

Basically, pulmonary infiltrative patterns can be categorized as follows: (a) lobar consolidation, (b) fluffy or patchy parenchymal infiltrates, (c) streaky or wedge-shaped opacities, (d) parahilar-peribronchial infiltrates, (e) reticular or reticulonodular infiltrates, (f) hazy-to-opaque lungs, and (g) miliary opacities. In addition, some infiltrates tend to cluster around the hilar regions, while others are more peripheral or basal in distribution. Each pattern has its own list of differential diagnostic possibilities, and even though considerable overlap often occurs, it is of value to know which entities are most likely to produce the different patterns. Not only does this aid in directing immediate therapy, it also assists in unraveling difficult problems.

LOBAR CONSOLIDATION

A lobar consolidation results when the alveoli become full of fluid, and most commonly the fluid is a purulent exudate secondary to a bacterial infection (Fig. 1.67A and B). Overall, the commonest infection is pneumococcal pneumonia, but in children under 2 to 3 years of age, *Haemophilus influenzae* pneumonia is more common. Staphylococcal and then *Mycoplasma pneumoniae* infections are next most common as causes of lobar consolidations. Fungal infections generally do not produce isolated lobar consolidations, except perhaps for actinomycosis, and viral consolidations, if they exist, are very rare. Other bacterial infections also can produce consolidating pneumonias, including Gram-negative infections, but none are particularly common in children.

Radiographically, in any given case, the entire lobe eventually can become consolidated, but initially the opacification tends to begin in the periphery of the lobe. With mature consolidations, air in the bronchi stands out as an air bronchogram. Pleural effusions commonly are associated with bacterial pneumonia and, indeed, many times develop into frank empyemas. Most lobar consolidations are associated with only slight change of volume in the involved lobe. The rather uncommon *Klebsiella pneumoniae* can produce considerable expansion of the lobe and bulging of the adjacent fissures (see Fig. 1.41A), but, overall, minimal volume loss is the rule with consolidations. When volume loss is more pronounced, a problem arises in differentiating the findings from simple atelectasis (Fig. 1.68A and B). With consolidation, since the alveoli are full of exudate, there is no reason for significant volume loss to occur. However, as the pneumonia clears, atelectasis can develop. When atelectasis is the only, or predominant, problem, volume loss is more marked. In evaluating atelectasis, it is important to appreciate the characteristic fashion in which the various lobes collapse (Fig. 1.69). Furthermore, it is important to note that, not infrequently, atelectasis is more difficult to evaluate on one or the other of the two standards views of the chest.

The problem of differentiating consolidation from atelectasis is not academic. Indeed, in the assess-

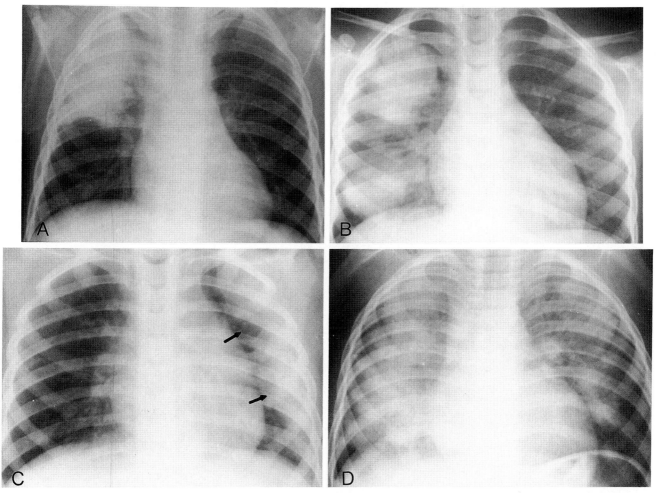

Figure 1.67. Consolidations. A. Typical, well-developed pneumonia of the right upper lobe. Note the central air bronchogram and the relatively normal position of the minor fissure. This indicates very little volume loss. **B.** Two more consolidations, within the lobes of the right lung. Note that there is little volume loss in the right lung. **C.** Peripheral consolidation on the left due to pulmonary contusion *(arrows)*. **D.** Bilateral consolidation due to bleeding into the lungs in idiopathic pulmonary hemosiderosis.

ment of respiratory infections in children, it is the commonest dilemma encountered. The reason for this is that viral infections are the most common lower respiratory tract infections in children, and atelectasis secondary to mucous plugging of a bronchus very commonly accompanies such infections. The same holds true for patients with asthma, which is also primarily a bronchial problem. In the end, in some cases differentiation of atelectasis and pneumonia will not be possible radiographically, and in such cases clinical correlation is essential. In this regard, patients with bacterial pneumonia usually are first seen with abrupt onset of high fevers and toxic symptoms. With viral infections (bronchitis-peribronchitis), although high fever can be seen in infants, the clinical appearance usually is milder and associated with problems such as coryza, nasal congestion, and croup.

In children with asthma, when an apparent consolidation is encountered and the patient exhibits clinical findings typical of an acute asthma attack (e.g., wheezing, little or no fever), the consolidation almost always is due to atelectasis; bacterial pneumonia seldom precipitates an acute asthma attack. Of course, pneumonia can occur in children with asthma, but when it does the clinical signs and symptoms are those of a bacterial infection and not those of an asthma attack. If confusion remains, a follow-up radiograph may be useful to demonstrate rapid clearance, which can only occur with atelectasis (Fig. 1.70).

Other conditions that might be seen with consoli-

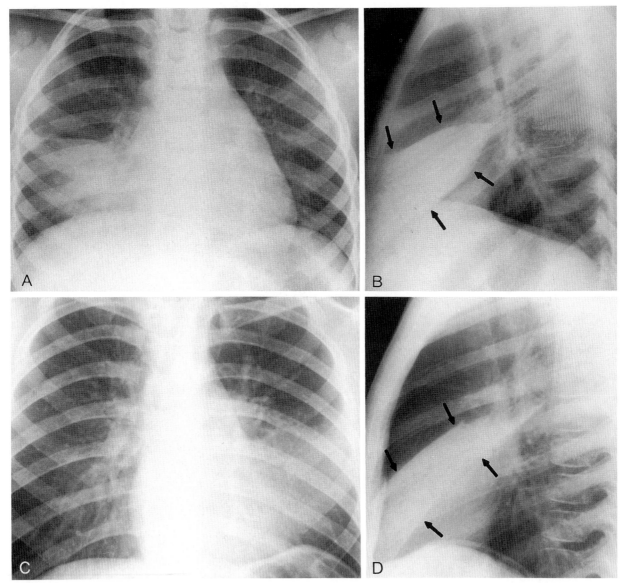

Figure 1.68. Consolidation: infiltrate or atelectasis? A. Consolidating pneumonia with volume loss. Note typical right middle lobe consolidation. Little volume loss is suggested. **B.** On lateral view, however, more than usual collapse of the right middle lobe is present *(arrows)*. Clinical correlation is most important here. The patient had a fever of 104°F and abrupt onset of cough and chest pain. This does not occur with atelectasis. **C. Atelectasis mimicking pneumonia.** Note the homogeneous opacity *on the left.* The fact that the left lung is smaller than the right and the left upper lobe appears blacker (due to compensatory emphysema) suggests that volume loss is present and that atelectasis should be the cause of the lingular opacity. Parahilar peribronchial infiltrates bilaterally belie the presence of a viral infection and/or asthma. **D.** Lateral view shows characteristic collapse of the lingula *(arrows)*. Such a profound degree of collapse usually does not occur with lobar pneumonias. This patient had asthma and was afebrile.

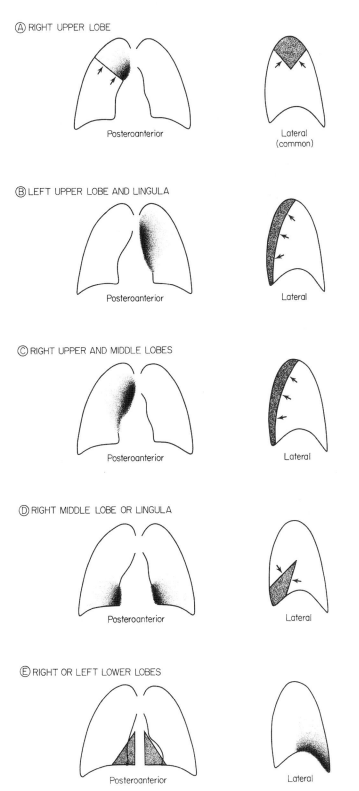

Figure 1.69. Atelectasis: varying configurations. A. Right upper lobe atelectasis. **B.** Left upper lobe and lingular atelectasis. **C.** Right upper lobe and right middle lobe atelectasis. **D.** Right middle lobe or lingular atelectasis. **E.** Right lower lobe or left lower lobe atelectasis. *Arrows* indicate direction of collapse and displacement of the involved major fissures. (From Swischuk LE: *Emergency Imaging of the Acutely Ill or Injured Child,* ed. 3. Baltimore: Williams & Wilkins, 1994:78.)

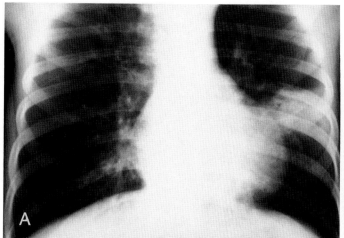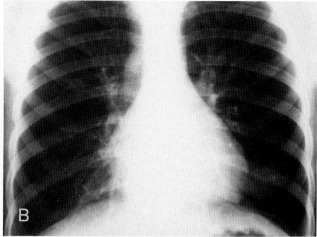

Figure 1.70. Atelectasis in a child with asthma. A. Note the peripheral area of consolidation in the left lung that suggests the presence of a pneumonia. However, this patient's initial clinical appearance consisted of an acute exacerbation of asthma with only a low grade fever. **B.** A follow-up film taken the next day showed that the previous opacity has cleared and was due to atelectasis.

dation of a lobe include pulmonary contusion (Fig. 1.67C), pulmonary infarction, bleeding into the lung from idiopathic pulmonary hemosiderosis (Fig. 1.67D) or from a lesion such as an arteriovenous malformation, or pulmonary vein atresia localized to one lobe (36). In the latter condition, consolidation results from pulmonary edema, either secondary to elevated venous pressure or from pulmonary infarction. However, all of these conditions, with the exception of pulmonary contusion, are rare in childhood.

Finally, it might be noted that the normally large thymus gland in an infant can mimic an upper lobe consolidation, particularly if the radiograph is obtained with the patient in a slightly rotated position. This problem occurs more commonly on the right and in some cases gives the false impression of a complete right upper lobe consolidation.

FLUFFY OR PATCHY INFILTRATES

These infiltrates can be scattered diffusely throughout both lungs or localized to one lobe. In either case, they are rather nonspecific (Figs. 1.71 and 1.72). Basically, these infiltrates have ill-defined margins, and, for the most part, they reflect alveolar disease, where the alveoli are full of inflammatory exudate, edema fluid, or blood. When these infiltrates are bilateral, most commonly they are the result of infection; staphylococcal infections notoriously produce this pattern, but they are also seen with *H. influenzae, M. pneumoniae,* and streptococcal infections. As a rule, however, they do not occur with pneumococcal pneumonia.

Other, less common conditions producing patchy alveolar infiltrates include aspiration pneumonia, immunologic disease, fungal infections, sarcoidosis, milk allergy (3, 6, 11), visceral larva migrans (43), idiopathic pulmonary hemosiderosis (in its active, bleeding stage) (21, 30) (Fig. 1.71A), uremic lung with edema or bleeding, allergic lung (due to inhaled or ingested materials) (18, 38), Loeffler's allergic pneumonia, hydrocarbon pneumonitis, near-drowning (40), lipoid pneumonia (14), and lung hemorrhage.

Patchy, indeed, fluffy-appearing opacities also can be seen with segmental atelectasis, and while this is not common with bacterial infections, it is very common with viral or *M. pneumoniae* infections. The reason for this is that these infections involve the bronchi and peribronchial interstitium more than the alveoli. This being the case, these infections are associated with considerable bronchospasm and mucus secretion, and, together, these factors lead to bronchial obstruction and atelectasis. When extensive, atelectasis can be difficult to differentiate from patchy pneumonia, but a clue is that such atelectasis tends to cluster around the hilar regions (Fig. 1.72A). The peripheral lung fields remain relatively clear, a distribution quite different from the more diffuse pattern seen with bacterial infiltrates (Fig. 1.71B). Nonetheless, in many cases, it is not until repeat films are obtained that one is convinced that atelectasis only is the problem (Fig. 1.72B). In addition, it should be reiterated that clinical correlation is of the utmost importance in such cases, for often the radiographs in these children appear much worse than would be expected based on the child's clinical

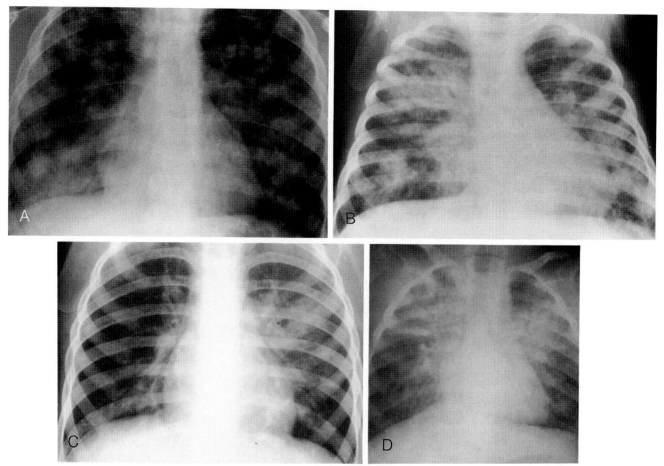

Figure 1.71. Patchy or fluffy infiltrates. A. Note widespread patchy infiltrates in this patient with idiopathic pulmonary hemosiderosis (acute episode with pulmonary hemorrhage and edema). **B.** Another infant with similar infiltrates due to staphylococcal pneumonia. **C. Patchy infiltrates in one lobe.** Note the patchy, hazy opacity in the left upper lobe and lingula. On this view, this opacity could be due either to bacterial pneumonia or atelectasis. On lateral view, however, there was no evidence of volume loss. Under these circumstances, atelectasis is unlikely and pneumonia, usually due to a bacterial or *Mycoplasma* infection, should be suspected. **D.** Bilateral fluffy infiltrates representing pulmonary edema resulting from the massive aspiration of acidic gastric contents (Mendelson syndrome).

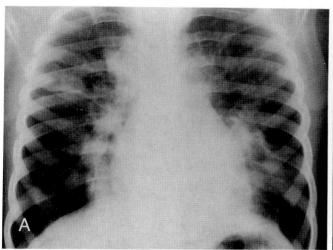 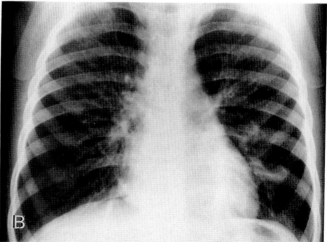

Figure 1.72. Patchy atelectasis mimicking pneumonia. A. Note widespread patchy infiltrates in both lungs. However, they are clustered toward the hilar regions of the lung, and this should favor segmental atelectasis over bacterial pneumonia. **B.** Less than 24 hours later, almost all of the apparent infiltrates have disappeared. Only a few vertical streaks of atelectasis remain in the lung bases. (From Swischuk LE: *Emergency Imaging of the Acutely Ill or Injured Child,* ed. 3. Baltimore: Williams & Wilkins, 1994:16.)

condition. Similar findings are seen in pertussis infection, for initially this also is a bronchial problem (2). Only later with superimposed infection does true alveolar involvement occur. Patchy infiltrates localized to one lobe usually are the result of bacterial or *M. pneumoniae* infections (Fig. 1.71C).

STREAKS AND WEDGES

Thin streaks commonly occur with fluid accumulations in the pleural fissures, or as Kerley A and B lines in interstitial pulmonary edema (Fig. 1.73C).

When the streaks are more wedge-shaped or triangular, segmental atelectasis should be the problem (Fig. 1.73A and B). Occasionally, fluid accumulations in the interlobar fissures can be somewhat wedge-shaped, but their fissural location should be a clue to the correct diagnosis. Fibrotic streaking in the lungs generally is uncommon in children, except as seen with healed tuberculosis, and in these cases, often a calcified hilar lymph node or peripheral Ghon lesion accompany the fibrotic streak. Fibrotic streaks resulting from other pulmonary infections generally are uncommon, except in aspiration pneumonia.

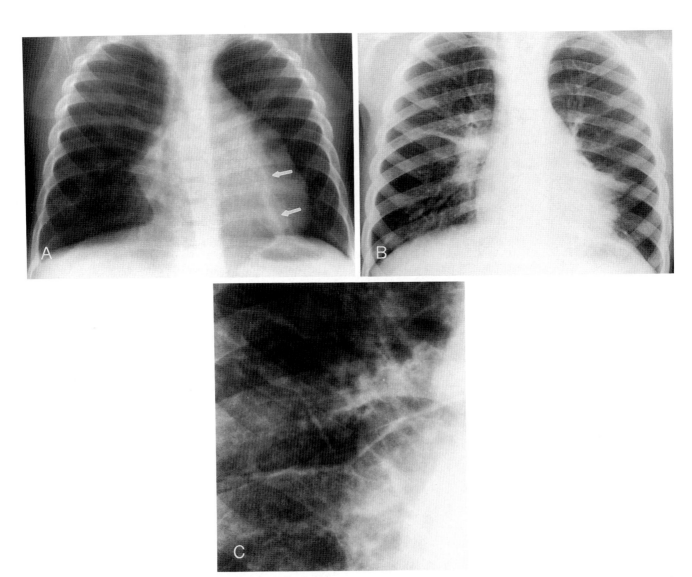

Figure 1.73. Streaks and wedges. A. Note typical vertical streak of discoid atelectasis *(arrows)* behind the left side of the heart. This infant had a viral lower respiratory tract infection. **B.** Another patient with early atelectasis of the right upper lobe *(arrows)*. This patient had asthma (note extensive parahilar-peribronchial infiltrates). **C.** Numerous streaks secondary to interstitial pulmonary edema. These represent distended lymphatics and edema along interlobular septa; the longer lines are referred to as Kerley A lines, while the shorter ones are Kerley B lines.

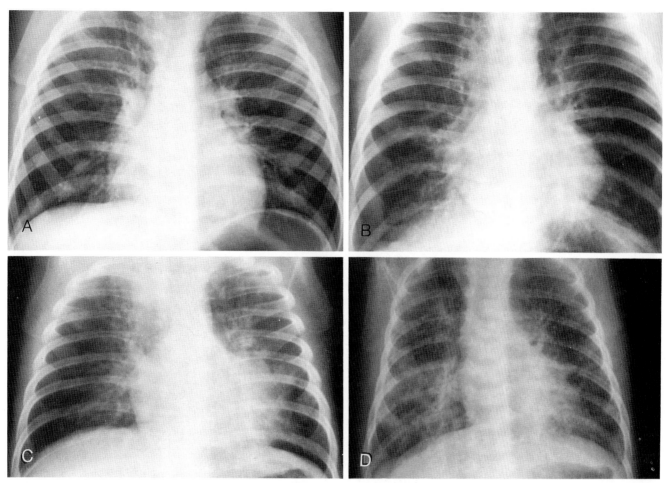

Figure 1.74. Parahilar-peribronchial infiltrates. A. Typical appearance of radiating parahilar-peribronchial infiltrates, associated with hilar adenopathy in viral lower respiratory tract infection. **B.** Extensive parahilar-peribronchial infiltrates, associated with marked overaeration in an infant with cystic fibrosis. **C.** Parahilar-peribronchial infiltrates, with a more ragged interstitial pattern in an infant with pertussis. **D.** Another infant with similar infiltrates due to *Chlamydia*.

PARAHILAR-PERIBRONCHIAL INFILTRATES

The term "parahilar-peribronchial infiltrate" refers to poorly defined opacities that surround the bronchi and radiate outward from the hilar regions. The hilar opacities are due to parahilar inflammation and sometimes adenopathy, and overall the chest has a "ragged" or "dirty" appearance. The presence of such infiltrates infers that bronchial infection or inflammation exists, and in some cases actual thickening of the bronchial wall can be seen. Most commonly, parahilar-peribronchial infiltrates are seen with viral lower respiratory tract infection (4, 25, 32), and in many cases, are associated with bilateral hilar adenopathy (Fig. 1.74A). The outward radiating pattern of the infiltrates attests to their peribronchial distribution, but at the same time, mimics

the radiating pattern of passive vascular congestion. This is not surprising, for the peribronchial space is interstitial, and when passive vascular congestion occurs, it first occurs in this same interstitial compartment. *M. pneumoniae* infections also commonly produce this pattern of infiltration (10, 13, 28), but the pattern is not produced by the standard bacterial infections of childhood.

Other conditions where parahilar-peribronchial infiltrates are seen include chronic asthma (especially with superimposed viral bronchitis), cystic fibrosis, immunologic deficiency states, interstitial pulmonary edema, pertussis, and *Chlamydia* infections (Fig. 1.74C and D). Pertussis infection predominantly causes bronchitis, and it is only later that parenchymal infiltrates develop secondary to superimposed bacterial infection (2). The parahilar-peribronchial pattern of early pertussis infection has led

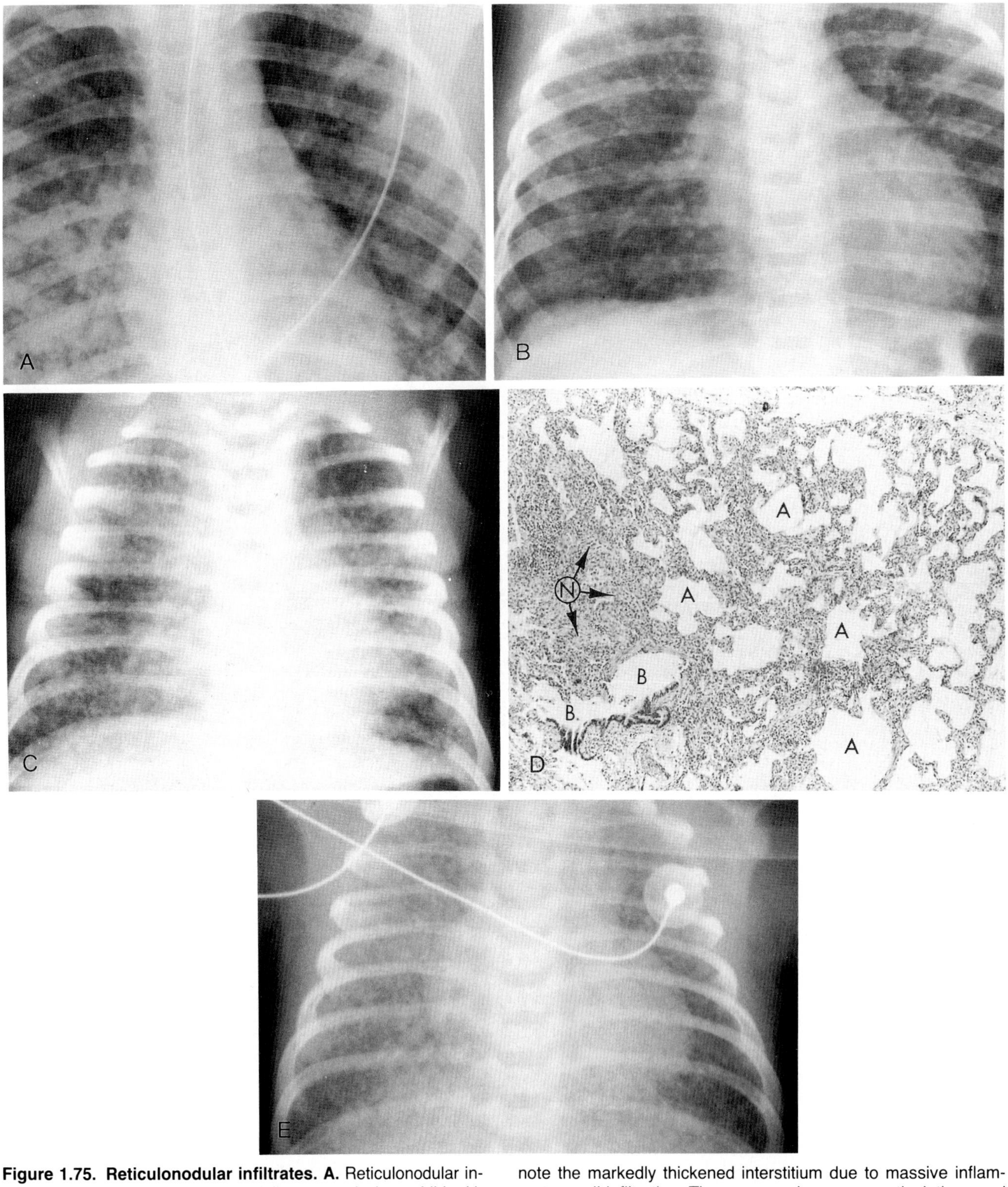

Figure 1.75. Reticulonodular infiltrates. A. Reticulonodular infiltrates due to *Pneumocystis carinii* pneumonia in a child with AIDS. **B.** Reticulonodular infiltrates in histiocytosis-X. **C.** Nodular infiltrates in infant with viral interstitial pneumonia. **D.** Histologic material from infant in part **C.** Note the clear alveoli *(A)*, but also note the markedly thickened interstitium due to massive inflammatory cell infiltration. These areas show up as reticulations and the more pronounced area of infiltration as nodules *(N)*. Peripheral bronchiole *(B)*. **E.** A newborn infant with pneumonia appearing as a reticulonodular pattern.

to the descriptive term "shaggy heart," but this pattern is much more commonly seen with viral lower respiratory tract infection.

RETICULAR, NODULAR, AND RETICULONODULAR INFILTRATES

These patterns intertwine, but all basically reflect interstitial pulmonary disease (Figs. 1.75 and 1.76). In most cases the reticulonodularity is relatively delicate, but in some cases the nodules may be larger and may coalesce to erroneously suggest the presence of alveolar (acinar) infiltrates (Fig. 1.77). In addition, with pulmonary edema and in certain inflammatory conditions, fluid that is initially confined to the interstitial space can eventually seep into the alveoli. Even so, it is important to appreciate that interstitial disease predominates.

The commonest cause of reticular or reticulonodular infiltrates in children is viral pulmonary infection, followed closely by *M. pneumoniae* infection. This pattern is sometimes seen with primary tuberculosis or fungal infections, especially histoplasmosis, but is quite uncommon with the ordinary bacterial pneumonias. An exception to this statement is neonatal pneumonia, which can have a broad spectrum of radiographic patterns, including reticulonodular infiltrates (Fig. 1.75E). In immunocompro-

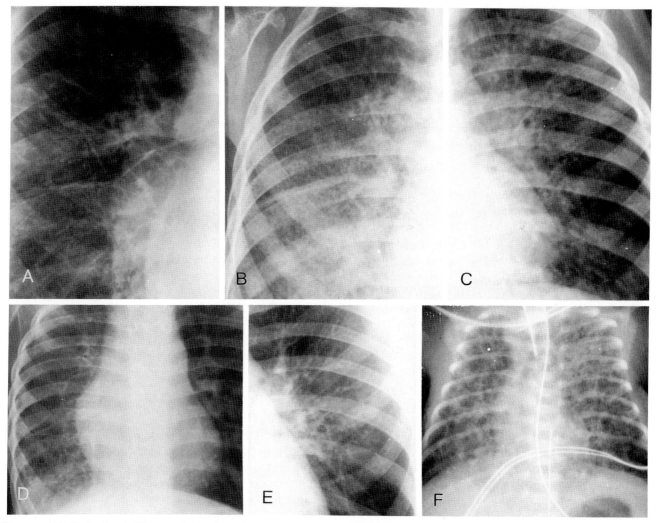

Figure 1.76. Reticular infiltrates. A. Reticularity, in a patient with interstitial pulmonary edema secondary to profound heart failure from thyrotoxicosis. The small transverse lines are Kerley B lines, while the long, oblique lines are Kerley A lines. **B.** Fine reticularity, in a patient with Niemann-Pick disease. **C.** Reticular infiltrates in a patient with immunologic disease. **D.** Unilateral reticularity, especially well seen in the right lower lobe, in a generally small right lung. These findings are quite typical of unilateral pulmonary vein atresia. **E.** Reticular infiltrate in left upper lobe secondary to *Mycoplasma pneumoniae* infection. **F.** A coarse reticular pattern in a premature infant with advanced bronchopulmonary dysplasia.

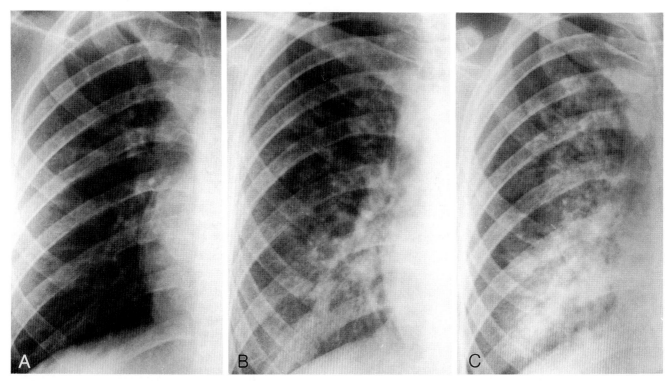

Figure 1.77. Reticulonodular infiltrates: progressing to alveolar pattern. A. Normal chest in patient with renal failure. **B.** Early reticular infiltrates secondary to uremic pneumonitis. **C.** Advanced reticulonodular infiltrates seen the next day. This represents even more extensive interstitial involvement and thickening and, probably, some alveolar spillover.

mised children, reticular or reticulonodular infiltrates are a common presentation for opportunistic pulmonary infections, such as *Pneumocystis carinii*. In the early stages of *Pneumocystis* infections, the infiltrates are primarily interstitial, although patchy scattered alveolar opacities can develop later. In children with the acquired immunodeficiency syndrome (AIDS), *P. carinii,* cytomegalovirus, and mycobacteria infections all can be associated with this type of lung pattern. In addition, a group of chronic lymphocytic infiltrative disorders can also occur and have an identical radiographic appearance (42) (Fig. 1.75A). Lymphocytic infiltrates also have been associated with juvenile rheumatoid arthritis (19) and hypersensitivity reactions (41).

Pulmonary edema, when confined to the interstitial space, also can lead to a reticular or reticulonodular lung pattern. Pulmonary edema can be cardiac or noncardiac in origin, and in children probably more often is noncardiac. Examples of noncardiac pulmonary edema include acute glomerulonephritis (17, 19), where the problem is fluid and electrolyte retention, and the collagen vascular diseases, where the edema is due to vasculitis. Pulmonary edema can also occur as a complication of acute upper airway obstruction in children (15, 26, 34). Finally, it might

be added that the Kerley A and B lines of congestive heart failure (12) are in fact examples of peripheral reticular infiltrates. They result from dilated septal lymphatics and interstitial edema, and most commonly are seen with lesions of the left cardiac valves or myocardium leading to congestive heart failure. However, they can be seen with any cause of pulmonary edema, as outlined in Table 1.14.

Other conditions causing reticular or reticulonodular infiltrates include pulmonary lymphangiectasia or hemangiomatosis (31), pulmonary vein atresia, idiopathic pulmonary hemosiderosis (chronic stage), Henoch-Schönlein purpura (hemorrhage and/or edema) (24), pulmonary fibrosis, the reticuloendothelioses, lymphoma, sarcoidosis (22), leukemia, metastatic disease (lymphangitic spread), tuberous sclerosis, chronic aspiration, immunologic disease, and cystic fibrosis. In most conditions, the infiltrative pattern extends throughout both lungs, but when it is localized to one lobe, *M. pneumoniae* infection should be one's diagnosis of choice (Fig. 1.76E). Such focal reticulation seldom, if ever, is seen with bacterial infection.

In the newborn infant, a diffuse reticular or reticulonodular pattern can be seen in the early stages of the Wilson-Mikity or bronchopulmonary dysplasia

Table 1.14
Pulmonary Edema

Cardiac causes		
Left-side cardiac failure		
Myocardial disease	}	Common
Valvular disease (obstruction, insufficiency)		
Vascular obstructive disease (e.g., coarctation)	}	Uncommon
Hyperkinetic cardiac failure		
Left-to-right shunt, admixture lesions	}	Common
Anemia		
Arteriovenous fistula	}	Rare
Thyrotoxicosis		
Noncardiac causes		
Kidney disease		
Acute glomerulonephritis		
Chronic renal failure	}	Common
Iatrogenic fluid overload		
Near-drowning		Moderately
Neurogenic (increased intracranial pressure)	}	common
Lung toxicity		
Rheumatic pneumonitis		
Allergic lung		
Toxic inhalants	}	Uncommon
Vasculitis		
Collagen vascular diseases		
Idiopathic hemosiderosis		
Pulmonary vein obstruction (acquired or congenital)	}	Rare
Drug abuse		

syndromes (Fig. 1.76F). Although the radiographic appearance of these conditions is similar, their pathogenesis probably differs. Bronchopulmonary dysplasia occurs primarily in infants who have undergone oxygen therapy and positive pressure ventilation, whereas the Wilson-Mikity syndrome often occurs in the absence of these conditions. In addition, pulmonary hypertension and pulmonary fibrosis are uncommon in the Wilson-Mikity syndrome but are quite common with bronchopulmonary dysplasia. In general, infants with bronchopulmonary dysplasia have a poorer survival rate.

Honeycombing of the lung represents the most severe form of the reticular pattern, but it is uncommon in children. In the strictest sense, a honeycomb pattern probably represents a combination of interstitial and air space disease, and it is most characteristic of conditions that result in pulmonary fibrosis. In the pediatric age group, idiopathic pulmonary fibrosis is rare, and more often fibrosis occurs

secondary to viral interstitial pneumonia, idiopathic pulmonary hemosiderosis (21, 30), chemotherapeutic agent or drug toxicity (1, 27), neurofibromatosis, scleroderma, tuberous sclerosis, storage diseases, chronic pulmonary infection, chronic aspiration, immunologic deficiency states, and oxygen toxicity (9).

HAZY-TO-OPAQUE INFILTRATES

This pattern of infiltration also reflects interstitial disease, and is characterized by a diffuse, homogeneous haziness of the lungs. In more profound cases, haziness may be so dense that the lungs are nearly opaque. Most commonly, this pattern of infiltration is seen with pulmonary edema (cardiac or noncardiac) (8, 17, 20), viral interstitial pneumonitis, and *P. carinii* pneumonia (5) (Fig. 1.78). In more advanced cases, air bronchograms are clearly visible, and probably result from the fact that the interstitium is so thickened that it compresses the alveoli. In doing so, lung aeration is reduced to the point where alveolar disease is mimicked. Of course, in some of these cases the disease process may extend into the alveoli (i.e., edema fluid spills into the alveoli or inflammatory cells are extruded into the alveoli), but it is important to remember that interstitial disease still is the predominant problem (Fig. 1.78C and D).

Hazy lungs also can be seen with pulmonary fibrosis, idiopathic pulmonary hemosiderosis (fibrotic stage), lipoid pneumonia, shock lung, pulmonary hemorrhage (including Goodpasteur's syndrome), near-drowning, hemolytic uremic syndrome, and collagen vascular diseases (i.e., vasculitis with pulmonary edema). In the newborn infant, hazy opacity of the lungs commonly reflects clearing alveolar fluid as seen in the neonatal retained fluid syndrome (35, 39). Rapid clearance of such fluid, usually within 24 to 48 hours, is the rule (Fig. 1.79A and B). In the premature neonate, hazy lungs are most often seen with lung immaturity, pneumonia, pulmonary hemorrhage, and the preliminary, edematous stages of bronchopulmonary dysplasia (Fig. 1.79C).

MILIARY OPACITIES

Miliary opacities are interstitial opacities, and the small dots visualized result from the summation of numerous fine reticulations crossing one over the other. They are most characteristic of miliary tuberculosis (Fig. 1.80A) (29), but also can be seen with viral lower respiratory tract infection (viral pneumo-

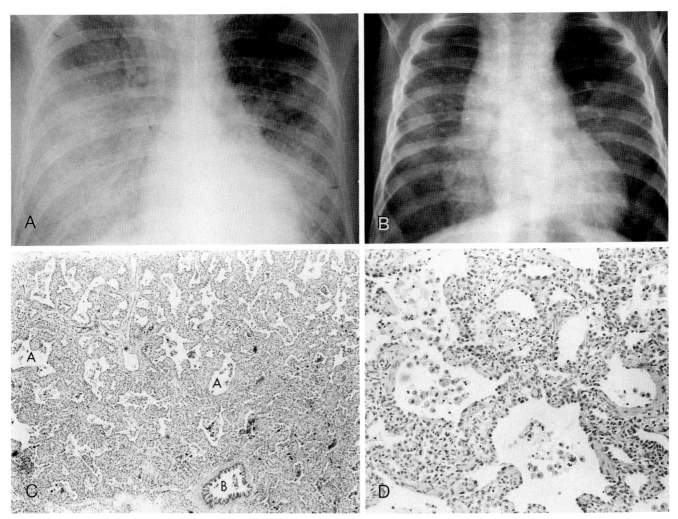

Figure 1.78. Hazy infiltrates. A. Typical diffuse hazy infiltrates of *Pneumocystis carinii* pneumonia. **B.** An infant with interstitial pneumonitis due to parainfluenza virus producing hazy infiltrates in both lungs. **C.** Histologic material from the infant seen in part **B.** Note the very thickened interstitium secondary to diffuse inflammatory cell infiltrate. Note that in some areas, the alveoli *(A)* still are open, but in others, they are completely compressed by the impinging interstitial thickening. Bronchiole *(B)*. **D.** Higher power demonstrating that the alveoli contained only a few inflammatory cells, but that the interstitium is packed with inflammatory cells. On trichrome stain, early interstitial fibrosis also was present.

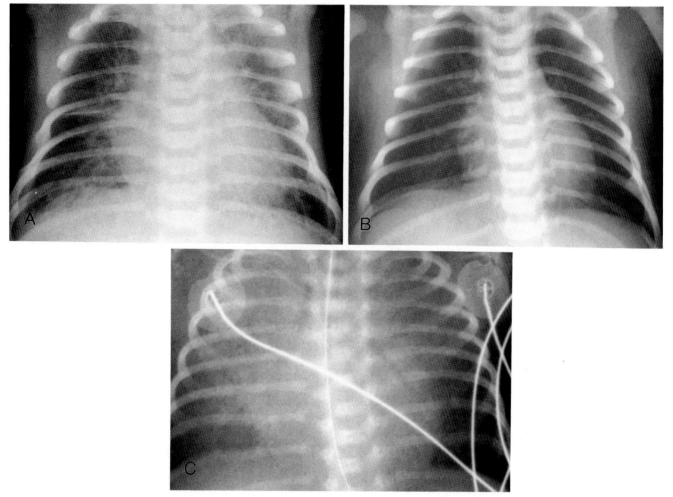

Figure 1.79. Hazy lungs in the newborn infant. A. Note the diffuse haziness of the lungs, accompanied by parahilar streaks and small bilateral pleural effusions. **B.** The same infant 24 hours later shows complete clearing of the lung and pleural fluid. **C.** Diffuse lung haziness in a premature infant with the early edematous stage of bronchopulmonary dysplasia.

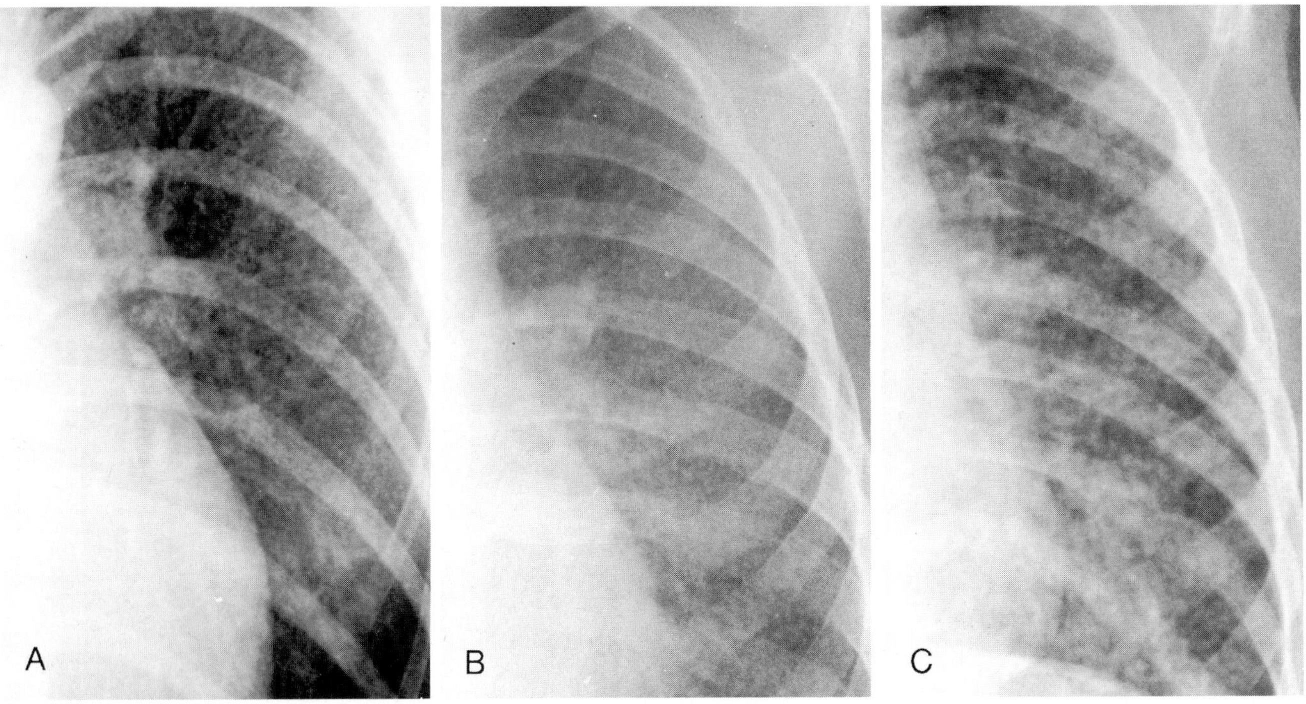

Figure 1.80. Miliary opacities. A. Typical fine miliary nodules of tuberculosis. **B.** Slightly larger nodules in another infant with miliary tuberculosis. **C.** Fine miliary opacities in idiopathic pulmonary hemosiderosis (chronic phase with interstitial fibrosis).

nitis), idiopathic pulmonary hemosiderosis (Fig. 1.80C), metastatic disease to the lungs, lymphoma, leukemia, aspirated foreign matter (16), and sarcoidosis. When miliary infiltrates become larger, a more reticulonodular pattern of infiltration results. This latter phenomenon is common with miliary tuberculosis in infants (Fig. 1.80B).

BASAL INFILTRATES

Basically, basal infiltrates either are homogeneous and hazy, or fluffy and patchy (Fig. 1.81). This latter pattern most commonly occurs with aspiration pneumonias, including hydrocarbon aspiration (23). The basal and medial distribution of these infiltrates attests to the fact that aspiration occurred in the upright position. Diffuse, hazy infiltrates in the lung bases (Fig. 1.81A) reflect interstitial disease and most commonly occur with viral pulmonary infections, desquamative interstitial pneumonia, or lipoid interstitial pneumonia. The etiology of desquamative interstitial pneumonia is unknown, but lymphocytic interstitial pneumonia is known to accompany AIDS in children. A similar basal distribution also commonly is seen with cardiac and noncardiac pulmonary edema and the vasculitis of collagen vascular disease (Fig. 1.81A). Just why these infiltrates

favor the lung bases is not known, but one possibility is that since most of these diseases lead to increased capillary permeability (i.e., severe damage to the interstitium and its vessels), gravity tends to favor the accumulation of the transudate (i.e., edema fluid) in the lower lobes. This may be enhanced by the normally greater flow of blood to the lower lobes.

DENSE CENTRAL INFILTRATES

Some of the conditions producing basal infiltrates also produce dense central infiltrates, and such infiltrates can be streaky or more homogeneous. Streaky, reticular infiltrates infer interstitial disease and have been dealt with in the section on parahilar-peribronchial disease (see Fig. 1.72). Dense, central homogeneous infiltrates usually signify alveolar disease but also can be seen with extensive interstitial disease. Pulmonary edema is the most common cause of such infiltration (Fig. 1.81D), but dense central infiltrates also can be seen with the hemolytic uremic syndrome, pulmonary alveolar proteinosis, lipoid pneumonia, uremia, chronic aspiration and rheumatic pneumonia (33).

In conclusion, although many infiltrative patterns are nonspecific, with an organized approach, one still

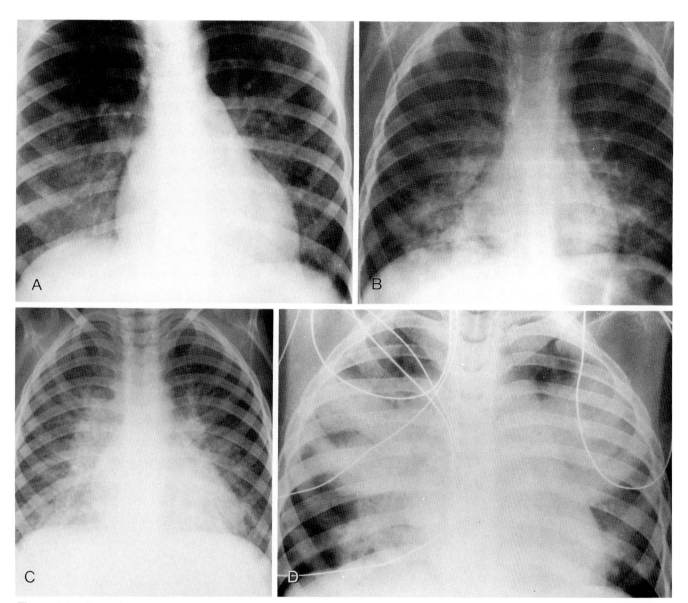

Figure 1.81. Basal infiltrates. A. Note diffuse, basal haziness due to interstitial bleeding and edema in a patient with periarteritis nodosa. **B.** Typical fluffy and ragged, medial basal infiltrates due to hydrocarbon aspiration. **C. Basal and central infiltrates.** Typical distribution of reticular infiltrates in patient with pulmonary edema secondary to glomerulonephritis. The infiltrates are both central and basal. **D.** Dense **central infiltrates** due to iatrogenic fluid overload and pulmonary edema. Edema, at this stage, is alveolar. Note sparing of the apices and basal portions of the lungs.

Table 1.15
Pulmonary Infiltrate Patterns—Infections

	Type of Infiltrate									
	Pneumococcus	*Staphylococcus*	*Haemophilus*	*Streptococcus*	*Pertussis (early)*	*Mycoplasma*	*Virus*	*Tuberculosis*	*Fungus*	*Pneumocystis carinii*
Consolidation	+++	++	+++	+	+/-	+++	-	+	+[a]	+/-
Atelectasis (lobar)	-	-	-	-	+	+++	+++	+++	+	-
Patchy, fluffy										
Bilateral, diffuse	-	+++	+	+	+[b]	+[b]	+[b]	-	+++	++
Lobar	+/-	+++	+	++	-	++	-	-	+	+
Basal, bilateral	-	-	-	-	-	-	+/-[b]	-	-	-
Parahilar-peribronchial	-	-	-	-	+++	+++	+++	-	-	-
Reticulonodular	-	-	-	-	+	+++[c]	+++	+[d]	++	++
Honeycombed	-	-	-	-	-	-	-	-	-	-
Hazy to opaque	-	-	-	-	-	+/-	+	-	-	+++
Hazy (basal)	-	-	-	-	-	+	++	-	-	+
Miliary	-	-	-	-	-	+/-	+	+++	+	-
Diffuse streaks and wedges[b]	-	-	-	-	+	+++	+++	-	-	-

Legend: +++, commonly seen in the condition; ++, moderately common in the condition; +, occasionally seen in the condition; +/-, rarely seen in the condition; -, never, or nearly never, seen in the condition.
[a] Especially actinomycosis.
[b] Atelectasis usually.
[c] Often one lobe only.
[d] Usually nodular.

can present the referring physician with a reasonable list of diagnostic possibilities for each pattern encountered. The more common conditions producing these patterns are summarized in Tables 1.15 and 1.16.

REFERENCES

1. Alvarado CS, Boat TF, Newman AJ: Late onset pulmonary fibrosis and chest deformity in two children treated with cyclophosphamide. *J Pediatr* 92:443–445, 1978.
2. Barnhard HJ, Kniker WT: Roentgenologic findings in pertussis: with particular emphases on the "shaggy heart" sign. *AJR* 84:445–450, 1960.
3. Chang CH, Wittig HJ: Heiner's syndrome. *Radiology* 92:507–508, 1969.
4. Conte P, Heitzman ER, Markarian B: Viral pneumonia, roentgen pathological correlations. *Radiology* 95:267–272, 1970.
5. Dee P, Winn W, McKee K: *Pneumocystis carinii* infection of the lung: radiologic and pathologic correlation. *AJR* 132:741–746, 1979.
6. Diner WC, Knicker WT, Heiner DC: Roentgenologic manifestations in the lungs in milk allergy. *Radiology* 77:564–572, 1961.
7. Eggleston PA, Ward BH, Pierson WE, Bierman CW: Radiographic abnormalities in acute asthma in children. *Pediatrics* 54:442–449, 1974.
8. Felman AH: Neurogenic pulmonary edema: observations in 6 patients. *AJR* 112:393–396, 1971.
9. Glauser FL, Smith WR: Pulmonary interstitial fibrosis following near-drowning and exposure to short-term high oxygen concentrations. *Chest* 68:373–375, 1975.
10. Guckel C. Benz-Bohm G, Widemann B: Mycoplasia pneumonias in childhood: roentgen features, differential diagnosis and review of literature. *Pediatr Radiol* 19:499, 1989.
11. Heiner DC, Sears JW, Knicker WT: Multiple precipitins to cow's milk in chronic respiratory disease: a syndrome involving poor growth, gastrointestinal symptoms, evidence of allergy, iron deficiency anemia, and pulmonary hemosiderosis. *Am J Dis Child* 103:634–654, 1962.
12. Heitzman ER, Ziter FM, Markarian B, McClennan BL, Sherry HS: Kerley's interlobar septal lines: roentgen pathologic correlation. *AJR* 100:578–582, 1967.
13. Herbert DH: The roentgen features of Eaton agent pneumonia. *AJR* 98:300–304, 1966.
14. Hugossan CO, Riff EJ, Moore CCM, Akhtar M, Tufenkeji HT: Lipoid pneumonia in infants: a radiological-pathological study. *Pediatr Radiol* 21:193, 1991.
15. Izsak E: Pulmonary edema due to acute upper airway ob-

Table 1.16
Pulmonary Infiltrate Patterns—Noninfections

	Pulmonary edema	Pulmonary Hemosiderosis	Allergic lung	Sarcoidosis	Aspiration pneumonia	Pulmonary fibrosis	Pulmonary contusion	Pulmonary hemorrhage	Reticuloendotheliosis	Leukemia-lymphoma	Asthma	Cystic fibrosis	Lymphangiectasia hemangiomatosis
Consolidate	+	−	−	−	++	−	+++	+	−	−	+[a]	+[a]	−
Atelectasis (lobar)	−	−	−	−	+++	−	−	−	−	−	+++	+++	−
Patchy													
Bilateral	+	+++	+++	+	+++	−	−	+++	+++	−	+/−[b,c]	++	−
Lobar	−	−	+/−	−	+++	−	−	+++	−	−	+++[c]	++[c]	−
Basal	−	−	−	−	+++	−	−	−	−	−	−	−	−
Parahilar-peribronchial	++	−	−	+	+++	−	−	−	+	−	+++	+++	−
Reticulonodular	++	+++	+	++	+	+++	−	−	++	++	+/−[b]	++	+++
Honeycombed	−	+	−	+	−	+++	−	−	+++	−	−	+++[d]	+
Hazy to opaque	+++	++	−	+/−	+	+/−	−	++[e]	−	−	−	−	−
Hazy (basal)	++	+	−	−	−	+++	−	−	−	−	−	−	−
Miliary	−	++	−	−	−	−	−	−	−	+	−	−	−
Diffuse streaks and wedges[c]	−	−	−	−	++	−	−	−	−	−	+++[c]	+++[c]	−

Legend: + + +, commonly seen in the condition; + +, moderately common in the condition; +, occasionally seen in the condition; +/−, rarely seen in the condition; −, never, or nearly never, seen in the condition.
[a] With superimposed bacterial infection only.
[b] With superimposed virus infection.
[c] Atelectasis usually.
[d] Large honeycomb due to cystic change.
[e] Usually opaque.

struction for aspirated foreign body. *Pediatr Emerg Care* 2:235–237, 1986.

16. Kaplan SL, Gnepp DR, Katzenstein A, Feigin RD: Miliary pulmonary nodules due to aspirated vegetable particles. *J Pediatr* 92:448–450, 1978.

17. Kirkpatrick JA, Fleisher DS: Roentgen appearance of chest in acute glomerulonephritis in children. *J Pediatr* 64:492–498, 1964.

18. Levin DC: The P.I.E. syndrome-pulmonary infiltrates with eosinophilia: a report of 3 cases with lung biopsy. *Radiology* 89:461–465, 1967.

19. Lovell D, Lindsley C, Langston C: Lymphoid interstitial pneumonia in juvenile rheumatoid arthritis. *J Pediatr* 105:947–949, 1984.

20. Macpherson RI, Banerjee AJ: Acute glomerulonephritis: a chest film diagnosis? *J Can Assoc Radiol* 25:58–64, 1974.

21. Matsaniotis N, Karpouzas J, Apostolopoulou E, Messaritakis J: Idiopathic pulmonary hemosiderosis in children. *Arch Dis Child* 43:307–309, 1968.

22. Merten DF, Kirks DR, Grossman H: Pulmonary sarcoidosis in childhood. *AJR* 135:673–679, 1980.

23. Neuhauser EBD, Griscom NT: Aspiration pneumonitis in children. *Prog Pediatr Radiol* 1:265–293, 1967.

24. Olson JC, Kelly KJ, Pan CG, Worthmann DW: Pulmonary disease with hemorrhage in Henoch-Schönlein purpura. *Pediatrics* 89:1177–1181, 1992.

25. Osborne D: Radiologic appearance of viral disease of the lower respiratory tract in infants and children. *AJR* 13:29–33, 1978.

26. Oudijhane K, Bowen A, Oh KS, Young LW: Pulmonary edema complicating upper airway obstruction in infants and children. *J Can Assoc Radiol* 43:278, 1992.

27. Patel AR, Shah PC, Rhee HL, Sassoon H, Rao K: Cyclophosphamide therapy and interstitial pulmonary fibrosis. *Cancer* 38:1542–1549, 1976.

28. Putman CE, Curtis A McB, Simeone JF, Jensen P: *Mycoplasma* pneumonia: clinical and roentgenographic patterns. *AJR* 124:417–422, 1975.

29. Reed MH, Pagtahan RD, Zylak C, Berg T: Radiologic features of miliary tuberculosis in children and adults. *J Can Assoc Radiol* 28:175–181, 1977.

30. Repetto G, Lisboa CM, Emparanza E, Ferretti R, Neira N, Etchart M, Maneghello J: Idiopathic pulmonary hemosiderosis. *Pediatrics* 40:24–32, 1967.

31. Rowen M, Thompson JR, Williamson RA, Wood BJ: Diffuse pulmonary hemangiomatosis. *Radiology* 127:445–451, 1978.

32. Scanlon GA, Unger JD: The radiology of bacterial and viral pneumonias. *Radiol Clin North Am* 11:317–338, 1973.

33. Serlin SP, Rimsza ME, Gay JH: Rheumatic pneumonia: the need for a new approach. *Pediatrics* 56:1075–1077, 1975.

34. Shumaker D, Kottamasu S, Preston G, Treloar D: Acute pulmonary edema after near strangulation. *Pediatr Radiol* 19:59–60, 1988.

35. Swischuk LE: Transient respiratory distress of the newborn—TRDN: a temporary disturbance of a normal phenomenon. *AJR* 108:557–563, 1970.

36. Swischuk LE, L'Heureux P: Unilateral pulmonary vein atresia or stenosis (diagnostic roentgenographic and clinical features). *Am J Roentgenol Radium Ther Nucl Med* 136:667–672, 1980.

37. Teixidor HS, Rubin E, Novick GS, Alonso DR: Smoke inhalation: radiologic manifestations. *Radiology* 149:383–387, 1983.

38. Unger GF, Scanlon GT, Fink JN, Unger JD: A radiologic approach to hypersensitivity pneumonias. *Radiol Clin North Am* 11:339–356, 1973.

39. Wesenberg RL, Graven SN, McCabe EB: Radiological findings in wet-lung disease. *Radiology* 98:69–74, 1971.

40. Wunderlich P, Ruprecht E, Treffz F, Thomsen H, Burkhardt J: Chest radiographs of near-drowned children. *Pediatr Radiol* 15:297–299, 1985.

41. Wolf SJ, Stillerman A, Weinberger M, Smith W: Chronic interstitial pneumonitis in a 3-year-old child with hypersensitivity to dove antigens. *Pediatrics* 79:1027–1029, 1987.

42. Zimmerman BL, Haller JO, Price AP, Thelmo WL, Fikrig S: Children with AIDS: is pathologic diagnosis possible based on chest radiographs? *Pediatr Radiol* 17:303–307, 1987.

43. Zinkham WH: Visceral larva migrans. *Am J Dis Child* 132:627–633, 1978.

PULMONARY VASCULARITY

In the normal individual, the pulmonary artery and its branches diminish in caliber as they travel from their origin in the hilar regions to the periphery of the lungs. Indeed, in the outer third of the lungs, they become so small that generally they are invisible (Fig. 1.82). Centrally, the vessels have reasonably distinct walls and are relatively straight. Also, the size and number of pulmonary vessels are usually symmetrical in the lungs of a normal child. Any deviation from this pattern of pulmonary vascularity should suggest abnormality, and the abnormal patterns that can be encountered are: (a) increased vascularity (large dilated arteries) or vascular congestion (edema), (b) decreased vascularity or lung oligemia, (c) prominent central arteries with diminutive peripheral branches (pulmonary hypertension), and (d) unequal blood flow to the two lungs (Table 1.17). The latter pattern was discussed earlier in the section dealing with unequal lung size, and is not discussed here.

INCREASED VASCULARITY OR VASCULAR CONGESTION

The term "vascular congestion," as applied radiographically, probably conjures different images for different individuals. This is because the term is used to describe both active and passive congestion, although the two appear quite different and have a different etiology. **Active vascular congestion** (increased vascularity) results from more blood than usual passing through the pulmonary circulation. For this to occur, there must be a communication between the systemic and pulmonary circulations. Because systemic pressures are higher than pulmonary pressures, some of the blood from the systemic circulation is diverted to the pulmonary circulation. Classically, this occurs with congenital heart lesions in which a left-to-right shunt (i.e., ventricular septal defect, atrial septal defect, patent ductus arteriosus, aorticopulmonary window), or cardiac admixture lesion (e.g., transposition, truncus arteriosus, single ventricle, total anomalous pulmonary venous return) is present.

Radiographically, with active congestion, the pulmonary artery branches become visualized well into the outer third of the lungs (Fig. 1.82*B*). They become more tortuous and meandering, but their walls remain relatively distinct. It is interesting that, even though the pulmonary veins clearly also must enlarge and dilate, they seldom are seen as distinct structures. Perhaps this occurs because their walls are thinner than those of the arteries. Generally, increased pulmonary blood flow does not become radiographically detectable until the shunt ratio reaches approximately 2.5 to 1. In other words, the right ventricular output must be more than two and one-half times the left ventricular output before one can appreciate increased pulmonary blood flow (1, 2, 4).

With **passive vascular congestion**, excessive flow of blood through the lungs does not occur, but rather there is obstruction to the passage of blood through the lungs. This can result from obstructing lesions of the pulmonary veins, left side of the heart, or proximal aorta, and left-side myocardial disease. Left-sided cardiac obstructing lesions leading to passive congestion include aortic stenosis, mitral stenosis, coarctation of the aorta, and cor triatriatum. Because the left ventricle can withstand increased pressures for a considerable length of time, it is unusual for patients with obstructive lesions of the left ventricle or aorta to be initially seen with passive congestion in infancy or early childhood. In the neonatal period, severe passive congestion can occur with pulmonary vein atresia, total anomalous pulmonary venous return below the diaphragm (type III), and the hypoplastic left heart syndrome (including premature closure of the foramen ovale). In any age group, the most common myocardial abnormalities leading to passive congestion are myocarditis (usually viral) and a variety of cardiomyopathies.

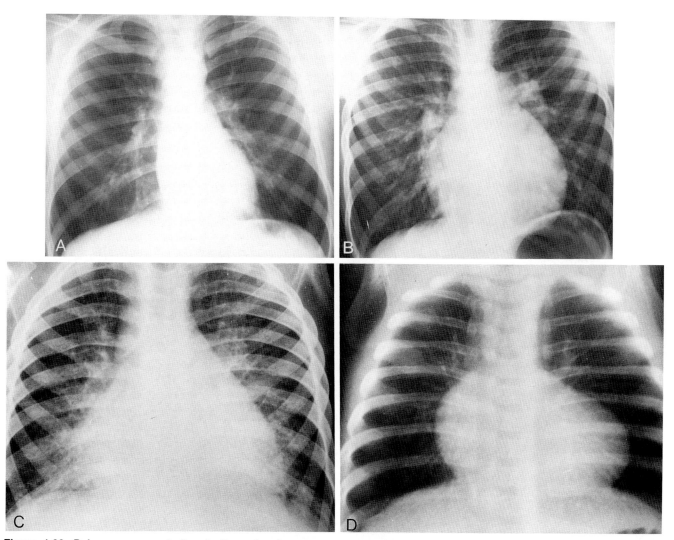

Figure 1.82. Pulmonary vascularity. A. Normal pulmonary vascularity. Note that the vessels taper uniformly and become invisible in the outer third of the lungs. **B. Increased vascularity: active congestion.** Note how much larger the individual vessels (pulmonary artery branches) appear. They also are more nodular, and are visible into the outer third of the lungs. This patient had an atrial septal defect. **C. Increased vascularity: passive congestion.** Note the hazy or fuzzy appearance of the pulmonary vascularity. Individual vessels are not visualized and streaks of interstitial fluid are seen. This patient had myocarditis. **D. Decreased pulmonary vascularity.** Note marked radiolucency of the lungs. Also note that individual pulmonary artery branches are hard to find; they are thin and stringy. This patient had tetral-

Table 1.17
Pulmonary Vascular Patterns

Increased vascularity		
Active		
Left-to-right shunt	}	Common
Cardiac admixture lesion		
Systemic arteriovenous fistula	}	Rare
Passive		
Left heart failure (myocardial disease)	}	Common
Acute glomerulonephritis (fluid overload)		
Left heart failure (vascular or valvular disease)	}	Moderately common
Fluid overload (iatrogenic, chronic renal failure)		
Neurogenic pulmonary edema		
Decreased vascularity		
Right outflow tract obstruction (congenital)		
Acidosis-hypoxia	}	Common
Hypovolemia (dehydration)		
Obstructive emphysema		
Right outflow tract obstruction (acquired)	}	Rare
Hypovolemia (blood loss)		

These include hypertrophic cardiomyopathy, restrictive cardiomyopathy, dilated cardiomyopathy, and endocardial fibroelastosis. A transient hypertrophic cardiomyopathy occurs in infants of diabetic mothers, and secondary cardiomyopathies also can be seen with glycogen storage disease (primarily Pompe disease), thyrotoxicosis, and hypothyroidism. In addition, the condition of aberrant left coronary artery also usually leads to myocardial ischemia and left-sided heart failure, and thus often is conveniently included in this group of diseases.

In all of these conditions, the radiographic findings are similar, for as blood backs up in the pulmonary veins, it causes intraluminal pressures to rise and transudation of fluid into the interstitium. First, this leads to haziness of the medial lung fields and a general fuzziness or indistinctness of the pulmonary artery walls. Thereafter, as more fluid accumulates in the interstitium, fuzziness and indistinctness become more profound, and eventually fluid seeps into the alveolar spaces and classic pulmonary edema is seen (Fig. 1.82C).

If pulmonary venous pressures rise gradually over a long period of time, redistribution of blood flow to the upper lobes of the lungs occurs. Classically, this is seen with mitral stenosis, but mitral stenosis, either congenital or acquired, is rare in children. Indeed, the most common lesion of rheumatic heart disease in childhood is mitral insufficiency and not mitral stenosis. Thus, in the pediatric age group, one does not witness the phenomenon of redistribution of blood flow as often as in adulthood.

Other causes of passive vascular congestion of the lungs, on a noncardiac basis, include iatrogenic fluid overload, neurogenic pulmonary edema, chronic or acute renal failure, acute glomerulonephritis (fluid and electrolyte retention), inappropriate antidiuretic hormone secretion, and systemic arteriovenous fistulae. In addition, any left-to-right shunt or cardiac admixture lesion can cause the heart to fail, leading to passive congestion superimposed on an initial picture of active congestion.

DECREASED PULMONARY VASCULARITY

When pulmonary blood flow to the lungs is decreased, the lungs become more radiolucent (blacker) than normal. The reason, of course, is that the "solid tissue to air" ratio of the lungs is altered in favor of air. On a congenital basis, this most often occurs with lesions that obstruct the right side of the heart and are associated with an obligatory right-to-left shunt. As a result of the right-to-left shunt, the patient is usually cyanotic, and the best known example of this phenomenon is tetralogy of Fallot. In this condition, right ventricular outflow tract obstruction (i.e., infundibular and, many times, valvular pulmonary stenosis) is accompanied by a high ventricular septal defect. The right ventricular outflow tract obstruction results in preferential shunting of blood from the right ventricle, through the ventricular septal defect, into the right ventricle, and out the overriding aorta. Therefore, the severity of cyanosis is dependent on the degree of right ventricular outflow obstruction. In addition to the findings of diminished peripheral pulmonary vascularity, the main pulmonary artery segment is usually concave (Fig. 1.82D). The aortic arch is right-sided in approximately 25% of cases. Other congenital conditions that are associated with decreased pulmonary vascularity include the hypoplastic right heart syndrome (i.e., tricuspid atresia, pulmonary atresia, hypoplastic right ventricle), trilogy of Fallot (ASD with valvular pulmonary stenosis), Ebstein's anomaly, and the rare Uhl's disease (parchment right ventricle).

Acquired obstruction of the pulmonary blood flow most often is seen with reactive pulmonary arteriolar spasm secondary to hypoxia and acidosis. Pulmonary embolus is uncommon in infants and children, as is obstruction of the pulmonary artery by adjacent tumors, masses, or mediastinal inflammatory processes. In all of these cases, the lungs are quite hyperlucent and the pulmonary arteries difficult to visualize, especially in the lung periphery where the vessels become very thin, wispy, and almost invisible.

Decreased pulmonary blood flow also is seen with obstructive emphysema of the lungs (i.e., asthma, cystic fibrosis, and centrally obstructing endotracheal or paratracheal lesions). In these patients hypoxia and acidosis often coexist, and these factors, as they induce vascular spasm, cause a further decrease in blood flow through the already compressed and decreased pulmonary arteries. Hypovolemia is another cause of decreased pulmonary blood flow in the pediatric age group and is especially common in infants. Most often, it is secondary to severe vomiting or diarrhea (3), but massive blood loss also is a cause.

PULMONARY HYPERTENSION

Pulmonary hypertension, when demonstrable radiographically, has an initial appearance of enlarged central pulmonary arteries that abruptly taper to relatively diminutive peripheral pulmonary artery branches. The transition point is between the inner one-third and outer two-thirds of the lungs (see Fig. 1.60B). Pulmonary hypertension usually develops in patients with long-standing left-to-right shunts or cardiac admixture lesions, in which the continuous flow of excessive volumes of blood through the pulmonary circulation gradually leads to hypertrophy of the peripheral pulmonary arterial walls. Pulmonary hypertension also can be seen in conditions associated with chronic overdistension of the lungs, such as asthma, cystic fibrosis, and α-1 antitrypsin deficiency. It also can be seen with multiple pulmonary emboli, but the commonest cause, by far, is an underlying congenital heart lesion with a left-to-right shunt or cardiac admixture problem.

REFERENCES

1. Chen JTT, Capp MR, Johnsonrude IS, Goodrich JK, Lester RG: Roentgen appearance of pulmonary vascularity in the diagnosis of heart disease. *Am J Roentgenol Radium Ther Nucl Med* 112:559–570, 1971.
2. Simon M: The pulmonary vasculature in congenital heart disease. *Radiol Clin North Am* 6:303–318, 1968.
3. Swischuk LE: Microcardia: uncommon diagnostic problem. *AJR* 103:115–118, 1968.
4. Swischuk LE: *Plain Film Interpretation in Congenital Heart Disease,* ed 2. Baltimore: Williams & Wilkins, 1979: 16–28.
5. Swischuk LE, Stansberry SD: Pulmonary vascularity in pediatric heart disease. *J Thorac Imag* 4:1–6, 1989.

Great Vessel Configurations

Although the aorta and pulmonary artery usually are clearly visible in the child, in the infant they often are obscured by the overlying thymus gland. Nonetheless, much as in the adult, either great vessel can be too large or too small (1, 12), and the aorta can be on the left or on the right (Tables 1.18 and 1.19). When it is on the right, it can provide a significant clue to the presence of certain congenital heart problems.

Large Aorta

The normal aorta in a child is relatively smaller than its counterpart in an adult. Therefore, **prominence of the aorta in an infant or child should raise one's suspicion of an underlying abnor-**

Table 1.18
Aortic Configurations

Large aorta	
Aortic stenosis (valvular) Patent ductus arteriosus	Common
Coarctation of aorta Systemic hypertension Tetralogy of Fallot Persistent truncus arteriosus	Moderately common
Pseudocoarctation Aortitis Aortic aneurysm Aorticopulmonary window	Rare
Small aorta	
Ventricular septal defect Atrial septal defect Endocardial cushion defect	Common
Supravalvular aortic stenosis Interrupted aortic arch (infant) Hypoplastic left heart (neonate) TAPVR and other intracardiac left-to-right shunts[a]	Relatively rare
Right aortic arch	
Isolated anomaly (no ring, no heart disease)	Common
With vascular ring With tetralogy of Fallot With truncus arteriosus	Moderately common
With other congenital heart disease	Relatively rare

[a]TAPVR, total anomalous pulmonary venous return.

Table 1.19
Pulmonary Artery Configuration

Large (convex) pulmonary artery	
Pulmonary valve stenosis Left-to-right shunts Cardiac admixture lesions	Common
Pulmonary hypertension	Moderately common
Pulmonary insufficiency Hypoplastic left heart (neonate) Interrupted aortic arch (infant) Infantile coarctation aorta (infant) Idiopathic dilation (adolescent) Post-tetralogy of Fallot repair	Uncommon
Aneurysm Absent pulmonary valve	Rare
Small (concave or flat) pulmonary artery	
Infundibular pulmonary stenosis (tetralogy of Fallot)	Common
Hypoplastic right heart syndrome (neonate) Ebstein's anomaly Transposition of great vessels Truncus arteriosus	Moderately common
Tricuspid insufficiency Uhl's disease	Rare
Unequal pulmonary artery branches	
Tetralogy of Fallot Truncus arteriosus Hypoplastic pulmonary artery and lung	Common
Acquired hypoplastic lung (Swyer-James) Pulmonary valve stenosis (in childhood)	Uncommon
Unilateral pulmonary vein atresia Hemitruncus arteriosus	Rare

mality. Aortic enlargement in children most often involves the aortic knob and ascending aorta. Enlargement of the descending aorta is uncommon but can be seen with systemic hypertension, some forms of aortitis, aortic aneurysm, and coarctation of the aorta (poststenotic dilation).

The commonest cause of enlargement of the ascending and transverse (aortic knob) portions of the aorta is congenital valvular aortic stenosis.

subvalvular aortic stenosis generally is not associated with an enlarged aorta but, occasionally, the aorta may dilate with membranous subvalvular aortic stenosis. In such cases, the location of the hole in the subvalvular membrane is such that it acts as if it were a stenosed aortic valve. In either case, the resultant jet of blood, under pressure, causes the aorta to dilate (Fig. 1.83A). With supravalvular aortic stenosis, the aorta is underdeveloped and small.

Less common causes of proximal aortic enlargement include aortic insufficiency or systemic hypertension. In the latter condition, the aorta dilates because of increased peripheral vascular resistance, while with aortic insufficiency, enlargement is due to the propulsion of increased volumes of blood into the aorta from the left ventricle. The volume of blood ejected from the left ventricle is increased because, during systole, blood that would ordinarily pass out into the systemic circulation during systole is dumped back into the left ventricle in diastole. This then causes the left ventricle to dilate.

Still another cause of aortic enlargement is increased blood flow associated with a left-to-right shunt at the great vessel level. Most often, the problem is patent ductus arteriosus, but it also can be seen with the much rarer aorticopulmonary window. In both of these lesions, the excessive volumes of blood flowing through the lungs (because of the left-to-right shunt) are delivered back to the left side of the heart, and since in most cases there are no associated intracardiac communications, this same increased volume is ejected out the aorta and causes it to enlarge.

In persistent truncus arteriosus, an enlarged aortic shadow is also seen. In this condition, the pulmonary artery originates from the aorta (truncus) rather than from the right ventricle. Blood in the right ventricle must empty through an associated ventricular septal defect into the left ventricle, and then all of the heart's blood goes out the persistent truncus causing it to enlarge (Fig. 1.83A). In approximately one-third of these patients, the aortic arch is right-sided. The aorta also can enlarge when the pulmonary artery is obstructed to a profound degree. Classically, this occurs in severe tetralogy of Fallot (see Fig. 1.87), where, in essence, the aorta must handle the output from both ventricles. Enlargement of the aorta due to aortic wall disease is relatively rare in children but, when seen, usually is due to Marfan syndrome, homocystinuria, Takayasu's aortitis, traumatic or mycotic aortic aneurysm (Fig. 1.83B), or the mucocutaneous lymph node syndrome (Kawasaki disease). The aorta also can dilate in coarctation of the aorta, and the notch at the site of coarctation combined with adjacent prestenotic and poststenotic dilation of the aorta constitute the classic figure "3" sign (Fig. 1.84A and B). MRI is useful for both preoperative and postoperative evaluation of this condition (2, 5, 11) (Fig. 1.84C). In the condition known as "pseudocoarctation," or "congenital kinking" of the aorta (6), the aorta is dilated, somewhat higher in position than normal, and severely kinked. During cardiac catheterization, no pressure gradient

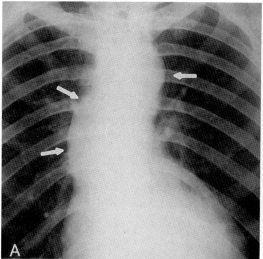
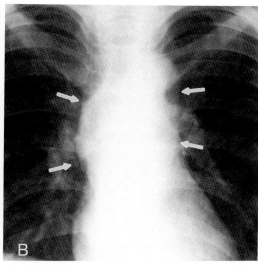

Figure 1.83. Large aorta. A. Patient with persistent truncus arteriosus. *Arrows* denote the very large aorta (actually the persistent truncus). Also note the concave pulmonary artery and, in this case, decreased pulmonary vascularity. More commonly, such aortic enlargement is seen with aortic stenosis, aortic insufficiency, and systemic hypertension. **B.** Dilated aorta due to mycotic aneurysm *(arrows)*.

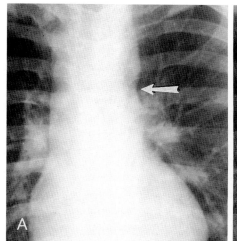
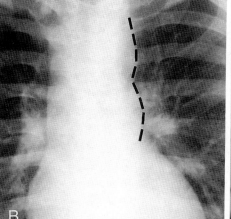
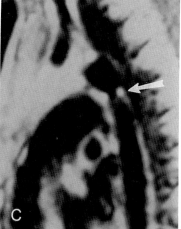

Figure 1.84. Coarctation of the aorta. A. Note the notch and "figure 3" sign *(arrow)* caused by the prominent pre- and poststenotic portions of the descending aorta. **B.** Diagrammatic representation of the figure 3 sign. **C.** MRI demonstrating the coarctation in the upper descending aorta *(arrow)*.

across the apparent narrowing is demonstrable. With true coarctation, of course, actual stenosis and a pressure gradient are present.

SMALL AORTA

A small aorta can be seen with hypoplasia or underdevelopment of the aorta, or with lesions where less than normal volumes of blood flow through the aorta. The latter is much more common and usually results from an intracardiac left-to-right shunt (i.e.,

atrial septal defect or ventricular septal defect). In both conditions, since systemic pressures are higher than pulmonary pressures, blood is shunted from the left to the right side of the heart before it reaches the aorta. Therefore the aorta is never required to handle a normal volume of blood and becomes smaller than normal (Fig. 1.85A). Conversely, if the left-to-right shunt occurs at the great vessel level (i.e., patent ductus arteriosus, aorticopulmonary window), the aorta is of normal size or enlarged. In these cases, no intracardiac shunt is present, and

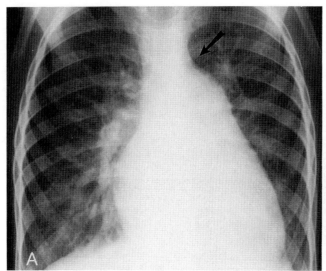
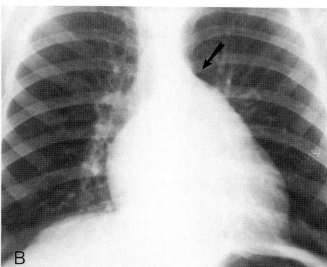

Figure 1.85. Small aorta. A. Note the small aorta *(arrow)* in this patient with an atrial septal defect. The pulmonary artery, just below it, is enlarged (usual for this condition). **B.** Note the almost invisible aorta *(arrow),* secondary to hypoplasia as a part of supravalvular aortic stenosis. This patient had the infantile hypercalcemia syndrome (Williams syndrome).

thus all of the extra blood leaving the left side of the heart passes through the proximal aorta and causes it to enlarge.

Smallness of the aorta due to actual hypoplasia is relatively uncommon and, when seen, usually occurs in infants with lesions such as the hypoplastic left heart syndrome (i.e., mitral atresia, aortic atresia), interrupted aortic arch (4, 8), and supravalvular aortic stenosis. This latter condition usually is associated with the infantile hypercalcemia syndrome (Williams syndrome) (3, 7), and is the only one of these lesions that may go undetected beyond infancy (Fig. 1.85B). Smallness of the aorta also occurs in long-standing mitral stenosis, but this situation is uncommon in children. Smallness of the aorta, in these cases, probably is related to decreased blood flow through the left side of the heart.

RIGHT AORTIC ARCH

A right aortic arch can exist under three conditions: as an isolated anomaly, with a true vascular ring, or with an underlying congenital heart lesion. Most often it occurs as an isolated anomaly, and next most commonly it accompanies a congenital heart lesion. In the latter case, the most commonly associated conditions are tetralogy of Fallot (in about 25% of cases) and persistent truncus arteriosus (in about 33% of cases). The presence of a right-side aortic arch in these conditions is a valuable clue to their diagnosis, for the incidence of right aortic arch in any other congenital heart lesion is less than 5%.

Least common is right aortic arch as part of a vascular ring, and virtually always the ring will consist of either a double aortic arch or a right-side aorta with aberrant left subclavian artery and an encircling ductus arteriosus or ligamentum arteriosum (12).

Radiographically, a right-side aortic arch should be suspected when there is absence of the normal left aortic knob and fullness, or a definite bulge (bump) in the right paratracheal region (see Fig. 1.93B). In most cases, the bump (aortic knob) is located just a little above where it would be if it were normal and on the left. On barium swallow, there is concomitant right-side indentation on the esophagus, and both the trachea and esophagus can also be compressed from behind. When a vascular ring is present, barium swallow reveals a reverse "S" or opposing double indentations of the esophagus (see Fig. 1.2C).

LARGE PULMONARY ARTERY

Enlargement of the pulmonary trunk is most commonly seen with pulmonary valve stenosis and in a variety of conditions associated with increased pulmonary blood flow. In pulmonary valve stenosis, the jet of blood ejected through the stenotic valve is directed toward the walls of the main pulmonary artery, causing it to enlarge (Fig. 1.86). In some cases, the left pulmonary artery also is involved and enlarges.

Increased pulmonary blood flow usually occurs with left-to-right shunts or cardiac admixture lesions where intracardiac communications allow abnormal

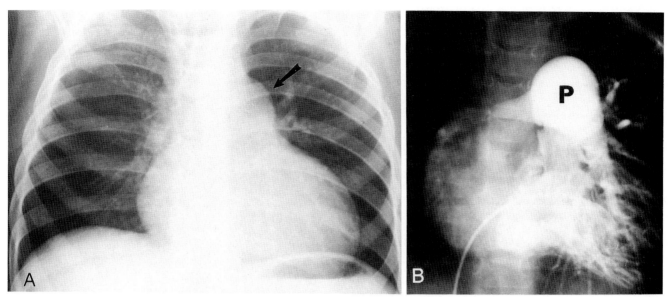

Figure 1.86. Large pulmonary artery. A. Note the large pulmonary artery *(arrow)* in this patient with pulmonary valve stenosis and an atrial septal defect (i.e., tetralogy of Fallot). **B.** Pulmonary angiogram showing the large size of the poststenotically dilated pulmonary artery *(P)*.

shunting of blood from the left to the right side of the heart (see Fig. 1.85*A*). However, it also occurs (although far less often) with pulmonary valve insufficiency, because blood regurgitated into the right ventricle during diastole results in a greater than normal volume of blood being ejected into the pulmonary artery during systole. As a consequence, the pulmonary artery enlarges, and when insufficiency is due to absence of the pulmonary valve, enlargement can be marked. Tetralogy of Fallot commonly is associated with this latter lesion and, in most cases, the proximal right and left pulmonary artery branches also enlarge (9, 10). Indeed, they may erroneously suggest the presence of hilar masses (see Fig. 1.60*C*), for the peripheral pulmonary artery branches are underdeveloped and "pruned" in their appearance.

A final cause of increased flow of blood through the pulmonary artery is severe left-side obstruction. However, the conditions leading to this problem are not common and tend to be seen in the neonate or young infant. They include the hypoplastic left heart syndrome (e.g., mitral atresia, aortic atresia), interrupted aortic arch, and infantile coarctation of the aorta.

The pulmonary artery also dilates with pulmonary hypertension (see Fig. 1.60*B*) and, rarely, with mycotic aneurysms of the pulmonary artery. The pulmonary artery also can dilate after repair of tetralogy of Fallot. In some cases this is due to iatrogenically produced pulmonary insufficiency, while in others it is due to dilation of the patch used for correction of the infundibular stenosis (see Fig. 1.94*C*). Idiopathic pulmonary artery dilation is uncommon in the pediatric age group, except in adolescent girls. Consequently, if one sees a dilated pulmonary artery in an infant or young child, it is quite unlikely that it is due to idiopathic pulmonary artery dilation, and one should look for some other cause.

SMALL PULMONARY ARTERY

A small pulmonary artery occurs because of primary underdevelopment, decreased pulmonary artery blood flow, or apparent smallness because it is located in an abnormal position. For the most part, this latter problem occurs with complete transposition of the great vessels and persistent truncus arteriosus. In the latter lesion, especially, the pulmonary artery may appear quite small (see Fig. 1.83*A*). Primary underdevelopment occurs with infundibular pulmonary stenosis (i.e., tetralogy of Fallot) (Fig. 1.87), the hypoplastic right heart syndrome (i.e., pulmonary valve atresia, tricuspid atresia, tricuspid stenosis), and Ebstein's anomaly. It also can occur with tricuspid insufficiency and Uhl's disease.

ASYMMETRY OF PULMONARY ARTERY SIZE AND BLOOD FLOW

This problem, for the most part, has been discussed in the section on unequal aeration of lungs

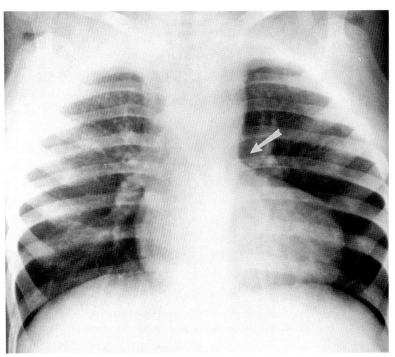

Figure 1.87. Small pulmonary artery. Note the small pulmonary artery *(arrow)* producing the appearance of a concave pulmonary artery segment. This patient had tetralogy of Fallot with infundibular pulmonary stenosis. The aorta is left sided and a little enlarged.

(see p. 7). Basically, however, one pulmonary artery enlarges when the other is absent or hypoplastic, and the phenomenon can occur on a congenital basis or with acquired pulmonary disease such as the Swyer-James lung. In addition, a large left pulmonary artery can be seen in some cases of pulmonary valve stenosis, and a small left pulmonary artery often is seen with tetralogy of Fallot. Smallness of either pulmonary artery is quite common in persistent truncus arteriosus, and, finally, the pulmonary artery may be small, along with its lung, in primary or acquired lung hypoplasia.

REFERENCES

1. Castellanos A, Hernandez FA: Size of ascending aorta in congenital cardiac lesions and other heart diseases. *Acta Radiol* 6:49–64, 1967.
2. Fletcher BD, Jacobstein MD: MRI of congenital abnormalities of the great arteries. *AJR* 146:941–948, 1986.
3. Garcia RE, Friedman WF, Kaback MM, Rowe RD: Idiopathic hypercalcemia and supravalvular aortic stenosis: documentation of a new syndrome. *N Engl J Med* 271:117–120, 1964.
4. Gokcebay TM, Batillas J, Pinck RL: Complete interruption of the aorta at the arch. *Am J Roentgenol Radium Ther Nucl Med* 114:362–370, 1972.
5. Gomes AS, Lois JF, George B, Alpan G, Williams RG: Congenital abnormalities of the aortic arch: MR imaging. *Radiology* 165:691–695, 1987.
6. Hoeffel JC, Henry M, Mentre B, Louis JP, Pernot C: Pseudocoarctation or congenital kinking of the aorta: radiologic consideration. *Am Heart J* 89:428–436, 1975.
7. Jones KL, Smith DW: The Williams elfin facies syndrome. *J Pediatr* 86:718–723, 1975.
8. Moller JH, Edwards JE: Interruption of aortic arch: anatomic patterns and associated cardiac malformations. *Am J Roentgenol Radium Ther Nucl Med* 95:557–572, 1965.
9. Pernot C, Hoeffel JC, Henry M, Worms AM, Stehlin H, Louis JP: Radiological patterns of congenital absence of the pulmonary valve in infants. *Radiology* 102:619–622, 1972.
10. Osman MZ, Meng CCL, Girdany BR: Congenital absence of the pulmonary valve: report of eight cases with review of the literature. *Am J Roentgenol Radium Ther Nucl Med* 106:58–69, 1969.
11. Rees S, Somerville J, Ward C, Martinez J, Mohiaddin RH, Underwood R, Longmore DB: Coarctation of the aorta: MR imaging in late postoperative assessment. *Radiology* 173:499–502, 1989.
12. Swischuk LE: *Plain Film Interpretation in Congenital Heart Disease,* ed 2. Baltimore: Williams & Wilkins, 1979:23–28, 205–221.

Cardiac Abnormalities of Size

The radiographic evaluation of cardiac size in children requires some degree of experience, and we have found the cardiothoracic ratio to be of little

Table 1.20
Cardiac Size Abnormalities

Large cardiac silhouette		
Congenital heart disease	}	
Acquired heart disease	}	Common
Pericardial fluid	}	
Extracardiac causes	}	Uncommon
Cardiac or pericardial tumors	}	Rare
Small cardiac silhouette (microcardia)		
Dehydration	}	
Stretched mediastinum (emphysema)	}	Common
Severe blood loss	}	Uncommon
Cardiac atrophy	}	Rare

value. Aberrations of cardiac size largely consist of a heart that is too large, and the presence of cardiomegaly generally implies a cardiac abnormality (Table 1.20).

LARGE CARDIAC SILHOUETTE

Usually, if one can exclude a large thymus gland and/or a poor inspiratory effort causing apparent cardiomegaly, a large heart infers the presence of cardiac disease. The abnormality can be pericardial, myocardial, or valvular, and in the pediatric age group, heart disease most often is congenital. Thereafter one might consider a variety of acquired myocardial or valvular abnormalities, and leading the list are rheumatic heart disease and viral myocarditis. These latter conditions also are the most common causes of a pericardial effusion, but pericardial fluid also can be seen with bacterial infections, generalized edema (anasarca), chronic or acute renal diseases with fluid retention, and the collagen vascular diseases. Metastatic disease of the pericardium is a rare cause of pericardial effusion, and effusion secondary to tuberculosis and fungal infections is also quite rare. Hemopericardium also is rare in children, except when associated with chest trauma. Bleeding into the pericardial space can occasionally occur with bleeding disorders and metastases to the pericardial sac. Similarly, chyle in the pericardium is very rare.

Distinguishing cardiac silhouette enlargement due to pericardial fluid collections from enlargement resulting from actual cardiomegaly can be accomplished on plain chest films, but usually an effusion is best evaluated with ultrasonography (Fig. 1.88B). On chest films, with pericardial effusions, the heart is rather globular, the vascularity is not congested, and the superior mediastinum is wider than normal.

This is due to the fact that fluid, as it accumulates in the pericardial sac, slowly envelops the roots of the great vessels (Fig. 1.88A). With true cardiac enlargement, the superior mediastinum often is not as wide and the vessels tend to be congested, either on a passive or active basis.

Cardiomegaly that is not associated with primary cardiac disease occurs less commonly. Such cardiac enlargement can occur as the result of fluid and electrolyte retention (e.g., chronic renal disease, acute glomerulonephritis, inappropriate antidiuretic hormone secretion), peripheral arteriovenous fistulae, severe anemia, and metabolic disease (e.g., hypothyroidism, hypocalcemia). Tumors are a rare cause of cardiomegaly, and they often cause eccentric enlargement or bumps projecting off the cardiac silhouette. The most common primary cardiac tumor in infants and children is rhabdomyoma, and a large percentage of these tumors are seen in patients with tuberous sclerosis. Teratomas and fibromas of the heart are less common. Malignant cardiac tumors are primarily metastatic (e.g., lymphoma, osteosarcoma).

SMALL CARDIAC SILHOUETTE

A small cardiac silhouette, or microcardia, is surprisingly common in the pediatric age group. For the most part, three causes of microcardia exist: (a) markedly decreased intravascular fluid volume, (b) stretching and compression of the mediastinum, and (c) cardiac atrophy (3). Fluid loss is by far the commonest cause and most frequently is seen with vomiting, diarrhea, and dehydration (Fig. 1.88C). A less common cause is severe blood loss. After hypovolemia due to profound fluid or blood loss, the next most common cause of a small cardiac silhouette is stretching and compression of the mediastinum by diffuse obstructive emphysema. Most commonly, this is encountered in asthma and cystic fibrosis, but it can be seen with other causes of overaeration. Actual cardiac atrophy is relatively rare and is seen with the cachexia associated with malignant tumors or chronic infections (3). In addition, some degree of cardiac atrophy occurs with adrenal insufficiency (Addison's disease), but this is quite uncommon in the pediatric age group. The cause probably is disuse atrophy of the cardiac muscle because of the chronic hypotension present in these patients.

REFERENCES

1. Chan HS, Sonley MJ, Moes CA, Daneman A, Smith CR, Martin DJ: Primary and secondary tumors of childhood in-

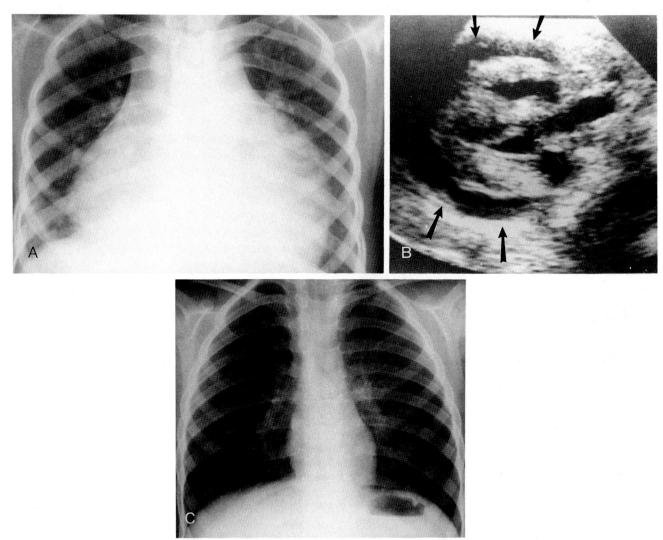

Figure 1.88. Cardiac silhouette size abnormalities. A. Enlargement. In this patient, the heart is globular in shape, and the superior mediastinum is widened due to pericardial fluid accumulating in the portion of the pericardial sac that extends to the bases of the great vessels. Small bilateral pleural effusions also are present in this patient with lupus erythematosus. **B.** Ultrasound verifies pericardial fluid *(arrows)* in another patient with myocarditis. **C. Microcardia.** Note the very small heart in this child who had severe burns. Microcardia resulted from hypovolemia. For microcardia secondary to overdistension of the lungs, see Figure 1.1.

volving the heart, pericardium, and great vessels: a report of 75 cases and review of the literature. *Cancer* 56:825–836, 1985.

2. Harding CO, Pagon RA: Incidence of tuberous sclerosis in patients with cardiac rhabdomyoma. *Am J Med Genet* 37:443–446, 1990.

3. Swischuk LE: Microcardia: an uncommon diagnostic problem. *AJR* 103:115–118, 1968.

Superior Mediastinal Widening

Superior mediastinal widening can be bilateral or unilateral (Table 1.21), and often the same conditions cause either configuration. In all cases, however, superior mediastinal widening is due to increased soft tissue bulk, and can result from dilated vascular structures, inflammatory diseases of the mediastinum, or primary or secondary tumors.

Table 1.21
Superior Mediastinal Widening[a]

Bilateral and relatively symmetric		
Normal thymus gland	}	Common
Adenopathy (inflammatory, tumoral)		
Mediastinal tumor		Moderately common
Dilated aorta		
Persistent LSVC		
Vein of Galen aneurysm		
TAPVR-type I ("snowman" or "figure 8")		
Mediastinitis		
Thyroiditis		Uncommon
Mediastinal hematoma		
Goiter		
Mediastinal fat		
Dilated esophagus		
Bilateral upper lobe agenesis		
Aneurysm of great veins		Rare
Unilateral		
Thymus, normal (R or L)	}	Common
Superior vena cava (R)		
Dilated ascending aorta (R)		
Upper lobe atelectasis (R)		
Adenopathy (R or L)		Moderately common
Mediastinal tumor, cyst (R or L)		
Right-side aorta (R)		
Dilated esophagus (R or L)		
Persistent LSVC[b]		
Mediastinal hematoma (R or L)		Rare
Goiter (R or L)		
Mediastinal fat (R or L)		

[a]LSVC, left superior vena cava; TAPVR, total anomalous pulmonary venous return.
[b]Usually causes bilateral widening because of normal inferior vena cava on right.

BILATERAL SUPERIOR MEDIASTINAL WIDENING

In infancy and through the age of 2 or 3 years, the commonest cause of bilateral superior mediastinal widening, by far, is the normal thymus gland. The configurations of the normal thymus gland are endless, and it is not uncommon for one side of the gland to be more prominent than the other (Fig. 1.89). After the normal thymus gland, tumor or mediastinal lymph node enlargement should be considered (Fig. 1.90A and B). Mediastinal lymphadenopathy can be either inflammatory or neoplastic (i.e., lymphoma, leukemia, or metastatic disease). Primary tumors in the mediastinum include thyroid neoplasms, teratoma, thymoma, cystic hygroma, neurofibroma, neuroblastoma (ganglioneuroma), germ cell tumor, and hemangioma, but all occur far less frequently than do the other causes of superior mediastinal widening.

Vascular abnormalities producing mediastinal widening are rather common, but most often, the widening they produce is unilateral. Nonetheless, when the aorta dilates in both its ascending and descending portions, superior mediastinal widening can result, and this occurs most commonly with aortic stenosis or aortic insufficiency. However, it also occurs with persistent truncus arteriosus (see Fig. 1.83A) and aortic wall disease as seen in Marfan syndrome, homocystinuria, and Takayasu's disease. Occasionally, similar widening can be seen with systemic hypertension, but more often it is the aortic knob and descending aorta that dilate in this condition.

Another uncommon but characteristic cause of superior mediastinal widening resulting from dilation of blood vessels is the "snowman" or "figure 8" heart of total anomalous pulmonary venous return (3, 5, 8). In the type I form of the condition, the so-called "vertical" vein on the left, the innominate vein on top, and the superior vena cava on the right produce an abnormal inverted U-shaped vessel that causes the widening (Fig. 1.90C and D). Other vascular conditions producing superior mediastinal widening include persistence of the left superior vena cava (2) and, rarely, aneurysms of the great vessels. In newborns and young infants with intracranial arteriovenous malformations (e.g., vein of Galen aneurysm), the arteries and veins of the neck and superior mediastinum can become markedly enlarged and also cause superior mediastinal widening (9).

Inflammatory mediastinitis, thyroiditis, benign goiter, mediastinal hematoma (due to trauma, bleeding disorders, catheter-related injury), mediastinal

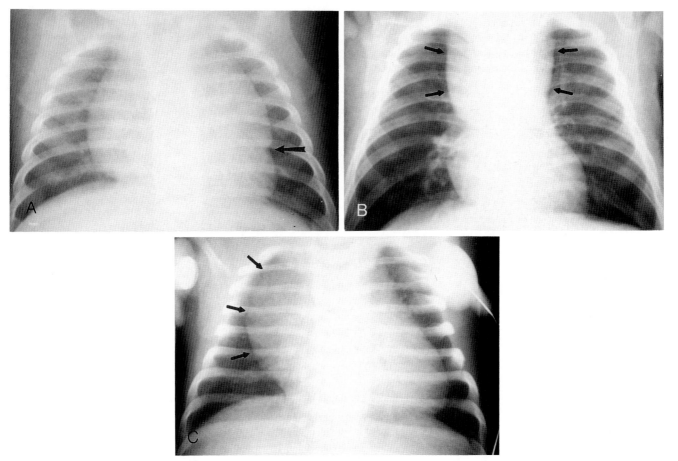

Figure 1.89. Normal thymus gland. A. Note prominence of the superior mediastinum due to the large normal left and right lobes of the thymus. A notch is seen on the left at the junction of the thymus gland and the left cardiac border *(arrow)*. **B.** Note the high position of this normal thymus gland *(arrows)*. **C.** In this infant, the right lobe of the thyroid *(arrows)* is more prominent than the left.

fat accumulation with steroid therapy, a dilated, obstructed esophagus, and the very rare bilateral upper lobe pulmonary agenesis complete the list of causes of bilateral superior mediastinal widening of childhood.

UNILATERAL SUPERIOR MEDIASTINAL WIDENING

Overall, unilateral superior mediastinal widening is more common on the right, largely due to the presence of the superior vena cava. The superior vena cava can dilate idiopathically (1, 6) (Fig. 1.91*A*), with heart failure (i.e., increased central venous pressure), with increased blood flow such as occurs with total anomalous pulmonary venous return to the superior vena cava, and with obstruction secondary to thrombosis, mediastinal tumors, or intracardiac tumors. Primary intracardiac tumors are rare,

and more commonly the problem is venous and intracardiac extension of Wilms tumor of the kidney. In addition to the foregoing causes of superior vena caval prominence, the superior vena cava can be displaced to the right by an enlarged ascending aorta, a right-sided aortic arch, or a tumor or cyst located between the vena cava and the trachea.

Other common causes of unilateral right-side superior mediastinal widening include an asymmetrically prominent thymus gland (see Fig. 1.89*C*), adenopathy, and right upper lobe atelectasis (Fig. 1.91*B*). Such atelectasis can occasionally be associated with a tracheal or anomalous apical bronchus (7) (Fig. 1.91*B*). Rounding out the causes of right-side superior mediastinal widening are dilation of the ascending aorta (as seen in aortic stenosis, aortic insufficiency, and primary aortic wall diseases) and unilateral mediastinal tumors and cysts (Fig. 1.91*C* and *D*).

The most common causes of left-side mediastinal

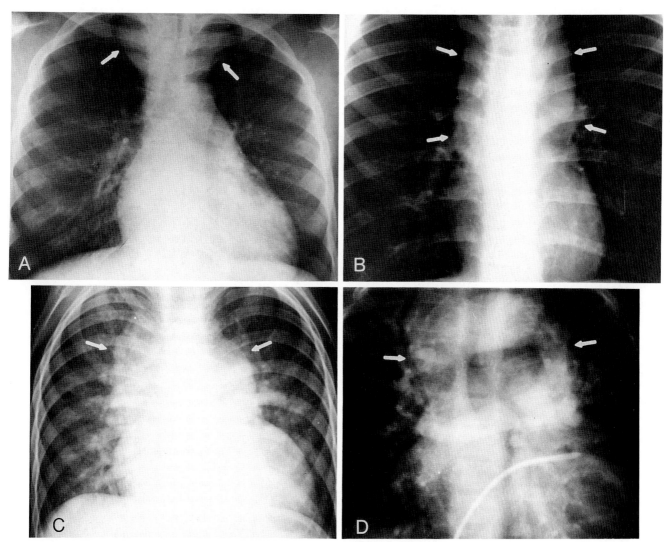

Figure 1.90. Superior mediastinal widening. A. Note marked superior mediastinal widening due to an **enlarged thyroid gland** *(arrows)*. There is associated tracheal compression. **B.** Mediastinal widening due to **lymphoma** *(arrows)*. **C.** Mediastinal widening due to **total anomalous pulmonary venous return** *(arrows)*. Also note that the heart is enlarged and the vascularity engorged. **D.** Cardioangiogram demonstrating the abnormal **inverted U-shaped vessel** that causes the superior mediastinal widening *(arrows)*. All of the blood from both lungs is collected by this vessel and then emptied into the superior vena cava. The vessel lies anterior to the trachea.

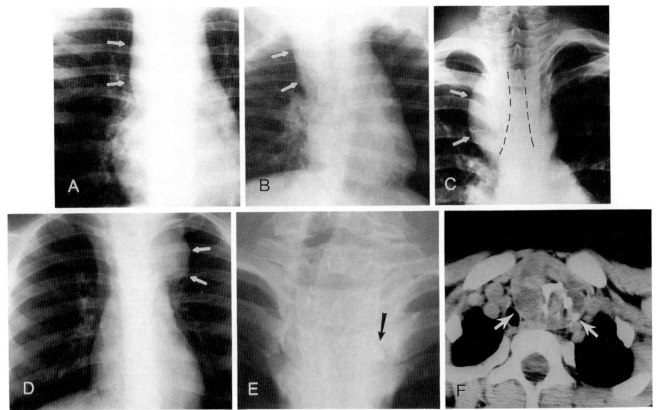

Figure 1.91. Unilateral superior mediastinal widening. A. Unilateral right side widening due to **idiopathic dilation of the superior vena cava** *(arrows).* **B.** Right side widening due to **right upper lobe collapse** *(arrows)* associated with a tracheal bronchus. **C.** Right-side widening due to an **asymptomatic esophageal duplication cyst** *(arrows).* **D.** Left-side superior mediastinal widening caused by **adenopathy** in a child with his-tiocytic lymphoma *(arrows).* **E.** Mild widening of the superior mediastinum is accompanied by deviation of the trachea to the right. Note the formed calcification *(arrow)* within this **teratoma. F.** CT of the same patient shows the large complex mass displacing the trachea to the right *(arrows).* (Parts **E** and **F** courtesy of C. Keith Hayden, Jr., M.D.)

widening are a unilaterally prominent thymus gland and unilateral adenopathy (Fig. 1.91*D*). Left-side prominence also can be seen with dilation of the aorta above a coarctation or persistence of the left superior vena cava (2). Finally, it is possible that any of the tumors, cysts, or tumor-like conditions producing bilateral superior mediastinal widening could produce unilateral widening on either side. The position of the trachea is important in differentiating such lesions from the thymus gland, because the thymus gland usually does not deviate the trachea, while tumors and tumor-like conditions frequently do (Fig. 1.91*E* and *F*).

REFERENCES

1. Bell MJ, Guiterrez JR, DuBoise JJ: Aneurysm of the superior vena cava. *Radiology* 95:317, 1970.
2. Cha EM, Khoury GH: Persistent left superior vena cava. Radiologic clinical significance. *Radiology* 103:375–381, 1972.
3. Darling RC, Rothney WB, Craig JM: Total pulmonary venous drainage into the right side of the heart: report of 17 autopsied cases not associated with other major cardiovascular anomalies. *Lab Invest* 6:44–65, 1957.
4. Heil BJ, Felman AH, Talbert JL, Hawkins IF, Garmica A: Idiopathic dilatation of the superior vena cava. *J Pediatr Surg* 13:193, 1978.
5. Paster SB, Swensson RE, Yabek SM: Total anomalous pulmonary venous connection. *Pediatr Radiol* 6:132–140, 1977.
6. Polansky S, Gooding CA, Potter B: Idiopathic dilation of the superior vena cava. *Pediatr Radiol* 2:167, 1974.
7. Siegel MJ, Shackelford GD, Francis RS, McAlister WH: Tracheal bronchus. *Radiology* 130:353–355, 1979.
8. Swischuk LE: *Plain Film Interpretation in Congenital Heart Disease,* ed 3. Baltimore: Williams & Wilkins, 1986:118.
9. Swischuk LE: Large vein of Galen aneurysms in the neonate (a constellation of diagnostic chest and neck radiologic findings). *Pediatr Radiol* 6:4–9, 1977.

Mediastinal Bumps

Mediastinal bumps usually first are recognized on frontal views of the chest, and in assessing these bumps, it is helpful to consider them by location (Fig. 1.92). Basically, these locations include: (a) right paratracheal, (b) left paratracheal, (c) upper left cardiac border, (d) lower left cardiac border, (e) right cardiac border, and (f) paraspinal gutters (Table 1.22). Lumps caused by hilar masses are discussed elsewhere (see p. 55).

LOCATION 1: RIGHT PARATRACHEAL

A lump in the right paratracheal region most commonly is caused by an enlarged lymph node or a vascular structure (Fig. 1.93A). Adenopathy usually is inflammatory in nature and most often is caused by tuberculous or fungal infection. Next most common is adenopathy secondary to metastatic disease, and least common is isolated adenopathy due to lymphoma or leukemia. When these latter diseases involve the mediastinal lymph nodes, involvement usually is massive and presentation is that of a superior mediastinal mass. As far as vascular structures

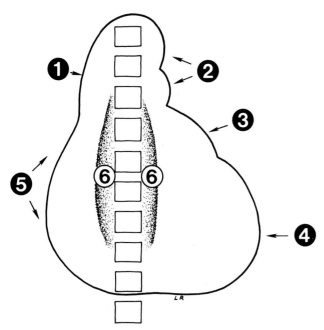

Figure 1.92. Mediastinal bumps and bulges: diagrammatic representation. Lumps, bumps, and bulges along the mediastinum can be considered according to location: *location 1*—right paratracheal; *location 2*—left paratracheal; *location 3*—high left upper cardiac border; *location 4*—lower left cardiac border; *location 5*—entire right cardiac border; and *location 6*—paraspinal areas.

Table 1.22
Discrete Mediastinal Bumps

Location 1
Normal azygous vein / Lymph node	Common
Right-side aorta / Tumor, cyst / Compressed thymus with anterior pneumothorax	Moderately common
Dilated azygous vein	Uncommon

Location 2
Large aorta / Ductus bump in neonate	Common
Tumor, cyst / Compressed thymus with anterior pneumothorax	Moderately common
Postcoarctation patch / Hemiazygous vein enlarged / Aorta, pulmonary artery, ductus aneurysm	Rare

Location 3
Thymus / Left atrial appendage	Common
Congenital corrected transposition / Ebstein's anomaly	Uncommon
Partial absence of pericardium / Single ventricle with transposition / Coronary artery aneurysm / Juxtaposition of R atrial appendage / Post-op conduits / Dilated patch of repaired tetralogy of Fallot	Rare

Location 4
Left ventricular hypertrophy / Right ventricular hypertrophy	Common
Tumor (cardiac, pericardial) / Congenital aneurysm of heart	Rare

Location 5
Enlarged right atrium / Displacement of right atrium by large heart	Common
Mesoversion / Large thymus	Uncommon
Tumor (cardiac or pericardial) / Congenital aneurysm of the heart / Coronary artery aneurysm (upper border) / Pericardial defect (upper border)	Rare

Location 6
Long stripes — Normal aorta	Common
Pleural fluid / Dilated aorta	Moderately common
Localized bulge — Paraspinal abscess / Compression fracture with hematoma	Common
Spinal or paraspinal tumor / Adenopathy; inflammation, tumor	Uncommon
Extramedullary hematopoiesis / Neuroenteric cyst	Rare

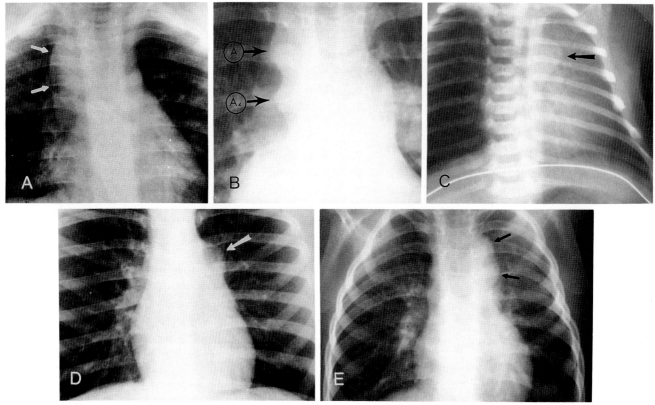

Figure 1.93. Mediastinal bumps: locations 1 and 2—right and left paratracheal. A. Note the large right paratracheal lump produced by enlarged lymph nodes *(arrows)*. On the left, note the normal aortic knob *(A)*. **B.** Right aortic arch and azygous vein. Note typical appearance of a right aortic arch *(A)* and just below it, the normal azygous vein *(Az)*. **C.** Note the dilated infun-

dibular remnant (ductus bump) of the recently closed ductus arteriosus in this newborn infant *(arrow)*. **D.** Dilated hemiazygous vein *(arrow)* in a patient with congenital absence of the inferior vena cava and hemiazygous continuation. **E.** Note the dilated patch angioplasty *(arrows)* in a child with repaired coarctation of the aorta.

are concerned, the two that regularly produce lumps in this area are a right aortic arch and the azygos vein (Fig. 1.93B). The right aortic arch bump is located higher than the one caused by the azygos vein, and the azygos vein bump, when normal, is rarely more than 1 cm in diameter. When it becomes enlarged, however, it can be very prominent, and most often this occurs with total anomalous pulmonary venous return to the azygos vein (16) or absence of the inferior vena cava with azygos continuation (1, 3, 4, 18). In these latter cases, since systemic blood cannot get back to the heart via the inferior vena cava, it does so through the azygos vein, by way of the paravertebral plexus. On lateral view of the chest, absence of the normal inferior vena cava, just at the bottom of the cardiac silhouette, can provide a valuable clue to diagnosis. Acquired obstruction of the inferior vena cava can produce similar enlargement of the azygos vein, and occasionally the vein can enlarge with heart failure. Remaining causes of

a bump in this region include a variety of mediastinal tumors or cysts.

LOCATION 2: LEFT PARATRACHEAL

Vascular structures account for most of the bumps seen in this area, because both the aortic knob and main pulmonary artery are located here. Enlargement of both of these structures has been covered previously (see Figs. 1.83 and 1.86), and the only other vascular structure that can enlarge here with any frequency is a patent ductus arteriosus. However, beyond the neonatal period, the ductus is seldom seen as an isolated structure, and, indeed, usually it blends with the concomitantly enlarged aorta and pulmonary artery to form the so-called "aorticoductal" infundibular complex (15). In the neonate, the dilated infundibular ductal remnant (after spontaneous closure) commonly is seen as the normal ductus bump (5) (Fig. 1.93C). However, it disappears after the first month or so of life and, thereafter, if ductal dilation is suspected, one should consider the rather rare ductal aneurysm (12, 14).

Other causes of a lump in this region include lymph node enlargement, mediastinal tumors, or, rarely, a dilated hemiazygous vein (Fig. 1.93D). The hemiazygous vein can enlarge if the inferior vena cava is absent or obstructed (6), and the problem is the same as that which occurs when blood is diverted into the azygos vein on the right. Mediastinal tumors, aortic or pulmonary artery aneurysms, and dilated aortic coarctation patch repairs (Fig. 1.93E) also can produce lumps in this area.

LOCATION 3: UPPER LEFT CARDIAC BORDER

In this area, one can encounter discrete bumps or just a generalized fullness, and the commonest cause of the latter is normal thymus, followed by an enlarged left atrial appendage. Most commonly, left atrial appendage enlargement occurs with rheumatic mitral valve disease (Fig. 1.94A), for although left atrial enlargement also occurs with ventricular septal defect and patent ductus arteriosus, associated enlargement of the left atrial appendage is not as common. However, fullness in this area, not due to enlargement of the left appendage, does occur with certain other congenital heart lesions. For example, in congenitally corrected transposition of the great vessels, the bulge is due to the abnormal left-sided position of the inverted aorta and right ventricle (Fig. 1.94B). A similar configuration can be seen with single ventricle, where congenitally corrected transposition of the great vessels is a common associated lesion.

Fullness along the upper left cardiac border also can be produced by the rudimentary right ventricle seen in Ebstein's anomaly. In Ebstein's anomaly, the tricuspid valve is displaced forward into the right ventricle, and most of the right ventricle is incorporated into the right atrium. That which remains usually is located high along the upper left cardiac border and, in many cases, produces a discrete bump or step-like fullness (2) (see Fig. 1.97A).

Other relatively rare causes of generalized fullness along the upper left cardiac border include dilation of the patch utilized for correction of infundibular stenosis in tetralogy of Fallot (Fig. 1.94C) and juxtapositioning of the right and left atrial appendages. Normally, the right atrial appendage lies on the right, but in certain complicated congenital

heart lesions, it becomes inverted and lies on the left, just above, or in juxtaposition to the normal left atrial appendage. Together, these structures produce bulging of the upper left cardiac border.

A **discrete bump** along the upper left cardiac border occasionally can be caused by left atrial appendage enlargement, but more often it is due to herniation of the left atrial appendage through a partial pericardial defect (7, 17, 20), or to a coronary artery aneurysm (Fig. 1.95). Both conditions are rather rare. In children, aneurysms of the coronary artery most often occur with the mucocutaneous lymph node syndrome (8, 13) or periarteritis nodosa (11). More recently, postoperative pulmonary artery conduits also have been seen to produce bulges here (20).

LOCATION 4: LOWER LEFT CARDIAC BORDER

Fullness or bulging in this location is due, almost always, to a cardiac abnormality and usually is caused by left or right ventricular hypertrophy. Hypertrophy of the right ventricle tends to produce a more discrete or nose-like bulging (i.e., coeur en sabot), and the former, a more generalized bulging or rounded fullness (Fig. 1.96A and B). The *coeur en sabot* configuration (boot-shaped heart), of course, is classic for tetralogy of Fallot, although it is not seen in all cases. Left ventricular hypertrophy is seen with lesions producing obstruction to the flow of blood from the left side of the heart (e.g., aortic stenosis, coarctation of the aorta). Rarely, bumps or fullness in this region can be caused by cardiac tumors or aneurysms (Fig. 1.96C).

It also should be noted that generalized bulging or prominence of the left cardiac border occurs with any form of cardiomegaly, and is not limited to right or left ventricular hypertrophy. However, in these cases, generalized enlargement of the heart is present and prominence of the left cardiac border is less specific.

LOCATION 5: RIGHT CARDIAC BORDER

Localized bulging of the upper portion of the right cardiac border is uncommon, because isolated right atrial appendage enlargement, herniation of the right atrial appendage through a focal defect of the pericardium, and coronary artery aneurysms all are rare. Overall, then, it is bulging of the lower right cardiac border that is usually of concern, and the commonest cause of such bulging is enlargement of

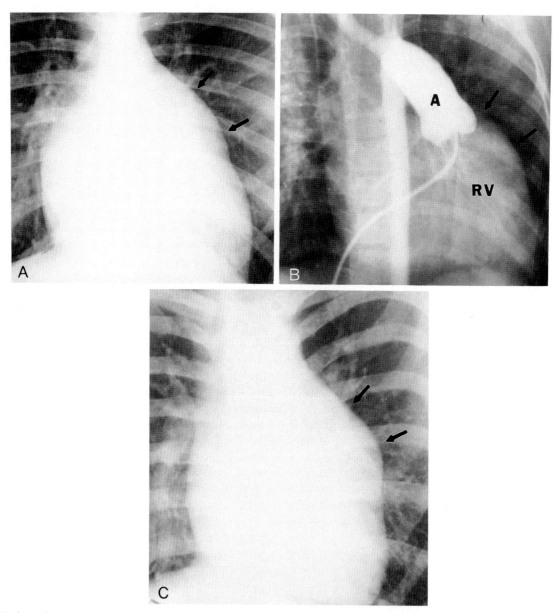

Figure 1.94. Location 3: upper left cardiac border—generalized fullness. A. Note fullness of the upper left cardiac border due to left atrial appendage enlargement *(arrows)* in rheumatic heart disease. **B.** Congenitally corrected transposition of the great vessels. Note position of the right ventricle *(RV)* and the aorta *(A)*. The aorta is inverted, and together the aorta and right ventricle produce fullness of the upper left cardiac border *(arrows)*. A similar bump can be seen in Ebstein's anomaly (see Fig. 1.97*A*). **C.** Note bulging of the upper left cardiac border due to the dilated patch used for correction of infundibular stenosis in tetralogy of Fallot.

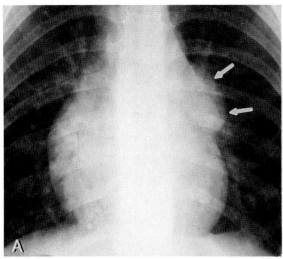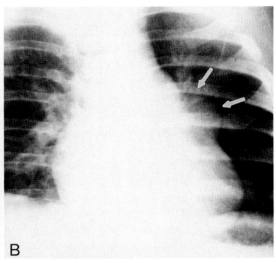

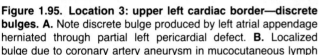

Figure 1.95. Location 3: upper left cardiac border—discrete bulges. A. Note discrete bulge produced by left atrial appendage herniated through partial left pericardial defect. **B.** Localized bulge due to coronary artery aneurysm in mucocutaneous lymph node syndrome. (From Cook A, L'Heureux P: Radiographic findings in the mucocutaneous lymph node syndrome. *AJR* 132:107–109, 1979.)

the right atrium (Fig. 1.97A). This can result from tricuspid insufficiency, tricuspid stenosis, tricuspid atresia, or from the delivery of extra volumes of blood to the right atrium. The latter problem occurs with atrial septal defect and anomalous pulmonary venous return (either total or partial) to the right atrium. Tricuspid valve stenosis or atresia usually is a part of the hypoplastic right heart syndrome. Tricuspid valve insufficiency, although occasionally occurring on an isolated basis, usually is seen with pulmonary valve atresia (type II, with relatively large right ventricle remaining), Ebstein's anomaly, Uhl's disease of the myocardium, and trilogy of Fallot. When massive, the right atrial curve extends high into the mediastinum (Fig. 1.97A).

The right atrium also is displaced to the right when the remainder of the heart enlarges, even though the atrium itself is not enlarged. This can occur even if it is the left side of the heart that enlarges, and an excellent example of this phenomenon is prominence of the right cardiac border caused by hypertrophy of the left ventricle in conditions such as aortic stenosis. Similar pseudoenlargement of the right atrium occurs with the cardiac malposition known as mesocardia. Mesocardia represents a milder degree of dextroversion of the heart (i.e., less rotation of the heart to the right), and the result is that the heart seems to sit exactly in midline. This causes the right atrial region to appear more prominent than usual (Fig. 1.97B). Rarely, right cardiac border prominence is due to a pericardial or cardiac tumor and, even more rarely, a cardiac aneurysm.

LOCATION 6: PARASPINAL LUMPS AND THICKENINGS

The only normal paraspinal stripe that is regularly visualized on an upright view in the pediatric age group is the one caused by the descending aorta on the left (Fig. 1.98A). This normal stripe can become more prominent with systemic hypertension or poststenotic dilation in coarctation of the aorta (Fig. 1.98B). When the aorta is right-sided and descends on the right, a similar but perhaps slightly more slanted stripe, occurs on the right. The presence of this stripe provides a significant clue to the presence of the right-side aortic arch (Fig. 1.98D). The next most common paraspinal stripe is the one caused by the accumulation of pleural fluid against the spine, usually on the left (Fig. 1.98C).

Other causes of diffuse paraspinal widening of the soft tissues are those that occur with underlying pathologic processes of the spine such as osteomyelitis (paraspinal abscess), fractures (hematoma), spinal and spinal cord tumors, paraspinal lymphoma or leukemia, and fibrotic pleural thickening (Fig. 1.98E). In many of these conditions, however, thickening is more localized than diffuse and, indeed, localized bumps or areas of thickening along the spine usually are accounted for by the presence of paraspinal accumulations of pus, fluid, blood (Fig. 1.98F), or tumor. In such cases, it is essential that one inspect the adjacent vertebral bodies and intervening disc spaces for clues to the proper diagnosis. This is best accomplished on lateral view, and when both

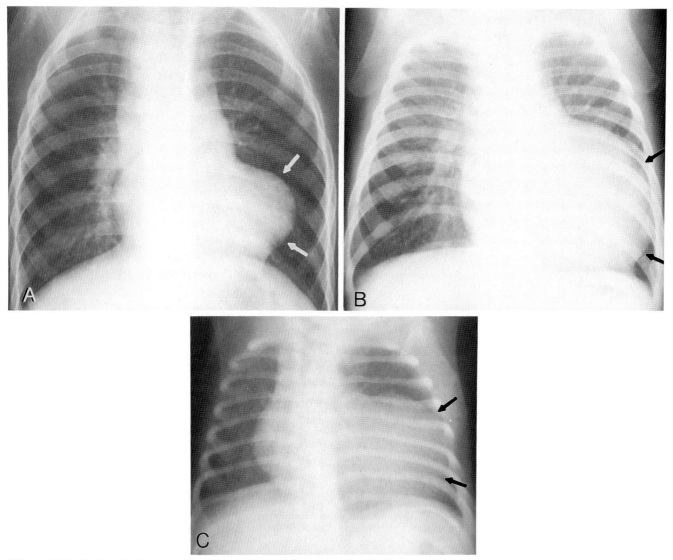

Figure 1.96. Mediastinal bumps: location 4—lower left cardiac border. A. Note typical coeur en sabot configuration of right ventricular hypertrophy *(arrows)* in tetralogy of Fallot. **B.** Profound roundness and generalized bulging of the left cardiac border *(arrows)* due to marked left ventricular hypertrophy. The patient had coarctation of the aorta. **C.** Very marked bulging of the left lower cardiac border *(arrows)* due to a cardiac tumor. (Part **C** courtesy of M. Wagner, M.D., and E. B. Singleton, M.D., Houston, Texas.)

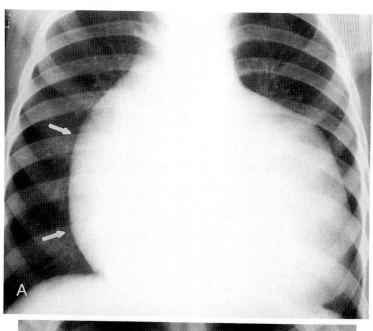

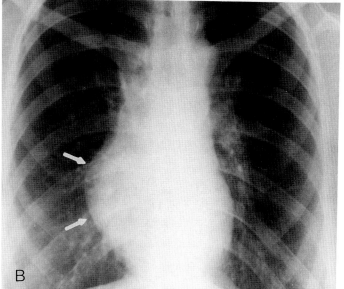

Figure 1.97. Mediastinal bumps: location 5—right cardiac border. A. Marked right atrial enlargement *(arrows)* in patient with tricuspid insufficiency secondary to Ebstein's anomaly of the tricuspid valve. Note how high the right atrial curve extends into the superior mediastinum. Also note the typical shoulder or bump along the upper left cardiac border (a location 3 bulge). The pulmonary vascularity is decreased and the pulmonary artery is small and concave. **B.** Apparent bulging of the right cardiac border *(arrows)* suggests right atrial enlargement, but is due, in fact, to partial cardiac rotation to the right (i.e., mesocardia).

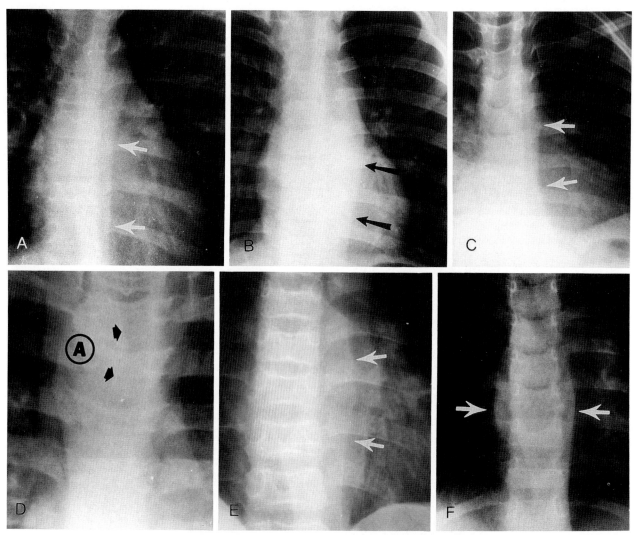

Figure 1.98. Paraspinal stripes and bumps: location 6. A. Note the normal left paraspinal stripe *(arrows)* produced by the normal descending aorta. **B.** Markedly dilated descending aorta *(arrows)* in patient with coarctation. **C.** Left paraspinal stripe *(arrows)* secondary to fluid accumulation in a patient with nephrotic syndrome. A subpulmonic pleural effusion also was present on the left, and an extensive pleural effusion was present on the right. **D.** Note the aorta *(A)* on the right producing deviation of the trachea *(arrows)*. The aorta descends on the right, causing the slanted paraspinal stripe just below the aortic knob. **E.** Paraspinal stripe *(arrows)* due to pleural thickening in a patient with sickle cell disease and repeated pneumonias with empyema. **F.** Bilateral localized paraspinal bulging *(arrows)* secondary to bleeding from a pathologic fracture of a vertebra involved with eosinophilic granuloma.

vertebrae and interventing disc are destroyed, osteo-myelitis is the most likely possibility. With other conditions, the disc spaces remain intact, but with most infections, except for some fungal infections, the disc space is narrowed.

Paraspinal hematomas most commonly are seen with thoracic spine injury, but accidental trauma to the thoracic spine is not particularly common in childhood. Indeed, more often than not, the problem is a pathologic compression fracture of the vertebral body(ies), occurring with conditions such as metastatic disease, histiocytosis-X (Fig. 1.98F), leukemia,

and lymphoma. Pathologic vertebral fractures also occur with the demineralized spine of rickets, steroid therapy, Cushing syndrome, osteogenesis imperfecta, and hyperparathyroidism.

Other causes of paraspinal bulging include primary bony tumors of the spine (somewhat rare in childhood) and neurogenic tumors such as neuroblastoma, ganglioneuroma, and neurofibroma. The latter is the least common of the three. Other less common causes of widening of the paraspinal stripe include extramedullary hematopoiesis, neurenteric cysts (usually associated with anterior vertebral body defects), aneurysms of the aorta, and dilated azygos or hemiazygous veins with obstruction of the superior vena cava after repair of transposition of the great vessels (19).

REFERENCES

1. Abrams HL: Vertebral and azygos venous systems, and some variations in systemic venous return. *Radiology* 69:508–526, 1975.
2. Amplatz K, Lester RG, Schiebler GL, Adams P Jr, Anderson RC: The roentgenologic features of Ebstein's anomaly of the tricuspid valve. *Am J Roentgenol Radium Ther Nucl Med* 81:788–794, 1959.
3. Anderson RC, Adams P Jr, Burke B: Anomalous inferior vena cava with azygos continuation (infrahepatic interruption of inferior vena cava): report of 15 cases. *J Pediatr* 59:370–383, 1961.
4. Berdon WE, Baker DH: Plain film findings in azygos continuation of the inferior vena cava. *Am J Roentgenol Radium Ther Nucl Med* 104:452–457, 1968.
5. Berdon WE, Baker DH, James LS: The ductus bump (a transient physiologic mass in chest roentgenograms of newborn infants). *AJR* 95:91–98, 1965.
6. Brodelius A, Johansson BW, Sievers J: Anomalous inferior vena cava with azygous and hemiazygous continuation. *Acta Paediatr Scand* 51:331–336, 1962.
7. Chang CV, Leigh TF: Congenital partial left pericardial defect associated with herniation of the left atrial appendage. *Am J Roentgenol Radium Ther Nucl Med* 86:517–520, 1961.
8. Cook A, L'Heureux P: Radiographic findings in the mucocutaneous lymph node syndrome. *AJR* 132:107–109, 1979.
9. Deutsch V, Wexler L, Blieden LC, Yahini JH, Neufeld HN: Ebstein's anomaly of tricuspid valve: critical review of roentgenological features and additional angiography signs. *AJR* 125:395–411, 1975.
10. Elliott LP, Hartmann AF Jr: The right ventricular infundibulum in Ebstein's anomaly of the tricuspid valve. *Radiology* 89:694–700, 1967.
11. Glanz S, Bittner SJ, Berman MA, Dolan TF Jr, Talner NS: Regression of coronary-artery aneurysms in infantile polyarteritis nodosa. *N Engl J Med* 249:939–941, 1976.
12. Heikkinen ES, Similä S: Aneurysm of ductus arteriosus in infancy: report of two surgically treated cases. *J Pediatr Surg* 7:392–397, 1972.
13. Kato H, Koike S, Yamamoto M, Ito Y, Yano E: Coronary aneurysms in infants and young children with acute febrile mucocutaneous lymph node syndrome. *J Pediatr* 86:892–898, 1975.
14. Kirks DR, McCook TA, Serwer GA, Oldham, NH Jr: Aneurysm of the ductus arteriosus in the neonate. *AJR* 134:573–576, 1980.
15. Klatte EC, Burko H: The roentgen diagnosis of patent ductus arteriosus. *Semin Roentgenol* 1:87–101, 1966.
16. Möes CAF, Fowler RS, Trusler CA: Total anomalous pulmonary venous drainage into the azygos vein. *AJR* 98:378–387, 1966.
17. Nogrady MB, Nemec J: Partial congenital pericardial defect in childhood: report of four cases. *J Can Assoc Radiol* 21:116–119, 1970.
18. Petersen RW: Infrahepatic interruption of inferior vena cava with azygos continuation (persistent right cardinal vein). *Radiology* 84:304–307, 1965.
19. Polansky SM, Culham JAG: Paraspinal densities developing after repair of transposition of the great arteries. *AJR* 134:394–396, 1980.
20. Swischuk LE, Alexander A, Hayden CK Jr, Sapire DW: Postoperative lumps and bumps in congenital heart disease: their significance. *Perspect Radiol* 3:45–52, 1990.
21. Tabakin BS, Hanson JS, Tampas JP, Caldwell EJ: Congenital absence of left pericardium. *Am J Roentgenol Radium Ther Nucl Med* 94:122–128, 1965.

Miscellaneous Mediastinal Abnormalities

MEDIASTINAL SHIFT

The commonest cause of mediastinal shift is volume loss or gain on one or the other of the lungs. This problem has been discussed earlier (see Aeration Disturbances), but, basically, with volume loss the mediastinum shifts towards the involved lung, while with volume gain it shifts away from the involved lung. The commonest cause of volume loss is atelectasis, and the commonest cause of volume gain is obstructive emphysema. However, volume gain also can be seen with large pleural fluid collections and large unilateral chest masses, and volume loss can be associated with unilateral pulmonary hypoplasia or agenesis (Table 1.23).

Other causes of mediastinal shift, without evidence of primary lung size discrepancy, include pectus excavatum and absence of the left pericardium (1, 2). The latter condition is rare but, when seen, tends to be associated with prominence of the aorta and pulmonary artery. Pectus excavatum is much more common than absence of the left pericardium and, radiographically, the findings are rather characteristic. In addition to shift of the mediastinal structures to the left, findings include increased prominence of the vascular markings of the right lung, especially those adjacent to the spine, a more

Table 1.23
Mediastinal Shift

Unilateral atelectasis Unilateral obstructive emphysema Unilateral pleural fluid	Common
Unilateral mediastinal mass Unilateral pulmonary hypoplasia Pectus excavatum	Uncommon
Absence of pericardium (unilateral) Agenesis of one lung	Rare

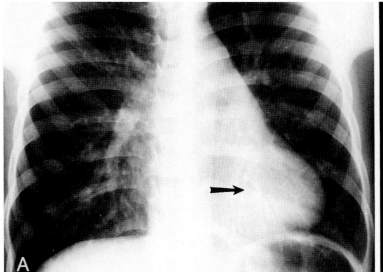

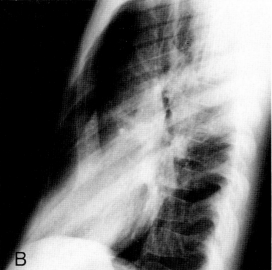

Figure 1.99. Mediastinal shift. A. Pectus excavatum. Note typical shift of the mediastinal structures to the left *(arrow)*, accentuation of the right lung vascularity, nonvisible cardiac silhouette to the right of the spine, horizontally oriented posterior ribs, and deeply slanting anterior ribs. **B.** Lateral view showing degree of pectus excavatum deformity. Similar shift can be seen with absence of the pericardium, but on lateral view the "depressed sternum" deformity, of course, is not present.

horizontal posture of the posterior ribs, and deeply slanted anterior ribs (Fig. 1.99).

RETROCARDIAC OPACITIES

Most commonly retrocardiac opacities are seen on the left, primarily because there is more heart on the left. The commonest causes of the finding are pneumonia or atelectasis and, depending on the extent of the problem, the opacity can be focal or diffuse, and can even involve the entire cardiac silhouette (Fig. 1.100A and B). When left lower lobe collapse is the problem, the edge of the collapsed lung frequently can be seen through the cardiac silhouette (Fig. 1.100C).

Other causes of increased opacity behind the heart include hiatus hernia (usually on the left), pulmonary sequestration (on either side, but more commonly on the left), pleural fluid (usually on the left), and other posterior mediastinal masses (either side). With sequestration, one may see vessels supplying and/or draining the lesion (Fig. 1.100D). Very rarely, pleural fluid accumulations or masses anterior to the heart can produce increased density of the cardiac silhouette.

REFERENCES

1. Dimich I, Grossman H, Bowman FD Jr, Griffith SP: Congenital absence of the left pericardium. *Am J Dis Child* 110:309–314, 1965.

2. Tabakin BS, Hanson JS, Tampas JP, Caldwell EJ: Congenital absence of the left pericardium. *Am J Roentgenol Radium Ther Nucl Med* 94:122–128, 1965.

Lung Masses

For the most part, this section deals with true intrapulmonary masses and, in childhood, they are not particularly common (Table 1.24). Actually, the most common mass is a pseudomass due to consolidating pneumonia (8). In these cases, the consolidation is caught just at the stage where it mimics a mass (Fig. 1.101A). The next most common cause of a pulmonary mass is a solid pulmonary abscess and then, less commonly, one can encounter a number of acquired or congenital pulmonary cysts. Cysts tend to have a sharp edge to their outer circumference, while abscesses are more apt to have indistinct mar-

Table 1.24
Lung Masses

Pneumonia pseudomass Pulmonary abscess Cysts (acquired or congenital)	Common
Loculated pleural fluid Pulmonary neoplasm Postinflammatory pseudotumor	Uncommon

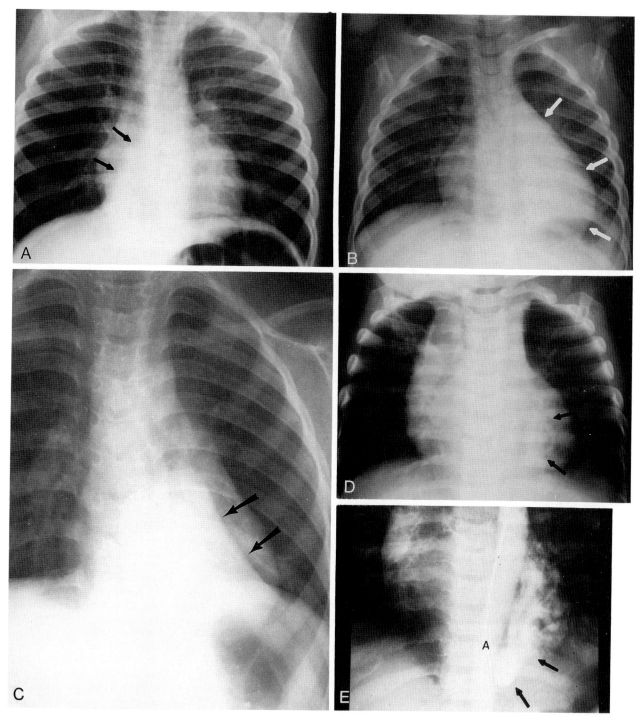

Figure 1.100. Retrocardiac opacities. A. Note the irregular opacity behind the right side of the heart *(arrows),* due to an early consolidating pneumonia. **B.** Generalized increased opacity of the entire left side of the heart (compare to normal radiolucency of right side), due to an extensive consolidating pneumonia, completely hidden by the heart. **C.** Typical configuration of left lower lobe atelectasis, producing a triangle of increased opacity behind the left side of the heart *(arrows).* **D.** Note irregular opacity behind the left side of the heart *(arrows).* Draining or supplying vessels also appear to be present, which suggests a sequestration. **E.** Aortogram in the same patient demonstrating the aorta *(A)* and the systemic vessels *(arrows)* to the sequestration.

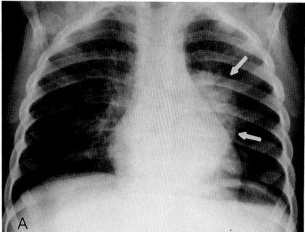 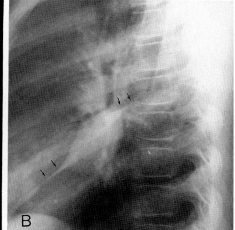

Figure 1.101. Pulmonary pseudomasses. A. Apparent mass *(arrows)* due to consolidating pneumonia. **B.** Interlobar pleural ef- fusion producing pulmonary mass. Note the characteristic taper- ing edges *(arrows)*.

gins. Of course, when a lung cyst becomes infected, it may look just like an abscess.

Primary pulmonary tumors are rare in infants and children, but probably the best known of these tumors is pulmonary blastoma. Pulmonary blastoma is thought by some to arise from primitive pulmonary blastema and contains both mesenchymal and epithelial components. This tumor can vary in appearance from a small peripheral nodule to a large mass that can occupy almost the entire hemithorax. In some cases, pulmonary blastoma can arise in preexisting cystic lung disease (2). Other rare primary lung malignancies include sarcomas (e.g., leiomyosarcoma, rhabdomyosarcoma), primitive neuroectodermal tumor (Askin tumor), and squamous cell carcinoma (sometimes associated with disseminated tracheobronchial juvenile papillomatosis). Solitary metastases can occur in the lungs and are probably more common than any of the primary pulmonary malignant tumors. Benign primary lung neoplasms include pulmonary choristoma (13), congenital mesenchymoma, hemangioma, hamartoma, teratoma (7), and plasma cell granuloma (6).

Rounding out the causes of intrapulmonary mass are loculated pleural effusions and postinflammatory pseudotumors. Postinflammatory pseudotumors result from previously consolidating infections (9), but generally are uncommon in the pediatric age group. However, they can occur with atypical measles pneumonia (4, 5, 14, 15) and occasionally with other pneumonias. Loculated pleural effusions can be quite large, but in most cases they are somewhat oblong or oval in configuration. In addition, their usually tapering, spindle-shaped ends attest to their interlobar fissure location (Fig. 1.101*B*). Because they tend to resolve spontaneously, they often are referred to as "vanishing tumors."

REFERENCES

1. Hartman GE, Schochat SJ: Primary pulmonary neoplasms of childhood: a review. *Ann Thorac Surg* 36:108–119, 1983.
2. Hedlung GL, Bisset GS III, Bove KE: Malignant neoplasms arising in cystic hamartomas of the lung in childhood. *Radiology* 173:77–70, 1989.
3. Kovanlikaya A, Pirnar T, Olqun N: Pulmonary blastoma: a rare case of childhood malignancy. *Pediatr Radiol* 22:155, 1992.
4. Margolin FR, Gandy TK: Pneumonia of atypical measles. *Radiology* 131:653–655, 1979.
5. Mitnick J, Becker MH, Rothberg M, Genieser NB: Nodular residua of atypical measles pneumonia. *AJR* 134:257–260, 1980.
6. Monzon CM, Gilchrist GS, Burgert EM Jr, O'Connell EJ, Telander RL, Hoffman AD, Li C-Y: Plasma cell granuloma of the lung in children. *Pediatrics* 70:268–274. 1982.
7. Morgan DE, Sanders C, McElvein RB, Nath H, Alexander Cb: Intrapulmonary teratoma: a case report and review of the literature. *J Thorac Imag* 7:70-77, 1992.
8. Rose RW, Ward BH: Spherical pneumonias in children simulating pulmonary and mediastinal masses. *Radiology* 106:179–182, 1973.
9. Schwartz EE, Katz SM, Mandell GA: Post-inflammatory pseudotumors of the lung: fibrous histiocytoma and related lesions. *Radiology* 136:609–613, 1980.
10. Senac MO Jr, Wood BP, Isaacs H, Weller M: Pulmonary blastoma: a rare childhood malignancy. *Radiology* 179:743–746, 1991.
11. Soloman A, Rubinstein ZJ, Rogoff M, Rozenman J, Urbach D: Pulmonary blastoma. *Pediatr Radiol* 12:148–149, 1992.
12. Sumner TE, Phelps CR II, Crowe JE, Poolos SP, Shaffner LD: Pulmonary blastoma in a child. *AJR* 133:147–148, 1979.

13. Wat K, Toomey F, Wat BY, Reiber N: Pulmonary choristoma in a neonate. *AJR* 139:377–379, 1982.
14. Wood BP, Bernstein RM: Pulmonary nodular "pneumonia" during the acute atypical measles illness. *Ann Radiol* 21:193–198, 1978.
15. Young LW, Smith DI, Glasgow LA: Pneumonia of atypical measles, residual nodular lesions. *Am J Roentgenol Radium Ther Nucl Med* 110:439–448, 1970.

Diaphragmatic Leaflet Position and Contour Abnormalities

Normally, the right diaphragmatic leaflet is a little higher than the left. Occasionally, the left can be elevated because of an underlying distended stomach or splenic flexure, but generally the right remains higher than the left. In addition, it should be noted that normally the diaphragmatic leaflets have a sharp outline, and if the outline becomes indistinct, an adjacent infiltrate or area of atelectasis should be suspected. The insertion of the normal major fissures can cause similar obliteration, but usually the cause is pneumonia or atelectasis. Position and contour abnormalities of the diaphragmatic leaflets are best considered on a unilateral or bilateral basis (Table 1.25).

UNILATERALLY ELEVATED DIAPHRAGMATIC LEAFLET

The commonest causes of a unilaterally elevated diaphragmatic leaflet are atelectasis of the ipsilateral lung or splinting of the diaphragmatic leaflet secondary to pneumonia, rib injury, or subdiaphragmatic injuries and inflammations. On the left, a distended stomach or splenic flexure also are common causes of an elevated diaphragmatic leaflet, but on the right, since the liver lies directly beneath the diaphragm, such causes are uncommon.

Other moderately common causes of unilateral elevation of a diaphragmatic leaflet are phrenic nerve palsy, eventration, an underlying abdominal mass or abscess, and subpulmonic pleural effusion. With subpulmonic effusions, the diaphragmatic leaflet often, but not always, appears somewhat flat medially and squared off laterally (Fig. 1.102*A* and *B*). On lateral view, in these cases, one usually can see a fluid meniscus in the posterior costophrenic angle, and decubitus views clearly demonstrate the presence of such fluid. Subpulmonic effusions occur most commonly with the nephrotic syndrome, acute glomerulonephritis, and intrathoracic or intraabdominal lymphoma. Relatively rare causes of a unilaterally

Table 1.25
Diaphragmatic Leaflet Position Abnormalities

Unilateral elevated	
Atelectasis Splinting Distended stomach or splenic flexure (L)	Common
Phrenic paralysis Eventration Abdominal mass Abdominal abscess	Moderately common
Diaphragmatic hernia (common in neonate) Diaphragmatic tumor Agenesis or hypoplasia of lung	Rare
Unilateral flattened	
Empyema or other fluid Obstructive emphysema	Common
Tension pneumothorax	Moderately common
Bilateral elevated	
Poor inspiration	Common
Ascites Peritonitis Hemoperitoneum Abdominal mass Neuromuscular disease	Moderately common
Bilateral eventration Laryngotracheal foreign body	Rare
Agenesis (newborn)	Very rare
Bilateral depressed	
Asthma Viral infection (bronchiolitis)	Common
Cystic fibrosis Overaeration with acidosis	Moderately common
Air hunger Bilateral tension pneumothorax Bilateral pleural fluid Other obstructive emphysema	Rare
Localized bulging	
Diaphragmatic hernia Eventration	Common

elevated diaphragmatic leaflet include congenital or acquired (posttraumatic) diaphragmatic hernia (except in the neonate where the congenital form is common), diaphragmatic tumor, hypoplasia or aplasia of the diaphragm, and hypoplastic lung. In this latter condition, the diaphragmatic leaflet is ele-

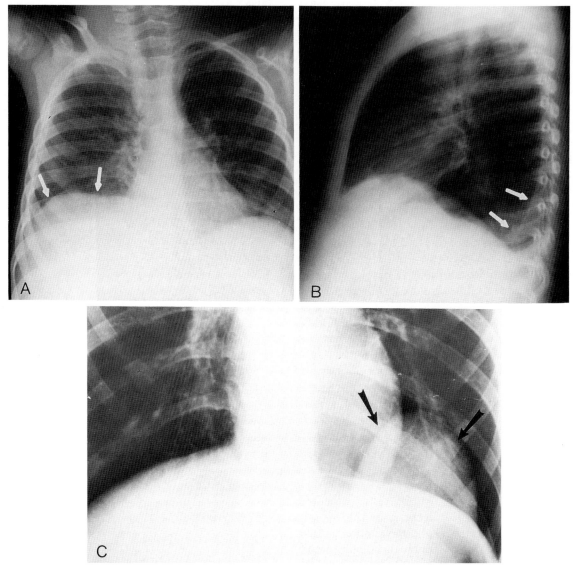

Figure 1.102. Elevated diaphragmatic leaflets. A. Subpulmonic effusion. Note characteristic squared-off and somewhat flat appearance of the apparently elevated right diaphragmatic leaflet. This is characteristic of a subpulmonic pleural effusion. A subpulmonic effusion also is present on the left, but the apparently elevated diaphragmatic leaflet appears nearly normal in configuration. Note, however, that there is a paraspinal collection of fluid (i.e., left paraspinal stripe). **B.** Lateral view in the same patient demonstrating typical posterior menisci of pleural fluid *(arrows)*. This patient had nephrotic syndrome. **C. Diaphragmatic leaflet bump.** This bump *(arrows)* was due to a kidney projecting through a congenital posterior diaphragmatic opening.

vated because of loss of volume of the hypoplastic lung.

UNILATERALLY DEPRESSED DIAPHRAGMATIC LEAFLET

A diaphragmatic leaflet becomes depressed because of a space-occupying problem in the ipsilateral hemithorax. For this reason, it almost always is a secondary finding, and can be seen with conditions such as unilateral obstructive emphysema, tension pneumothorax, and massive pleural fluid accumula-

tions. With fluid or air (pneumothorax) accumulations, if the volume is massive, the diaphragmatic leaflet not only is depressed, but also is inverted.

BILATERALLY ELEVATED DIAPHRAGMATIC LEAFLETS

Undoubtedly the commonest cause of bilaterally elevated diaphragmatic leaflets is simple underaeration of the chest secondary to a poor inspiratory effort. Thereafter, one should consider intraabdominal space-occupying problems such as ascites, peritonitis, and large abdominal masses as causes of elevation of the diaphragmatic leaflets. Other conditions to be considered include diaphragmatic weakness with neuromuscular disease, bilateral eventration, or the very rare, diaphragmatic agenesis (a neonatal problem). Another uncommon cause of bilaterally elevated leaflets is a central tracheal or laryngeal obstructing foreign body. These foreign bodies usually are located at or below the level of the larynx, but above the carina. Because they produce inspiratory obstruction, the lungs never are fully inflated, and the diaphragmatic leaflets constantly are higher in position than normal. However, it requires an astute observer and one who has knowledge of the problem to appreciate the finding.

BILATERALLY DEPRESSED DIAPHRAGMATIC LEAFLETS

As with the unilaterally depressed diaphragmatic leaflet, some intrathoracic space-occupying problem must exist to produce this phenomenon. Most commonly, this occurs with obstructive emphysema as seen with asthma and viral lower respiratory tract infections (especially bronchiolitis in the infant). However, it is also seen with other causes of obstructive emphysema, and these include cystic fibrosis, α-1 antitrypsin deficiency, congenital cutis laxa, central or bilateral foreign bodies, vascular rings and anomalies, intratracheal lesions, and paratracheal masses and cysts.

Overaeration of the lungs with bilateral leaflet depression also is commonly seen with acidosis and dehydration. In these patients, in an attempt to blow off CO_2 the lungs become hyperinflated and the leaflets become depressed. The findings can mimic obstructive emphysema, for, at the same time, dehydration leads to loss of fluid, hypovolemia, and diminished pulmonary vascularity. Air hunger, as seen with severe cyanotic congenital heart disease and even noncyanotic heart disease, can lead to similar overaeration of the lungs. Bilateral pleural effusions or pneumothoraces that are large enough to produce bilateral diaphragmatic leaflet depression are not particularly common, but can occur. The cause for diaphragmatic depression, in these cases, is obvious.

LOCALIZED BULGES ON DIAPHRAGMATIC LEAFLETS

The commonest discrete bulge of a diaphragmatic leaflet is caused by a focal diaphragmatic hernia with some organ protruding through the defect (Fig. 1.102C). Posteriorly, the organ is usually the kidney,

while anteriorly the spleen, liver, or omentum may be involved. In any of these cases, the bulge is located toward midline. Small eventrations also can produce somewhat localized bulging, but other than these two conditions, localized bulging of the diaphragmatic leaflets is uncommon in children. Certainly, diaphragmatic or pleural tumors in this area are rare.

Mediastinal Masses: Diagnostic Approaches

In considering mediastinal masses, it is customary to consider them as occurring in the anterior, middle, and posterior mediastinal compartments (Table 1.26). In the **anterior compartment,** the most com-

Table 1.26
Mediastinal Masses

Anterior		
Normal thymus (infants)	}	Common
Lymphoma	}	Relatively
Teratoma		common
Cystic hygroma	}	
Hemangioma		
Germ cell tumor		
Enlarged thyroid (goiter, tumor)		Uncommon
Vascular anomaly, aneurysm		
Morgagni hernia		
Thymoma	}	
Thymic cyst		Rare
Histiocytosis-X		
Middle		
Lymphoma, leukemia	}	
Lymphadenopathy (inflammatory)		Common
Lymphadenopathy (metastatic)	}	
Enlarged vessels		Uncommon
Duplication cyst		
Hiatus hernia		
Pericardial cyst/tumor	}	Rare
Cardiac tumor/aneurysm		
Posterior		
Neuroblastoma/ganglioneuroma	}	Common
Pulmonary sequestration	}	Moderately
Bochdalek hernia		common
Neurofibroma	}	
Neuroenteric cyst		
Anterior/lateral meningocele		Rare
Teratoma, sarcoma		
Extramedullary hematopoesis		
Spinal tumor/infection/fracture		

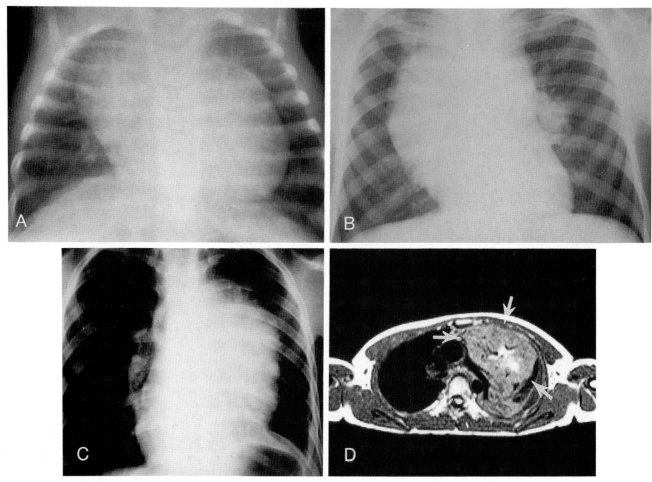

Figure 1.103. Anterior mediastinal masses. A. A large normal thymus gland in an infant. Note that the trachea is in a normal position. **B.** An abnormally enlarged thymus gland in an older child with **Hodgkin's lymphoma. C.** A large **germ cell tumor** was the cause of this anterior mediastinal mass. **D.** MRI of the patient in part **C** shows the large, heterogenous mass in the anterior mediastinum *(arrows)*.

mon mass is the normal thymus gland, and one of its distinguishing features is that it does not displace the trachea (Fig. 1.103A). Only when the gland is unusually high in position or if it is associated with a thymic cyst does displacement occur. Thymic tumors are quite rare, but other masses occurring in the anterior mediastinum include thyroid tumors, goiter, thyroiditis, teratoma (often with calcification and usually in infants), cystic hygroma (usually extending from neck), hemangioma, Langerhans cell histiocytosis (4) and lymphoma. Actually, lymphomatous involvement of the anterior mediastinum is quite common in children (3) and represents an extension of the same process originating in the middle mediastinum. Such mass formation can take the form of lymph node enlargement or infiltration of the thymus gland by the lymphoma (Fig. 1.103B), and a similar phenomenon can occur with leukemia. MRI

is an excellent modality for evaluating the thymus gland and other anterior mediastinal masses (6) (Fig. 1.103C and D), but CT and ultrasound have also been used. Mediastinal cysts are rare in the anterior mediastinum. Another relatively uncommon anterior superior mediastinal mass is the one caused by the dilated, inverted U-shaped vessel, the "snowman" or "figure 8" heart configuration in type I total anomalous pulmonary venous return (see Fig. 1.90C and D). Finally, it might be noted that destructive or tumoral lesions of the sternum can result in retrosternal masses projecting into the superior mediastinum.

Inferiorly, in the anterior mediastinum, one can encounter diaphragmatic hernias, and occasionally these can extend into the pericardial sac. Those located just to either side of midline are termed Morgagni hernias.

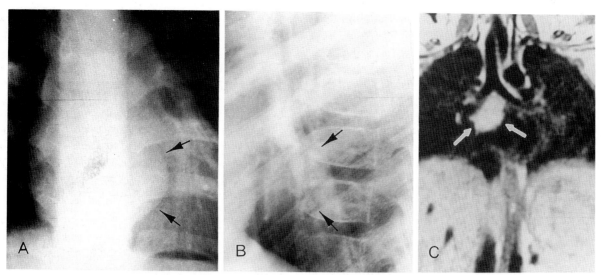

Figure 1.104. Middle mediastinal mass. A. Spherical retrocardiac mass *(arrows)* due to an **esophageal duplication cyst. B.** Lateral view shows the retrocardiac (middle mediastinum) position of the mass *(arrows).* **C. Bronchogenic cyst** in a typical subcarinal location *(arrows).* Note the high signal intensity on the T$_1$-weighted MRI image due to the proteinaceous fluid within the cyst.

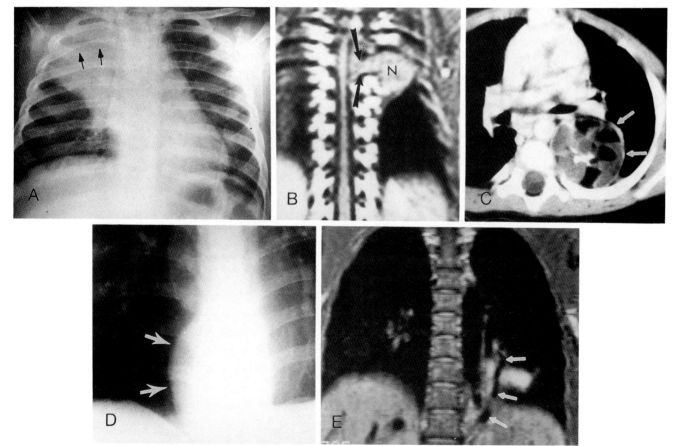

Figure 1.105. Posterior mediastinal masses. A. Posterior mediastinal mass due to **neuroblastoma.** The presence of rib erosion *(arrows)* indicates the posterior mediastinal location of this mass. **B.** Another child with a left posterior mediastinal neuroblastoma *(N)* that extends into the spinal canal *(arrows).* **C.** CT of an unusual teratoma of the posterior mediastinum *(arrows).* (Courtesy of C. Keith Hayden, Jr., M.D.) **D.** Nonspecific retrocardiac mass *(arrows)* that on barium swallow was found to be a **hiatus hernia.** More often, hiatus hernias are central or left-sided. **E.** MRI of a **pulmonary sequestration.** Note the bright signal of the sequestered lung tissue and the abnormal supplying vessel extending from the aorta *(arrows).*

In the **middle mediastinum,** the commonest mass is that associated with lymphoma or leukemia and, as noted in the preceding paragraph, these masses frequently extend into the anterior mediastinum. Duplication cysts of the esophagus also occur in this compartment (Fig. 1.04A and B) and can be seen anywhere along the course of the esophagus. Bronchogenic cysts, on the other hand, tend to occur in the upper middle compartment, very often, just around the carina (Fig. 1.104C). Enlarged vessels such as the superior vena cava, aorta, or pulmonary artery also can produce middle mediastinal masses. Lymphadenopathy is a relatively common cause of a middle mediastinal mass and can be either inflammatory or neoplastic (usually leukemia or lymphoma) in nature.

In the **posterior mediastinal compartment,** one is dealing primarily with neurogenic tumors and cysts, and very often associated erosive changes in the vertebrae and ribs provide clues to the proper diagnosis (Fig. 1.105A). In this regard, most often one is dealing with a neuroblastoma or ganglioneuroma (1), for these tumors can produce adjacent rib erosion, and even involve the spinal canal in "dumbbell" fashion (Fig. 1.105B). In such cases, pedicular widening, posterior vertebral body scalloping, and sometimes calcification of the tumor can be seen. Neurofibromas, occurring alone or as part of generalized neurofibromatosis, are rather uncommon in children but, except for the absence of calcifications, produce changes similar to those described for neuroblastoma and ganglioneuroma. Neurenteric cysts and lateral or anterior meningoceles also are rare, but, when seen, are associated with anterior vertebral body defects and abnormal spinal curvatures. Other primary tumors (e.g., teratoma, sarcoma) are quite uncommon in the posterior mediastinum (Fig. 1.105C).

In the **lower portion of the posterior mediastinum,** one can encounter foramen of Bochdalek hernias, enteric cysts, hiatus hernias (Fig. 1.105), pancreatic pseudocyst extensions into the chest, extramedullary hematopoiesis (due to hereditary anemias such as thalassemia or hereditary spherocytosis), and pulmonary sequestrations. In the neonate, Bochdalek hernias are most common, but in the older child pulmonary sequestration and hiatus hernia are the most common. For the diagnosis of a suspected pulmonary sequestration, ultrasound and CT have been used, but MRI or angiography is best suited for demonstrating the abnormal vessels supplying the sequestration (Fig. 1.105E).

In addition to these problems, one may see a posterior mediastinal mass arising as part of, or secondary to, infection, trauma, or neoplasm of the spine or spinal cord.

REFERENCES

1. Adams GA, Schochat SJ, Smith EI, Shuster JJ, Joshi VV, Altshuler G, Hayes FA, Nitschke R, McWilliams N, Castleberry RP: Thoracic neuroblastoma: a pediatric oncology group study. *J Pediatr Surg* 28:372–378, 1993.
2. Han BK, Babcock DS, Oestreich AE: Normal thymus in infancy: sonographic characteristics. *Radiology* 170:471–474, 1989.
3. King RM, Telander RL, Smithson WA, Banks PM, Han MT: Primary mediastinal tumors in children. *J Pediatr Surg* 17:512–520, 1982.
4. Odagiri K, Nishihira K, Hatekeyama S, Kobayashi K: Anterior mediastinal masses with calcifications on CT in children with histiocytosis-X (Langerhans cell histiocytosis): report of two cases. *Pediatr Radiol* 21:550, 1991.
5. Oliphant L, McFadden RG, Carr TJ, Mackenzie DA: Magnetic resonance imaging to diagnose intralobar pulmonary sequestration. *Chest* 91:500–502, 1987.
6. Siegel MJ, Glazer HS, Wiener JI, Molina PL: Normal and abnormal thymus in childhood: MR imaging. *Radiology* 172:367–371, 1989.
7. Wernecke K, Vassallo P, Rutsch F, Peters PE, Potter R: Thymic involvement in Hodgkin's disease: CT and sonographic findings. *Radiology* 181:375–383, 1991.

CHAPTER

2

FACE, SINUSES, MASTOIDS, AND NECK

Neck-Upper Airway

TONGUE SIZE ABNORMALITIES

Determination of the size of the tongue, radiographically, is not always practical, but in certain conditions, tongue size changes are an important point in diagnosis (Table 2.1). A small tongue is rare and usually accompanies underdevelopment of the mandible. Enlargement of the tongue is more common and most often occurs with hypothyroidism. Less often, it is seen in trisomy-21 and rare conditions such as the Beckwith-Wiedemann syndrome (2, 5), a variety of developmental cysts of the tongue (4), and tumors such as hemangiomas, lymphangiomas, rhabdomyomas, and rhabdomyosarcomas (3, 6), and aggressive fibromatosis (1).

REFERENCES

1. Chen PC, Ball WS Jr, Towbin RB: Aggressive fibromatosis of the tongue: MR demonstration. *J Comput Assist Tomogr* 13:343–345, 1989.
2. Filippi G, McKusick VA: Beckwith-Wiedemann syndrome: exomphalos-macroglossia: report of two cases and review of literature. *Medicine* 49:279–298, 1970.
3. Liebert PS, Stool SE: Rhabdomyosarcoma of the tongue in an infant: results of combined radiation and chemotherapy. *Ann Surg* 178:621, 1973.
4. Lister J, Zachary RB: Cystic duplications in the tongue. *J Pediatr Surg* 3:491–493, 1968.
5. McNamara TO, Gooding CE, Kaplan SL, Clark RE: Exomphalos-macroglossia-gigantism (visceromegaly) syndrome: the Beckwith-Wiedemann syndrome. *AJR* 114:264–267, 1972.

Table 2.1
Abnormalities of Tongue Size

Large tongue		
Hypothyroidism	}	Common
Trisomy-21		
Beckwith-Wiedemann syndrome	}	Uncommon
Tumor	}	Rare
Cyst		
Small tongue		
Aglossia	}	Rare
Hypoglossia		

6. Solomon MP, Tolete-Velcek F: Lingual rhabdomyoma (adult variant) in a child. *J Pediatr Surg* 14:91–94, 1979.

NASOPHARYNGEAL SOFT TISSUES

During childhood, the soft tissues of the posterior nasopharynx are prominent due to normal adenoidal lymphoid hypertrophy (Fig. 2.1). However, before the age of 3 months, adenoidal tissue is sparse and not visible radiographically (3). After 3 months of age, the adenoids become progressively thicker, and $1/2$ to 1 inch thicknesses of tissue in this region are not unusual in normal children and adolescents. In infants and young children, normal adenoidal hypertrophy can produce airway obstruction. In older children, airway obstruction often is less pronounced, but adenoid enlargement can be a cause of mouth breathing or snoring. The underlying cause of adenoidal hypertrophy usually is repeated respiratory

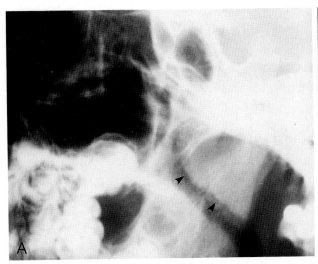
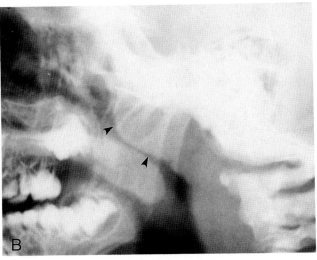

Figure 2.1. Normal adenoids and retropharyngeal lymphoid tissue. A. Note abundant adenoidal tissue in the nasopharynx *(arrows)*. Also note the normal air gap between the anterior surface of the adenoidal mass and the posterior wall of the maxillary sinuses. **B.** Another patient demonstrating adenoidal and retropharyngeal lymphoid tissue enlargement *(arrows)* erroneously suggesting a pathologic retropharyngeal mass. The soft palate is a little enlarged in this patient because of associated pharyngitis.

tract infection in a patient with an inherant tendency to produce an overabundance of lymphoid tissue.

A less common cause of increased thickness of the nasopharyngeal soft tissues is juvenile angiofibroma (5, 7). This tumor usually occurs in adolescent boys who are first seen with epistaxis and/or sinusitis. Lateral radiographs of the airway reveal a soft tissue mass that fills the nasopharynx, obliterating the air gap that normally exists between the anterior surface of the adenoids and the pterygomaxillary plate (6) (Fig. 2.2A). Such massive enlargement of the nasopharyngeal soft tissues is uncommon with adenoidal hypertrophy. CT reveals a markedly enhancing mass that expands the pterygopalatine fossa (Fig. 2.2B), and angiography demonstrates the hypervascularity of the mass (Fig. 2.2C). Angiomatous polyps can also occur in this region; however, such masses are usually smaller and do not demonstrate the intense enhancement that is seen with the angiofibroma.

Rhabdomyosarcoma is the most common primary malignant tumor of the nasopharynx (4). Rounding out the list of causes of nasopharyngeal masses are lymphoma (Fig. 2.2D), lymphoepithelioma (2), and a smattering of tumors such as neurofibroma, neuroblastoma, teratoma (1), cystic hygroma, chordoma of the clivus (9), hairy polyp (8) and basal encephalocele (Table 2.2).

As has been noted earlier, decreased thickness of the nasopharyngeal soft tissues is normal in infants less than 3 months of age, but when lymphoid tissue is absent in older children one should consider surgical removal of the adenoids or underdevelopment with immunologic deficiency states such as hypogammaglobulinemia and the ataxia telangiectasia syndrome (10).

Table 2.2
Nasopharyngeal Soft Tissues

Increased thickness	
Normal or hypertrophied adenoids ⎫ Infection ⎬	Common
Nasal polyp ⎫ Nasopharyngeal tumors ⎬ Nasolacrimal duct mucocele ⎭	Uncommon
Basal encephalocele ⎫ Base of skull tumors ⎬	Rare
Decreased thickness	
Small, normal (< 3 months)	Common
Surgical removal	Moderately common
Hypo- or agammaglobulinemia ⎫ Ataxia telangiectasia syndrome ⎬	Uncommon

REFERENCES

1. Alter AD, Cove JK: Congenital nasopharyngeal teratoma: report of a case and review of the literature. *J Pediatr Surg* 22:179–181. 1987.
2. Bass IS, Haller JO, Berdon WE, Barlow B, Carsen G, Khakoo Y: Nasopharyngeal carcinoma: clinical and radiographic findings in children. *Radiology* 156:651–654. 1985.
3. Capitanio MA, Kirkpatrick JA: Nasopharyngeal lym-

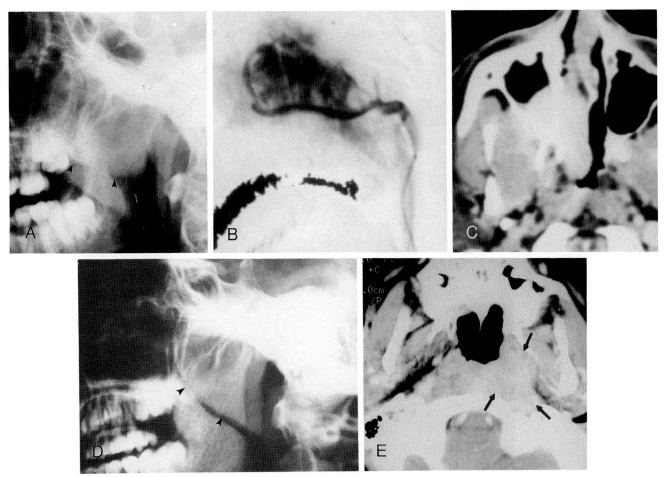

Figure 2.2. Nasopharyngeal masses. A. Juvenile angiofibroma. Note the mass *(arrows)* filling the nasopharynx. Also note that there is no air gap in front of the mass (compare with normal adenoidal enlargement in Figure 2.1*A*). **B.** Angiogram demonstrating vascularity typical of a juvenile angiofibroma *(arrows)*. **C.** Contrast-enhanced CT demonstrates an enhancing mass in the right nasopharynx extending into the maxillary sinus.

D. Enlargement of the adenoidal tissue mass secondary to lymphoma *(arrows)*. Again, note that the anterior air gap has been obliterated. Such obliteration occurs with simple adenoidal hyperplasia only in a few very severe cases. **E. Lymphoepithelioma.** Note the enhancing mass in the posterior nasopharyngeal soft tissues on the left *(arrows)*.

phoid tissue: roentgen observations in 257 children two years of age or less. *Radiology* 96:389–391, 1970.

4. Cunningham MJ, Myers EN, Bluestone CD: Malignant tumors of the head and neck in children: a twenty-year review. *Int J Pediatr Otorhinolaryngol* 13:279–292, 1987.
5. Fitzpatrick PJ: The nasopharyngeal angiofibroma. *Clin Radiol* 18:62–68, 1967.
6. Gonsalves CG, Briant TDR: Radiologic findings in nasopharyngeal angiofibromas. *J Can Assoc Radiol* 29:209–215, 1978.
7. Holman CB, Miller WE: Juvenile nasopharyngeal fibroma: roentgenologic characteristics. *AJR* 94:292–298, 1965.
8. Kochanski SC, Burton EM, Seidel FG, Chanin LR, Hensley S, Acker JD: Neonatal nasopharyngeal hairy polyp: CT and MR appearance. *J Comput Assist Tomogr* 14:1000, 1990.
9. Nolte K: Malignant intracranial chordoma and sarcoma of the clivus in infancy. *Pediatr Radiol* 8:1–6, 1979.
10. Ozonoff MB: Ataxia-telangiectasia: chronic pneumonia sinusitis, and adenoidal hypoplasia. *AJR* 120:297–299, 1974.

PALATE ABNORMALITIES

Underdevelopment of the uvula, soft palate, and, occasionally, the hard palate, is seen with congenital cleft palate. The small palate is readily demonstrable radiographically and, during phonation, may not elevate to its normal right-angle posture (Fig. 2.3*A*)as it apposes the posterior pharyngeal wall (2). Enlargement of the uvula most commonly is due to pharyngitis (see Fig. 2.1*B*), but occasionally can be seen with angioneurotic edema and, very rarely, with a tumor or cyst of the palate. The hard palate can be deformed or deviated secondary to a tumor arising above it, but this is an uncommon situation (1).

REFERENCES

1. Frech RS, McAlister WH: Teratoma of the nasopharynx producing depression of the posterior hard palate. *J Can Assoc Radiol* 20:204–205, 1969.
2. Swischuk LE, Smith PC, Fagan CJ: Abnormalities of the pharynx and larynx in childhood. *Semin Roentgenol* 9:283–300, 1974

HYPOPHARYNGEAL MASSES

Although any mass arising from the glottis, aryepiglottic folds, retropharynx, or nasopharynx can extend into the hypopharynx, this section deals with the masses that occur in the hypopharynx proper. The most common such mass is the enlarged, inflamed palatine tonsil or tonsils. Enlarged tonsils are often encountered in asymptomatic children (Fig. 2.3A), but, occasionally, the tonsils can be so large that they contribute to airway obstruction. Furthermore, calcifications within the tonsils can be seen occasionally (1). The next most common cause of a hypopharyngeal mass is a pseudomass due to projection of the inferior portion of a prominent uvula over the palatine tonsils. A rare cause of a mass in the hypopharynx is a tumor or cyst arising in the hypophar-

ynx, and a still rarer cause is an antrochoanal polyp, extending from the maxillary sinus on a long stalk into the hypopharynx (Fig. 2.3B). These polyps arise in the maxillary sinuses (2), and as they dangle into the hypopharynx, may cause a child to have difficulties with breathing or swallowing.

REFERENCES

1. Thomas DP: Tonsilloliths—a common cause of pharyngeal calcification. *Australas Radiol* 18:287–291, 1974.
2. Towbin R, Dunbar JS, Bove K: Antrochoanal polyps. *AJR* 132:27–31, 1979.

Retropharyngeal Soft Tissue Thickening

Thickening of the retropharyngeal space can be due to blood, edema, pus, or tumor (6) (Table 2.3), but the commonest cause is pseudothickening due to buckling of the airway when the neck is flexed and the film is obtained during expiration. Once this pitfall is appreciated, it becomes obvious that the retropharyngeal soft tissues should be evaluated only with the airway distended in full inspiration and the neck held in slight extension (Fig. 2.4). In addition to

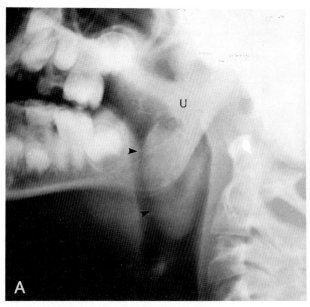

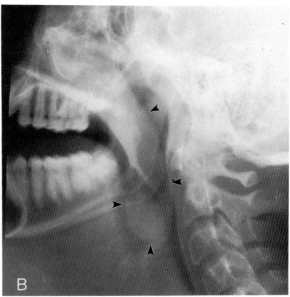

Figure 2.3. Hypopharyngeal masses. A. Note the **enlarged palatine tonsils** *(arrows)*. Such tonsilar enlargement is common in children, with or without tonsilar infection and, thus, cannot be used as a barometer of tonsillitis. Also note the position and size of the normal uvula *(U)*. It is in a phonating position (i.e., crying), characteristically at a right angle to the adenoidal pad, closing the nasopharyngeal air space. **B.** Mass due to an *antrochoanal polyp (arrows)*. These polyps originate in the maxillary sinus and dangle into the nasopharynx.

Table 2.3
Retropharyngeal Soft Tissue Thickening

Buckling of airway (pseudothickening) Inflammation (adenopathy) Retropharyngeal abscess	Common
Edema with C-spine injury Retropharyngeal tumor	Moderately common
Noninflammatory adenopathy Osteomyelitis of C-spine Tumors of C-spine	Uncommon
Myxedematous thickening Edema with obstructed superior vena cava Vein of Galen aneurysms Enteric cyst Goiter	Rare

this misleading configuration of the retropharyngeal soft tissues, one can encounter true, but still innocuous, thickening due to normally abundant lymphoid tissue. Indeed, the "thickening" or "mass" so produced often appears lumpy and worrisome (see Fig. 2.4C), but in fact the lumpy configuration favors normal lymphoid tissue. With pathologic thickening, the mass produced usually shows a smooth anterior margin and displaces the airway forward in a continuous arc (Fig. 2.5).

Pathologic thickening of the retropharyngeal tissues can be due to tumor, cyst, inflammation, abscess, edema, or massive lymph node enlargement. In addition to the arc-like anterior displacement of the airway, the normal stepoff of the air column at the level of the larynx is effaced (Fig. 2.5). Normally, with full inspiration, the soft tissues below the level of the larynx are approximately two times as thick as those above, and the reason for this is that the esophagus is located in this region. Radiographically, this produces a stepoff of the air column, a finding which is present even in those children with prominent, normal lymphoid tissue (see Fig. 2.4). With a pathologic mass, the stepoff usually is totally obliterated, even in less than florid cases (Fig. 2.5). In milder cases, a barium esophagram may be required to demonstrate displacement of the esophagus from the cervical spine.

The commonest cause of pathologic retropharyngeal soft tissue thickening is retropharyngeal inflammatory adenopathy (viral or bacterial) with or without abscess formation. If an abscess develops, air may be seen in the thickened soft tissues, but once again beware of expiratory films, for air trapped in the hypopharynx can give a similar appearance (3)

(Fig. 2.4A and B). Most commonly, retropharyngeal abscess occurs secondary to suppurative (pyogenic) adenitis. Occasionally, an abscess develops after perforation of the pharynx by a foreign body or during endotracheal intubation. Regardless of the cause, the inflammation is accompanied by muscle spasm and straightening of the cervical spine. In some cases, actual hyperflexion of the spine leads to an erroneous appearance of subluxation at C_1–C_2 and C_2–C_3. Inflammatory adenopathy in this region also can be seen with tuberculosis (scrofula), tularemia (9), and fungal diseases (e.g., histoplasmosis). Ultrasound is often useful to distinguish lymphadenopathy from an abscess (2), but CT or MRI may be required when planning drainage of an abscess (4).

Moderately common causes of retropharyngeal soft tissue thickening include prevertebral edema or hematoma secondary to cervical spine injury, noninflammatory lymphadenopathy, and a variety of retropharyngeal tumors. The most common retropharyngeal "tumor" is cystic hygroma, followed by neuroblastoma, ganglioneuroma, neurofibroma (7), hemangioma, and an occasional teratoma. Other causes of noninflammatory adenopathy include histiocytosis-X (Fig. 2.5B), leukemia, lymphoma, and sinus histiocytosis (1).

Thickening of the retropharyngeal space is seen uncommonly with underlying cervical spine osteomyelitis, primary cervical spine tumors, retropharyngeal goiter, myxedematous thickening in hypothyroid infants (5), duplication cysts, edema secondary to obstruction of the superior vena cava, and enlargement of the jugular veins and carotid arteries associated with vein of Galen aneurysm or other large intracranial arteriovenous malformations (8).

REFERENCES

1. Bankaci M, Morris RF, Stool SE, Paradise JL: Sinus histiocytosis with massive lymphadenopathy: report of its occurrence in two siblings with retropharyngeal involvement in both. *Ann Otol Rhinol Laryngol* 87:327–331, 1978.
2. Ben-Ami T, Yousefzadeh DK, Aramburo MJ: Pre-suppurative phase of retropharyngeal infection: contribution of ultrasonography in the diagnosis and treatment. *Pediatr Radiol* 21:23, 1990.
3. Currarino G, Williams B: Air collection in the retropharyngeal soft tissues observed in lateral expiratory films of the neck in 9 infants. *Pediatr Radiol* 23:186–188, 1993.
4. Glasier CM, Stark JE, Jacobs RF, Mancias P, Leithiser RE Jr, Seibert RW, Seibert JJ: CT and ultrasound imaging of retropharyngeal abscesses in children. *AJNR* 12:1191, 1992.
5. Grunebaum M, Moskowitz G: The retropharyngeal soft tissues in young infants with hypothyroidism. *AJR* 108:543–545, 1970.

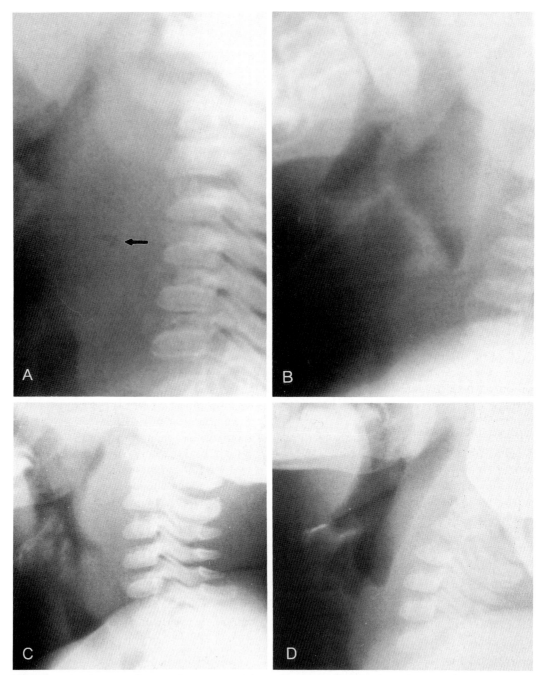

Figure 2.4. Normal retropharyngeal pseudomasses and thickenings. A. A film obtained in incomplete inspiration shows mass-like thickening of the retropharyngeal soft tissues. A small bubble of air within the tissues *(arrow)* could be mistaken for air in a retropharyngeal abscess. **B.** With deep inspiration, the airway is fully distended and the abnormal findings have disappeared. The previously noted air collection was actually due to air within the hypopharynx. **C.** Another infant with retropharyngeal thickening, suggesting a lumpy retropharyngeal mass. The lumpiness rules in favor of lymphoid tissue, but is not absolutely diagnostic. **D.** Note that with proper technique the mass has all but disappeared; only the central pad of lymphoid tissue still projects into the posterior aspect of the distended hypopharynx. However, note that the lateral recesses of the hypopharynx are normally distended, and that because of this, the normal stepoff between the posterior hypopharyngeal wall and the upper trachea is retained. When a true retropharyngeal mass is present, the lateral recesses usually are not distended and the stepoff is obliterated.

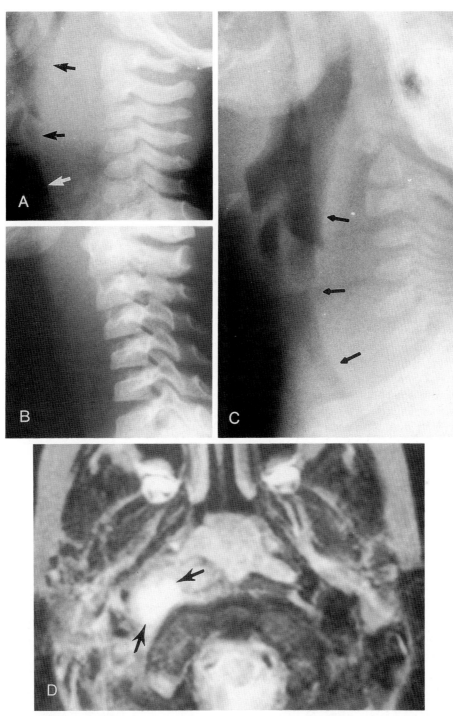

Figure 2.5. Abnormal retropharyngeal soft tissues. A. Young child with **retropharyngeal cellulitis** (i.e., preabscess) producing marked anterior displacement of the airway *(arrows).* In contrast to the infant shown in Figure 2.4*D,* this infant demonstrates displacement of the upper trachea from the spine and obliteration of the stepoff between the posterior pharyngeal air column and upper tracheal air column. The end result is that the entire airway is pushed forward in a continuous arc, a configuration not usually seen with normal lymphoid tissue. **B.** Similar findings, but more marked, in a patient with **massive adenopa-**thy in Letterer-Siewe disease. **C. Retropharyngeal cellulitis and adenitis** produce straightening of the spine, anterior displacement of the upper trachea, thickening of the retropharyngeal soft tissues, and obliteration of the stepoff between the hypopharyngeal and tracheal air columns (arrows). **D. Retropharyngeal abscess.** T$_2$-weighted MRI shows the high intensity fluid collection *(arrows)* in the retropharyngeal soft tissues on the right. (Courtesy of Phillip Tirman, M.D., San Francisco, California.)

6. McCook TA, Felman AH: Retropharyngeal masses in infants and young children. *Am J Dis Child* 133:41–43, 1979.
7. Steichen FM, Einhorn AF, Fellini A, Feind CR: Congenital retropharyngeal neurofibroma causing laryngeal obstruction in a newborn. *J Pediatr Surg* 6:480–483, 1971.
8. Swischuk LE, Crowe JE, Mewborne EB Jr: Large vein of Galen aneurysms in the neonate: a constellation of diagnostic chest and neck radiologic findings. *Pediatr Radiol* 6:4–9, 1977.
9. Umlas S-L, Jaramillo D: Massive adenopathy in oropharyngeal tularemia: CT demonstration. *Pediatr Radiol* 20:483, 1990.

Abnormalities of the Epiglottis and Aryepiglottic Folds

For the most part, abnormalities of the epiglottis consist of enlargement, for only occasionally will one see it to be smaller than normal (hypoplastic) or deformed. The usual cause of deformity is scarring after corrosive agent (usually lye) burn and, as far as enlargement is concerned, the commonest cause, by far, is epiglottitis (Table 2.4) (1, 6, 7). This infection is usually caused by the bacterium *Haemophilus influenzae,* and associated symptoms include dysphagia, drooling, fever, and dyspnea or respiratory distress. The epiglottis is usually very thick and edematous (Fig. 2.6A and B), and this thickening virtually always extends into the aryepiglottic folds. Milder

cases must be differentiated from the omega epiglottis, a normal variant in which the lateral flaps of the epiglottis fold down farther than usual, so that on lateral view of the neck the epiglottis appears thickened (Fig. 2.6C). In such cases, the aryepiglottic folds will remain thin.

When evaluating the aryepiglottic folds, one must be sure that the lateral neck radiograph is obtained in an adequate degree of inspiration, with the neck slightly extended. Neck flexion or suboptimal degrees of inspiration result in buckling and foreshortening of the aryepiglottic folds, making it difficult to differentiate the fold from the prominent shadow caused by the arytenoid cartilage at the base of the folds (Fig. 2.7). The folds should be assessed at a site as close as possible to the epiglottis in order to avoid

Table 2.4
Epiglottic and Aryepiglottic Fold Enlargement

Epiglottitis	}	Common
Angioneurotic edema	}	Uncommon
Corrosive burns		
Face and neck edema		
Tumor		
Aryepiglottic fold cyst	}	Rare
Sarcoidosis		
Hemorrhage (hemophilia)		
Radiation		

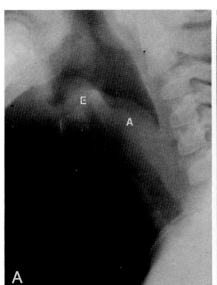 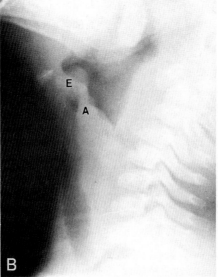 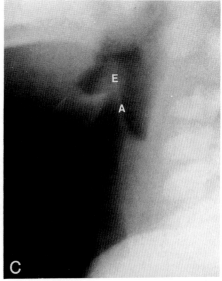

Figure 2.6. Epiglottic thickening. A. Typical thickening of the epiglottis *(E)* and aryepiglottic folds *(A)* in **epiglottitis.** Compare with the normal epiglottis and aryepiglottic folds in Figure 2.8A. **B.** Moderate epiglottic *(E)* and aryepiglottic fold *(A)* swelling in another patient with less severe epiglottitis. **C. Normal omega epiglottis.** The epiglottis *(E)* appears bulky, similar to those of the previous two patients with epiglottitis. Note, however, that the aryepiglottic folds *(A)* are thin in this normal patient.

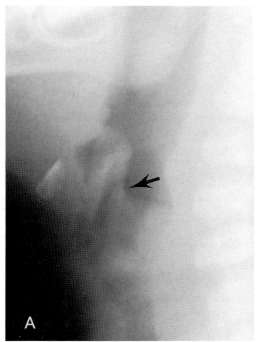
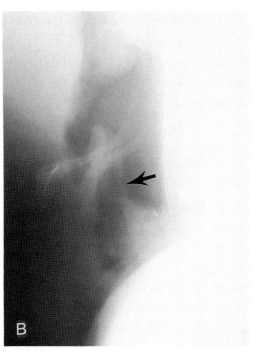

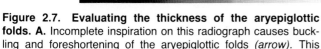

Figure 2.7. Evaluating the thickness of the aryepiglottic folds. A. Incomplete inspiration on this radiograph causes buckling and foreshortening of the aryepiglottic folds *(arrow)*. This makes them difficult to evaluate and gives the false impression of thickening. **B.** View of the same patient in full inspiration reveals that the folds are in fact quite thin and normal *(arrow)*.

mistaking the prominent arytenoid cartilage shadow for fold thickening (3).

Other causes of epiglottic edema may also be associated with aryepiglottic fold thickening, and include angioneurotic edema (8), corrosive agent ingestion (i.e., chemical burns), and other inflammatory conditions that cause acute edema of the face and neck (2, 4). Very rarely, the epiglottis and aryepiglottic folds can be enlarged as a result of laryngeal sarcoidosis (5), hemorrhage due to hemophilia, hemangioma or lymphangioma, or an aryepiglottic fold cyst (1).

REFERENCES

1. Dunbar JS: Upper respiratory tract obstruction in infants and children. *AJR* 109:225–247, 1970.
2. Herman TE, McAlister WH: Epiglottic enlargement: two unusual causes. *Pediatr Radiol* 21:139–140, 1991.
3. John SD, Swischuk LE, Hayden CK Jr, Freeman DH Jr: Aryepiglottic fold width in patients with epiglottitis: where should measurements be obtained? *Radiology* 190:123–125, 1994.
4. McCook TA, Kirks DR: Epiglottic enlargement in infants and children: another radiologic look. *Pediatr Radiol* 12:227, 1982.
5. McHugh K, deSilva M, Kilham HA: Epiglottic enlargement secondary to laryngeal sarcoidosis. *Pediatr Radiol* 23:71, 1993.
6. Poole CA, Altman DH: Acute epiglottitis in children. *Radiology* 80:798–805, 1963.
7. Swischuk LE, Smith PC, Fagan CJ: Abnormalities of the pharynx and larynx in childhood. *Semin Roentgenol* 9:283–300, 1974.
8. Watts FB Jr, Slovis TL: The enlarged epiglottis. *Pediatr Radiol* 5:133–136, 1977.

Vocal Cord Abnormalities

The vocal cords are visible on both lateral and frontal views of the neck and, indeed, frequently are visible at the top of regular chest films. Abnormalities of the vocal cords include indistinctness of their margins, thickening or increase in their bulk, fixation in the midline, and nodular growths. Any of these findings can be bilateral or unilateral (Table 2.5).

INDISTINCT-THICKENED CORDS ON LATERAL VIEW

The vocal cords can appear indistinct and thickened because of edema or spasm and in some cases both problems coexist. This certainly is true in croup, the commonest cause of indistinct vocal cords visible on lateral view (Fig. 2.8A). A similar appearance can be seen with vocal cord paralysis, vocal cord infiltration (see next section), and laryngeal trauma. Trauma most commonly is iatrogenic, secondary to endotracheal intubation. Rarely, the cords can have a similar appearance with laryngeal webs. Such webs, however, must involve the cords proper to cause any degree of fixation. Most laryngeal webs do not involve the cords directly.

THICKENED OR FIXED CORDS ON FRONTAL VIEW

Once again, croup is the commonest cause of this finding. In this condition, the spastic, edematous cords form a funnel or slit-like glottic opening (Fig. 2.8B). Similar fixation of the cords occurs with vocal cord paralysis (Fig. 2.9A and B) and, occasionally, with epiglottitis (2). Vocal cord paralysis usually occurs with neurologic conditions such as hydrocephalus, Arnold-Chiari malformation, cerebral agenesis, meningomyelocele, and encephalocele (3, 6). In the neonate, however, the most common cause is anoxic damage to the brainstem.

Trauma to the larynx also can cause the vocal cords to appear thickened and fixed on frontal view,

Table 2.5
Vocal Cord Abnormalities

Indistinct, fuzzy on lateral view		
Croup	}	Common
Paralysis	}	Moderately common
Trauma Storage diseases Lipoid proteinosis	}	Rare
Bilateral cord thickening and/or fixation		
Croup	}	Common
Trauma (iatrogenic) Paralysis Epiglottitis	}	Moderately common
Trauma (noniatrogenic) Laryngeal web	}	Uncommon
Storage diseases Lipoid proteinosis	}	Rare
Unilateral thickening and/or fixation		
Paralysis	}	Common
Iatrogenic trauma Subglottic hemangioma	}	Moderately common
Laryngeal web (unilateral)	}	Rare
Nodules		
Papillomatosis	}	Common
Postintubation granuloma	}	Uncommon
Benign and malignant tumors	}	Rare

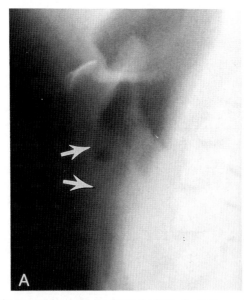 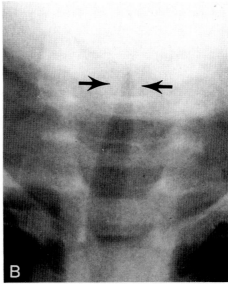

Figure 2.8. Indistinct vocal cords on lateral view. A. Note the indistinct vocal cords *(arrows)* in this patient with croup. The prominent, air-filled ventricle is common with croup. Similar cord indistinctness can be seen with edema secondary to trauma and fixation of the cords with vocal cord paralysis. Note the normal, thin aryepiglottic folds and their stout triangular base as a result of the arytenoid cartilages. **B.** Frontal view of the same patient, demonstrating typical funnel-shaped configuration of the inferior aspect of the vocal cords and subglottic portion of the trachea *(arrows)*. This finding is characteristic of croup, but can be seen in some cases of epiglottitis.

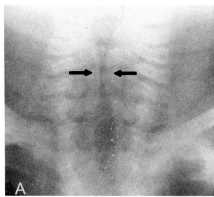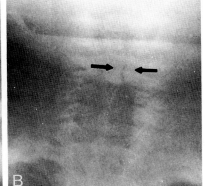

Figure 2.9. Vocal cord paralysis. A. Inspiratory view demonstrating bilateral vocal cord fixation *(arrows)*. Normally, during inspiration the vocal cords should fall away from midline to result in a glottic opening that is nearly the same width as the trachea. **B.** Expiration (phonation) view demonstrating slightly wavy (corrugated) but still adducted vocal cords *(arrows)* and overdistension of the obstructed trachea. The degree of cord excursion between resting and phonation is far below normal and signifies cord fixation. On lateral view, the findings in this patient were very similar to those of the infant with croup in Figure 2.8*A*.

and often the cords are lumpy and asymmetric. Other causes of thickening of the vocal cords include the various storage diseases and lipoid proteinosis (5). Tumors of the cords are quite rare, except for juvenile laryngeal papillomatosis and infantile subglottic hemangioma, but in these conditions thickening, most often, is unilateral. Laryngeal webs, when they involve the vocal cords directly, also can produce fixation of the cords, mimicking the findings of vocal cord paralysis.

UNILATERAL THICKENING OR FIXATION OF THE VOCAL CORDS

The commonest cause of unilateral fixation or apparent thickening of the vocal cords is vocal cord paralysis, and the commonest cause of such paralysis is stretching of the recurrent laryngeal nerve by an aneurysm or anomaly of position of the aorta or pulmonary artery. Similar stretching can be caused by critically located mediastinal cysts or masses, however, and, in the neonatal period, injury to this nerve can occur with stretching of the neck during difficult deliveries. Unilateral vocal cord paralysis generally results in a weak or abnormal cry, but stridor can develop when the patient is agitated. The radiographic findings are characteristic, because on frontal view the involved cord remains midline in position both with quiet breathing and with phonation. The other cord moves freely and in time may hypertrophy in a compensatory fashion. Unilateral thickening of the vocal cords also can occur when a subglottic hemangioma extends into the cords (4) (see

Fig. 2.12*B*) and in some cases of juvenile papillomatosis of the cords (1, 3). Rarely, when a laryngeal web involves one cord only, unilateral fixation can occur.

NODULES OF VOCAL CORDS

By far, the commonest cause of nodular masses on the vocal cords is the condition known as juvenile papillomatosis (1). The cause of this condition is presumed to be viral (i.e., human papillomavirus), and a maternal history of condyloma acuminatum is common. The papillomas develop in young children, who are examined for insidious onset of hoarseness and cough. Demonstration of nodules on or around the vocal cords is characteristic and usually best visualized on lateral view (Fig. 2.10). A much less common cause of vocal cord nodules is a postinflammatory granuloma secondary to long-term endotracheal intubation. Neoplasms, both benign and malignant, are quite rare in infants and children.

REFERENCES

1. Oleske JM, Kushnick T: Juvenile papilloma of the larynx. *Am J Dis Child* 121:417–419, 1971.
2. Slovis TL, Arcinue E: Subglottic edema in acute epiglottitis in children. *AJR* 132:500–504, 1979.
3. Snow JB Jr, Rogers KA: Bilateral adductive paralysis of vocal cords secondary to Arnold-Chiari malformation and its management. *Laryngoscope* 25:316, 1965.
4. Sutton TJ, Nogrady MB: Radiologic diagnosis of subglottic hemangioma in infants. *Pediatr Radiol* 1:211–215, 1973.
5. Weidner WA, Wenzi JE, Swischuk LE: Roentgenographic

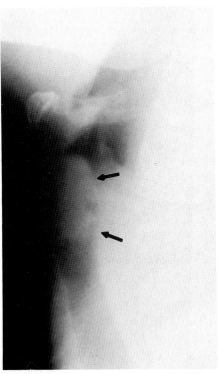

Figure 2.10. Vocal cord nodules: laryngeal papillamatosis. Note the lumpy, nodular appearing vocal cords *(arrows)*. The findings are characteristic of laryngeal papillomatosis.

findings in lipoid proteinosis: a case report. *Am J Radiol Radium Ther Nucl Med* 110:457–461, 1970.
6. Williams JL, Capitanio MA, Turtz MG: Vocal cord paralysis: radiologic observations in 21 infants and young children. *AJR* 128:649–651, 1977.

Table 2.6
Subglottic Tracheal Narrowing

Circumferential		
Croup	}	Common
Subglottic stenosis	⎫	
Paradoxic collapse with other glottic obstruction	⎬	Moderately common
Eccenteric	⎭	
Subglottic hemangioma	⎫	Moderately common
Posttracheostomy fibrosis	⎬	
Intratracheal thyroid	⎫	
Subglottic mucocele		
Histiocytoma	⎬	Rare
Papilloma		
Intratracheal thymus	⎭	

Subglottic Tracheal Narrowing

This section deals with narrowing of the trachea just below the glottis. The length of such narrowing seldom is greater than 1.5 cm, and the narrowing can be circumferential or eccentric (Table 2.6).

CIRCUMFERENTIAL SUBGLOTTIC TRACHEAL NARROWING

The commonest cause of such narrowing is that which occurs with viral croup (acute laryngotracheobronchitis) (Fig. 2.11*A* and *B*). Although such viral infections can effect the entire tracheobronchial tree, the predominant symptoms of croup (stridor, barking cough, and respiratory distress) are the result of laryngeal inflammation, edema, and obstruction. It has been shown that glottic or paraglottic obstruc-

tion causes air flow velocity to increase in the glottis, resulting in negative intratracheal pressures and paradoxical collapse of the subglottic trachea during inspiration (4). With expiration, the area of apparent narrowing frequently returns to normal. If there is considerable associated edema, however, some narrowing will persist. This situation most often occurs when croup is bacterial rather than viral in origin, and such cases may be associated with inflammatory membranes visible just below the cords (5) (see Fig. 2.12*C*).

A less common cause of subglottic tracheal narrowing is congenital subglottic stenosis (2). On the inspiratory view, the findings are indistinguishable from those of croup, but differentiation can be accomplished on the expiratory view. On expiration, with subglottic stenosis, subglottic narrowing remains fixed, unlike the situation with croup (Fig. 2.11*C* and *D*). Because of the more frequent use of endotracheal intubation in newborn infants, acquired subglottic stenosis now is more common than the congenital form and can produce a similar configuration. It might be noted that not all cases of acquired subglottic stenosis are smooth and circumferentially stenotic (7). Indeed, membranes, granulomas, and a variety of eccentric narrowings also occur.

Bilateral vocal cord paralysis is a relatively common cause of laryngeal obstruction in the newborn and young infant, resulting in circumferential, paradoxical inspiratory narrowing of the subglottic trachea identical to that seen with croup. The paralysis may be the result of injury to the cords during endotracheal intubation or to the recurrent laryngeal nerve during thoracic surgery, or may accompany a congenital disorder of the nervous system such as hydrocephalus or Arnold-Chiari malformation. Clinically, these patients usually have alteration of the

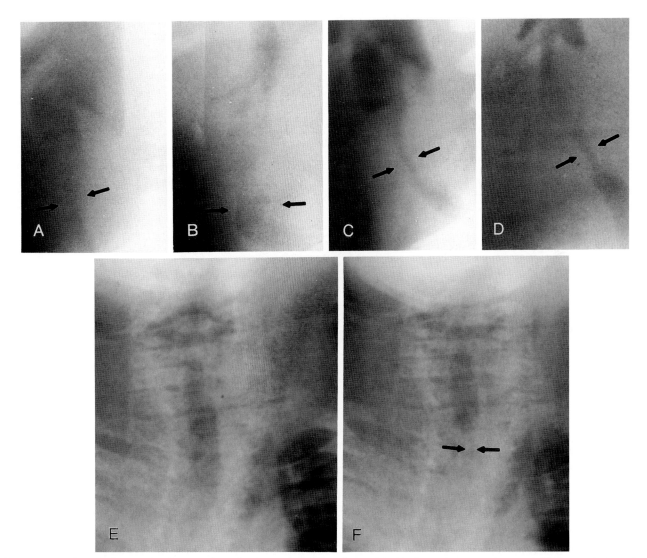

Figure 2.11. Subglottic tracheal narrowing. A. *Croup.* Inspiratory view demonstrating typical subglottic narrowing *(arrows),* overdistension of the hypopharynx, fuzziness of the vocal cords, and a prominent ventricle. **B.** Expiratory view demonstrates overdistension of the trachea and opening of the previously narrowed subglottic portion of the trachea to almost a normal diameter *(arrows).* This is common in croup. **C. Subglottic stenosis.** Inspiratory view. Note the typical subglottic narrowing *(arrows)* indistinguishable from that seen in croup. **D.** An expiratory view, however, demonstrates that the subglottic narrowing persists *(arrows).* This is characteristic of subglottic stenosis. **E.** *Focal tracheomalacia* in an infant born with esophageal atresia. During inspiration, the entire trachea is widely patent. **F.** With expiration, the upper trachea remains open, but the distal trachea collapses *(arrows).*

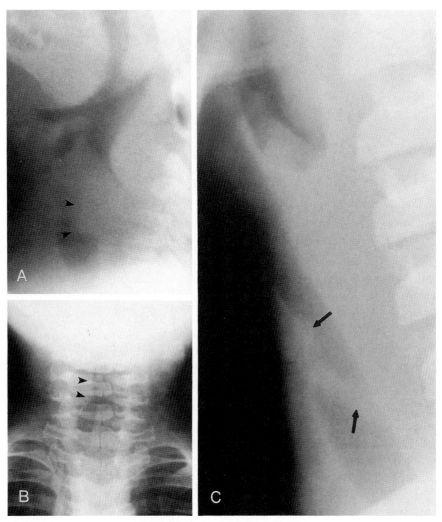

Figure 2.12. Eccentric subglottic masses and narrowings. **A.** Posterior subglottic mass secondary to subglottic hemangioma *(arrows)*. **B.** Another patient with a subglottic hemangioma producing eccentric lateral wall narrowing of the subglottic portion of the trachea *(arrows)*. **C.** *Membranous tracheitis*. Note the eccentric, anterior narrowing of the subglottic trachea, associated with a band-like defect due to intratracheal exudate *(arrows)*. (Courtesy of Robin Gaupp, M.D., Santa Fe, New Mexico).

voice or cry. Fluoroscopy or ultrasound are the best methods for demonstrating the abnormal motion of the vocal cords.

A relatively rare cause of paradoxical inspiratory subglottic collapse is a congenital laryngeal web. Such webs are usually located immediately below the vocal cords and cause some degree of fixation of the cords. Once again, plain radiography and fluoroscopy will demonstrate findings similar to those seen in croup, identifying the glottis as the site of obstruction. There are no definitive radiographic findings, however, and the final diagnosis is usually established with endoscopy. Rarely, extensive extratracheal neck masses can encircle the trachea (e.g., hemangioma, cystic hygroma), causing fixed concentric subglottic narrowing.

Excessive narrowing of the trachea during expiration is seen with tracheomalacia, a condition causing to focal or generalized weakening of the tracheal wall. Focal tracheomalacia often is the result of lesions that compress the trachea in utero, such as vascular anomalies or the dilated pouch of esophageal atresia (Fig. 2.11*E* and *F*). Generalized tracheomalacia is uncommon, but has been reported in association with polychondritis.

ECCENTRIC SUBGLOTTIC TRACHEAL NARROWING

When subglottic tracheal narrowing is eccentric, the cause is usually an intratracheal mass. The most common mass in the subglottic trachea is a subglottic hemangioma. These benign vascular tumors characteristically produce stridor in the first few weeks of life and most often occur on the lateral or posterior walls of the subglottic trachea (Fig. 2.12A and B). Other less common tracheal masses include ectopic thyroid tissue (4), subglottic mucoceles (1), postinflammatory histiocytomas (8), juvenile papillomas, and intratracheal thymus (6). Tracheal narrowing due to acquired subglottic stenosis can also sometimes appear eccentric.

REFERENCES

1. Dagan R, Leiberman A, Strauss R, Bar-Ziv J, Hirsch M: Subglottic mucocele in an infant. *Pediatr Radiol* 8:119–121, 1979.
2. Grunebaum M: The roentgenologic investigation of congenital subglottic stenosis. *AJR* 125:877–880, 1975.
3. Han BK, Dunbar JS, Striker TW: Membranous laryngotracheobronchitis (membranous croup). *AJR* 133:53–58, 1979.
4. Hardwick DF, Cormode EJ, Riddell DG: Respiratory distress and neck mass in a neonate intratracheal thyroid. *J Pediatr* 89:591–605, 1976.
5. John SD, Swischuk LE: Stridor and upper airway obstruction in infants and children. *RadioGraphics* 12:625–643, 1992.
6. Martin KW, McAlister WH: Intratracheal thymus: a rare cause of airway obstruction. *AJR* 149:1217–1218, 1987.
7. Scott JR, Kramer SS: Pediatric tracheostomy: I.Radiographic features of normal healing. *AJR* 130:887–891, 1978.
8. Siegel MJ, McAlister WH: Tracheal histiocytoma: an inflammatory pseudotumor. *J Can Assoc Radiol* 29:273–274, 1978.
9. Sutton TJ, Nogrady MB: Radiographic diagnosis of subglottic hemangioma in infants. *Pediatr Radiol* 1:211–215, 1973.

Calcification of Upper Airway Cartilage

Calcification of the tracheobronchial cartilage is rare in the children, and when seen is usually idiopathic (1, 3). Tracheobronchial cartilage calcification also can be associated with chondrodysplasia punctata (stippled epiphyses), idiopathic hypercalcemia (4), and the Keutel syndrome (2). Tracheobronchial calcification has also been observed in several children who received warfarin sodium therapy following mitral valve replacement (5).

REFERENCES

1. Russo PE, Coin CG: Calcification of the hyoid, thyroid, and tracheal cartilages in infancy. *AJR* 80:440–442, 1958.
2. Carmode EJ, Dawson M, Lowery RB: Keutel syndrome: clinical report and literature review. *Am J Med Genet* 24:289, 1986.
3. Santos JMG: Laryngotracheobronchial cartilage calcification in children: a case report and review of the literature. *Pediatr Radiol* 21:377–378, 1991.
4. Shiers JA, Neuhauser EBD, Bowman JR: Idiopathic hypercalcemia. *AJR* 78:19–29, 1957.
5. Taybi H, Capitanio MA: Tracheobronchial calcification: an observation in three children after mitral valve replacement and warfarin sodium therapy. *Radiology* 176:728, 1990.

Mandibular Abnormalities

SMALL MANDIBLE (MICROGNATHIA)

A small mandible most commonly is seen as part of the following syndromes: Pierre Robin syndrome, Treacher Collins syndrome (mandibulofacial dysostosis), trisomy-13, 18, and 22, and the cat-cry syndrome (chromosome 5p-syndrome). In these conditions, the entire mandible is hypoplastic. In the Goldenhar syndrome, the hypoplasia is predominantly unilateral (hemifacial microsomia). A small mandible also can be seen with cerebrocostomandibular syndrome, cleidocranial dysostosis, DiGeorge syndrome, Hallermann-Streiff syndrome, hypoglossia-hypodactyly, pyknodysostosis, some of the chondrodystrophies, and a variety of other rare syndromes.

LARGE MANDIBLE

The commonest cause of isolated enlargement of the mandible is cherubism (familial fibrous dysplasia of the jaw) (see Fig. 2.14C). The mandible also can enlarge with acromegaly, but of course such enlargement is not isolated to the mandible. Enlargement of the mandible also can occur with primary bony tumors, lymphoma (Burkett), metastatic disease, histiocytosis-X, and cysts in the mandible.

DESTRUCTIVE LESIONS OF THE MANDIBLE

Destruction of the mandible can be seen with infection (Fig. 2.13A), histiocytosis-X, and tumor. Bone destruction in histiocytosis-X may be so widespread and "clean" that the teeth seem to float in an invisible matrix. This "floating teeth" sign (Fig. 2.13B) is occasionally seen with other destructive lesions such as leukemia, lymphoma, and metastatic disease. A rarer cause of floating teeth is mandibular destruc-

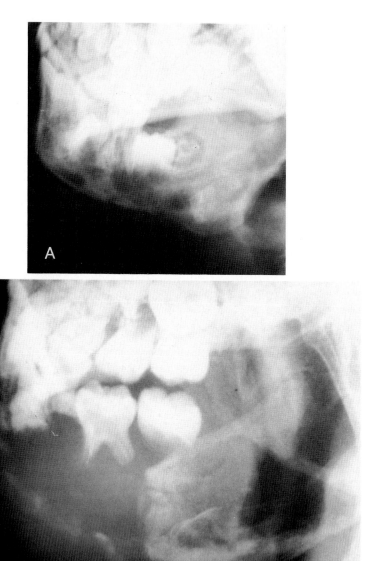

Figure 2.13. Destructive lesions of the mandible. A. Widespread destruction due to osteomyelitis. **B.** Typical floating teeth due to widespread destruction in histiocytosis-X.

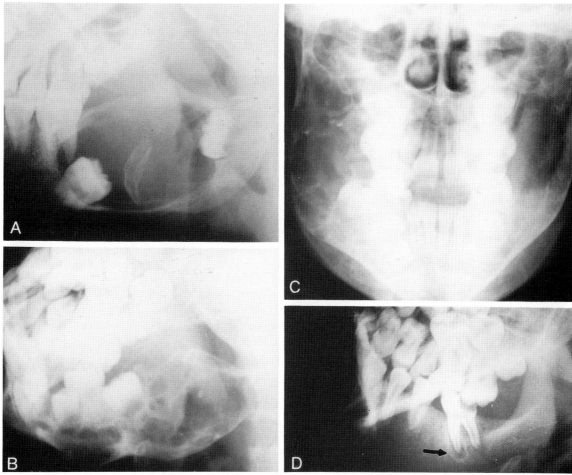

Figure 2.14. Cystic lesions of the mandible. A. Typical, well-demarcated, large dentigerous cyst in an 11-year-old child. Note the characteristic, ectopic tooth anteriorly. The posterior tooth is a normal, unerupted molar. **B.** Multiloculated lesion due to reparative granuloma of jaw in an 8-year-old child. This lesion often also is called a giant cell tumor. Similar multiloculation can be seen with ameloblastomas. **C.** Fibrous dysplasia producing a multiloculated lesion on the right, and a more diffusely lytic lesion on the left. Note that the mandible is enlarged (cherubism). **D.** Periapical abscess or so-called "radicular" cyst *(arrow)* of a molar with a large carie.

tion secondary to hemangioma or lymphangioma of the mandible. Primary bone malignancies such as fibrosarcoma, osteosarcoma, and Ewing sarcoma of the mandible are rare. Reparative granulomas (5) can produce nonspecific destruction of the mandible but more often produce a multiloculated cystic lesion (see Fig. 2.14B). In addition to these findings, the teeth often also are destroyed with any of these lesions.

CYSTS OF THE MANDIBLE

The most common cyst of the mandible is the dentigerous cyst. It is solitary, of variable size, demarcated by a sharp sclerotic margin, and associated with an ectopic tooth (Fig. 2.14A). Such cysts have a definite association with the Gorlin (basal cell nevus) syndrome (3, 6). With the possible exception of the radicular cyst, other cysts are rather uncommon (7). The radicular cyst is not a true cyst, but rather an abscess cavity around a tooth root. Usually it is small and has indistinct margins (Fig. 2.14D). Occasionally, ameloblastoma or reparative granuloma (1, 5) can produce a solitary cystic lesion, but most often both of these lesions produce multilocular cysts (Fig. 2.14B). The commonest cause of a multilocular cyst, however, is fibrous dysplasia (Fig. 2.14C). Giant cell tumors also produce multiloculated cystic lesions, but currently most of these are believed to be reparative granulomas (5). Aneurysmal bone cysts can also occur in the mandible of children.

SCLEROTIC LESIONS OF THE MANDIBLE

The commonest cause of **diffuse sclerosis** of the mandible is Caffey disease, or infantile cortical hyperostosis (periosteal new bone deposition). Sclerosis also can be seen with osteoblastic bone dysplasias such as osteopetrosis, pyknodysostosis, infantile hypercalcemia, and fibrous dysplasia. Fibrous dysplasia also can produce **focal sclerosis,** and other causes of focal sclerosis include histiocytosis-X (healing phase) (4), chronic osteomyelitis, reactive periostitis with adjacent soft tissue infection (i.e., adenitis), and sclerosing tumors such as hemangiomas and odontomas. Osteomas of the mandible and maxilla are commonly associated with familial adenomatous polyposis (2).

Abnormalities of the Maxilla

For the most part, causes of cysts, tumors, destruction, or increased sclerosis of the maxilla are the same as for the mandible. By the same token, a small or large maxilla occurs for the same reasons as does a small or large mandible, and consequently almost anything that can be said for the mandible can be said for the maxilla.

REFERENCES

1. Bhaskar SN: Oral tumors of infancy and childhood: a survey of 293 cases. *J Pediatr* 63:195–210, 1963.
2. Carl W, Sullivan MA: Dental abnormalities and bone lesions associated with familial adenomatous polyposis: report of cases. *J Am Dent Assoc* 119:137–139, 1989.
3. Gorlin RJ, Goltz RN: Multiple nevoid basal-cell epithelioma, jaw cysts and bifid ribs: syndrome. *New Engl J Med* 262:908, 1960.
4. Herman TE, Shackelford GD, Borders JL, Dehner LP: Unusual manifestations of Langerhans cell histiocytosis of the head and neck: case report with pseudoaneurysm of external carotid artery, tracheal, mandibular, and sphenoid involvement. *Pediatr Radiol* 23:41–43, 1993.
5. Jaffe HL: Giant cell reparative granuloma, traumatic bone cyst, and fibrous (fibro-osseous) dysplasia of the jaw bones. *Oral Surg* 6:159–175, 1953.
6. Rater CJ, Selke AC, Van Epps EF: Basal cell nevus syndrome. *AJR* 103:589–594, 1968.
7. Shafer WG: Cysts, neoplasms, and allied conditions of odontogenic origin. *Semin Roentgenol* 6:403–413, 1971.

HYPOPLASIA OF THE TEETH

Hypoplasia or absence of the teeth can occur with the hypoglossia-hypodactyly syndrome, cleidocranial dysostosis, Ellis-van Creveld syndrome, pyknodysostosis, ectodermal dysplasia (anhidrotic type) (1, 2), the otopalatodigital syndrome, hypoparathyroidism, and osteogenesis imperfecta (odontogenesis imperfecta) (2).

REFERENCES

1. Capitanio MA, Chen JTT, Arey JB, Kirkpatrick JA: Congenital anhidrotic ectodermal dysplasia. *AJR* 103:168–172, 1968.
2. Taybi H, Lachman RS: *Radiology of Syndromes.* 3d ed. Chicago: Year Book Medical Publishers, 1990.

LAMINA DURA ABNORMALITIES

The normal lamina dura is seen as a thin white line surrounding the tooth root or bud. In some normal children it is exceptionally dense (Fig. 2.15A). It

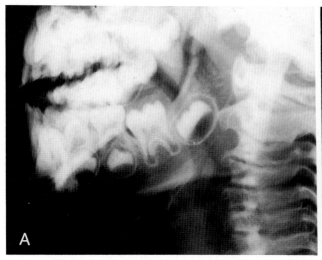 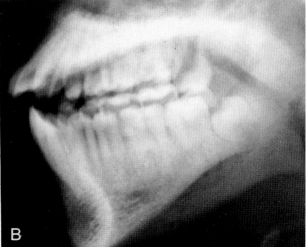

Figure 2.15. Lamina dura abnormalities. A. Extremely dense lamina dura, occasionally seen in a normal child. **B.** Virtually invisible lamina dura in a patient with severe rickets.

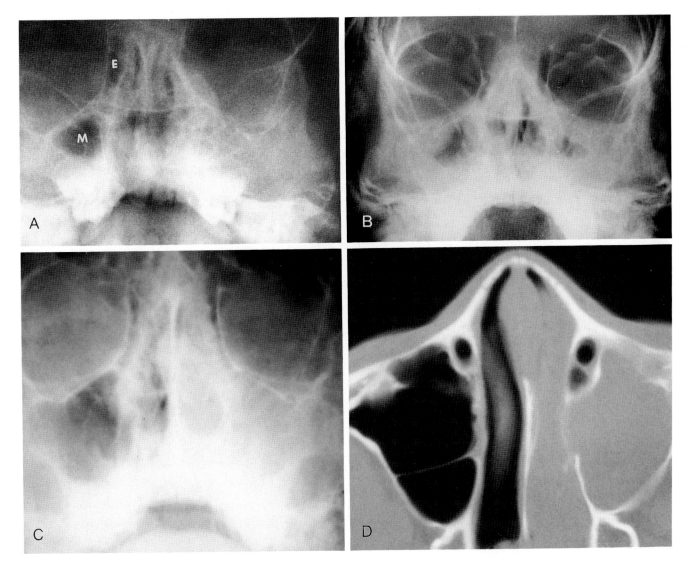

Figure 2.16. Paranasal sinus opacification. A. The maxillary *(M)* and ethmoid *(E)* sinuses *on the right* are normal. *On the left* they are totally obliterated by inflammatory change. If they were obliterated on both sides, one might erroneously conclude that they did not exist. **B.** Note mucosal thickening of the right maxillary sinus and an air-fluid level *on the left.* **C.** Note complete opacification of the left maxillary sinus and the left nasal cavity. **D.** CT of the patient in part C reveals obliteration of the left maxillary sinus and nasal cavity by a large antrochoanal polyp.

also may become more dense in hypoparathyroidism. When it is indistinct, the most likely problems are hyperparathyroidism or severe rickets (Fig. 2.15B), but it also becomes somewhat indistinct with any cause of severe demineralization.

Paranasal Sinuses

The paranasal sinuses develop at different times, but ethmoid and maxillary sinus development occurs first. These sinuses are present at birth, but they are very small in the first 6 months of life, making them difficult to visualize and assess. Closely behind eth-

moid and maxillary sinus development is sphenoid sinus development; then, between 7 and 10 years of age, the frontal sinuses appear. All of these facts are important in the assessment of sinus disease in children, but it is especially important to note that maxillary and ethmoid sinus development occurs early, and that sinusitis is not uncommon in infants.

OPACIFICATION OF THE SINUSES

Normally, the paranasal sinuses are aerated and radiolucent, and when they appear opacified, they are diseased (1, 3). Opacification most often is due to mucosal thickening or fluid accumulation (Fig. 2.16A and B). The commonest fluid is the inflammatory exudate associated with acute sinusitis, while mucosal thickening can occur with allergy, infection, or cystic fibrosis. Very often, with allergy mucosal thickening is circumferential, while with acute sinusitis, on upright view, air-fluid levels may be seen. Opacification of the sinuses also can occur with polyps, either on a sporadic allergic basis or in association with cystic fibrosis. Allergic aspergillosis of the sinuses can cause diffuse opacification, and expansion and erosion of the sinus walls (5). Rarely, one can encounter an antrochoanal polyp (9), which arises in the maxillary sinus, causes it to be opacified, and then extends, indeed dangles, into the nasopharynx (Fig. 2.16C and D). Opacification by blood usually occurs with trauma to the face and nose, but occasionally can be seen with a bleeding disorder or even a severe infection.

Opacification of the sinuses by tumors arising within them is quite rare in children. Actually, it is more common for the tumor to arise from the bones around the sinus cavity. This is especially true of the maxillary and sphenoid cavities, and such tumors often turn out to be extensions of a soft tissue sarcoma or a tumor of the lymphoma-leukemia group. Metastatic disease can also develop in the paranasal sinuses, and, rarely, the tumors may be odontogenic in origin.

Angiofibromas of the nasopharynx also can involve the sinuses and, depending on the size of the lesion, the maxillary, ethmoid, and sphenoid sinuses may be involved. These tumors may present with sinusitis and epistaxis, and the radiographic findings (especially the angiographic ones) are rather characteristic (see Fig. 2.2A–C). After angiofibroma, the next most common tumor arising in the nasopharynx is lymphoepithelioma, but sinus involvement with this tumor is less common. Opacification of the sinuses also can occur with mucoceles (8) and, rarely, with Wegener granulomatosis (6).

SINUS WALL DESTRUCTION

Destruction of the paranasal sinus walls occurs primarily with infection and tumor, and, of course, most often the sinus cavity itself is opacified. Tumor destruction probably is more common, and the tumor usually is a sarcoma (especially rhabdomyosarcoma), lymphoma, leukemia, or metastatic disease. Rarely, hemangiomas, lymphangiomas, or odontogenic tumors can produce destruction. Destruction also can occur with mucoceles, which are uncommon in children but sometimes occur with cystic fibrosis (7). Sinus destruction also occurs with Wegener granulomatosis (6) and histiocytosis-X.

PARANASAL SINUS MASSES

The commonest mass seen in a paranasal sinus is a mucus retention cyst. Most commonly, this cyst occurs in the maxillary sinuses, often along the floor (Fig. 2.17A and B). Cysts usually are smooth-edged, round, or half-moon-shaped, and not associated with bony destruction. They result from the postinflammatory blockage of mucus glands. Less commonly, one can encounter mucoceles of the paranasal sinuses, either inflammatory or posttraumatic in origin. These lesions result from the blockage of the main draining ducts of the sinuses and characteristically produce opacification and expansion of the sinus. Ethmoid and sphenoid sinus involvement is most common in children (4). Odontogenic cysts are uncommon masses that can arise from the floor of the maxillary sinus and cause erosion and remodeling of the sinus walls. The presence of the displaced molar tooth within the cyst is characteristic. Antrochoanal polyps arise within the maxillary sinus and frequently extend through the sinus ostium into the nasopharynx. Sinus tumors are uncommon and include rhabdomyosarcoma (Fig. 2.17D), lymphoma, hemangioma, ossifying fibroma, and inverted papilloma (2).

Finally, a very specific mass occurring in the maxillary sinus is that associated with a blowout fracture of the orbit. In these cases, blunt trauma to the orbit forces intraorbital contents through the thin floor of the orbit (i.e., the roof of the maxillary sinus), and the soft tissues so displaced project as a mass (tear drop) from the roof of the maxillary sinus (Fig. 2.17C). CT or MRI is most helpful in demonstrating these and other mass lesions of the sinus cavities.

ASYMMETRY OF SINUS CAVITIES

Asymmetry can involve size, density, or configuration. Normally, the frontal sinuses are very asymmetric both in terms of size and radiolucency. The ethmoid and maxillary sinus cavities usually are symmetrical in all respects, although maxillary antrum asymmetry can occur. With the frontal sinuses, unequal but normal unilateral thickening of the bone overlying the sinus cavities can lead to apparent asymmetry of aeration, but with the other sinus cavities, if asymmetry of density exists, underlying disease should be suspected (e.g., infection, trauma, tumors, polyps).

A pitfall to avoid in the assessment of sinus size asymmetry, especially with the maxillary sinus cavities, is not to interpret a sinus cavity as being congenitally small when actually it just appears that

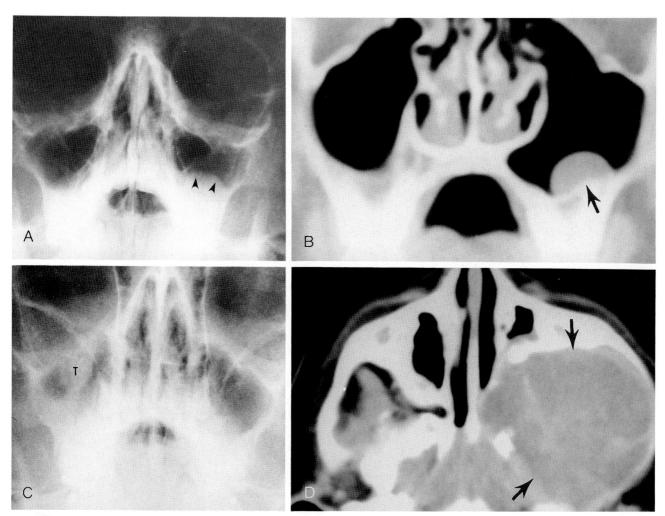

Figure 2.17. Paranasal sinus masses or destruction. A. Mucus retention cyst. Note the convex soft tissue mass arising from the floor of the left maxillary sinus *(arrows)*. **B.** CT of a similar maxillary retention cyst *(arrow)*. **C.** Partially obliterated right maxillary sinus and teardrop *(T)* configuration of a *blowout fracture* of the orbit. **D. Rhabdomyosarcoma** involving the left maxillary sinus *(arrows)*.

way because the air has been replaced by fluid or mucosal thickening. Indeed, because in most of these cases associated demineralization of the sinus wall (common with infection and inflammation) renders it indistinct, it is easy to erroneously interpret the sinus cavity as small or absent rather that present and abnormal.

Enlargement of a sinus on one side can be seen with expanding lesions such as mucoceles, large polyps, odontogenic cysts, and tumors. Distortion of sinus shape can be seen with trauma, neurofibromatosis, or, less commonly, with deforming tumors of the face.

REFERENCES

1. Arruda LK, Mimica IM, Sole D, Wecky, LL. M. Schoettler J, Heiner DC, Naspitz CK: Abnormal maxillary sinus radiographs in children: do they represent bacterial infection? *Pediatrics* 85:553–558, 1990.
2. Buetow PC, Smirniotopoulos JG, Wenig BM: Pediatric sinonasal tumors. *Appl Radiol* 22:21–28, 1993.
3. Kogutt MS, Swischuk LE: Diagnosis of sinusitis in infants and children. *Pediatrics* 52:121–124, 1973.
4. Ledesma-Medina J, Osman MZ, Girdany BR: Abnormal paranasal sinuses in patients with cystic fibrosis of the pancreas: radiological findings. *Pediatr Radiol* 9:61–64, 1980.
5. Manning SC, Vuich F, Weinberg AG, Brown OE: Allergic aspergillosis: a newly recognized form of sinusitis in the pediatric population. *Laryngoscope* 99:681–685, 1989.
6. Orlowski JP, Clough JD, Dyment PG: Wegener's granulomatosis in the pediatric age group. *Pediatrics* 61:83–90, 1978.
7. Schulte T, Buhr W, Brassel F, Emons D: Mucocele of paranasal sinuses in a young infant with cystic fibrosis. *Pediatr Radiol* 20:600, 1990.
8. Siegel MJ, Shackelford GD, McAlister WH: Paranasal sinus mucoceles in children. *Radiology* 133:623–626, 1979.
9. Towbin R, Dunbar JS, Bove K: Antrochoanal polyps. *AJR* 132:27–31, 1979.

Soft Tissues of the Neck

The soft tissues of the anterior and lateral parts of the neck seldom are examined radiographically, but increased soft tissue bulk is not uncommon and can be seen with cervical adenopathy and a variety of soft tissue tumors. Distinct masses anterior, or lateral, to the trachea can be seen with lesions such as thyroid cysts, sublingual thyroid (Fig. 2.18A), and branchial cleft cysts. **Calcifications of the soft tissues of the neck** most often occur in inflamed lymph nodes, but occasionally can be seen with chronic infections of the salivary glands. Very rarely, they may be seen in an underlying cervical teratoma or neuroblastoma.

Table 2.7
Neck Masses

Cystic		
Abscess	}	Common
Branchial cleft cyst		
Thyroglossal duct cyst	}	Moderately common
Cystic hygroma		
Hematoma (resolving)		Uncommon
Solid		
Lymphadenopathy	}	Common
Fibromatosis colli		
Hemangioma		
Lymphoma	}	Moderately common
Rhabdomyosarcoma		
Neuroblastoma		
Teratoma		
Metastases	}	Uncommon
Thyroid neoplasm		
Lipoma		

Although the diagnostic possibilities for a cervical soft tissue mass are numerous, ultrasound is very useful for narrowing the differential diagnosis (Table 2.7) and in some cases is diagnostic (2, 3). Sonography easily identifies cysts and masses with cystic components. A simple cyst in the neck usually represents a developmental cyst such as a branchial cleft or thyroglossal duct cyst (Fig. 2.18B). Cystic hygroma results from anomalous development of the lymphatic system in the neck and appears as a multiseptate cyst (4) (Fig. 2.18C and D). These lesions frequently are complicated by hemorrhage, causing increased echogenicity within the cyst fluid. An abscess or resolving hematoma can also appear cystic, although both tend to be less well defined and more heterogeneous than developmental cysts.

The most common solid soft tissue mass found in the neck is lymphadenopathy, and inflammatory causes predominate. Lymph nodes are usually easy to identify with ultrasound, appearing as hypoechoic round or oval masses that are frequently multiple and clustered (Fig. 2.18E). Ultrasound cannot reliably differentiate inflammatory lymph nodes from tumoral lymphadenopathy. Another solid neck mass that has a characteristic ultrasound appearance is fibromatosis colli, a fibrous mass-like lesion that occurs in the sternocleidomastoid muscle in young infants and is associated with torticollis. Enlargement of the sternocleidomastoid muscle is seen (Fig. 2.18F), but the echotexture can vary from hyper- to slightly hypoechoic. For the most part, other solid soft tissue masses of the neck cannot be reliably distinguished by ultrasound alone; however, the physical characteristics of the mass can be helpful. Hem-

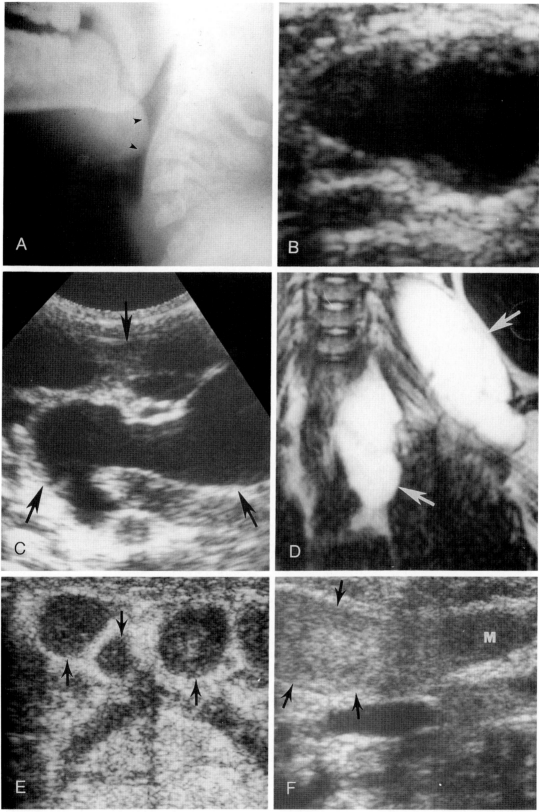

Figure 2.18.   Neck masses. A. Sublingual thyroid. Note the large sublingual mass *(arrows)* projecting into the hypopharynx. (Courtesy of M. H. Schreiber, M.D., Galveston, Texas). **B. Branchial cleft cyst.** Ultrasound shows a thin-walled, simple cyst that was found in the lateral neck. **C. Cystic hygroma.** Ultrasound shows a characteristic multiloculated cystic mass *(arrows)* with relatively thin septations and only a small amount of internal solid material. **D.** MRI of another patient with a cystic hygroma of the left neck. This T_2-weighted image shows the high intensity, multiloculated cystic mass extending down into the superior mediastinum *(arrows).* **E. Lymphadenopathy.** Note the multiple, round, hypoechoic lymph nodes *(arrows)* in a child with cat-scratch fever. **F. Fibromatosis colli.** Note the slightly echogenic, mass-like enlargement of the sternocleidomastoid muscle *(arrows).* Normal muscle *(M).*

angiomas and lipomas tend to feel soft upon palpation, and differ sonographically. Lipomas have a homogeneous echogenic texture, whereas hemangiomas tend to be more heterogeneous and frequently show small hypoechoic or cystic areas with evidence of blood flow on color Doppler imaging. Solid neck masses that are firm on palpation include a variety of soft tissue tumors. The most common malignant tumors found in the neck are lymphoma and rhabdomyosarcoma. Less common neck neoplasms include neuroblastoma (1), teratoma, sarcoma, metastatic malignancy, and thyroid tumors. When any of the soft tissue neck masses are large, MRI or CT are useful for defining the extent of the lesion and its effect on surrounding neck structures (5).

REFERENCES

1. Abramson SJ, Berdon WE, Ruzai-Shapiro C, Stolar C, Garvin J: Cervical neuroblastoma in eleven infants—a tumor with favorable prognosis: clinical and radiologic (US, CT, MRI) findings. *Pediatr Radiol* 23:253–257, 1993.
2. Glasier CM, Seibert JJ, Williamson SL, Seibert RW, Corbitt SL, Rodgers AB, Lange TA: High resolution ultrasound characterization of soft tissue masses in children. *Pediatr Radiol* 17:233–237, 1987.
3. Kraus R, Han BK, Babcock DS, Oestreich AE: Sonography of neck masses in children. *AJR* 146:609, 1986.
4. Sheth S, Nussbaum AR, Hutchins GM, Sanders RC: Cystic hygromas in children: sonographic-pathologic correlation. *Radiology* 162:821–824, 1987.
5. Siegel MJ, Glazer HS, St Amour TE, Rosenthal DD: Lymphangiomas in children: MR imaging. *Radiology* 170:467–470, 1989.

CHAPTER
3
ABDOMEN

Abdominal Masses

Abdominal masses are common in pediatric patients, and frequently more than one imaging modality will be used to identify and diagnose a given abdominal mass. Plain radiographs of the abdomen remain an important component of the early investigation of an abdominal mass, primarily for the purpose of detecting calcifications and the effect of the mass on surrounding structures such as the bones or the gastrointestinal tract. A general idea of the possible organ of origin can be gleaned if the mass is visible radiographically (Fig. 3.1). However, more detailed analysis of abdominal masses requires some type of sectional imaging. Ultrasound can quickly provide important information regarding the organ of origin and allows some degree of tissue characterization. Therefore, it is usually the screening procedure of choice for abdominal masses in children. The main drawbacks of ultrasound are that it is operator dependent and that abdominal gas can interfere with the quality of images. Nevertheless, in many cases ultrasound will establish the diagnosis, and if the mass is small, further imaging may not be necessary. For larger, ill-defined, or poorly visualized masses, CT or MRI can be helpful. Both modalities provide superior delineation of the margins and extent of abdominal masses. Vascular involvement is best demonstrated with ultrasound or MRI. Gastrointestinal contrast studies may be used for masses arising from the stomach or intestines, but if the lesion is believed to be in the mesentery, CT, MRI, or ultrasound are more productive. Intravenous urography and angiography now are seldom used for the investigation of pediatric abdominal masses.

When evaluating an abdominal mass with plain radiographs, one must be aware of certain common pseudomasses. The commonest of these are the fluid-filled stomach or urinary bladder (Fig. 3.2A–C). Another pseudomass commonly seen in infancy is an umbilical hernia (Fig. 3.2D), which can appear bubbly when the hernia contains air-filled intestine. A similar central pseudomass can be seen in infants with a meningocele or meningomyelocele, and in neonates with an umbilical stump. Less common causes of a pseudomass include fluid-filled loops of intestine, colostomy or ileostomy sites, and superficial skin lesions such as hemangiomas and neurofibromas.

A complete discussion of the imaging characteristics of pediatric abdominal masses is beyond the scope of this text, but the major differentiating findings for the more common masses are presented. The masses are grouped according to the findings that might be seen on radiographs or at ultrasound, specifically, the organ of origin and the degree of echogenicity.

Renal and Adrenal Masses

Tumors account for the majority of renal masses found in pediatric patients (Table 3.1). Although most are solid tumors, it is quite common for these masses to appear sonographically complex, exhibiting a variable degree of cystic change within the tumor. In the newborn and young infant the most common renal tumor is mesoblastic nephroma. This tumor is generally considered to be benign, but cases of metastasis have been reported (12). Sonographically, mesoblastic nephroma is seen as a well-defined intrarenal mass that is predominantly solid (Fig. 3.3A), although areas of hemorrhage and cystic de-

ZONES

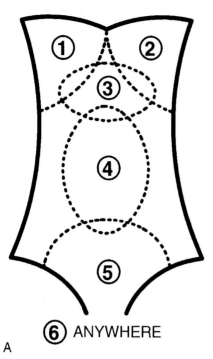

A

ABDOMINAL MASSES

ZONE	MOST LIKELY CAUSE OR ORGAN OF ORIGIN	
1	Liver	(++++)
	Gallbladder	(++++)
	Bile Duct	(++++)
	Duodenum	(++)
	Adrenal	(+)
2	Spleen	(++++)
	Stomach	(++++)
	Adrenal	(+)
3	Adrenal	(++++)
	Pancreas	(++++)
	Liver	(++++)
	Stomach	(++++)
	Kidney	(++)
4	Kidney	(++++)
	Adrenal	(++)
	Retroperit Tumor	(++++)
5	Bladder	(++++)
	Uterus-Vagina	(++++)
	Ovaries	(++++)
	Presacral Masses	(++++)
6	Mesenteric Cysts	(++++)
	Omental Cysts	(++++)
	Duplication Cysts	(++++)

B

Figure 3.1. Abdominal masses. The abdomen has been divided into zones. The most likely organs of origin are outlined for each zone.

generation within the mass are not uncommon (4, 5, 11). Calcification within the mass is a rare occurrence (9).

Wilms tumor is the most common renal neoplasm of childhood, and although it is a malignant tumor, its imaging characteristics are indistinguishable from those of mesoblastic nephroma. Wilms tumor is usually well encapsulated, and can be entirely solid or contain numerous cystic areas (Fig. 3.3B–D). The imaging workup of Wilms tumor should include a close inspection of the contralateral kidney, because bilateral tumors can occur in as many 5 to 10% of patients (Fig. 3.3E). Interesting clinical findings that have been associated with Wilms tumor in some patients are aniridia, hemihypertrophy, and the Beckwith-Weidemann syndrome. This tumor can extend through the renal vein into the inferior vena cava and even the right atrium, findings that are probably best evaluated with ultrasound.

Renal cell carcinoma is an uncommon renal tumor in children, although it is somewhat more common in older children and adolescents. Renal cell carcinoma carries a much graver prognosis than Wilms tumor. Clear cell sarcoma (14, 23) and malignant rhabdoid tumor of the kidney (21) are two rare but extremely aggressive neoplasms that occur in child-

hood. Leukemic or lymphomatous involvement of the kidneys most often results in diffuse infiltration and enlargement of the kidneys; however, occasionally a lymphoma can be seen as a solitary mass or as multiple nodules (25). Other renal tumors are extremely rare and include the benign juxtaglomerular cell tumor, angiomyolipoma (usually in patients with tuberous sclerosis) (18), lymphangioma, and teratoma.

Urinary tract infections are common in children and can diffusely or focally involve the renal parenchyma. Focal bacterial nephritis (acute lobar nephronia) causes a focal area of edema within the kidney that can be mistaken for a mass. Such focal infections must be differentiated from a renal abscess, which often requires drainage in addition to antibiotic therapy. Usually a renal abscess appears more cystic or complex than focal nephritis (Fig. 3.3F). Other cystic masses of the renal parenchyma include the benign multilocular cyst and its malignant counterpart, epithelial nephroblastoma. Both tumors appear as multiloculated, well-encapsulated, predominantly cystic lesions (Fig. 3.3G), although epithelial nephroblastoma is generally associated with a greater amount of solid, polypoid material within the cysts (3). Simple renal cysts are much less common in children than in adults but are probably more

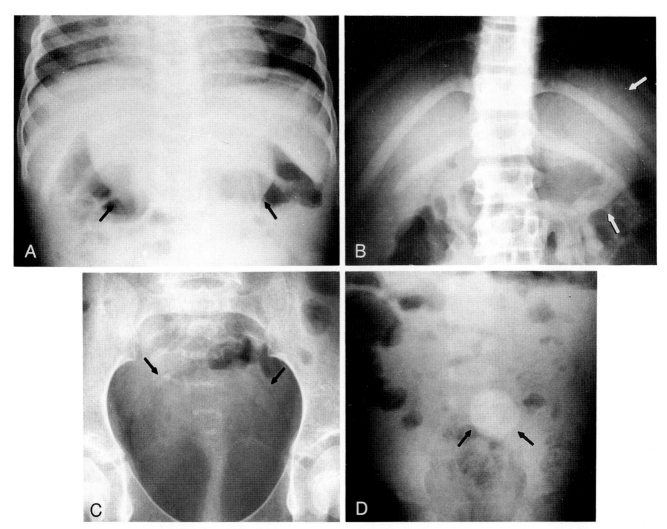

Figure 3.2. Abdominal pseudotumors. A. Fluid-filled stomach *(arrows),* in upright position, producing a pseudomass. **B.** Pseudomass produced by food in fundus of stomach *(arrows).* **C.** Pseudomass produced by distended normal urinary bladder *(arrows).* **D.** Pseudomass produced by umbilical hernia *(arrows).* A similar pseudomass can be seen with meningoceles.

Table 3.1
Renal Masses

Wilms tumor[a]	}	Common
Mesoblastic nephroma[a]		
Lobar nephronia[a]/abscess[b]	}	Moderately common
Simple cyst[b]		
Multilocular cyst[b]		
Epithelial nephroblastoma[b]	}	Uncommon
Renal cell carcinoma[a]		
Lymphoma[a]		
Rhabdoid tumor[a]		
Clear cell sarcoma[a]		
Angiomyolipoma[a]		
Juxtaglomerular cell tumor[a]	}	Rare
Lymphangioma[b]		
Teratoma[a]		

[a] Solid or complex.
[b] Cystic.

common than was previously suspected (17). Such cysts can occur in the peripheral renal cortex or in the peripelvic region of the kidney (Fig. 3.3*H*). As previously mentioned, both Wilms tumor and mesoblastic nephroma can be largely cystic and difficult to differentiate from benign multilocular cysts (3).

Suprarenal masses in infants and children most often originate in the adrenal gland (Table 3.2). In the newborn infant, hemorrhage is, by far, the most common cause of an adrenal enlargement or mass. In the early stages following hemorrhage, the hematoma has a characteristic echogenic appearance. During the following week, as the hematoma resolves, the mass becomes hypoechoic to anechoic and decreases in size (Fig. 3.4*A* and *B*). It is important to follow an adrenal hemorrhage until significant resolution is seen, because occasionally hemorrhage can

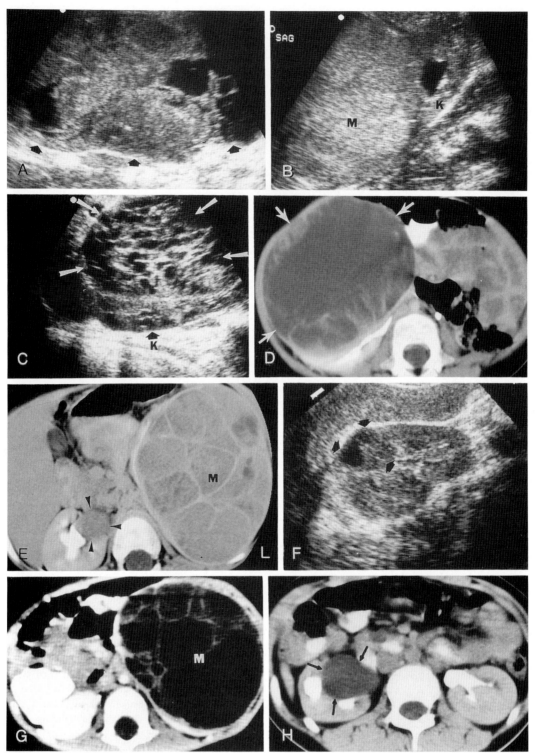

Figure 3.3. **Renal masses. A. Mesoblastic nephroma.** Ultrasound shows this mass to be predominantly solid with several internal cystic areas *(arrows)*. **B. Wilms tumor.** Note the large solid mass *(M)* arising from the kidney *(K)*. No clear plane is seen between the two structures, and the residual renal tissue wraps around the inferior edge of the mass ("claw" sign). **C.** A different Wilms tumor that demonstrates multiple cystic areas on ultrasound *(arrows)*. Kidney *(K)*. **D.** CT of the patient in Part **C** more clearly demonstrates the extent of the large, predominantly cystic tumor arising from the right kidney *(arrows)*. **E. Bilateral Wilms tumors.** Note the large, encapsulated mass arising from the left kidney *(M)*. This mass contains a number of internal lobules and several areas of cystic change. Also note the small tumor in the right kidney *(arrowheads)*. **F. Abscess.** Note the complex mass involving the upper portion of the kidney *(arrows)*. **G. Multilocular cyst.** Note the large, multiseptated cystic mass arising from the left kidney *(M)*. **H. Parapelvic renal cyst.** This large central simple cyst *(arrows)* resulted in partial obstruction of the collecting system and subsequent stone formation.

Table 3.2
Adrenal Enlargement/Mass

Adrenal hemorrhage Neuroblastoma/ganglioneuroma	} Common
Adrenal cortical hyperplasia	} Moderately common
Adrenocortical carcinoma Cortical adenoma Pheochromocytoma Congenital cyst Abscess Wolman disease	} Rare

occur in a neonatal adrenal tumor such as neuroblastoma. In such cases, adrenal enlargement will not resolve completely.

After the newborn period, masses in the adrenal gland represent an adrenal tumor, primarily one of the neuroblastoma-ganglioneuroma group of neoplasms. These tumors are of neural crest origin and exhibit a variable degree of malignancy. Although the benign ganglioneuroma tends to be more well-defined than the aggressive neuroblastoma, in general benign and malignant tumors cannot be reliably differentiated by their imaging characteristics. Neuroblastoma classically is a poorly defined, heterogeneous, echogenic mass (Fig. 3.4E). The presence of a distinct echogenic nodule at ultrasound has been suggested as a specific finding in neuroblastoma (1). Rarely, neuroblastoma will appear cystic at ultrasound (2, 6). Occasionally, a hydronephrotic upper pole moiety of a duplex kidney can mimic a cystic suprarenal mass. Other primary tumors of the adrenal gland are rare in children. Adrenal cortical carcinoma is usually a functional tumor that frequently results in virilization. The tumor tends to be highly aggressive and occasionally exhibits calcification (19, 20). Carcinomas are somewhat more common than adrenal adenomas, which have been reported in association with Gardner syndrome and multiple endocrine neoplasia type I. Pheochromocytomas and congenital adrenal cysts (Fig. 3.4F) are also rare in pediatric patients.

An enlarged but otherwise normal adrenal gland can be seen with adrenocortical hyperplasia. Usually the adrenal enlargement is bilateral (22) and the infant demonstrates genital ambiguity due to the adrenogenital syndrome. The adrenal can also appear enlarged when the ipsilateral kidney is congenitally absent or markedly hypoplastic (Fig. 3.4C). Both adrenal enlargement and hemorrhage have been reported in patients receiving corticotropin (ACTH) therapy for infantile spasms or inflammatory bowel disease (15, 16). Wolman disease is a rare hereditary

abnormality of lipid metabolism that causes enlarged and densely calcified adrenal glands. Adrenal abscesses are also quite rare but can develop in newborn infants with sepsis.

Other retroperitoneal masses are uncommon, except for lymph node involvement with leukemia or lymphoma. The retroperitoneum is one of the more common locations for a teratoma, but teratomas are more likely to occur in the sacrococcygeal region than in the upper retroperitoneum (8). Other benign neoplasms of the retroperitoneum include lipomas (10, 24), hemangiomas, lymphangiomas (7), and neurofibromas.

REFERENCES

1. Amundson GM, Trevenen CL, Mueller DL, Rubin SZ, Wesenberg RL: Neuroblastoma: a specific sonographic tissue pattern. AJR 148:943–945, 1987.
2. Atkinson GO Jr, Zaatari GS, Lorenzo RL, Gay BB Jr, Garvin AJ: Cystic neuroblastoma in infants: radiographic and pathologic features. AJR 146:113–117, 1986.
3. Beckwith JB, Kiviat NB: Multilocular renal cysts and renal tumors. AJR 136:435–436, 1981.
4. Berdon WE, Wigger HJ, Baker DH: Benign tumor to be distinguished from Wilms' tumor: report of 3 cases. AJR 118:18–27, 1973.
5. Christmann D, Becmeur F, Marcellin L, Dhaoui R, Roy E, Sauvage P, Walter JP: Mesoblastic nephroma presenting as a haemorrhagic cyst. Pediatr Radiol 20:553, 1990.
6. Croitoru DP, Sinsky AB, Laberge J-M: Cystic neuroblastoma. J Pediatr Surg 27:1320–1321, 1992.
7. Davidson AJ, Hartman DS: Lymphangioma of the retroperitoneum: CT and sonographic characteristics. Radiology 175:507–510, 1990.
8. Davidson AJ, Hartman DS, Goldman SM: Mature teratoma of the retroperitoneum: radiologic, pathologic, and clinical correlation. Radiology 172:421–425, 1989.
9. Fernbach SK, Schlesinger AE, Gonzalez-Crussi F: Calcification and ossification in a congenital mesoblastic nephroma. Urol Radiol 7:165–167, 1985.
10. Fisher MF, Fletcher BD, Dahms BB, Haller JO, Friedman AP: Abdominal lipoblastomatosis: radiographic, echographic, and computed tomographic findings. Radiology 138:593–596, 1981.
11. Grider RD, Wolverson MK, Jagannadharao B, Graviss ER, O'Conner DM: Congenital mesoblastic nephroma with cystic component. J Clin Ultrasound 9:43–45, 1981.
12. Heidelberger KP, Ritchey ML, Dauser RC, McKeever PE, Beckwith JB: Congenital mesoblastic nephroma metastatic to the brain. Cancer 72:2499–2502, 1993.
13. Iyer R, Efekhari F, Varma D, Jaffe N: Cystic retroperitoneal lymphangioma: CT, ultrasound and MR findings. Pediatr Radiol 23:305–306, 1993.
14. Khalil RM, Aubel S: Clear cell sarcoma of the kidney: a case report. Pediatr Radiol 23: 407–408, 1993.
15. Levin TL, Morton E: Adrenal hemorrhage complicating ACTH therapy in Crohn's disease. Pediatr Radiol 23:457–458, 1993.
16. Liebling MS, Starc TJ, McAlister WH, Ruzal-Shapiro CB, Abramson SJ, Berdon WE: ACTH induced adrenal en-

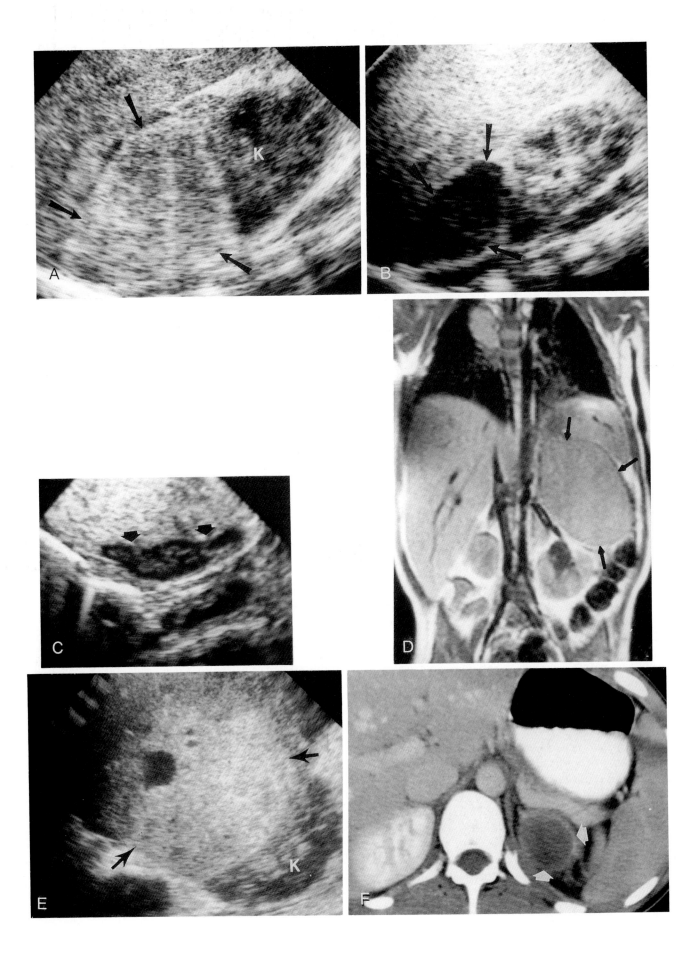

largement in infants treated for infantile spasms and acute cerebellar encephalopathy. *Pediatr Radiol* 23:454–456, 1993.

17. McHugh K, Stringer DA, Hebert D, Babiak CA: Simple renal cysts in children: diagnosis and follow-up with US. *Radiology* 178:383, 1991.

18. Narla LD, Slovis TL, Watts FB, Nigro M: The renal lesions of tuberous sclerosis (cysts and angiomyolipoma): screening with sonography and computerized tomography. *Pediatr Radiol* 18:205–209, 1988.

19. Prando A, Wallace S, Marins JL, Pereira RM, de Oliveira ER: Sonographic finding of adrenal cortical carcinomas in children. *Pediatr Radiol* 20:163–165, 1990.

20. Sabbaga CC, Avilla SA, Schulz C, Garbers JC, Blucher D: Adrenocortical carcinoma in children: clinical aspects and prognosis. *J Pediatr Surg* 28:841–843, 1993.

21. Sisler CL, Siegel MJ: Malignant rhabdoid tumor of the kidney: radiologic features. *Radiology* 172:211–212, 1989.

22. Sivit CJ, Hung W, Taylor GA, Catena LM, Brown-Jones C, Kushner DC: Sonography in neonatal congenital adrenal hyperplasia. *AJR* 156:141–143, 1991.

23. Sleight G, Lock MM: Clear cell sarcoma of the kidney: a renal tumor of childhood that metastasizes to bone. *AJR* 146:64–66, 1986.

24. Sullivan WG, Wesenberg RL, Lilly JR: Giant retroperitoneal lipoma in children. *Pediatrics* 66:123–125, 1980.

25. Weinberger E, Rosenbaum DM, Pendergrass TW: Renal involvement in children with lymphoma: comparison of CT with sonography. *AJR* 155:347–349, 1990.

Presacral Masses

Masses that are found in the presacral space often represent some form of neoplasm (Table 3.3). Sacrococcygeal teratoma is the most common tumor in this region and occurs primarily in the newborn and young infant. Teratomas (and dermoids) are complex masses that consist of elements of all three dermal layers. Calcifications can occur in as many as 60% of these tumors, and such calcifications frequently take the form of teeth or bones. Fat is also commonly

present within the mass and can be best shown with CT or MRI (Fig. 3.5). Neurogenic tumors (e.g., neuroblastoma, ganglioneuroma, neurofibroma) also occur in this location.

If the sacrum appears destroyed or deformed, the most likely possibilities are a tumor arising from the sacrum (e.g., chordoma) or an anterior sacral meningocele. Meningoceles in this location are frequently associated with anorectal abnormalities such as ectopic anus, and they sometimes occur in patients with neurofibromatosis. Neurenteric cysts occasionally occur in the presacral region and may also be accompanied by sacral defects.

Table 3.3
Presacral Masses

Sacrococcygeal teratoma Obstructed rectum with fecal material	Common
Abscess (ruptured appendix, regional enteritis) Neurogenic tumors Hematoma with trauma	Uncommon
Rhabdomyosarcoma Chordoma of sacrum Anterior meningocele Duplication cyst	Rare

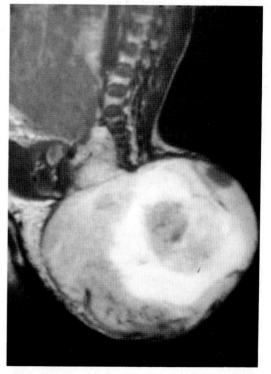

Figure 3.5. Presacral teratoma. This large mass extends from the presacral space and possesses variable areas of signal intensity due to the presence of fluid, calcification, and fat.

Figure 3.4. Adrenal masses or enlargement. A. Adrenal hemorrhage. Ultrasound of the abdomen of a 1-day-old neonate reveals a large echogenic mass *(arrows)* displacing and compressing the kidney *(K)*. This represents an acute adrenal hemorrhage. **B.** Ultrasound of the same infant 4 days later reveals that the hemorrhage has decreased in size and has become hypoechoic *(arrows)*. This is the characteristic appearance of a resolving hemorrhage. **C.** Apparent enlargement of an otherwise normal adrenal gland *(arrows)* in an infant with ipsilateral renal agenesis. **D. Neuroblastoma—MRI.** Note the large left upper quadrant mass *(arrows)* that displaces the kidney inferiorly. **E.** Ultrasound of another child with neuroblastoma shows a large, predominantly echogenic adrenal mass *(arrows)*, with a few small cystic areas. The kidney *(K)* is compressed by this mass, and renal invasion was found at surgery. **F. Adrenal cysts.** This 12-year-old girl presented with left upper quadrant pain, and CT revealed a partially cystic adrenal mass that at surgery was found to represent a hemorrhagic cyst.

Occasionally, fluid will collect between the rectum and the sacrum and give the appearance of a mass. Abscesses are not rare in this region and are usually associated with a ruptured appendix or regional enteritis. Presacral hematomas can occur following pelvic trauma.

Cystic Abdominal Masses

The list of causes of cystic masses within the abdomen is extensive (Table 3.4), and, again, one must rely on the general location of the mass within the abdomen to help make a diagnosis (see Fig. 3.1). Probably the most common cystic mass in the upper abdomen is actually a markedly hydronephrotic kidney. When hydronephrosis is severe, the renal parenchyma can be very thin and difficult to visualize (Fig. 3.6A). In most cases, the dilated, communicating collecting structures of a hydronephrotic kidney can be distinguished from the multiple noncommunicating cysts that occur in a multicystic dysplastic kidney (Fig. 3.6B). The latter condition is the result of ureteral obstruction during fetal development. The dysplastic renal tissue can be sparse and is usually interspersed between multiple variably sized cysts. Neoplasms of the kidney can undergo cystic degeneration, and in some cases may appear predominantly cystic (see Renal Masses).

Table 3.4
Cystic Abdominal or Pelvic Mass

Hydronephrosis (severe) Multicystic dysplastic kidney Ovarian cyst Abscess	Common
Parasitic cyst Enteric duplication cyst Mesenteric cyst Hydrops of gallbladder Choledochal cyst Urachal cyst Pancreatic pseudocyst Cerebrospinal fluid pseudocyst Teratoma/dermoid Lymphangioma Necrotic tumor Adrenal hemorrhage (resolving) Biloma Renal multilocular cyst	Uncommon
Mesenchymal hamartoma (liver) Cystic hepatoblastoma Cystadenoma (ovary, biliary) Papillary cystic and solid tumor (pancreas)	Rare

The hepatobiliary system is a relatively common site of origin of upper abdominal cysts in children. Massive distension of the gallbladder occurs in acute hydrops of the gallbladder. This condition probably results from transient cystic duct obstruction due to inflammation and frequently is a part of the mucocutaneous lymph node syndrome (4) and HIV infection. Transient distension fo the gallbladder can also occur in infants on parenteral nutrition (1). Choledochal cysts include a variety of types of cystic dilation of the common bile and hepatic ducts. Older children with choledochal cysts classically present with the clinical triad of jaundice, pain, and a right upper quadrant mass; however, the signs and symptoms can be quite variable, particularly in the newborn and young infant. Sonography typically shows a cystic mass in the porta hepatis separate from the gallbladder (Fig. 3.6C). Frequently, dilated intrahepatic bile ducts will also be seen. Tc[99m]-IDA scintigraphy can be used to verify that the cyst communicates with the biliary system. Cysts of the hepatic parenchyma may be congenital or acquired, and acquired cysts are usually the result of infection (e.g., echinococcal cysts, amebic abscess, bacterial abscess) (Fig. 3.6D) or trauma (i.e., resolving hematoma). Congenital hepatic cysts may be single or multiple. Solitary congenital cysts frequently are isolated lesions, and are rarely of clinical significance unless massive enlargement occurs (2). Multiple hepatic cysts are frequently seen in patients with autosomal dominant polycystic kidney disease.

Developmental cysts arising from the gastrointestinal tract or mesentery are not rare. Gastrointestinal duplication cysts characteristically demonstrate a wall that consists of an inner echogenic layer and a thin outer hypoechoic layer, which are analogous to the layers seen sonographically in the normal wall of the stomach or intestines (3). This may help to differentiate duplications from other simple walled cysts in the abdomen (Fig. 3.6E and F). Pancreatic pseudocysts (Fig. 3.6G) usually are the result of blunt abdominal trauma in children and frequently are a complication of child abuse (8). Other causes of pancreatitis in children include infections (10) (usually viral), steroid therapy, anomalies of the bile ducts, cystic fibrosis (9), hereditary pancreatitis (15), and, occasionally, idiopathic causes (11). Solid and cystic papillary tumor of the pancreas is a rare type of pancreatic tumor in children (Fig. 3.6H) (13). In children with ventriculoperitoneal shunts, adhesions within the abdomen can cause the cerebrospinal fluid to collect around the shunt tip, forming a multiseptated cyst (Fig. 3.6I).

The most common cysts arising in the pelvis are

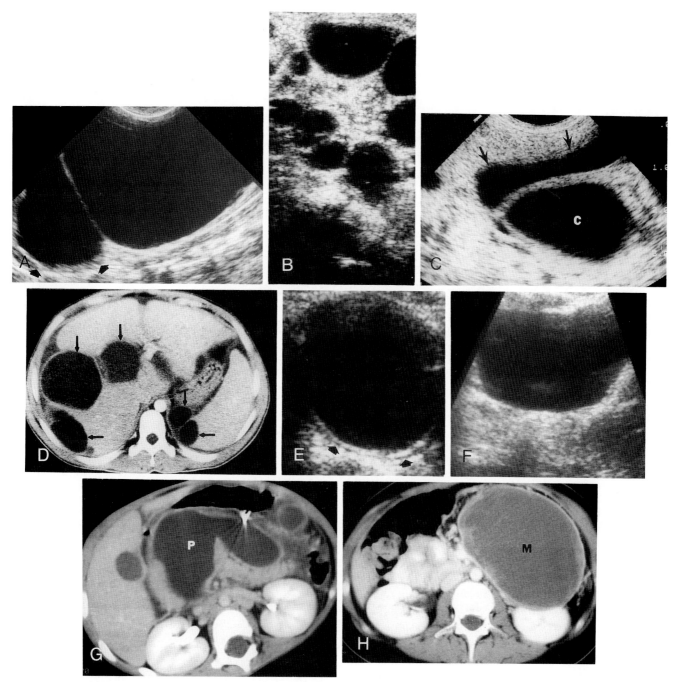

Figure 3.6. Cystic abdominal masses. A. Massive hydronephrosis in an infant with ureteropelvic junction obstruction. The markedly thinned renal parenchyma is barely visible over the upper pole *(arrows).* **B. Multicystic dysplastic kidney.** Note the multiple cysts of variable sizes with a small amount of intervening dysplastic renal tissue. **C. Choledochal cyst.** Note the large, oval cyst *(C),* adjacent to, but separate from, the gallbladder *(arrows).* **D.** Multiple cysts *(arrows)* in and around the liver and spleen, due to disseminated **echinococcal** disease following at-

tempted surgical drainage. **E. Intestinal duplication cyst.** Note the double layered appearance of the wall *(arrows).* **F. Mesenteric cyst.** Ultrasound shows a simple, single-layered wall in this cyst that was discovered incidentally after abdominal trauma. **G.** This large pancreatic pseudocyst *(P)* was the result of blunt abdominal trauma due to child abuse. The cyst was successfully drained percutaneously. **H. Cystic and solid papillary tumor of the kidney.** Note the large, predominantly cystic mass *(M)* that arose from the tail of the pancreas *(continued).*

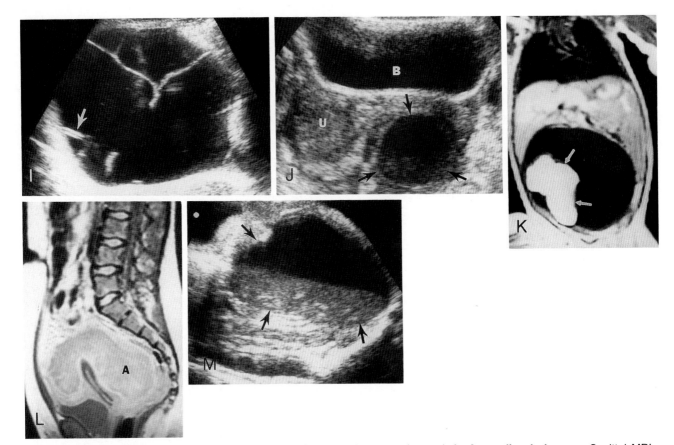

Figure 3.6. Cystic abdominal masses (continued). I. Cerebrospinal fluid pseudocyst. This multiseptated cyst formed around the abdominal tip of the ventriculoperitoneal shunt *(arrow)*. **J. Ovarian cyst.** The left adnexal cyst *(arrows)* shows internal echoes due to hemorrhage. Uterus *(U)*, bladder *(B)*. **K. Cystic teratoma.** MRI demonstrates the large, predominantly cystic abdominal mass. A large area of fat was also found within the tumor *(arrows)*. **L. Appendiceal abscess.** Sagittal MRI reveals a large complex mass surrounding the uterus that represented an indolent abscess following appendiceal perforation. This patient exhibited only minimal symptoms from this abscess. **M. Hydrometrocolpos.** Note the markedly enlarged, fluid-filled vagina *(arrows)*. A fluid/debris level can also be seen.

simple follicular cysts of the ovary. These occur most commonly in adolescents (Fig. 3.6*J*); however, they are also occasionally found in newborn infants, probably because of the influence of maternal hormones (12). Such cysts frequently resolve spontaneously (16), but in some cases rupture or undergo torsion (7). Teratomas and dermoids are the most common cystic neoplasms arising from the ovary (Fig. 3.6*K*) (6). These masses vary from completely cystic masses to very complex masses containing cystic and solid components, including formed calcifications (14) (see Fig. 3.14*A*). Cystadenomas of the ovary are much less common in children than in adults (5). Abscesses also can appear cystic (Fig. 3.6*L*). Hydrometrocolpos due to congenital vaginal obstruction can be encountered in the newborn period or around puberty (Fig. 3.6*L*). Often the dilated vagina and uterus are filled with blood, causing homogeneous echogenicity on ultrasound.

REFERENCES

1. Arad I, Peleg O, Udassin R, et al: Gallbladder distention in premature neonates receiving parenteral nutrition. *J Perinat Med* 17:337–340, 1989.
2. Athey PA, Lauderman JA, King DE: Massive congenital solitary nonparasitic cyst of the liver in infancy. *J Ultrasound Med* 5:585–587, 1986.
3. Barr LL, Hayden CK Jr, Stansberry SD, Swischuk LE: Enteric duplication cysts in children: are ultrasonographic wall characteristics diagnostic? *Pediatr Radiol* 20:326–328, 1990.
4. Bradford BF, Reid BS, Weinstein BJ, Oh KS, Girdany BR: Ultrasonographic evaluation of the gallbladder in mucocutaneous lymph node syndrome. *Radiology* 142:381–384, 1982.
5. Brown MF, Hebra A, McGeehin K, Ross AJ III: Ovarian masses in children: a review of 91 cases of malignant and benign masses. *J Pediatr Surg* 28:930–932, 1993.
6. Buy J-N, Ghossain MA, Moss AA, Bazot M, Doucet M, Hugol D, Truc JB, Poitout P, Ecoiffier J: Cystic teratoma of the ovary: CT detection. *Radiology* 171:697–701, 1989.
7. Currarino G, Rutledge JC: Ovarian torsion and amputa-

tion resulting in partially calcified, pedunculated cystic mass. *Pediatr Radiol* 19:395–399, 1989.

8. Dahman B, Stephens CA: Pseudocysts of the pancreas after blunt abdominal trauma in children. *J Pediatr Surg* 16:17–21, 1981.
9. Daneman A, Gaskin K, Martin DJ, Cutz E: Pancreatic changes in cystic fibrosis: CT and sonographic appearance. *AJR* 141:653–655, 1983.
10. Eichelberger MR, Hoelzer DJ, Koop CE: Acute pancreatitis: the difficulties of diagnosis and therapy. *J Pediatr Surg* 17:244–254, 1982.
11. Ghishan F, Greene HL, Avant G: Chronic relapsing pancreatitis in childhood. *J Pediatr* 102:514–518, 1983.
12. Nussbaum AR, Sanders RC, Hartman DS, Dudegon DL, Parmley TH: Neonatal ovarian cysts: sonographic-pathologic correlation. *Radiology* 168:817–822, 1988.
13. Ohtomo K, Furui S, Onoue M, Okada Y, Kusano S, Shiga J, Suda K: Solid and papillary epithelial neoplasm of the pancreas: MR imaging and pathologic correlation. *Radiology* 184:567–570, 1992.
14. Sisler CL, Siegel MJ: Ovarian teratomas: a comparison of the sonographic appearance in prepubertal and postpubertal girls. *AJR* 154:139–142, 1990.
15. Spencer JA, Lindsell DRM, Isaacs D: Hereditary pancreatitis: early ultrasound appearance. *Pediatr Radiol* 20:293–295, 1990.
16. Warner BW, Kuhn JC, Barr LL: Conservative management of large ovarian cysts in children: the value of serial pelvic ultrasonography. *Surgery* 112:749–755, 1992.

Liver Masses and Lesions

Liver masses in infants and children are uncommon but are by no means rare (Table 3.5) (2). In newborns and young infants, benign tumors predominate (11), and the most common of these are the hemangioendothelioma and hemangioma. These vascular neoplasms exhibit variable ultrasound characteristics, and diagnosis frequently requires that more than one imaging study be performed (Fig. 3.7A and B). CT, MRI, nuclear scintigraphy, or arteriography have all been used with variable degrees of success (9, 11). Hemangiomas and hemangioendotheliomas may be solitary or multiple, and when multiple or large, they occasionally result in high output cardiac failure. Mesenchymal hamartoma is a less common benign primary tumor of the liver that usually is primarily cystic but can sometimes be more complex (Fig. 3.7C) (4, 14, 16, 17). Hepatic adenomas occur infrequently in childhood, but can be found in association with glycogen storage disease type I or Fanconi's anemia. Angiomyolipomas in patients with tuberous sclerosis and focal nodular hyperplasia are rare lesions in the pediatric population.

In older infants and children, malignant liver tumors become more common than the benign neoplasms. Metastatic disease occurs more frequently than primary hepatic malignancies, and neuroblastoma is the most common childhood tumor to metastasize to the liver. The vast majority of primary hepatic malignant tumors consist of hepatoblastoma and hepatocellular carcinoma (6, 10). Hepatoblastoma occurs almost exclusively in children less than 3 years of age, whereas hepatocellular carcinoma occurs in older children with peaks at 4 years of age and in adolescence. Hepatoblastoma most commonly is seen as a large solitary mass, and hepatocellular carcinoma can be solitary but is more likely to be multicentric than hepatoblastoma. Preexisting liver disease (e.g., biliary atresia, glycogen storage disease, chronic hepatitis, and other causes of cirrhosis) predisposes children to the development of hepatocellular carcinoma, although this occurs much less frequently in children than in the adults. Fibrolamellar hepatocarcinoma is a subtype of hepatocarcinoma that occurs in children and is associated with a significantly better prognosis. Rare malignant neoplasms of the liver in children include embryonal sarcoma (Fig. 3.7D) (15), rhabdomyosarcoma of the bile ducts (1, 5), mixed mesenchymal sarcoma, and teratocarcinoma. Ultrasound, CT, and MRI are all excellent methods for identifying malignant neoplasms of the liver, but the imaging characteristics of these tumors are nonspecific and do not permit differentiation of one malignancy from another. Ultrasound is an excellent means of evaluating the hepatic and portal veins for signs of tumor invasion, which has been noted to occur more frequently in hepatocellular carcinoma. MRI is especially useful in

Table 3.5
Liver Masses and Lesions

Hemangioma/hemangioendothelioma Hepatoblastoma Infection/abscess Hematoma Metastases	Relatively common
Mesenchymal hamartoma Embryonal sarcoma Hepatocellular carcinoma Lymphoma/leukemia Biliary tract neoplasms	Uncommon
Adenoma Focal nodular hyperplasia Lipoma/angiomyolipoma Peliosis hepatis Rhabdomyosarcoma Mesenchymoma	Rare

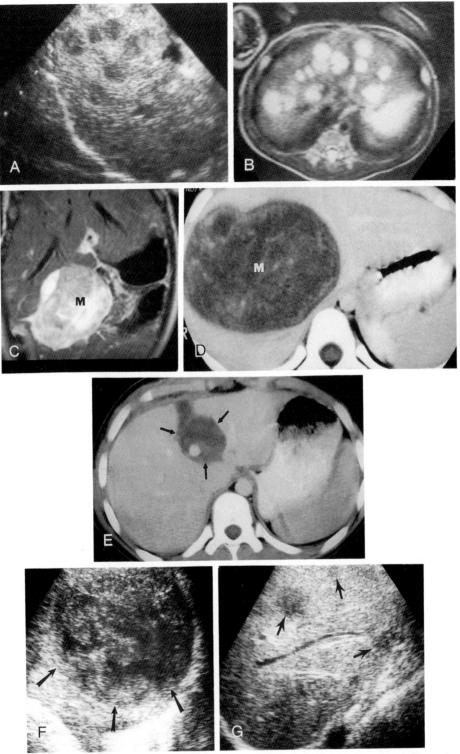

Figure 3.7. Liver masses. A. Hemangioendotheliomas. Ultrasound revealed multiple round, hypoechoic lesions within the liver of this young infant. **B.** On T$_2$-weighted MRI images, the lesions maintain very bright signal intensity. This is a characteristic appearance for hemangiomas and hemangioendotheliomas. **C.** T$_2$-weighted MRI in an 8-month-old infant with fetal alcohol syndrome revealed a large heterogenous mass *(M)* extending from the right lobe of the liver. This mass was found to be a pedunculated hepatic **hamartoma. D.** CT of a large undifferentiated **sarcoma** in a 4-year-old child. The large, well-defined, heterogenous mass *(M)* is nonspecific and could represent other types of malignant hepatic tumors. **E.** This low- attenuation lesion with a high-attenuation internal nodule *(arrows)* was encountered on CT obtained following blunt abdominal trauma. This was found to be a posttraumatic **biloma. F. Amebic abscess.** Note the large, round, complex hepatic mass *(arrows)*. **G. Cat-scratch disease.** Note several poorly defined hypoechoic lesions within the liver *(arrows)*. Similar lesions were also found within the spleen.

evaluating tumor resectability and for identifying postoperative tumor recurrence (3).

Hepatic trauma is common in childhood and can result in mass-like lesions within the liver due to hemorrhage or bile extravasation (Fig. 3.7*E*). Hepatic abscesses and inflammatory lesions in children are usually due to hematogenous infection. Pyogenic infections secondary to generalized sepsis are probably most common (Fig. 3.7*F*), and *Staphylococcus aureus* is the most frequently isolated organism (12). Echinococcal cysts and amebic abscesses (7, 8) are also quite common in endemic areas. Immunocompromised children commonly develop disseminated candidiasis and other fungal infections that can involve the liver. The spleen is often also involved, and similar hepatic and splenic lesions can be seen in children with cat-scratch disease (13) (Fig. 3.7*G*).

REFERENCES

1. Arnaud O, Boscq M, Asquier E, Michel J: Embryonal rhabdomyosaroma of the biliary tree in children: case report. *Pediatr Radiol* 17:250–251, 1987.
2. Boechat MI, Kangarloo H, Gilsanz V: Hepatic masses in children. *Semin Roentgenol* 23:185–193, 1988.
3. Boechat MI, Kangarloo H, Ortega J, Hall T, Feig S, Stanley P, Gilsanz V: Primary liver tumors in children: comparison of CT and Mr imaging. *Radiology* 169:727–732, 1988.
4. Federici S, Galli G, Sciutti R, Cuoghi O: Cystic mesenchymal hamartoma of the liver. *Pediatr Radiol* 22:307, 1992.
5. Goeffray A, Couanet D, Montagne JP: Ultrasonography and computed tomography for diagnosis and follow-up of biliary duct rhabdomyosarcomas in children. *Pediatr Radiol* 17, 127, 1987.
6. Giacomantonio M, Ein SH, Mancer K, Stephens CA: Thirty years of experience with pediatric primary malignant liver tumors. *J Pediatr Surg* 19:523–525, 1984.
7. Hayden CK, Jr., Toups M, Swischuk LE, Amparo EG: Sonographic features of hepatic amebiasis in childhood. *J Can Assoc Radiol* 35:279–282, 1984.
8. Juimo AG, Gervez F, Angwafo FF: Extraintestinal amebiasis. *Radiology* 182:181–183, 1992.
9. Klein MA, Slovis TL, Chang C-H, et al: Sonographic and Doppler features of infantile hepatic hemangiomas with pathologic correlation. *J Ultrasound Med* 9:619, 1990.
10. Miller JH, Greenspan BS: Integrated imaging of hepatic tumors in childhood. Part I: malignant lesions (primary and metastatic). *Radiology* 154:83–90, 1985.
11. Miller JH, Greenspan BS: Integrated imaging of hepatic tumors of childhood. Part II: benign lesions (congenital, reparative, and inflammatory). *Radiology* 154:91–100, 1985.
12. Oleszczuk-Raszke K, Cremin BJ, Fisher RM: Ultrasonic features of pyogenic and amebic hepatic abscesses. *Pediatr Radiol* 19:230–233, 1989.
13. Rappaport DC, Cumming WA, Ros PR: Case report. Disseminated hepatic and splenic lesions in cat-scratch disease: imaging features. *AJR* 156:1227–1228, 1991.
14. Ros PR, Goodman ZD, Ishak KG, Dachman AH, Olmsted WW, Hartman DS, Lichtenstein JE: Mesenchymal hamartoma of the liver: radiologic-pathologic correlation. *Radiology* 158:619–624, 1986.
15. Ros PR, Olmsted WW, Dachman AH, Goodman ZD, Ishak KG, Hartman DS: Undifferentiated (embryonal) sarcoma of the liver: radiologic-pathologic correlation. *Radiology* 161:141–145, 1986.
16. Rosenbaum DM, Mindell HJ: Ultrasonographic findings in mesenchymal hamartoma of the liver. *Radiology* 138:425–427, 1981.
17. Stanley P, Hall TR, Wooley MM, Diament MJ, Gilsanz V, Miller JH: Mesenchymal hamartomas of the liver in childhood: sonographic and CT findings. *AJR* 147:1035–1039, 1986.

Abdominal Calcifications and Other Opacities

Abdominal calcifications occur in both infants and children, and can be classified by shape as (a) irregular, amorphous, or flocculent, (b) curvilinear, (c) punctate, (d) stone or stonelike, and (e) formed (Table 3.6).

IRREGULAR AMORPHOUS OR FLOCCULENT CALCIFICATIONS

This type of calcification primarily is seen with tumor necrosis, infection, inflammation, venous thrombosis, hemorrhage, or infarction. Necrosis within a tumor is a common cause, and most often occurs with neuroblastoma and its benign counterpart, ganglioneuroma (Fig. 3.8*A*). These calcifications can be finely granular or more irregular and flocculent, and are found in as many as 60% of primary abdominal neuroblastomas. Much less frequently, amorphous calcifications are seen with other intraabdominal tumors (e.g., hepatoblastoma, hepatic hemangioma, dermoid or teratoma (Fig. 3.8*B* and *C*), Wilms tumor, and other adrenal tumors.

Postinflammatory irregular calcifications can occur in lymph nodes (Fig 3.8*E*) and in the liver (9) and spleen. Less commonly, they occur in the kidney and, rarely, in the prostate gland (12). Postinflammatory or catheterization-induced calcifications in the liver can be seen in neonates and can remain after the newborn period (1, 26, 27). Posthemorrhagic calcifications can occur in any organ, but most commonly are seen in the adrenal gland. Such hemorrhage occurs at birth and the resulting calcification often is discovered as an incidental finding. In some cases, the calcification can be curvilinear, outlining the triangular shape of the adrenal gland. These features, together with the characteristic location, virtually assure the diagnosis (Fig. 3.8*D*).

Table 3.6
Intraabdominal Calcifications and Opacities

Irregular-Flocculent

Tumors (esp. neuroblastoma)[a]	}	Common
Idiopathic adrenal[b]		
Foreign material (pica)[a]	}	Moderately common
Meconium peritonitis[a]		
Liver, postabscess, post-thrombus[b]		
Papillary necrosis (kidney)[b]	}	Uncommon
Lymph nodes[b]		
Infarct (spleen, liver, kidney, intestine)		
Bladder (schistosomiasis, cytoxan)		
Oxalosis (kidney)		
Hamartoma[b]		
Prostate	}	Rare
Necrotic bowel-old[b]		
Infarcted ovary[b]		
Infarcted abdominal testes[b]		
Pancreatitis[a]		

Curvilinear

Cystic tumors		
Posthemorrhagic outline of adrenal gland	}	Moderately common
Residual meconium peritonitis from neonate		
Hydronephrosis	}	Relatively rare
Cystic kidney or other cyst		
Renal cortical necrosis		

Stones or stone-like densities

Fecalith in appendix	}	Common
Urinary tract stones		
Gallstones	}	Moderately common
Ingested pebbles		
Granulomas in spleen, liver		
Phleboliths		
Medullary sponge kidney	}	Rare
Ingested mercury, chromium salts		

Formed calcification

Teratoma, dermoid	}	Common
Staghorn calculi	}	Rare
Fetus-in-fetu	}	Very rare

Miscellaneous-diffuse of organ

Milk of calcium gallbladder or hydronephrotic kidney		
Diffuse kidney (oxalosis, renal tubular acidosis, chronic glomerulonephritis)	}	Rare
Wolman disease (adrenal gland)		
Hemochromatosis (liver)		

[a]Generalized or focal.
[b]Focal.

Other irregular calcifications can be seen in conditions such as renal papillary necrosis (due to sepsis dehydration, collagen vascular disease, sickle cell disease, or diabetes), renal tubular acidosis (distal tubular type), and oxalosis (Fig. 3.9A and B) (5). In addition, intrarenal calcifications can occur with hypercalcemia in conditions such as hyperparathyroidism, hypervitaminosis D, severe osteoporosis, steroid therapy, milk-alkali syndrome, ileal dysfunction (16), and sarcoidosis.

Rarely, focal irregular calcifications can be seen with hamartomas of the liver or spleen, or as residual calcifications from perinatal intestinal ischemia, perforation, or meconium peritonitis. With meconium peritonitis, calcified meconium may be found anywhere in the abdomen as a result of intestinal rupture in utero (Fig. 3.9D). Such calcifications can be focal or diffuse, irregular or curvilinear, and occasionally are found in the scrotum or the thorax. Mobile calcifications can occur with idiopathically amputated ovaries in girls (9), and infarcted intraabdominal testes in infant boys also can calcify. Similar calcifications can occur after infarction in organs such as the liver, spleen, kidney, and intestine. Irregular calcifications of a more diffuse nature occur with chronic pancreatitis. Although this situation is quite rare in children, it can occur in association with cystic fibrosis (11) or hereditary pancreatitis, and the pancreatic distribution of the calcifications is a clue to the diagnosis (Fig. 3.9C). Calcifications secondary to thrombus of the portal vein, inferior vena cava, or renal vein are uncommon (1, 14, 25, 26) and tend to be bullet-shaped (Fig. 3.8D). Rarely, calcifications of the urinary bladder secondary to inflammation (e.g., schistomiasis) or infection (e.g., cytoxan cystitis) also can be encountered.

Although they are not true intraabdominal calcifications, certain ingested materials in the gastrointestinal tract can mimic calcifications. One of the most common causes is dirt eating or pica (6) (Fig. 3.10A), and similar densities can be seen with lead (i.e., paint chips), bismuth-containing medications, and mercury and chromium compounds. The latter two substances tend to form small globules within the gastrointestinal tract (Fig. 3.10B), and the finding is important because heavy metal ingestion can be associated with dire consequences.

CURVILINEAR CALCIFICATIONS

Curvilinear calcifications, apart from those seen with meconium peritonitis (Fig. 3.11C) in the neona-

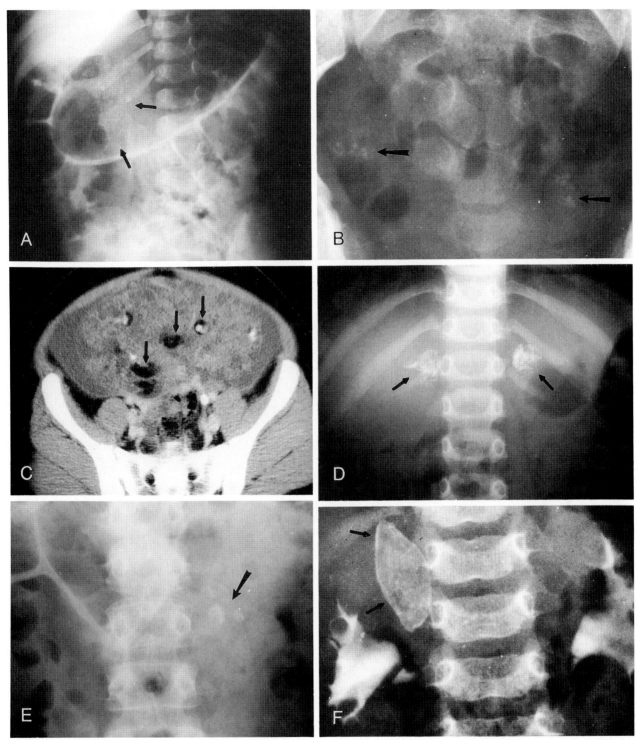

Figure 3.8. Irregular abdominal calcifications. A. Irregular amorphous calcifications within a **ganglioneuroblastoma** *(arrows)*. **B.** Irregular calcifications in bilateral ovarian **dermoids** *(arrows)*. **C.** CT of a large abdominal **teratoma** arising from the ovary. Note the punctate and irregular calcifications and scattered areas of fat *(arrows)* within the mass. **D.** Typical idiopathic (posthemorrhagic) adrenal calcifications *(arrows)*. Note the al-most triangular shape of the right gland. **E.** Irregular calcifications in old, inflamed abdominal lymph nodes *(arrow)*. **F.** Typical bullet-shaped calcification of venous **thrombus** in the inferior vena cava *(arrows)*. (Courtesy of Kassner EG, Baumstark A, Kinkhabwala MN, Ablow RC, Haller JO: Calcified thrombus in the inferior vena cava in infants and children. *Pediatr Radiol* 4:167–171, 1976.

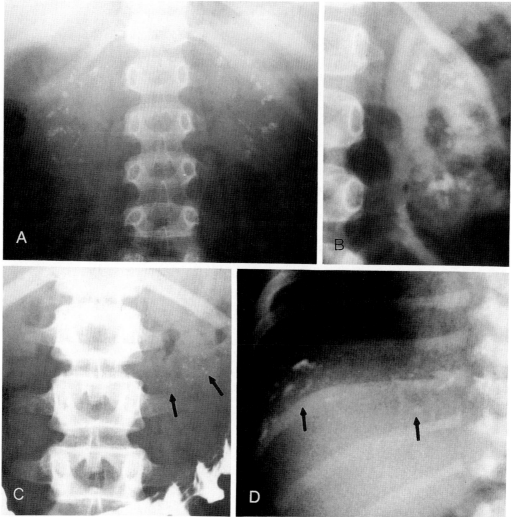

Figure 3.9. Irregular abdominal calcifications. A. Typical irregular calcifications in both kidneys due to **renal tubular acidosis. B.** Plain radiographs showing similar irregular calcifications in patient with **oxalosis.** Also, note diffuse, homogeneous parenchymal calcification of the kidney. **C.** Small scattered calcifications in the pancreas *(arrows)* in this 12-year-old girl with chronic **pancreatitis. D. Meconium peritonitis.** Note the cluster of irregular calcifications representing calcified meconium overlying the superior surface of the liver *(arrows).*

tal period, are quite rare. They can be seen along the periphery of resolving adrenal gland hemorrhages and, on rare occasions, in hydronephrotic or multicystic kidneys (17) (Fig. 3.11A). They also can occur with renal cortical necrosis (18) (Fig. 3.11D) and cystic abdominal tumors, especially adrenal cortical carcinoma (Fig. 3.11B). In renal cortical necrosis, if calcification is incomplete it may appear irregular. On the other hand, when it is extensive and surrounds the kidney, diffuse calcification of the renal parenchyma can be mimicked (Fig. 3.11D).

Very rarely, curvilinear calcifications can be seen in the wall of a urinary bladder due to schistosomiasis or hemorrhagic cystitis after cytoxan therapy.

Clearly, these latter two situations are rare, as are curvilinear calcifications within the blood vessels of the abdomen.

STONES, STONE-LIKE, AND PUNCTATE CALCIFICATIONS

Calcified stones occur in the urinary tract, biliary tract, appendix, and occasionally a Meckel's diverticulum (11). Fecaliths of the appendix are quite common in children and adolescents (Fig. 3.12A) and are often associated with appendicitis. Urinary tract calculi are not uncommon (Fig. 3.12B), and of these, re-

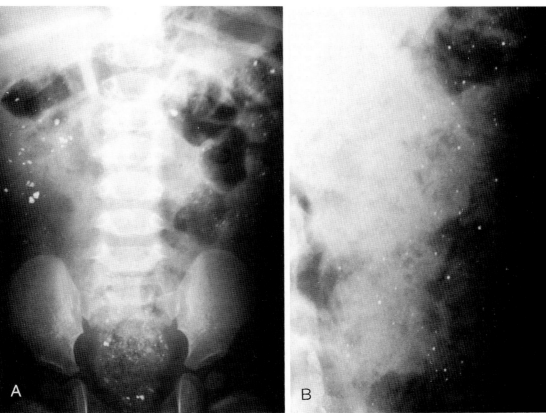

Figure 3.10. Scattered abdominal opacities. A. Diffuse opacities (dirt) scattered throughout the colon in this "dirt eater." Similar densities can be seen with lead paint chip ingestion and bismuth containing medications. **B.** Small globules in the gastrointestinal tract secondary to mercury ingestion.

nal and ureteral stones are the more common types. Bladder stones occur almost exclusively in chronically immobilized children (7) and frequently are quite large (Fig. 3.12C). Calculi in the upper urinary tract, on the other hand, tend to be small and difficult to detect. In children, the majority of renal stones are associated with pre-existing conditions such as congenital urinary tract obstruction and other anomalies, urinary tract infection, prolonged immobilization, or hypercalcemia due to metabolic abnormalities such as idiopathic hypercalcemia, hyperparathyroidism, hypervitaminosis D, milk alkali syndrome, oxalosis (5), and cystinosis (10). Nephrolithiasis is not uncommon in premature infants who receive prolonged diuretic therapy (4). In addition, idiopathic renal stones occur and are more common than generally was appreciated in the past.

Stones in the biliary tract most often are seen in patients with hemolytic anemias (e.g., sickle cell disease), in those receiving total parenteral nutrition, and in pregnant adolescents, but idiopathic cholelithiasis is also fairly common. Cholelithiasis (and more often uncalcified biliary sludge) is not uncommon in infancy, and in some cases resolves spontaneously (8, 15). The cause of gallstones in infants may be related to immature regulation of bile salt secretion. Rarely, gallstones are seen with chronic ileal disease or ileal resection (16), obesity, sepsis, and spinal cord disease. The characteristic location (anterior part of right upper quadrant), multiplicity, and often faceted nature of the stones are the keys to diagnosis (Fig. 3.13A). The diagnosis is easily confirmed with ultrasonography. Calcified pelvic phleboliths, which are so common in adults, rarely are seen in childhood. Actually, when a phlebolith is visualized, it most likely lies within hemangioma or arteriovenous malformation (Fig. 3.13C). The round, bullseye-like appearance of these stones is a strong clue to their origin.

Finally, it should be noted that ingested pebbles can mimic stones (Fig. 3.13B), as can ingested iron and calcium tablets. Iron tablets, when ingested in overdose, are especially important to detect, because they can result in severe gastritis and hemorrhage. Solitary or multiple, punctate calcified granulomas are relatively common in the liver or spleen, and

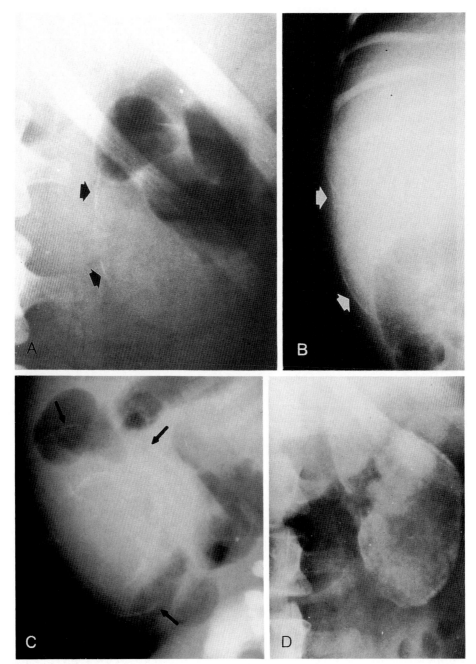

Figure 3.11. Curvilinear calcifications. A. Curvilinear calcification in a **multicystic dysplastic kidney** *(arrows)* in a 13-year-old child. **B.** Curvilinear rim-like calcification in the periphery of an **adrenocortical carcinoma** in a neonate *(arrows)*. **C.** Curvilinear calcifications due to **cystic meconium peritonitis** *(arrows)*. **D.** Curvilinear calcifications outlining the kidney in **renal cortical ne crosis.** Because the rim of calcification surrounds the entire kidney, the renal parenchyma appears almost homogeneously dense. (Part *B* courtesy of Charles Hendrick, M.D., Amarillo, Texas.)

usually are due to healed tuberculosis or histoplasmosis (Fig. 3.13*D*).

FORMED CALCIFICATIONS

Formed calcifications are those that take the form of an actual structure (e.g., bones, teeth). Such calcifications are not particularly common in childhood, but do occur in dermoids or teratomas. Most are located in the pelvis of females and arise from the ovaries (Fig. 3.14*A* and *B*), but they also can be presacral or higher in the retroperitoneum (Fig. 3.14*C*). Many times they also contain fat, and then the diagnosis can be established with confidence. Teeth are

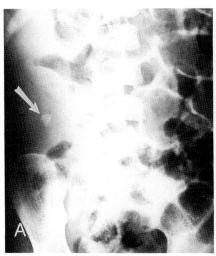
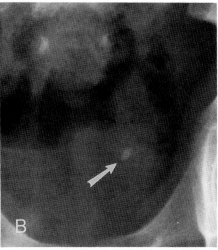
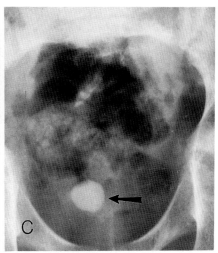

Figure 3.12. Stones and stone-like calcifications. A. Fecalith *(arrow)* in patient with perforated appendicitis. Note the surrounding soft tissue density (abscess) and associated small bowel obstruction. **B.** Ureteral stone *(arrow)* in a young male with renal colic. **C.** Large bladder stone *(arrow)* in a chronically immobilized child as a result of neurologic disease.

easily visualized on plain films, but the fat is better seen with MRI or CT (see Fig. 3.8C). Similar calcifications occur in the rare abdominal "tumor" known as fetus in fetu. This abnormality is believed to represent an aborted monozygotic twin, and can be differentiated from a teratoma when a recognizable vertebral segment or other mature bone is seen (2). Staghorn calculi, mimicking formed calcifications, are rare in children, and almost always occur in chronically immobilized patients or those with severe hypercalcemic states.

MISCELLANEOUS CALCIFICATIONS

Occasionally, very fine, diffuse, and virtually homogeneous calcifications occur. This occurs with milk of calcium in an obstructed, diseased gallbladder (3) and, very rarely, in a hydronephrotic kidney. Fine, diffuse, and homogeneous parenchymal calcifications of the kidney can be seen with oxalosis (see Fig. 3.9B). Similar fine, diffuse amorphous calcifications can occur in the liver in newborns as a result of herpes simplex virus infection (21). A final, peculiar calcification, often very dense, is that which occurs in the enlarged adrenal glands of the storage disease known as Wolman's disease (24).

REFERENCES

1. Ablow RC, Effman EL: Hepatic calcifications associated with umbilical vein catheterization in the newborn infant. *AJR* 114:380–385, 1972.
2. Al-Baghadadi R: Fetus in fetu in the liver: case report and review of the literature. *J Pediatr Surg* 27:1491–1492, 1992.
3. Beauregard WG, Ferguson WT: Milk of calcium cholecystitis. *J Pediatr* 96:876–877, 1980.
4. Blickman JG, Herrin JT, Cleveland RH, Jaramillo D: Co-existing nephrolithiasis and cholelithiasis in premature infants. *Pediatr Radiol* 21:363–364, 1991.
5. Carsen GM, Radkowski MA: Calcium oxalosis: a case report. *Radiology* 113:165–166, 1974.
6. Clayton RS, Goodman PH: Roentgenographic diagnosis of geophagia (dirt eating). *AJR* 73:203, 1955.
7. Conley SB, Shackelford GD, Robson AM: Severe immobilization hypercalcemia renal insufficiency and calcification. *Pediatrics* 63:142–145, 1979.
8. Debray D, Pariente D, Gauthier F, Myara A, Bernard O: Cholelithiasis in infancy: a study of 40 cases. *J Pediatr* 122:385–391, 1993.
9. Fletcher RM, Boat DKB, Karl SR, Gross GW: Ovarian torsion: an unusual cause of bilateral pelvic calcifications. *Pediatr Radiol* 18:172–173, 1988.
10. Gearhart JP, Herzberg GZ, Jeffs RD: Childhood urolithiasis: experiences and advances. *Pediatrics* 87:445–450, 1991.
11. Hirschy JC, Thorpe JJ, Cortese AF: Meckel's stones: a case report. *Radiology* 119:19–20, 1976.
12. Iannaccone G, Antonelli M: Calcification of the pancreas in cystic fibrosis. *Pediatr Radiol* 9:85–89, 1980.
13. Izzidien AY: Prostatic calcification in a 4-year-old boy. *Arch Dis Child* 55:963–968, 1980.
14. Kassner EG, Baumstark A, Kinkhabwala MN, Ablow RC, Haller JO: Calcified thrombus in the inferior vena cava in infants and children. *Pediatr Radiol* 4:167–171, 1976.
15. Keller MS, Markle BM, Laffey PA, Chawla HS, Jacir N, Frank JL: Spontaneous resolution of cholelithiasis in infants. *Radiology* 157:345–348, 1985.
16. Kirks DR: Lithiasis due to interruption of the enterohepatic circulation of bile salts. *AJR* 133:383–388, 1979.
17. Kutcher R, Schneider M, Gordon DH: Calcification in polycystic disease. *Radiology* 122:77–80, 1977.
18. Leonidas JC, Berdon WE, Griebetz D: Bilateral renal cortical necrosis in the newborn infant: roentgenographic diagnosis. *J Pediatr* 79:623–627, 1971.
19. Lester PD, McAllister WH: A mobile calcified spontane-

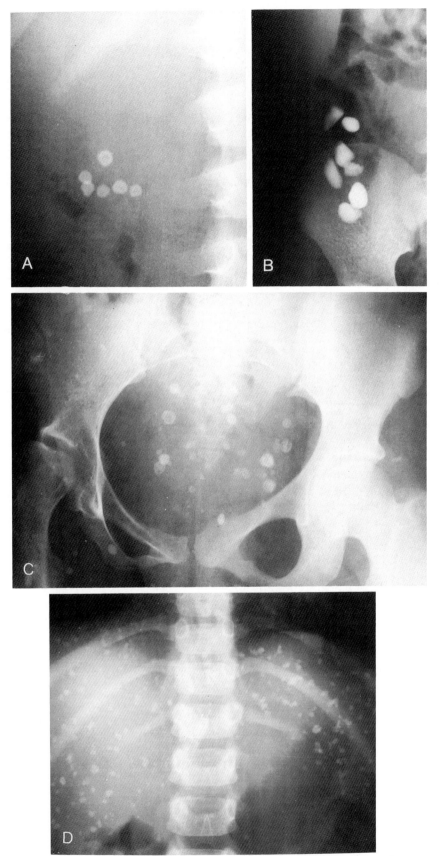

Figure 3.13. Stones, stone-like, and punctate calcifications.
A. Typical gallstones in a patient with sickle cell disease. **B.** Pebbles in the cecum mimicking pathologic calcifications. This patient was a dirt eater. **C.** Multiple phleboliths in an extensive hemangioma (Hasselbach-Merritt syndrome). Some of these calci- fications have a typical "bullseye" appearance. Also note associated bony deformity of the pelvis. This is characteristic of angiomatous tumors. **D.** Typical punctate calcifications in the liver and spleen in a patient with healed disseminated histoplasmosis.

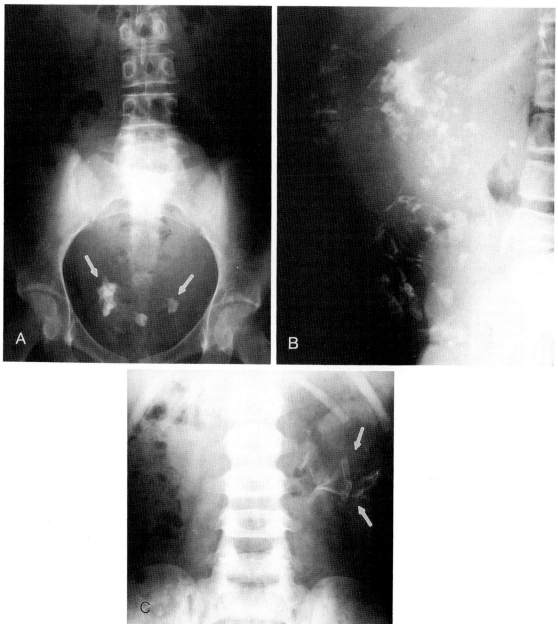

Figure 3.14. Formed calcifications. A. Note quite well-formed teeth in a teratoma of the ovary *(arrows)*. Also note the soft tissue mass of the tumor rising out of the pelvis. **B.** Lateral view in another patient with a very large teratoma containing both formed bone and teeth. **C.** Formed calcification (bone) in a retroperitoneal teratoma *(arrows)*.

ously amputated ovary. *J Can Assoc Radiol* 21:143–145, 1970.

20. Mannhardt W, Schumacher R: Progressive calcifications of lungs and liver in neonatal herpes simplex virus infection. *Pediatr Radiol* 21:236–237, 1991.

21. Marquis JR: The incidence of pelvic phleboliths in pediatric patients. *Pediatr Radiol* 5:211–212, 1977.

22. Partlow WF, Taybi H: Teratomas in infants and children. *AJR* 112:155–166, 1971.

23. Queloz JM, Capitanio MA, Kirkpatrick JA: Wolman's disease. Roentgen observations in 3 siblings. *Radiology* 104:357–359, 1972.

24. Reif S, Sloven DG, Lebenthal E: Gallstones in children.

Characterization by age, etiology, and outcome. *Am J Dis Child* 145:105–108, 1991.

25. Schullinger JN, Santulli TV, Berdon WE, Wigger HJ, MacMillan RW, Demartini PD, Baker DH: Calcific thrombi of the inferior vena cava in infants and children. *J Pediatr Surg* 13:429–434, 1978.

26. Schneider K, Hartl M, Fendel H: Umbilical and portal vein calcification following umbilical vein catheterization. *Pediatr Radiol* 19:468, 1989.

27. Shackelford GD, Kirks DR: Neonatal hepatic calcification secondary to transplacental infection. *Radiology* 122:753–757, 1977.

28. Staple TW, McAlister WH: Roentgenographic visualiza-

tion of iron preparation in the gastrointestinal tract. *Radiology* 83:1051, 1964.

Abnormal Organ and Tissue Densities

Normally, each organ or tissue in the abdomen has a specific density, i.e., air-containing structures are relatively black, fatty structures gray or radiolucent, and muscles and solid organs relatively white (i.e., water density). If any of these organs or tissues appear whiter or denser than normal, it is because they are enlarged (i.e., more tissue mass) or infiltrated with calcium or iron salts. The former, of course, is most common.

Diffuse excess calcium deposition usually affects the kidneys and can occur with any number of hypercalcemic states (i.e., hyperparathyroidism, severe osteoporosis, steroid therapy–induced osteoporosis, excess calcium intake, milk-alkali syndrome, idiopathic hypercalcemia, hypervitaminosis D, hyperparathyroidism-like states in hormonally active bone tumors, oxaluria, renal tubular acidosis). Generalized increased density of the liver usually occurs because of increased iron deposition, and most often this takes the form of hemosiderosis after repeated transfusions (1, 7). Hepatic iron deposition results in increased attenuation values on CT or decreased liver intensity on MRI (Fig. 3.15D). Similar excessive iron deposition has been described in abdominal lymph nodes after multiple transfusions in thalassemia (9), but idiopathic or primary hemochromatosis in children is very rare.

Decreased density, or abnormal radiolucency, of an organ is rather uncommon, except in the liver with marked fatty replacement (3, 8). Most commonly, such fatty degeneration occurs with severe protein malnutrition in cystic fibrosis or kwashiorkor. However, it also can be seen with toxic insult to the liver, Reye's syndrome, tyrosinemia (6), and diabetes mellitus. The finding of fatty liver in such cases often is readily demonstrable with plain films (Fig. 3.15A), but usually is more vivid on ultrasound (4) or CT (Fig. 3.15B and C).

A generalized increase in abdominal fat leads to radiolucency of the entire abdomen, and can be seen with lipomas of the abdomen (3, 10) or excessive accumulation of fat in the omentum, mesentery, or retroperitoneal space (2, 5). The latter situation most commonly occurs with exogenous obesity, but steroid therapy utilized for conditions such as the nephrotic syndrome or regional enteritis is probably just as common. Increased fatty tissue also can be seen with the Prader-Willi syndrome, Cushing syndrome, and the Laurence-Moon-Biedl syndrome. Increased radiolucency in the abdomen because of excessive fat content also is said to occur with chylous ascites and with chylous cysts, but the finding is difficult to appreciate on plain films.

Finally, it should be noted that fat frequently is present in dermoids or teratomas in the abdomen, and this finding, together with the frequently present formed bones or teeth, assures the diagnosis. Fat in these lesions, once again, is more readily demonstrable with CT or MRI, and although some of these lesions can occur in the retroperitoneal space, most occur in the pelvis.

REFERENCES

1. Franken EA Jr, Smith WL, Siddiqui A: Noninvasive evaluation of liver disease in pediatrics. *Radiol Clin North Am* 18:239–252, 1980.
2. Giubilei D, Cicia S, Nardia P, Patane E, Villani RM: Radiographic exhibit: lipoma of the omentum in a child. *Radiology* 137:357–358, 1980.
3. Griscom NT, Capitanio MA, Wagoner ML, Culham G, Morris L: The visibly fatty liver. *Radiology* 117:385–389, 1975.
4. Henschke CI, Goldman H, Teele RL: The hyperechogenic liver in children: cause and sonographic appearance. *AJR* 138:841–846, 1982.
5. Hernandez R, Poznaski AK, Holt JF, Weintraub W: Abnormal fat collections in the omentum and mesocolon of children. *Radiology* 122:193–196, 1977.
6. Macvicar D, Dicks-Mireaux C, Leonard JV, Wight DG: Hepatic imaging with computed tomography of chronic tyrosinaemia type I. *Br J Radiol* 63:605–608, 1990.
7. Smith WL, Quattromani F: Radiodense liver in transfusion hemochromatosis. *AJR* 128:316–317, 1977.
8. Swischuk LE: A new and unusual roentgenographic finding of fatty liver in infants. *AJR* 122:159–164, 1974.
9. Winchester PH, Cerwin R, Dische R, Canale V: Hemosiderin laden lymph nodes: an unusual roentgenographic manifestation of homozygous thalassemia. *AJR* 118:222–226, 1973.
10. Young LW, Severson MV, Burke EC, Hattery RR: Radiological case of the month—retroperitoneal lipoma in a child. *Am J Dis Child* 134:83–84, 1980.

Ascites

Ascites is a common problem throughout infancy and childhood and, as in adults, it can accompany a wide variety of conditions (Table 3.7) (4). Large amounts of ascites in the newborn infant probably most commonly occur as a part of the syndrome of

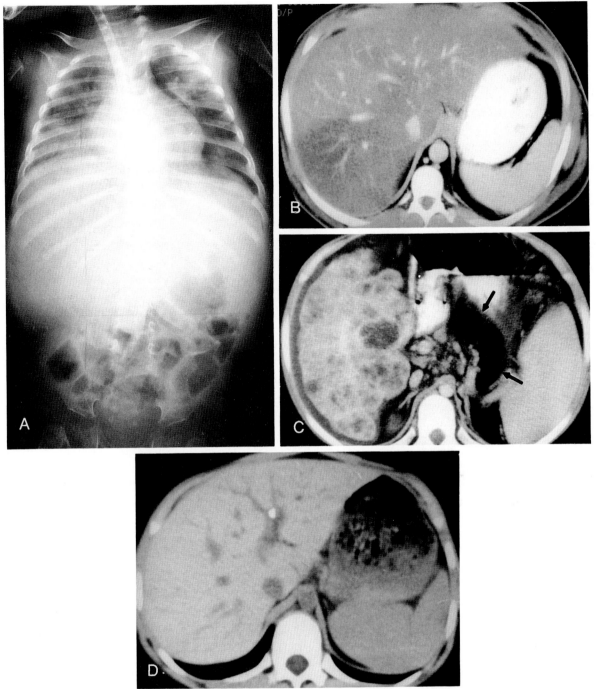

Figure 3.15. Fatty liver. A. Typical radiolucent appearance of a **fatty liver.** The liver is enlarged and displaces the intestines downward. Note that the spleen is whiter than the liver (they should have the same density). **B.** Fatty liver secondary to steroid therapy. The fat infiltration is uneven in this liver, causing patchy areas of decreased attenuation. **C.** A nodular fatty liver in a child with cystic fibrosis. Also note marked fatty replacement of the pancreas *(arrows).* (Courtesy of Jiles Perreault, M.D., Montreal.) **D.** CT demonstrates a dense liver due to **hemosiderosis** in a child with chronic anemia due to Diamond-Blackfan syndrome. Also note the calcified phlebolith within the portal vein.

Table 3.7
Ascites

Hydrops fetalis Liver disease Nephrotic syndrome Portal vein obstruction Hemorrhage	Common
Urinary tract obstruction Neonatal chylous ascites Hypoproteinemia Cardiac disease Peritonitis Ruptured cysts	Uncommon
Intestinal lymphangiectasia Pancreatitis Peritoneal metastasis Vascular emergencies Bile duct perforation Lysomal storage disease	Rare

hydrops fetalis. This condition is characterized by an excessive accumulation of fluid by the fetus and is usually associated with hemolysis and anemia. Although classically hydrops has been considered a complication of Rh incompatibility hemolytic disease, there are numerous causes, including other hemolytic anemias, cardiovascular abnormalities, vascular accidents, infections, and tumors. In newborn infants with urinary tract obstruction, large urine collections can be found in the abdomen. This most often occurs in male infants with posterior urethral valves. Chylous ascites in the newborn, like chylothorax, is probably the result of congenital hypoplasia or obstruction of the lymphatic system. In slightly older infants and young children, localized or generalized collections of bile in the abdomen may be the result of spontaneous perforation of the common bile duct (5). The precise cause of these perforations is unknown, but they may be due to bile duct obstruction or congenital or acquired weakness of the bile duct walls. Hepatobiliary scintigraphy is the study of choice for confirmation that the peritoneal fluid originated from the biliary tract (2). Complications of umbilical and other intravascular catheters in the newborn infant can also result in abnormal intraabdominal fluid collections.

In older infants and children, primary liver diseases and hepatic or portal vein obstruction are relatively common causes of ascites. Ascites can be seen with intestinal lymphangiectasia and other causes of hypoproteinemia. Pancreatitis is an uncommon cause of ascites in children; however, small amounts of intraperitoneal fluid are very common in children with gastrointestinal inflammatory conditions (e.g.,

appendicitis) and vascular problems (e.g., intussusception, Henoch-Schönlein purpura) (1, 7). Rarely, ascites can be one of the initial features noted in newborns with lysosomal storage disease (3).

Intraabdominal fluid collections are also present in patients with meconium peritonitis and other forms of peritonitis, and with hemoperitoneum. Although in some of these conditions the complexity of the fluid can be ascertained with ultrasound, in general, ultrasound provides poor specificity with regard to the type of fluid present. Also, ascites must be differentiated from large cystic masses such as mesenteric cysts or lymphangiomas that can mimic free fluid collections (6).

REFERENCES

1. Aveline B, Guimaraes R, Bely N, Salles J-P, Cugnenc P-H, Frija G: Intraabdominal serous fluid collections after appendectomy: a normal sonographic finding. *AJR* 161:71–73, 1993.
2. Banani SA, Bahador A, Nezakatgoo N: Idiopathic perforation of the extrahepatic bile duct in infancy: pathogenesis, diagnosis, and management. *J Pediatr Surg* 28:950–952, 1993.
3. Daneman A, Stringer D, Reilly BJ: Neonatal ascites due to lyosomal storage disease. *Radiology* 149:463–467, 1983.
4. Griscom NT, Colodny AH, Rosenberg HK, Fliegel CP, Hardy BE: Diagnostic aspects of neonatal ascites: report of 27 cases. *AJR* 128:961–969, 1977.
5. Haller JO, Condon VR, Berdon WE, Oh KS, Price AP, Bowen AD, Cohen HL: Spontaneous perforation of the common bile duct in children. *Radiology* 172:621–624, 1989.
6. Lugo-Olivieri CH, Taylor GA: CT differentiation of large abdominal lymphangioma from ascites. *Pediatr Radiol* 23:129–130, 1993.
7. Swischuk LE, Stansberry SD: Ultrasonographic detection of free peritoneal fluid in uncomplicated intussusception. *Pediatr Radiol* 21:350–351, 1991.

Extraintestinal Air

As in the adult, extraintestinal air can be located in the peritoneal cavity, retroperitoneal space, intestinal wall (i.e., pneumatosis cystoides intestinalis), biliary tract, portal veins, and, occasionally, in the kidney. In the latter case, air usually is present in the collecting systems of patients with ureteroileostomies (8). The finding actually is normal for these patients, but in other very rare patients (usually those with diabetes), air (gas) in the kidney is the result of severe gas-forming infection. Air in the biliary tract is very uncommon in the pediatric age group, and usually is the result of reflux into the biliary tract secondary to duodenal obstruction. Portal vein gas most commonly is seen in the neonate, either iatrogenically introduced by umbilical vein catheterization, or as a complication of necrotizing enterocolitis. Ultrasound can sometimes detect portal vein gas before it is radiographically visible (6). In older children, portal vein gas is much less common but can be seen with any cause of intestinal necrosis (Fig. 3.16A). Air in the liver parenchyma itself usually is the result of a liver abscess.

Intraperitoneal free air is much more common than retroperitoneal free air, and the causes and radiographic findings are much the same as in the adult. Most commonly, the problem is a perforated viscus, which can be the result of blunt abdominal trauma, gastrointestinal inflammation, or iatrogenic perforation with nasogastric or rectal tubes. Spontaneous rupture of the stomach usually occurs in the newborn infant and has been related to ulcer disease, hypoxia-induced focal necrosis, indomethacin therapy, and overinflation due to positive-pressure ventilation. When pneumoperitoneum is identified in an infant or child receiving ventilation, one must also consider the possibility that the air is the result

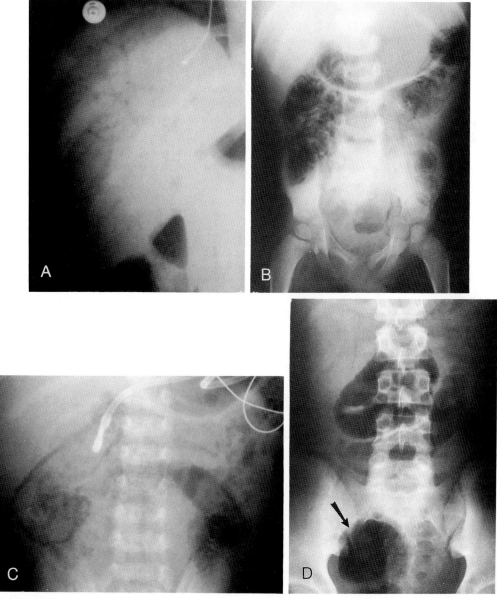

Figure 3.16. Extraintestinal gas. A. Massive air in the portal veins in a child with bowel ischemia. **B. Pneumatosis intestinalis.** Typical linear and curvilinear collections of gas in the wall of the intestine. **C.** An infant with necrotizing enterocolitis, demonstrating extensive linear and bubbly collections of air. **D.** Large collection of gas in a pelvic abscess *(arrow)*, secondary to perforated appendicitis. Also, note small bowel obstruction. On upright view, an air-fluid level was present in this abscess cavity.

of extension of a pneumomediastinum into the abdomen, even if a pneumomediastinum is not clearly visible.

Intramural air (pneumatosis intestinalis) is most commonly seen in the neonate and, when it is seen in association with dilated loops of intestine, is the hallmark of necrotizing enterocolitis. Beyond the newborn period, pneumatosis is rare but can be seen with intestinal overdistension, bowel ischemia, severe enterocolitis (2), collagen vascular disease (7), cystic fibrosis (3, 4), leukemia (5), steroid therapy (1), and, very rarely, secondary to a pneumomediastinum (9). When pneumatosis intestinalis is due to simple overdistension of the intestine, air enters the intestinal wall through mucosal tears, but with the other causes of intestinal disease, pneumatosis is a complication of intestinal ischemia and necrosis. The cause in patients with cystic fibrosis or steroid therapy is unknown. Radiographically, pneumatosis intestinalis can be seen as linear, curvilinear, or bubbly collections of gas in the intestinal wall (Fig. 3.16B and C).

Finally, it should be noted that free extraintestinal air can be seen loculated in abdominal abscesses. In some cases, these abscesses appear surprisingly thin walled, and the collection of air can be misinterpreted as a cyst or diverticulum (Fig. 3.16D).

REFERENCES

1. Bornes PF, Johnston TA: Indolent pneumatosis of the bowel wall associated with immune suppressive therapy. *Ann Radiol* 16:163–166, 1973.
2. Capitanio MA, Greenberg SB: Pneumatosis intestinalis in two infants with rotavirus gastroenteritis. *Pediatr Radiol* 21:361, 1991.
3. Djurhuus MJ, Lykkegaard E, Pock-Steen OC: Gastrointestinal radiological findings in cystic fibrosis. *Pediatr Radiol* 1:113–118, 1973.
4. Hernanz-Schulman M, Kirkpatrick J Jr, Schwachman H, Herman T, Schulman G, Vawter GF: Pneumatosis intestinalis in cystic fibrosis. *Radiology* 160:497–499, 1986.
5. Keats TE, Smith TH: Benign pneumatosis intestinalis in childhood leukemia. *AJR* 122:150–152, 1974.
6. Merritt CR, Goldsmith JP, Sharp MJ: Sonographic detection of portal venous gas in infants with necrotizing enterocolitis. *AJR* 143:1059–1062, 1984.
7. Oliveros MA, Herbst JJ, Lester PD, Ziter FA: Pneumatosis intestinalis in childhood dermatomyositis. *Pediatrics* 52:711–712, 1973.
8. Rittenberg GM, Warren D: Air in the pelvicalceal system: a normal finding in patients with ureteroileostomies. *AJR* 128:311–312, 1977.
9. Seaman WB, Fleming RJ, Baker DH: Pneumatosis intestinalis of the small bowel. *Semin Roentgenol* 1:234, 1966.

Abnormal Intestinal Gas Patterns

In the normal child, one usually can identify gas in the stomach and scattered in the small bowel and colon. Abnormal gas patterns include (a) isolated distension of the stomach, (b) distension of stomach and duodenum, (c) dilated loops of small bowel, (d) dilated colon and small bowel, (e) isolated colon dilation, (f) dilated transverse colon only, (g) one or two isolated loops of bowel (sentinel loops), and (h) airless intestine (Tables 3.8 and 3.9).

DISTENDED STOMACH

The commonest cause of a stomach distended with air is normal air swallowing in infants (Fig. 3.17A and B). However, if gastric dilation is severe or persistent, or if abdominal distension or vomiting occurs, gastric outlet obstruction should be considered. When isolated gastric dilation is seen in a newborn infant with little or no evidence of gas in the gastrointestinal tract distally, the obstruction usually lies in the distal gastric antrum or the proximal duodenum. Gastric atresia and antropyloric webs are the most common forms of congenital gastric outlet obstruction. These anomalies are thought to be due to an ischemic insult to the stomach in fetal life. Gastric atresia is easily diagnosed by plain radiographs alone, for no gas will be seen to pass into the duodenum and small bowel (Fig. 3.17C). Antropyloric membranes, however, are frequently incomplete and the degree of gastric outlet obstruction is variable (Fig. 3.17D). Ultrasound or contrast examinations are usually required for demonstrating these anomalies.

In the older infant, obstruction at the pylorus becomes more common and is most frequently due to pylorospasm or hypertrophic pyloric stenosis. Isolated pylorospasm is common in infants and young children. In the majority of patients, no precipitating etiology of the spasm is found, but occasionally the spasm is associated with peptic ulcer disease. Pylorospasm has also been encountered in patients with adrenal insufficiency and the adrenogenital syndrome. Hypertrophic pyloric stenosis is a developmental or acquired condition that usually occurs in infants between 2 and 8 weeks of age. The precise etiology is unknown, but factors such as prolonged spasm, hyperacidity, increased gastrin levels, and prolonged vagal stimulation have been implicated. This condition is characterized by circumferential hypertrophy of the pyloric muscle, resulting in a

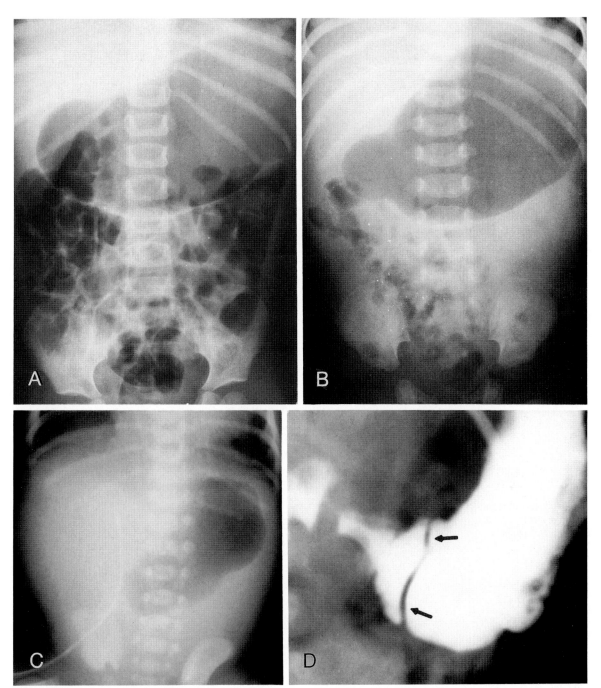

Figure 3.17.   Gastric distension. A. Note what at first appears to be a pathologically overdistended stomach. Such distension is common in normal infants and is due to air swallowing. This was a normal infant. Also note that the remainder of the gas pattern is normal. **B.** Another infant with a distended stomach and very little gas in the remainder of the gastrointestinal tract. Such a pattern can be seen with gastric outlet obstruction (e.g., pyloric stenosis) and, occasionally, with gastroenteritis. It also can be seen in normal infants, however, and this patient was normal. **C.** Complete gastric outlet obstruction due to **gastric atresia.** This infant also has epidermolysis bullosa, a known association. **D. Antral diaphragm.** Note the linear filling defect across the gastric antrum *(arrows),* which causes only minimal obstruction.

Table 3.8
Abdominal Gas Patterns

Distended stomach	
Normal (infants)	
Hypertrophic pyloric stenosis	Common
Pylorospasm	
Antropyloric membrane	
Gastric ulcer disease	
Gastroenteritis	Uncommon
Duodenal obstruction	
Antral foveolar hyperplasia (prostaglandin therapy)	
Duplication cysts (antrum)	Rare
Ectopic pancreas (antrum)	
Polyps, tumors (antrum)	
Small bowel obstruction (beyond neonatal period)	
Perforated appendicitis	
Intussusception	Common
Incarcerated hernia	
Postoperative adhesions	
Regional enteritis	Moderately common
Pseudo-obstruction in gastroenteritis	
Peritoneal bands	
Duplication cysts	
Midgut volvulus	Rare
Small bowel tumors	
Chronic pseudo-obstruction syndrome	
Dilated Colon (beyond neonatal period)	
Functional (psychogenic) megacolon	Common
Hirschsprung disease	
Colonic stenosis	
Hypothyroidism	
Chagas' disease	
Chronic immobilization	
Medication producing hypotonia	Rare
Neuronal intestinal dysplasia	
Plexiform neurofibromatosis of colon	
Segmental dilation of colon	

high-grade gastric outlet obstruction in the majority of patients. Although pylorospasm and hypertrophic pyloric stenosis can have a similar appearance clinically and on contrast examinations, ultrasound can be used to clearly differentiate the hypertrophied muscle mass of pyloric stenosis from the spastic pylorus without evidence of hypertrophied muscle.

Peptic ulcer disease occurs in children, but is a rather uncommon cause of gastric outlet obstruction in these patients. Postinflammatory strictures are rare. Other rare causes of gastric outlet obstruction include a variety of critically located masses, including gastrointestinal duplication cysts, ectopic pancreatic tissue, gastric polyps, or tumors of the stomach or duodenum. On contrast examination, such lesions tend to produce eccentric narrowing of the antropyloric region, and ultrasound can also be used to identify most masses in this region. Gastric outlet obstruction due to antral foveolar hyperplasia can develop in infants with cyanotic heart disease receiving prostaglandin therapy (7).

Isolated gastric distension also occasionally can occur with gastroenteritis and with postoperative paralytic ileus. In the latter instance, profound distension may occur and can lead to cardiorespiratory difficulty, probably due to mechanical pressure and vagal overstimulation. Similar acute distension can be seen in severely ill patients (i.e., in sepsis) and, occasionally, with excessive air swallowing that occurs with severe respiratory distress or a large tracheoesophageal fistula. Uncommonly, endotracheal tubes erroneously directed into the esophagus can result in severe gastric distension and even rupture.

Finally, it might be noted that with the patient in the supine position, duodenal obstruction can give the appearance of simple gastric overdistension due to gastric outlet obstruction. The reason for this is that in the supine position the descending duodenum may be filled with fluid. The stomach, of course, being more anterior, is filled with air and, consequently, one might erroneously conclude that the stomach alone is distended and obstructed. Decubitus, prone, or upright views can reveal the true nature of the obstruction in these cases.

SMALL BOWEL OBSTRUCTION

With mechanical obstruction of the small bowel, just as in the adult, distended intestinal loops tend to assume a more orderly configuration than normal and, on upright views, are seen as acute, inverted hairpin loops. The number of loops corresponds to the level of obstruction; i.e., if obstruction is located in the third or fourth portion of the duodenum, only the duodenal loop is distended, whereas if it is located in the jejunum or ileum, progressively increasing numbers of distended loops are seen. Following the progression of air in the previously gasless abdomen of the newborn infant will often provide the diagnosis when an obstruction is present in the duodenum or proximal jejunum. The classic "double bubble" sign (Fig. 3.18A), due to a dilated stomach and duodenal bulb, occurs when the obstruction is in the second portion of the duodenum. Obstruction at this site most commonly occurs with duodenal atresia, with or without annular pancreas. Duodenal diaphragms, and occasionally peritoneal bands, also can produce a high duodenal obstruction. Although these abnormalities usually are apparent in the newborn period, duodenal diaphragms and peritoneal bands occasionally can remain silent until later in childhood (14). Duodenal obstruction after the newborn period is relatively uncommon, but can be the result of duodenal hematomas, postoperative adhesions, or compression of the duodenum by adjacent neoplasms or cysts. The superior mesenteric artery syndrome is a controversial entity that probably occurs only in those patients who are quite thin and who remain in the supine position for prolonged periods of time. These patients include chronically ill children, neurologically impaired children, children with acute burns, and those in total body casts.

When the entire duodenal loop is distended and obstruction seems to be present at the junction of the third and fourth portions of the duodenum (Fig. 3.18B), the most likely cause of obstruction is peritoneal bands and/or midgut volvulus, problems associated with malrotation and abnormal fixation of the small intestine. Because of the threat of bowel ischemia in the presence of midgut volvulus, contrast studies should be performed for verification whenever obstruction is encountered at this level and immediate surgery is not contemplated. Less commonly, obstruction in the distal duodenum is due to a duodenal diaphragm, a compressing adjacent tumor or cyst, adhesions, or compression by the superior mesenteric artery. If three "bubbles" are seen, one can assume that the obstruction lies in the proximal jejunum (9) (Fig. 3.18C), and thereafter one can only imply an approximate level of obstruction by noting the number of distended loops present (Fig. 3.18D).

When multiple loops of dilated, organized, obstructed small bowel are seen, the obstruction may lie in the distal small bowel or colon. The most likely cause of a distal small bowel obstruction varies with the age of the child. In the newborn infant, meconium ileus and ileal atresia are the most common causes of a low small bowel obstruction. Rarely, a Meckel's diverticulum can cause small bowel obstruction in the newborn (2). After the newborn period through the first few months of life, incarcerated hernias (mainly inguinal) are the most likely cause of the small bowel obstruction (Fig. 3.18D). Between 6 months and 3 years of age, intussusception becomes the most common abnormality to result in a

small bowel obstruction; however, radiographic evidence of obstruction will not be seen in all cases. The degree of obstruction in intussusception depends on the length of time the intussusception has been present and, to some extent, on how far it has progressed into the colon. In about one-third of the cases, the head of the intussusceptum can be seen outlined by a crescent of air on the plain radiograph, but a nonspecific abdominal mass is a common appearance (8). In addition, absence of gas in the right abdomen and loss of visualization of the liver edge can provide helpful clues (Fig. 3.18G). When intussusception occurs in this age range of late infancy through early childhood, the intussusception is usually idiopathic, probably related to inflammatory changes such as mucosal edema or hypertrophied intestinal lymphoid tissue. When the condition occurs in the newborn or in older children, however, a leading lesion such as a polyp, tumor, or diverticulum usually is present.

Throughout the remainder of childhood and adolescence, the most common cause of a distal small bowel obstruction is perforated appendicitis (6). The obstructive pattern develops only after the inflamed appendix perforates, and is probably due to a combination of paralytic ileus with a partial intestinal obstruction due to the inflammatory mass in the ileocecal region (Fig. 3.18E and F). Less commonly, other inflammatory conditions involving the ileum and cecum can cause a similar pattern of obstruction. These conditions include regional enteritis and typhlitis in children with leukemia. Other uncommon causes of small bowel obstruction in children include postoperative adhesions, peritoneal bands, volvulus, compressing abdominal masses, pseudoobstruction chronic syndrome, and delayed meconium ileus in patients with cystic fibrosis (1). Intramural hematomas can occasionally grow large enough to cause a small bowel obstruction. These are usually the result of abdominal trauma or the vasculitis of Henoch-Schönlein purpura (Fig. 3.18H). Obstruction by small bowel tumors or polyps is rare, except when these masses act as a lead point for intussusception.

COLON OBSTRUCTION

Obstruction of the colon can be either structural or functional (Table 3.8). In the newborn infant, anorectal anomalies (imperforate anus, ectopic anus) are largely responsible for structural colonic obstruction. Colonic stenosis or atresia can occur at any site along the course of the colon and is probably secondary to an intrauterine vascular insult. Functional co-

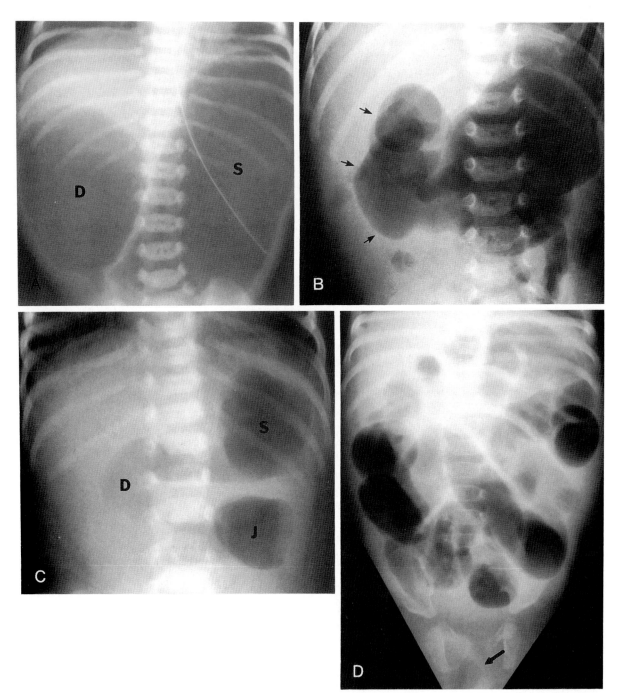

Figure 3.18. Intestinal obstruction: number of loops indicating level of obstruction. A. Typical double bubble of **duodenal atresia.** Stomach *(S)*, duodenum *(D)*. **B.** Distended stomach and duodenal loop *(arrows)* indicating obstruction at the third or fourth portion of the duodenum, due to **midgut volvulus. C.** Triple bubble representing the distended stomach *(S)*, duodenum *(D)*, and proximal jejunum *(J)* in a neonate with high **jejunal atresia. D.** Low small bowel obstruction with numerous distended loops of intestine due to an **incarcerated inguinal hernia.** Note the gas-filled loop of bowel in the left inguinal region *(arrow)*. **E.**

Low small bowel obstruction due to **perforated appendicitis.** Note dilated loops of small bowel, organized in a stepladder configuration typical of mechanical small bowel obstruction. **F.** Upright view in the same patient demonstrating numerous inverted U-shaped loops with short air-fluid levels. **G.** Infant with **intussusception** showing early small bowel obstruction (numerous distended loops of intestine) and typical paucity of gas on the right side. **H.** High-grade small bowel obstruction due to a large intramural hematoma in a patient with **Henoch-Schönlein purpura.**

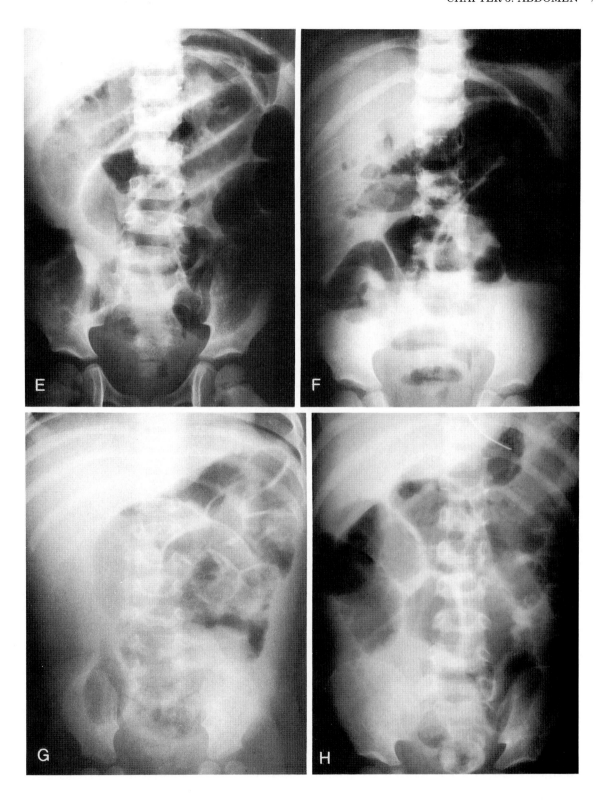

lonic obstruction is usually the result of ganglion cell abnormalities—either immaturity or absence. The meconium plug syndrome, the small left colon syndrome, and functional colonic immaturity of the premature infant are all similar functional disorders of the colon that are probably related to immaturity of the ganglion cells. Although the rectum is frequently normal in size in these conditions, in some patients the distal colon and rectum will appear contracted in a pattern that is virtually indistinguishable from

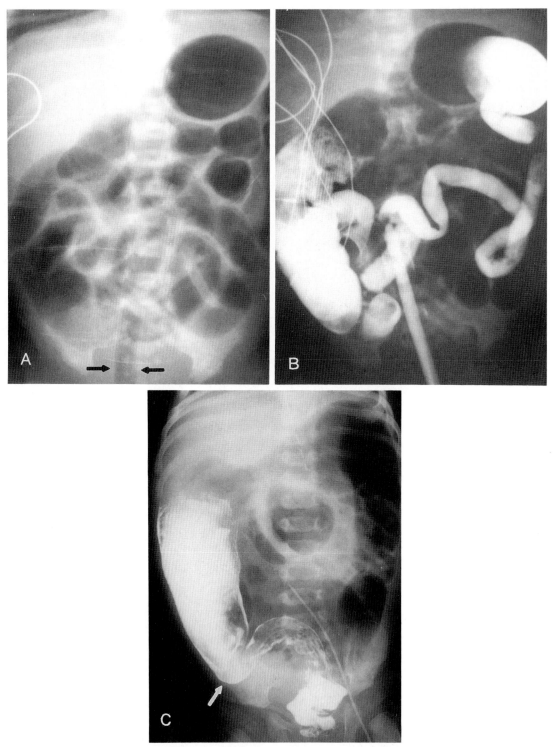

Figure 3.19. Colonic obstruction. A. Numerous loops of dilated bowel indicate a distal bowel obstruction. Note the narrow rectum *(arrows).* **B.** A contrast enema examination in the same patient reveals the small size of the left colon in this infant with **small left colon syndrome. C.** Note the contracted rectosigmoid colon with an abrupt transition to dilated proximal colon *(arrow)* in this infant with **Hirschsprung disease.**

that seen with Hirschsprung disease (Fig. 3.19A and B).

In Hirschsprung disease, the colonic ganglion cells are absent for a variable length of the colon, always including the rectum. The aganglionic segment is generally contracted (Fig. 3.19C) and sometimes demonstrates bizarre spasm, and the absence of peristalsis causes a functional obstruction. In patients with this condition, bowel obstruction frequently occurs in the newborn or in early infancy, but some patients present at an older age with complaints of chronic constipation. The major differentiating point between conditions due to colonic immaturity and Hirschsprung disease is that the meconium plug or small left colon syndromes can be successfully treated by rectal stimulation or water-soluble contrast enema, whereas patients with Hirschsprung disease require surgical correction. It should be noted that Hirschsprung disease in the newborn often fails to demonstrate the classic contrast enema findings that are seen in older infants and children. Therefore, a 24-hour delayed film is essential, for if delayed passage of contrast is encountered, Hirschsprung disease is the presumptive diagnosis.

Functional megacolon or constipation in childhood refers to a condition in which chronic constipation occurs in the presence of normal ganglion cells. The cause of this condition is poorly understood but is probably multifactoral, with contributions by both physical and psychological factors. This condition differs from Hirschprung disease in that symptoms are not present from birth, the rectum is filled with feces, and encopresis and emotional problems are frequently present. Other causes of colonic obstruction are rare, but include compression of the colon by eccentric masses or cysts, colonic tumors, peritoneal bands, volvulus, postinflammatory stricture, Chaga's disease, segmental dilation of the colon, neuronal intestinal dysplasia (10), neurofibromatosis, and functional obstruction such as might occur with fecal impaction or hypothyroidism.

PARALYTIC ILEUS

Paralytic ileus appears as numerous distended loops of both large and small bowel, and the picture is not nearly as orderly as that seen with mechanical obstruction. As a result, on upright view numerous "sluggish" loops of intestine with long air-fluid levels are seen. This is quite different from the acute hairpin, rather organized pattern seen with mechanical obstruction (Fig. 3.20). In the pediatric age group, the commonest cause of paralytic ileus is gastroenteritis (Table 3.9), and, thereafter, one should con-

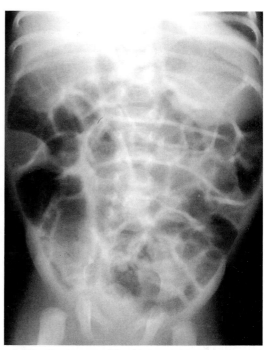

Figure 3.20. Gastroenteritis. Note numerous loops of distended intestine. Both large and small bowel are proportionately distended and the pattern has a "disorganized" appearance. This is characteristic of paralytic ileus.

Table 3.9
Abdominal Gas Patterns

Paralytic ileus		
Gastroenteritis	}	Common
Peritonitis		
Sepsis	}	Moderately common
Moribund patient		
Vascular insult		
Drug depression	}	Rare
Hypokalemia		
Dilated transverse colon (colon cutoff)		
Normal		
Perforated appendicitis	}	Common
Pancreatitis	}	Uncommon
Ischemia, infarct		
Toxic megacolon	}	Rare
Sentinal loop		
Appendicitis	}	Common
Paralytic ileus		
Pancreatitis	}	Moderately common
Isolated loop in gastroenteritis		
Normal, fortuitous	}	Uncommon
Closed loop obstruction		
Intestinal trauma		
Infarction	}	Rare

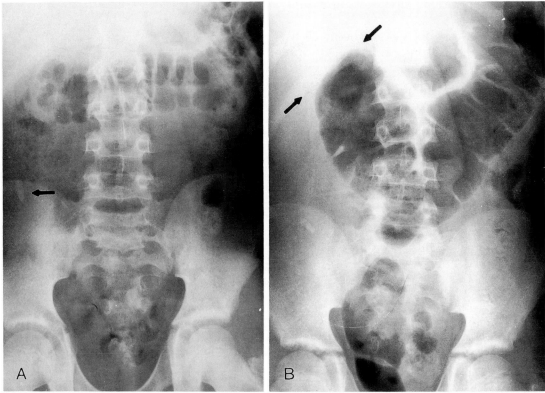

Figure 3.21. Dilated transverse colon. A. The transverse colon appears normal in this patient. The patient had acute abdominal pain and a fecalith on the right *(arrow)*. Ordinarily surgery would ensue, but symptoms resolved quickly and no surgery was performed at this time. **B.** Two years later, the patient had more severe abdominal symptoms, a markedly dilated transverse colon, and now a right side colon cutoff sign *(arrows)*. Note, specifically, that there is no air or fecal material in the cecum and ascending colon. This is quite different from the situation depicted in Part *A* and signifies **perforated appendicitis,** which was confirmed at surgery. Note that scoliosis, partial indistinctness of the right psoas shadow, and early small bowel obstruction also are present, and that the fecalith remains.

sider problems such as hypokalemia, hypocalcemia, peritonitis, meningitis, sepsis, prolonged immobilization, drugs such as valium or glucagon, and Ehlers-Danlos syndrome (3). Vascular insult to the intestines producing paralytic ileus is rather uncommon in children. Benign uniform gaseous distension of the small and large intestines is a common occurrence in small premature infants treated with nasal continuous positive-airway pressure (4). Aerophagia and immature bowel motility probably contribute to this condition, which can mimic paralytic ileus radiographically.

DILATED TRANSVERSE COLON

The transverse colon is a nondependent structure when the patient is examined in the supine position and, therefore, normally is filled with air (Fig. 3.21*A*). However, it also can be distended on a reflex basis with adjacent pancreatic inflammation or injury (11, 14) (Table 3.9). In these cases, the colon overlying the diseased pancreas is paralyzed and focally dilated, and the term "colon cut-off" often is applied to the configuration. A somewhat similar finding and one actually seen more often occurs with perforated appendicitis (Fig. 3.21*B*). As compared with the cut-off of the colon being on the splenic flexure side as in pancreatitis, in appendicitis the cut-off is on the hepatic flexure side (12). In these cases, the finding is believed to result from a combination of nonspecific, paralytic ileus of the transverse colon and lack of air in the cecum and ascending colon due to spasm. Dilation of the transverse colon due to ischemia or toxic megacolon in Hirschsprung disease, regional enteritis, or amebic colitis is relatively rare. It does occur, however, and often is associated with mural edema manifesting in thumbprinting due to intramural hemorrhage and edema.

SENTINEL LOOPS

Sentinel loops are focally distended loops of intestine that are distended because they (a) overlie inflamed or injured abdominal contents, (b) are involved in a closed loop obstruction, (c) are the first loops to be seen early in the course of regular intestinal obstruction (Fig. 3.22C and D), or (d) have suffered an ischemic insult (Table 3.9). Sentinel loops overlying inflamed or injured abdominal viscera are most common and usually occur in the right flank or right lower quadrant secondary to appendicitis (Fig. 3.22A and B). Sentinel loops seen elsewhere can result from infections such as cholecystitis, pancreatitis, pyelonephritis, and cystitis (13). Fortuitous, false sentinel loops can be seen in some normal individuals, and also with gastroenteritis. They tend to change from one view to another, whereas truly pathologic sentinel loops remain more fixed. Focally distended loops secondary to local intestinal ischemia are rather uncommon in the pediatric age group, except as seen in necrotizing enterocolitis of infancy. In this condition, an isolated, fixed, dilated loop of intestine is an ominous finding that suggests bowel necrosis and impending perforation.

Distension of the sigmoid colon mimicking sigmoid volvulus is quite common in normal children. Sigmoid volvulus is relatively rare in children, and cecal volvulus is even rarer (5). However, when sigmoid or cecal volvulus is seen it has an identical radiographic appearance to those conditions in the adult.

AIRLESS ABDOMEN

Normal infants and young children usually show considerable gas in the intestinal tract and, thus, when an airless abdomen is encountered, some abnormality should be suspected. Most often, the problem is severe vomiting and, for the most part, this occurs with acute gastroenteritis or appendicitis. Paucity of intestinal gas may also be seen with vomiting due to increased intracranial pressure and "cyclic" vomiting, decreased or depressed swallowing (e.g., moribund patients, obstructing nasopharyngeal tubes), and high gastrointestinal obstruction. Only occasionally is a totally airless abdomen an incidental normal finding.

REFERENCES

1. Edge WEB, Nuss D, Loening WEK: Late onset intestinal obstruction in cystic fibrosis. *S Afr Med J* 52:271–274, 1977.

2. Foyal MK, Bellah RD: Neonatal small bowel obstruction due to Meckel diverticulitis: diagnosis by ultrasonography. *J Ultrasound Med* 12:119–122, 1993.

3. Harris RD: Small bowel dilatation in Ehlers-Danlos syndrome: an unreported gastrointestinal manifestation. *Br J Radiol* 47:623–627, 1974.

4. Jaile JC, Levin T, Wung JT, Abramson SJ, Ruzal-Shapiro C, Berdon WE: Benign gaseous distension of the bowel in premature infants treated with nasal continuous airway pressure: a study of contributing factors. *AJR* 158:125–127, 1992.

5. Kirks DR, Swischuk LE, Merten DF, Filston HC: Cecal volvulus in children. *AJR* 136:419–422, 1981.

6. Melamed M, Melamed JL, and Rabushka SE: Appendicitis: "functional" bowel obstruction associated with perforation of the appendix. *AJR* 99:112–117, 1967.

7. Peled N, Dagan O, Babyn P, Silver MM, Barker G, Hellmann J, Scolnik D, Karen O: Please Gastric-outlet obstruction induced by prostaglandin therapy in neonates. *N Engl J Med* 327:505–510, 1992.

8. Ratcliffe JF, Fong S, Cheong L, O'Connell P: The plain abdominal film in intussusception the accuracy and incidence of radiographic signs. *Pediatr Radiol* 22:110–111, 1992.

9. Rathaus V, Grunebaum M, Ziv N, Kornreich L, Horev G: The bubble sign in the gasless abdomen of the newborn. *Pediatr Radiol* 22:106–109, 1992.

10. Scharli AF, Meier-Ruge W: Localized and disseminated forms of neuronal intestinal dysplasia mimicking Hirschsprung's disease. *J Pediatr Surg* 16:164–170, 1981.

11. Schwartz S, Nadelhaft J: Simulation of colonic obstruction at the splenic flexure by pancreatitis: roentgen features. *AJR* 78:607–616, 1957.

12. Swischuk LE, Hayden CK Jr: Appendicitis with perforation: the dilated transverse colon sign. *AJR* 135:687–690, 1980.

13. Young BR: Significance of regional or reflex ileus in roentgen diagnosis of cholecystitis, perforated ulcer, pancreatitis and appendiceal abscess, as determined by survey examination of acute abdomen. *AJR* 78:581–586, 1957.

14. Young LW: Pancreatic and/or duodenal injury from blunt trauma in childhood: radiopaque examinations and radiological review. *Ann Radiol* 18:377–390, 1975.

Thumbprinting

Thumbprinting can result either from thickening of the intestinal mucosa and submucosa (i.e., edema or infiltration) or simply from mucosal distortion secondary to intestinal spasm. When it is due to spasm, it is best demonstrated with a barium enema, but when due to edema or infiltration, a scalloped appearance of the affected loops sometimes can be appreciated on plain films. Spasm-produced thumbprinting can be seen in Hirschsprung disease and with intestinal inflammatory disease. When the problem is mural edema, ulcerative colitis usually is

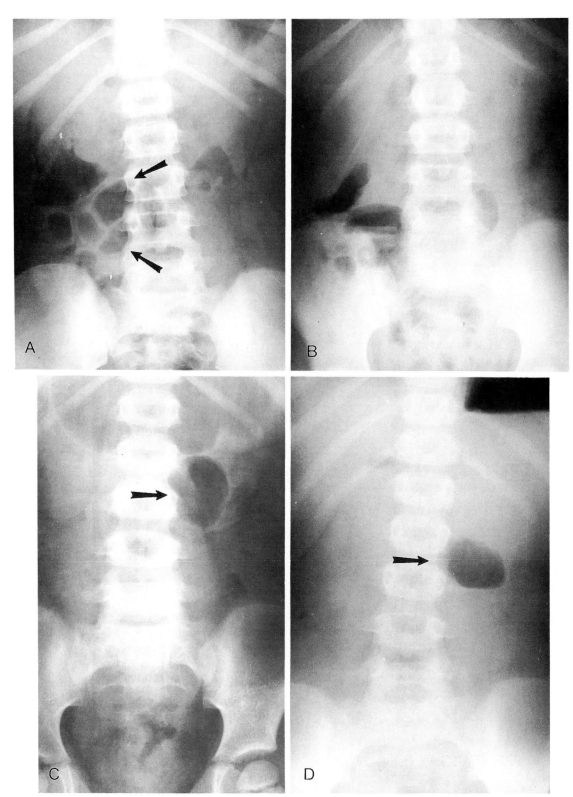

Figure 3.22. Sentinel loops. A. Typical collection of gas in the cecum and distal small bowel in a patient with early nonperforated appendicitis *(arrows).* **B.** Upright view demonstrates the same findings and also indistinctness of the ipsilateral psoas shadow and mild lumbar scoliosis. **C.** Localized loops of small bowel herald an early small bowel obstruction *(arrow).* **D.** Upright view confirms the findings and shows the same loops *(arrow).* Such fixed loops, no matter how small, should alert one to the presence of an obstruction, either an ordinary or closed loop obstruction.

the cause, but thumbprinting also can be seen with regional enteritis, pseudomembranous colitis, intestinal ischemia, amebic colitis, hemolytic uremic syndrome, eosinophilic (allergic) gastroenteritis (7), Henoch-Schönlein purpura (2), and intramural intestinal bleeding (4) due to trauma or blood dyscrasias. In most of these conditions, the finding is better demonstrated with barium studies. Nevertheless, ultrasound can be quite useful for identifying areas of intestinal edema and hemorrhage and for evaluating efficacy of therapy (1, 3, 5, 6).

REFERENCES

1. Alexander JE, Williamson SL, Seibert JJ, Golladay ES, Jimenez JF: Ultrasonographic diagnosis of typhlitis (neutropenic colitis). *Pediatr Radiol* 18:200–204, 1988.
2. Byrn JR, Fitzgerald JF, Northway JD, Anand SK, Scott JR: Unusual manifestations of Henoch-Schönlein syndrome. *Am J Dis Child* 130:1335–1337, 1976.
3. Couture A, Veyrac C, Baud C, Califer RB, Armelin I: Evaluation of abdominal pain in Henoch-Schönlein syndrome by high frequency ultrasound. *Pediatr Radiol* 22:12–17, 1992.
4. Grossman H, Berdon WE, Baker DH: Reversible gastrointestinal sign of hemorrhage and edema in the pediatric age group. *Radiology* 84:33, 1965.
5. Limberg B: Sonographic features of colonic Crohn's disease: comparison of in vivo and in vitro studies. *J Clin Ultrasound* 18:161, 1990.
6. Matsumoto T, Iida M, Sakai T, Kimura Y, Fujishima M: Yersinia terminal ileitis: sonographic findings in eight patients. *AJR* 156:965–967, 1991.
7. Teele RL, Katz AJ, Goldman H, Kettell RM: Radiographic features of eosinophilic gastroenteritis (allergic gastroenteropathy) of childhood. *AJR* 132:575–580, 1979.

Esophageal Stenosis

A focal area of narrowing within the esophagus is more likely to be an acquired condition than a congenital abnormality (Table 3.10). Such narrowing is most often the result of scarring due to a previous inflammatory process (Fig. 3.23B). Peptic esophagitis

Table 3.10
Esophageal Stenosis

Corrosive esophagitis Peptic esophagitis	} Common
Posttracheoesophageal fistula repair	} Moderately common
Congenital, tracheobronchial remnants Trauma, chronic foreign body Infectious esophagitis Epidermolysis bullosa Barrett esophagus Neoplasm	} Rare

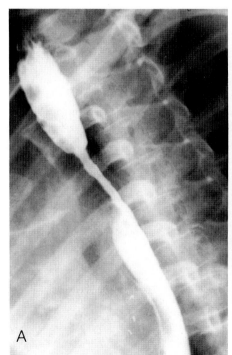
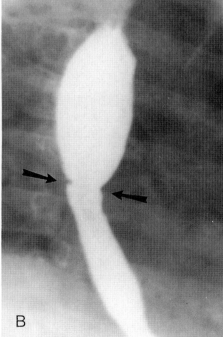
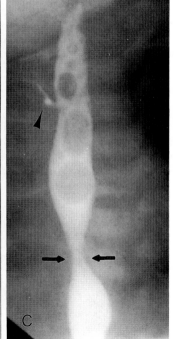

Figure 3.23. **Esophageal stenosis. A.** A long segment narrowing in the upper esophagus in a child with **Barrett esophagus** due to gastroesophageal reflux. **B. Esophageal web.** Note the band-like defect *(arrows)* representing an esophageal web due to reflux esophagitis in a 13-month-old child. **C.** Congenital stenosis of the distal esophagus *(arrows)* in an infant with repaired esophageal atresia. Note the small postoperative sinus tract *(arrowhead).*

due to gastroesophageal reflux is probably the most common cause of esophageal inflammation, although caustic ingestion is close behind and is associated with a much graver outcome. Infectious esophagitis is rare in children, except in immunodeficient patients (2). Esophagitis due to *Candida,* cytomegalovirus, and herpes virus are common in children with AIDS, but these infections rarely result in esophageal strictures after successful treatment. Postoperative narrowing can remain in the esophagus following repair of esophageal atresia and/or tracheoesophageal fistula. In addition, congenital stenosis of the distal esophagus may also occur in patients with tracheoesophageal fistula (Fig. 3.23C). Children with epidermolysis bullosa may develop bulla in the esophagus, which, with healing, can create a stricture. Other rare causes of esophageal stenosis are Barrett esophagus in children with prolonged gastroesophageal reflux (3) (Fig. 3.23A) and esophageal foreign bodies and trauma. Esophageal tumors are also quite rare in children. The majority are benign neoplasms such as hamartomas, hemangiomas, or leiomyomas (1). Esophageal carcinoma is very rare in children and usually arises in a pre-existing esophageal lesion (e.g., Barrett esophagus, caustic burn).

True congenital stenoses of the esophagus are rare. They can take the form of relatively long segments of circumferential narrowing or a thin membrane or web. Most congenital esophageal stenoses are thought to represent tracheobronchial remnants within the esophageal wall. Such strictures usually are found in the distal one-third of the esophagus.

REFERENCES

1. Rabushka LS, Fishman EK, Kuhlman JE, Hruban RH: Diffuse esophageal leiomyomatosis in a patient with Alport syndrome: CT demonstration. *Radiology* 179:176, 1991.
2. Renner WR, Johnson JF, Lichtenstein JE, Kirks DR: Esophageal inflammation and stricture: complication of chronic granulomatous disease of childhood. *Radiology* 178:189, 1991.
3. Yulish BS, Rothstein FC, Halpin TC Jr: Radiographic findings in children and young adults with Barrett esophagus. *AJR* 148:353–357, 1987.

Gastric Masses and Thickened Mucosal Folds

Gastric mucosal fold thickening is a relatively uncommon occurrence in infants and children (Table 3.11). The most common cause of gastritis in child-

Table 3.11
Gastric Masses[a] and Thickened Mucosal Folds[b]

Gastritis[a] Polyps[b] Ectopic pancreatic tissue[b] Caustic ingestion[a]	Moderately common
Foreign body, bezoar[b] Gastric duplication[b] Menetrier's disease[a] Crohn's disease[a] Neoplasm[b] Inflammatory pseudotumor[b]	Rare

hood is a viral infection, but such infections are seldom investigated radiographically. Peptic ulcer disease is much less common in children than in adults, but it is by no means rare (3). Other causes of gastric inflammation include ingestion of corrosive substances or medications, steroid-induced gastritis, eosinophilic (allergic) gastritis (6), and chronic granulomatous disease (1, 2). Marked mucosal fold thickening can be seen with Menetrier's disease, but this is quite rare in childhood (4).

Gastric masses can be mimicked by intraluminal contents such as bezoars and foreign bodies. Inflammatory pseudotumor is a benign proliferation of myofibroblasts and inflammatory cells that can rarely occur in the stomach and tends to have an aggressive appearance (5). True gastric neoplasms are uncommon. The same neoplasms that occur in the stomachs of adults can occur in children, although they occur much less frequently. In the newborn infant, teratoma is probably the most common gastric neoplasm. Gastric duplications can be visible as a mass, but the stomach is the least common location for a duplication within the gastrointestinal tract. Small nodules of ectopic pancreatic tissue can occur in the gastric antrum. A characteristic central umbilication representing a draining duct is sometimes seen in such nodules. Polyps of the stomach can be encountered in patients with polyposis syndromes such as Peutz-Jeghers syndrome, Gardner syndrome, and familial polyposis.

REFERENCES

1. Bowen A, Gibson MD: Chronic granulomatous disease with gastric antral narrowing. *Pediatr Radiol* 10:119–120, 1980.
2. Griscom NT, Kirkpatrick JA, Girdany BR, Berdon WE, Grand RJ, Mackie GG: Gastric antral narrowing in chronic granulomatous disease of childhood. *Pediatrics* 54:456–460, 1974.
3. Hayden CK, Swischuk LE, Rytting JE: Gastric ulcer disease in infants: US findings. *Radiology* 164:131–134, 1987.

4. Leonidas JC, Beatty EC, Wenner HA: Menetrier's disease and cytomegalovirus infection in childhood. *Am J Dis Child* 126:806–808, 1973.
5. Maves CK, Johnson JF, Bove K, Malott RL: Gastric inflammatory pseudotumor in children. *Radiology* 173:381–383, 1989.
6. Teele RL, Katz AJ, Goldman H, Kettell RM: Radiographic features of eosinophilic gastroenteritis (allergic gastroenteropathy) of childhood. *AJR* 132:575–580, 1979.

Thickened Intestinal Mucosal Folds

Thickened mucosal folds in the intestines can be the result of inflammation, generalized edema, hemorrhage, or infiltration of the intestinal wall (Table 3.12). In the small intestine, the pattern of fold thickening can vary from relatively straight folds to tortuous or nodular-appearing folds (3). Nodularity of the fold thickening tends to occur in conditions such as intestinal lymphangiectasia, parasitic infestation such as giardiasis (Fig. 3.24E), and cystic fibrosis (4) (Fig. 3.24A). Whipple's disease, which is rare in childhood, can also have this appearance. A finely nodular mucosal fold pattern that is similar to that seen in Whipple's disease can occur with *Mycobacterium avium-intracellulare* infections in children with AIDS. Enteropathic diarrhea and thickened mucosal folds frequently develop in these children, due to a wide variety of pathogens, including unusual organisms such as *Cryptosporidium, Isopora,* cytomegalovirus (1). Thickened but straight mucosal folds generally reflect intestinal edema, which can be seen in conditions such as nephrotic syndrome (Fig.

3.24F), gastroenteritis, eosinophilic or allergic enteritis (Fig. 3.24C), Zollinger-Ellison syndrome, celiac disease, protein-losing enteropathy, and other causes of generalized edema. When mucosal fold thickening is segmental, the most likely cause is intramural hemorrhage (e.g., blunt abdominal trauma, Henoch-Schönlein purpura) (Fig. 3.24B), infarction, or regional enteritis (2) (Fig. 3.24D).

REFERENCES

1. Haller JO, Cohen HL: Gastrointestinal manifestations of AIDS in children. *AJR* 162:387–393, 1994.
2. Stringer DA: Imaging inflammatory bowel disease in the pediatric patient. *Radiol Clin North Am* 25:93–113, 1987.
3. Swischuk LE: Mucosal patterns in diffuse disease in the small bowel. *Med Radiogr Photogr* 47:34–40, 1971.
4. Taussig LM, Saldino RM, di Sant Agnese PA: Radiographic abnormalities of the duodenum and small bowel in cystic fibrosis of the pancreas (mucoviscidosis). *Radiol* 106:369–376, 1973.

Microcolon

The term "microcolon" is generally used to describe a narrowed empty colon in a newborn infant. In most cases, this finding accompanies a distal small bowel obstruction, most commonly ileal atresia or meconium ileus. In these conditions, the volume of intestinal secretions and amniotic fluid that passes into the colon in fetal life is small, and therefore the colon does not become distended to a normal size. Following the treatment of these conditions, the size of the colon returns to normal. Functional problems involving the entire colon can also cause a microcolon appearance. This can occur with functional colonic obstruction of the premature and with the rare case of total colonic aganglionosis. Megacystis-microcolon-intestinal hypoperistalsis syndrome is an uncommon condition characterized by a massively distended bladder and a microcolon (1, 2). The intestines in these patients demonstrate poor peristalsis, but the ganglion cells within the intestines are normal or even increased. When only the distal portion of the colon is narrowed, conditions such as Hirschsprung disease, colon atresia, or the small left colon syndrome are the most likely causes.

Table 3.12
Thickened Small Bowel Mucosal Folds

Edema[a]
  Nephrotic syndrome
  Hypoproteinemia
  Portal vein obstruction
  Portal hypertension
Gastroenteritis[a]
Giardiasis[b]
Celiac disease[a]
	Common

Cystic fibrosis[b] Protein losing enteropathy[a] Regional enteritis[a]	Moderately common
Eosinophilic gastroenteritis[a] Intestinal lymphangiectasia[b] Zollinger-Ellison syndrome[a] Cardiac disease[a]	Relatively rare
Behcet syndrome[b]	Very rare

[a] Thick and straight.
[b] Thick and tortuous.

REFERENCES

1. Berdon WE, Baker DH, Blanc WA, Gay B, Santulli TV, Donovan C: Megacystis-microcolon-intestinal hypoperistalsis syndrome: a new cause of intestinal obstruction in the newborn. *AJR* 126:957–964, 1976.

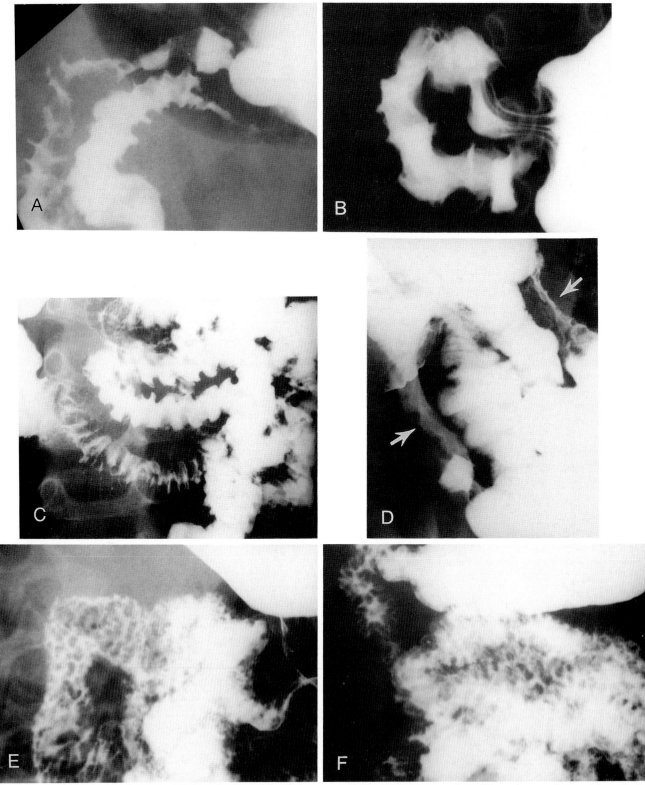

Figure 3.24. Thickened intestinal folds. A. Markedly thickened and irregular duodenal and jejunal mucosal folds in a child with **cystic fibrosis. B.** Thickened and irregular mucosal folds in the duodenum due to intramural hemorrhage with **Henoch-Schönlein purpura. C.** Thickened, but straight small bowel mucosal folds in a child with **eosinophilic gastroenteritis. D.** Note two separate segments of small bowel narrowing and irregularity *(arrows)* in a child with **regional enteritis. E.** Diffuse nodular thickening of the duodenal mucosal folds due to **giardiasis. F.** Thickened, nodular small bowel folds due to intestinal edema in a patient with **nephrotic syndrome.**

2. Krook OM: Megacystis-microcolon-intestinal hypoperistalsis syndrome in a male infant. *Radiology* 136:649–650, 1980.

Intestinal Masses and Nodules (Table 3.13)

Small nodules within the colon are rather common, and when multiple small sessile nodules are seen scattered throughout the colon, they usually represent a normal lymphoid follicular pattern or lymphoid hyperplasia (1). Usually this pattern is of no clinical significance in a child. A characteristic of these nodules is a small central umbilication. A rare form of focal lymphoid hyperplasia has been described that occurs as polypoid masses in the ileocecal region. The chronic form of this disease can result in pain, bleeding, weight loss, chronic anemia, and recurrent intussusception (3).

Polyps constitute the vast majority of masses that are found in the intestines of infants and children. The most common type of polyp is a nonadenomatous (juvenile) polyp that is thought to be related to either an inflammatory or hamartomatous process of the colon. These polyps are benign and frequently undergo self-amputation; however, they also can cause rectal bleeding, intussusception, or rectal prolapse. Juvenile polyps are most commonly single or few in number. When multiple intestinal polyps are found, one must consider the possibility of a polyposis syndrome (2). When innumerable polyps are seen extending through the colon, the most likely diagnosis is familial adenomatous polyposis; however, a rare familial form of juvenile polyposis can have a similar appearance (5). In the early stages of familial colonic polyposis, only a few polyps may be present, but eventually the colon becomes carpeted with numerous polyps. Because of the high risk of developing carcinoma within the polyps, this condition is treated by total colectomy. In Gardner syndrome, multiple colonic adenomatous polyps are associated with mesenchymal tumors of the bones and soft tissues. Turcot syndrome is a very rare condition in which adenomatous polyps of the colon and central nervous system tumors develop in the patient. Peutz-Jeghers syndrome is characterized by hamartomatous gastrointestinal polyps that are most common in the small intestine but can also arise in the colon, rectum, and stomach. These polyps frequently lead to chronic anemia and intussusception. The pseudopolyps that can develop in patients with inflammatory bowel disease are uncommon in childhood.

Intestinal tumors, in general, are relatively rare in infants and children. Benign small bowel neoplasms such as hamartomas and hemangiomas are most frequently seen in patients with disorders such as Klippel-Trenaunay-Weber syndrome, Sturge-Weber syndrome, neurofibromatosis, and tuberous sclerosis. Lymphoma is the most common primary malignancy of the small bowel, followed in frequency by carcinoma of the colon (4). Children with increased risk of an intestinal malignancy developing are those with adenomatous polyposis syndromes, chronic ulcerative colitis, children who have had a urinary diversion procedure, and some children who have received chemotherapy and radiation therapy for other malignancies. Fatty tumors and smooth muscle tumors are rare in children.

Table 3.13
Intestinal Masses and Nodules

Normal fecal material Lymphoid hyperplasia (colon)	Common
Lymphoid hyperplasia (small bowel) Juvenile polyps: inflammatory, sporadic	Moderately common
Pseudopolyps-ulcerative colitis, regional enteritis Familial polyposis	Uncommon

Other polyposis syndromes
  Peutz-Jeghers syndrome (small bowel)
  Canada-Cronkhite syndrome (colon, stomach)
  Gardner syndrome
Juvenile polyps, inflammatory-familial
Neoplasm
	Rare

REFERENCES

1. Capitanio MA, Kirkpatrick JA: Lymphoid hyperplasia of the colon in children. *Radiology* 94:323–327, 1970.
2. Erbe RW: Inherited gastrointestinal-polyposis syndromes [review article]. *N Engl J Med* 294:1101–1104, 1976.
3. Jana JZ, Belin R, Burke JA: Lymphoid hyperplasia of the bowel and its surgical significance in children. *J Pediatr Surg* 11:997–1006, 1976.
4. Lamego CM, Torloni H: Colorectal adenocarcinoma in childhood and adolescent: report of 11 cases and review of the literature [review article]. *Pediatr Radiol* 19:504–508, 1989.
5. Schwartz AM, McCauley RGL: Juvenile gastrointestinal polyposis. *Radiology* 121:441–444, 1976.

Renal Size Abnormalities

Renal enlargement is a common occurrence in infants and children, and although the list of causes is

Table 3.14
Large Kidneys

Nephrotic syndrome[a] Acute glomerulonephritis[a] Hydronephrosis Duplication anomaly	Common
Compensatory hypertrophy[b] Fused ectopy[b] Infant of diabetic mother[a] Infantile polycystic kidney[a] Adult polycystic kidney[a] Multicystic dysplastic kidney[b] Leukemia-lymphoma[a] Hemolytic-uremic syndrome[a] Henoch-Schönlein purpura[a] Intrarenal abscess, hematoma[b]	Moderately common
Renal vein thrombosis (acute)[b] Glycogen storage disease[a] Tuberous sclerosis[a] Beckwith-Wiedemann syndrome[a] Sickle cell disease[a]	Uncommon
Nephroblastomatosis[a] Bile nephrosis[a]	Rare

[a] Usually bilateral.
[b] Usually unilateral.

lengthy (Table 3.14), ultrasound can identify the cause in the majority of cases. Enlarged but otherwise normal-appearing kidneys occur with conditions that cause generalized organomegaly (e.g., Beckwith-Wiedemann syndrome, infant of diabetic mother) and with compensatory hypertrophy of the kidney due to nonfunction or absence of the contralateral kidney. Partially duplicated kidneys can appear enlarged and can usually be recognized by discontinuity of the central renal echoes (Fig. 3.25A). A solitary enlarged kidney may also be due to crossed fused ectopia.

One of the most common causes of renal enlargement is hydronephrosis. A complete discussion of the conditions resulting in hydronephrosis is beyond the scope of this text, but the most common cause of marked hydronephrosis is some form of ureteral or bladder outlet obstruction. Such obstructions include congenital ureteropelvic junction obstruction, ectopic ureterocele, and posterior urethral valves. Hydronephrosis due to vesicoureteral reflux is also fairly common, and although the hydronephrosis and renal enlargement tend to be less severe in this problem, in some cases marked hydronephrosis can occur (especially in patients with neurogenic bladder). Calyceal dilation due to conditions such as papillary necrosis or congenital megacalyces is uncommon.

Marked hydronephrosis must be differentiated from the enlarged, multicystic, dysplastic kidney (see Cystic Abdominal Masses).

A variety of diffuse renal parenchymal diseases can occur in children and result in renal enlargement. Most of these conditions are associated with edema of the kidney, and on ultrasound some of these kidneys will show increased renal parenchymal echogenicity and distortion of the normal architecture (Fig. 3.25B) (6). These findings are especially likely to occur in vascular problems such as renal vein thrombosis, hemolytic uremic syndrome (9), and Henoch-Schönlein purpura. Ultrasound is not particularly sensitive to renal changes in pyelonephritis, but in some patients renal enlargement, loss of the normal architecture, and thickening of the renal pelvis may be seen (12).

Renal cystic disease is a moderately common cause of enlarged kidneys. Multicystic dysplastic kidney is most commonly a unilateral process. When bilateral enlarged and cystic kidneys are seen, the most likely cause is one of the forms of polycystic kidney disease. The most common form of this disease to be encountered in infancy and childhood is the autosomal recessive (infantile or juvenile) form. In this condition, the kidneys are markedly enlarged and echogenic, and close inspection reveals numerous small cysts and tubular structures that represent the dilated, ectatic collecting tubules (Fig. 3.25C). Frequently, a thin sonolucent rim can be seen outlining the kidney (7). Visualization of the ectatic tubules is virtually a pathognomonic finding, both on ultrasound and intravenous urography, and differentiates this condition from the autosomal dominant (adult) form. The ectatic tubules are most easily visible in the infantile form of polycystic kidney disease. In juvenile polycystic kidney disease (which is also autosomal recessive and probably the same disease), the renal findings are similar but the ectatic tubules may be less distinct (8). In these patients, hepatic fibrosis and portal hypertension are commonly the problems that initially bring the patient to see the physician, rather than the renal disease.

Autosomal dominant (adult) polycystic kidney disease most commonly appears in early adulthood, but it may also be encountered in infancy and childhood. When this form is seen in a neonate, the appearance can be very similar to that of infantile polycystic kidney disease. In infants and children, however, the kidneys are enlarged but are not as echogenic as in the newborn. Multiple round cysts of variable sizes will be seen scattered throughout the kidneys (Fig. 3.25D), and similar cysts can also be found in the liver and pancreas. This condition can be differenti-

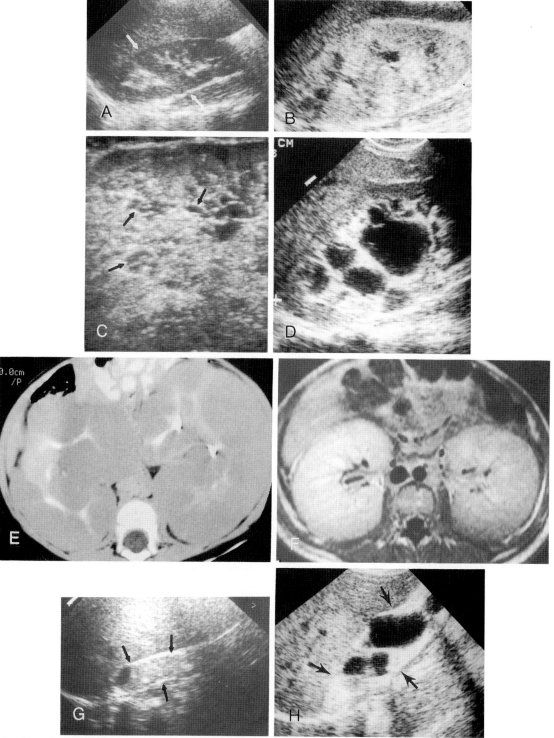

Figure 3.25. Renal size abnormalities. A. Duplex kidney. Note the interrupted central renal fat *(arrows)*, representing the separation of the renal collecting structures. **B. Nephrotic syndrome.** The kidney is enlarged and echogenic with loss of the normal architecture. Both kidneys were effected. **C. Autosomal recessive polycystic kidney disease.** Note the enlarged, distorted, and echogenic kidney. The multiple linear anechoic structures represent the ectatic tubules *(arrows)*. **D. Autosomal dominant polycystic kidney disease.** Note the multiple anechoic cysts of variable sizes. The contralateral kidney showed minimal cyst formation. **E. Nephroblastomatosis.** Massive lobular enlargement of the kidneys is seen bilaterally, with stretching and displacement of the collecting structures. **F.** Marked bilateral renal enlargement due to infiltration in an adolescent with **leukemia. G.** Small echogenic kidneys due to familial nephronophthesis *(arrows)*. **H.** Scarred fibrotic kidneys in a child with a history of posterior urethral valves *(arrows)*.

Table 3.15
Small Kidneys

Chronic pyelonephritis[a] Chronic glomerulonephritis[a] Congenitally hypoplastic[b]	Common
Renal vein thrombosis (chronic with atrophy)[b] Atrophy after obstructive uropathy[a] Reflux nephropathy[a] Renal artery stenosis, occlusion[b]	Moderately common
Postirradiation[b] Papillary necrosis (late)[a] Ask-Upmark kidney[b] Juvenile nephronophthisis (medullary sponge)[a]	Rare

[a]Often or usually bilateral.
[b]Usually unilateral.

ated from multicystic dysplastic kidney because it is generally bilateral and the renal parenchyma intervening between the multiple cysts has a less dysplastic appearance. Glomerulocystic disease is a rare disease characterized by cystic dilation of Bowman's spaces that can also appear as cortical macrocysts and increased echogenicity of the renal parenchyma. Renal cysts may also be encountered in a variety of syndromes (e.g., tuberous sclerosis (11), Zellweger syndrome (10), asphyxiating thoracic dysplasia, Ehlers-Danlos syndrome, and certain trisomies). In most of these conditions, the cysts are small and the kidneys are not particularly enlarged. Bile nephrosis (renal tubular ectasia with bile casts) is a rare cause of enlarged echogenic kidneys that occurs in children with liver or obstructive biliary tract disease (1).

An uncommon cause of renal enlargement in children is infiltration of the kidney. This most often occurs with neoplasms, in particular, leukemia and lymphoma (Fig. 3.25F). Nephroblastomatosis is a condition in which the primitive nephrogenic blastema persists within the kidney after fetal life (3, 4, 13). In these patients, the kidneys are usually markedly enlarged, with lobular thickening of the renal parenchyma (Fig. 3.25E). Some of the storage diseases can also infiltrate and enlarge the kidneys.

Small kidneys are usually the result of scarring that can follow a wide variety of renal abnormalities (Table 3.15). Such scarring most commonly follows chronic or recurrent infection or chronic glomerulonephritis. Small kidneys also can be the product of obstructive uropathy (Fig. 3.25H), postreflux nephropathy, or renal vascular occlusion. Renal atrophy or infarction is not an uncommon finding in children with neuroblastoma (2). Juvenile nephronophthesis is a condition characterized by abnormali-

ties of the medullary collecting tubules. In some patients with this condition, the kidneys are small and echogenic, and occasionally a few small cysts will be seen within the medullary pyramids (5) (Fig. 3.25G). Congenital hypoplasia of the kidneys is a relatively common cause of a small kidney. The usually unilateral condition is thought to result from a vascular insult in utero.

REFERENCES

1. Bruno MA, Spear GS, Dietrich RB, Pugh PA: Bile nephrosis in a neonate: sonographic findings of rapid kidney enlargement and increased echogenicity. *AJR* 159:628, 1992.
2. Day DL, Johnson RT, Odrezin GT, Woods WG, Alford BA: Renal atrophy or infarction in children with neuroblastoma. *Radiol* 180:493, 1991.
3. Fernbach SK, Feinstein KA, Donaldson JS, Baum ES: Nephroblastomatosis: comparison of CT with US and urography. *Radiology* 166:153–156, 1988.
4. Franken EA Jr, Yiu-Chiu V, Smith WL, Chiu LC: Nephroblastomatosis: clinicopathologic significance and imaging characteristics. *AJR* 138:950–952, 1982.
5. Garel LA, Habib R, Pariete D, Broyer M, Sauvegrian J: Juvenile nephronophthisis: sonographic appearance in children with severe uremia. *Radiol* 151:93–96, 1984.

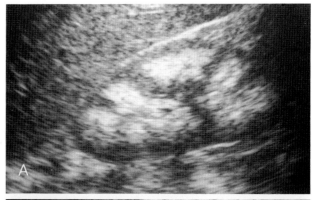

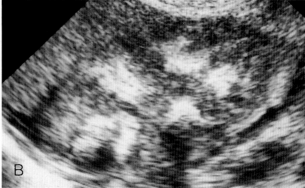

Figure 3.26. Echogenic renal pyramids. A. Prominent and echogenic renal pyramids in a child with idiopathic nephrocalcinosis. **B.** Acute tubular necrosis (medullary) in a 4-week-old infant. Note the markedly echogenic appearance of the pyramids.

6. Hayden CK Jr, Santa-Cruz FRM, Amparo EG, Brouhard B, Swischuk LE, Ahrendt DK: Ultrasonographic evaluation of the renal parenchyma in infancy and childhood. *Radiology* 152:413–417, 1984.
7. Hayden CK Jr, Swischuk LE, Smith TH, Armstrong EA: Renal cystic disease in childhood. *RadioGraphics* 6:97–116, 1986.
8. Kaariainen H, Jaaskelainen J, Kivisaari L, Koskimies O, Norio R: Dominant and recessive polycystic kidney disease in children: classification by intravenous pyelography, ultrasound, and computed tomography. *Pediatr Radiol* 18:45–50, 1988.
9. Kenney PJ, Brinsko RE, Patel DW: Sonography of the kidneys in hemolytic uremic syndrome. *Radiology* 21:547, 1986.
10. Luisiri A, Sotelo-Avila C, Silberstein MJ, Graviss GR: Sonography of the Zellweger syndrome. *J Ultrasound Med* 7:169–173, 1988.
11. Mitnick JS, Bosniak MA, Hilton S, Raghavendra BN, Subramanya BR, Geniesser NB: Cystic renal disease in tuberous sclerosis. *Radiol* 147:85–87, 1983.
12. Sty JR, Wells RG, Starshak RJ, Schroeder BA: Imaging in acute renal infection in children. *AJR* 148:471–477, 1987.
13. White KS, Kirks DR, Bove DR, Bove KE: Imaging of nephroblastomatosis: an overview. *Radiology* 182:1–5, 1992.

Echogenic Renal Medullary Pyramids

In normal infants and children, the medullary pyramids of the kidney are hypoechoic in relation to the rest of the renal parenchyma. Increased echogenicity of the medullary pyramids is not an uncommon occurrence and has a long list of causes (11). Transient idiopathic echogenicity of the pyramids can occur in neonates (10), but in many other patients the finding is related to hypercalcemia and hypercalciuria (Fig. 3.26A). One of the most common causes of hypercalciuria in infants is the use of long-term furosemide therapy in premature infants and in neonates with congestive heart failure and neonatal asphyxia (2, 5, 7). Exogenous steroid administration can also result in medullary nephrocalcinosis. Renal tubular acidosis is relatively common in childhood and, as in adults, can be associated with increased calcium phosphate salts in the urine, which can be deposited in the medullary pyramids. Other causes of hypercalciuria in children include hyperparathyroidism, Bartter syndrome (8, 9), medullary sponge kidney, Williams syndrome, prolonged immobilization (11), and glycogen storage disease type 1A (4).

The medullary pyramids can also appear echogenic in conditions that are not associated with elevated calcium levels. This can be a transient phenomenon in some normal newborn infants (1). Pyramidal hyperechogenicity has also been noted in some infants with autosomal recessive polycystic kidney disease (6). Children with sickle cell disease may demonstrate increased renal echogenicity, either diffuse or localized to the medullary pyramids (3, 12), which may be related to papillary necrosis. Medullary hyperechogenicity has also been described in children with Lesch-Nyhan syndrome, achondroplasia, and Hurler's mucopolysaccharidosis. Acute tubular necrosis and Tamm-Horsfall proteinuria can also result in echogenic pyramids (Fig. 3.26B). Rarely, renal hyperechogenicity in infants with autosomal recessive polycystic kidney disease can be confined to the medullary pyramids (6).

REFERENCES

1. Avni EF, Spechl-Robberecht M, Lebrun D, Gomes H, Garel L: Transient acute tubular disease in the newborn: characteristic ultrasound pattern. *Ann Radiol* 26:175–182, 1983.
2. Downing GJ, Egelhoff JC, Daily DK, Alon U: Furosemide-related renal calcifications in the premature infant: a longitudinal ultrasonographic study. *Pediatr Radiol* 21:563, 1991.
3. Ecbert DE, Jonutis AJ, Davidson, AJ: The incidence and manifestations of urographic papillary abnormalities in patients with S hemoglobinopathies. *Radiology* 113:59–63, 1974.
4. Fick JJA, Beek JFA: Echogenic kidneys and medullary calcium deposition in a young child with glycogen storage disease type 1A. *Pediatr Radiol* 22:72, 1992.
5. Glasier CM, Stoddard RA, Ackerman NB Jr, McCurdy FA, Null DM Jr, deLemos RA: Nephrolithiasis in infants:

Table 3.16
Abnormal Bladder Size

Small bladder	
Spastic neurogenic Chronic bladder outlet obstruction (hypertrophy)	Common
Severe cystitis (infection, drug-induced) Bladder diversion	Uncommon
Congenital small Surrounding tumor	Rare
Large bladder	
Neurogenic	Common
Prune-belly syndrome Chronic diuretic therapy	Moderately common
Diabetes insipidus Psychogenic water drinking Megacystis-microcolon syndrome Bartter syndrome	Rare

association with chronic furosemide therapy. *AJR* 140:107–108, 1983.

6. Herman TE, Siegal MJ: Pyramidal hyperechogenicity in autosomal recessive polycystic kidney disease resembling medullary nephrocalcinosis. *Pediatr Radiol* 21:270, 1991.

7. Kenney IJ, Aiken CG, Lenney W: Furosemide-induced nephro-calcinosis in very low birth weight infants. *Pediatr Radiol* 18:323–325, 1988.

8. Matsumoto J, Han BK, de Rovetto CR, Welch TR: Hypercalciuric Bartter syndrome: resolution of nephrocalcinosis with indomethacin. *AJR* 152:1251–1253, 1989.

9. Ohlsson A, Sieck U, Cumming W, Akhtar M, Serenius R: A variant of Bartter's syndrome: Bartter's syndrome associated with hydramnios, prematurity, hypercalciuria and nephrocalcinosis. *Acta Paediatr Scand* 73:868–874, 1984.

10. Riebel TW, Abraham K, Wartner R, Mueller R: Transient renal medullary hyperechogenicity in ultrasound studies of neonates: is it a normal phenomenon and what are the causes? *J Clin Ultrasound* 21:25–31, 1993.

11. Shultz PK, Strife JL, Strife CF, McDaniel JD: Hyperechoic renal medullary pyramids in infants and children. *Radiology* 181:163–167, 1991.

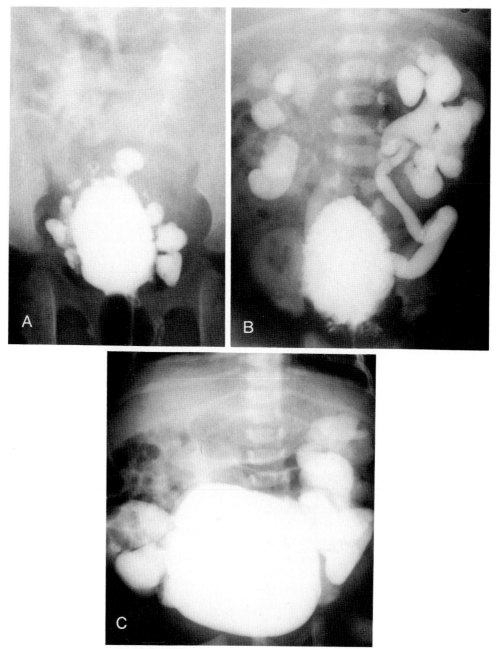

Figure 3.27. Bladder size abnormalities. A. Note the small and markedly trabeculated bladder, the result of urethral obstruction due to **posterior urethral valves. B.** Another infant with posterior urethral valves, showing a trabeculated bladder with bilateral vesicourethral reflux. **C.** A large bladder with reflux into markedly dilated ureters in an infant with **prune-belly syndrome.**

12. Zinn D, Haller JO, Gohen HL: Focal and diffuse increased echogenicity in the renal parenchyma in patients with sickle hemoglobinopathies: an observation. *J Ultrasound Med* 12:211–214, 1993.

Bladder Size Abnormalities

Abnormalities of the size of the urinary bladder are most often due to neurologic conditions or to bladder outlet obstruction (Table 3.16). A neurogenic bladder can take a variety of forms. A large atonic bladder is most commonly seen with nerve root and peripheral neuropathy, whereas spinal cord and brain abnormalities tend to produce a thick-walled, trabeculated, small bladder. In childhood, neurogenic bladder is frequently associated with spina bifida or meningomyelocele deformities. Other causes of a neurogenic bladder include anorectal anomalies with hypoplasia or absence of the sacrum (2), anterior sacral meningocele, presacral masses (e.g., teratomas), and intraspinal abnormalities such as diastematomyelia, cysts, and tumors. Chronic bladder outlet obstruction in children is most often the result of posterior urethral valves in infant boys. The chronic obstruction leads to muscular hypertrophy, resulting in a thick-walled and markedly trabeculated bladder (Fig. 3.27A). Severe hydronephrosis and hydroureter usually accompanies this condition (Fig. 3.27B).

Bladder abnormalities are virtually always present in patients with the prune-belly (Eagle-Barrett) syndrome. In some infants with this condition, urethral atresia or posterior urethral valves are present, which cause a small, hypertrophied bladder. More commonly, however, no cause of urethral obstruction is found. In these patients, the bladder is markedly enlarged and floppy and demonstrates poor emptying (Fig. 3.27C). Large urachal remnants are frequently present, as well as marked hydronephrosis and hydroureter. A massively enlarged, poorly functioning bladder is also a part of the megacystis-microcolon-intestinal hypoperistalsis syndrome (1). Some degree of bladder enlargement commonly occurs in conditions associated with chronic diuresis, including diabetes insipidus, chronic diuretic therapy, and psychogenic water drinking.

The most common cause of a small bladder is, once again, a spastic neurogenic bladder or a hypertrophied bladder due to chronic bladder outlet obstruction. When urinary diversion has been performed, the bladder frequently atrophies and becomes small. A scarred bladder can be the result of previous infection or drug-induced hemorrhagic cystitis. Congenital smallness of the bladder is quite rare.

REFERENCES

1. Berdon WE, Baker DH, Blanc WA, Gay B, Santulli TV, Donovan C: Megacystis-microcolon-intestinal hypoperistalsis syndrome: a new cause of intestinal obstruction in the newborn. *AJR* 126:937–964, 1976.
2. Koff SA, Derrider PA: Patterns of neurogenic bladder dysfunction in sacral agenesis. *J Urol* 118:87–89, 1977.

4

BONES AND
SOFT TISSUES

Generalized Bone Density Changes

For the most part, generalized bone density increase (i.e., whiter bones) infers excess calcium deposition and decreased density (lucent bones) represents loss or decreased deposition of calcium. Generally, conditions considered in this section are those where the bones are more or less normal in configuration. They are either more dense or less dense, but their overall configuration is still basically normal. Although many bony dysplasias and dystrophies may show changes in mineralization, they are not included in this section, because the bone density changes are more incidental than specific. In addition, bony problems manifesting in focal density changes are not considered.

Increased Bone Density

Excess calcium deposition leading to increased bone density can occur on a metabolic basis, with certain hematologic disorders, and inherently in some syndromes and bony dysplasias (Table 4.1). In terms of the **dysplasias,** the one best known is osteopetrosis, or Albers-Schönberg disease. In this condition, except in very mild cases, the changes of markedly white bones, with virtual obliteration of the medullary canal and widening of the metaphyses, are easy to detect (Fig. 4.1A). Other changes may include a bone-within-bone appearance and

transverse fractures of the chalk-like skeleton. Associated anemia and hepatosplenomegaly are common and are important in differentiating the condition from other conditions associated with increased bone density. These include entities such as pyknodysostosis (12, 16), idiopathic hypercalcemia (Williams) syndrome, Robinow-Silverman-Smith syndrome (11), and generalized sclerostenosis (4). This latter condition is similar, if not related, to van Buchem disease. Craniometaphyseal dysostosis appears similar to van Buchem disease except that the long bones, rather than being sclerotic, are osteoporotic and somewhat ballooned.

In pyknodysostosis, certain clinical (i.e., dwarfism, shortened extremities, frontal bossing) and roentgenographic (terminal phalangeal underdevelopment, biparietal bossing, Wormian bones) features cause confusion with cleidocranial dysostosis. In the latter, however, absence or hypoplasia of the clavicles and pubic bones is seen and no bony sclerosis occurs. Pyknodysostosis also can be confused with osteopetrosis, but with pyknodysostosis no hematologic disturbances are present and, thus, there is no hepatosplenomegaly. In addition, the "bone-within-bone" appearance and metaphyseal changes such as splaying and transverse banding are absent. Williams syndrome is associated with an abnormal facial appearance (often termed "elfin facies") and, in many cases, vascular abnormalities such as supravalvular aortic stenosis, peripheral pulmonary artery coarctations, and systemic artery stenoses. The bones, although increased in density, are not deformed or shortened to the extent that an obvious dysplasia is

Table 4.1
Increased Bone Density (Generalized)

Osteopetrosis Chronic renal disease[a]	Common
Idiopathic osteosclerosis of newborn Neonatal intrauterine infections Hypothyroidism Heavy metal intoxication Old periosteal bone deposition	Moderately common
Idiopathic hypercalcemia Storage diseases	Relatively rare
Pyknodysostosis Myelofibrosis Fluorosis Hypervitaminosis D Sclerosteosis and Van Buchem disease Kenny-Caffey syndrome Sarcoidosis Robinow-Silverman-Smith syndrome Pyle disease	Rare

[a] Treated.

suggested. Overall, however, the condition is not that common, and most cases actually show normal bone density. Even more rare is the Robinow-Silverman-Smith syndrome, a form of middle-segment dwarfism where, in addition to sclerotic bones (11), hypoplastic genitalia and spinal anomalies are seen.

In the neonatal period, all of the three preceding conditions can be confused with "transient osteosclerosis of the newborn" (13). In these patients it is believed that more compact bone than usual is present and causes the bones to become dense. The condition is temporary and the findings usually resolve by 2 or 3 months.

Increased bone density also is seen in the neonate with intrauterine infections. The cause of this phenomenon is unknown, but most likely there is impaired turnover of bone secondary to the infection. Vasculitis is the basic problem in these infants, and it may be that impaired blood supply leads to the bone density. Whatever the cause, the bones can appear quite sclerotic and the finding is most profound with rubella infections. However, it is also fre-

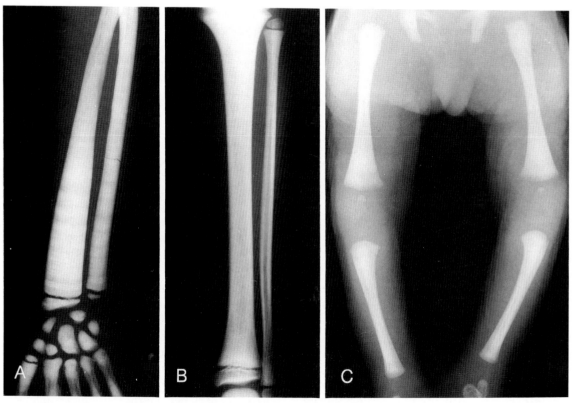

Figure 4.1. Increased bone density. A. Typical appearance of bony sclerosis in osteopetrosis. Also note diametaphyseal widening and multiple transverse, trophic bands. **B.** Generalized osteosclerosis in granulocytic leukemia. **C.** Osteosclerosis in neonatal syphilis.

quently seen with congenital syphilis (Fig. 4.1C). It is less commonly seen with cytomegalovirus infections.

Bony sclerosis also can be seen in certain **hematologic** diseases, but is relatively uncommon and occurs primarily with myelofibrosis, either primary or secondary. The latter usually is seen with conditions such as leukemia (Fig. 4.1B) (14), but also has been documented with congenital neutropenia (1).

Metabolic causes of increased bone density include the previously mentioned idiopathic hypercalcemia or Williams syndrome, dialyzed patients with chronic renal disease (9) (usually in the healing phase of renal osteodystrophy), hypervitaminosis D (increased calcium and phosphorus deposition), and hypothyroidism. In hypothyroidism, it is not known why the bones appear dense, but it may be because of slow bone metabolism leading to a lack of normal turnover of calcium in the bones. This is conjecture only, but whatever the cause, the abnormal density decreases with treatment.

Other causes of increased bone density include chronic lead and other heavy metal intoxication, fluorosis, the rare case of sarcoidosis (15), pseudo- and pseudopseudohypoparathyroidism, and the Kenny-Caffey syndrome (3, 7). In the latter condition, sclerosis is associated with stenosis of the medullary canals. As a result, the bones are quite thin, yet their cortices are thick and dense. With heavy metal poisoning and fluorosis the main problem is thickening of the trabeculae, but actual deposition of the heavy metal also occurs.

Before leaving the subject of increased bone density, it might be noted that under certain conditions only the diaphyses of long bones become dense and sclerotic. This occurs with certain bony dysplasias where increased diaphyseal bone deposition occurs and also with any condition where periosteal new bone deposition is seen (see Table 4.42). With most of these conditions, however, the fact that the bone shows increased density is more an associated finding than one used for primary diagnosis.

Decreased Bone Density

Decreased bone density results from decreased calcium content of the bones, and the finding occurs both with osteoporosis and osteomalacia (Table 4.2). With osteoporosis, however, there is concomitant decrease in bone matrix (i.e., osteoid), whereas with osteomalacia, bone matrix is normal. In osteomalacia

Table 4.2
Decreased Bone Density

Osteoporosis	
Disuse[a] Nutritional	Common
Chronic anemia Osteogenesis imperfecta Steroid therapy Collagen vascular diseases Hyperemia with infection, inflammation, arteriovenous fistula[b] Storage diseases	Moderately common
Idiopathic hypocalcemia Cushing syndrome Idiopathic juvenile osteoporosis Turner syndrome Hyperthyroidism Sudeck atrophy[b]	Relatively rare
Scurvy Sarcoidosis Progeria Ehlers-Danlos syndrome Homocystinuria Phenylketonuria Fibrogenesis imperfecta	Rare
Osteomalacia	
Rickets[c] Hyperparathyroidism Renal osteodystrophy	Commonest
Hypophosphatasia, pseudohypophosphatasia Fibrogenesis imperfecta Gangliosidosis[d] Jansen metaphyseal dysostosis[d] Mucolipidosis II (I cell disease)[d]	Relatively rare

[a] Immobilization.
[b] Single bone.
[c] All types.
[d] In infancy, changes resemble hyperparathyroidism.

the bone matrix simply is never adequately mineralized. Indeed, in time it actually becomes overabundant. This leads to bone softening, bending, and fracturing. These fractures may be overt, or of the Looser type, that is, a green-stick fracture due to chronic bending. With osteoporosis, bone bending is not a particular problem, but since the bones are structurally weak and brittle they tend to fracture easily.

The decrease in bone matrix in **osteoporosis** can result from primary lack of its formation or loss after normal deposition. The former occurs with scurvy

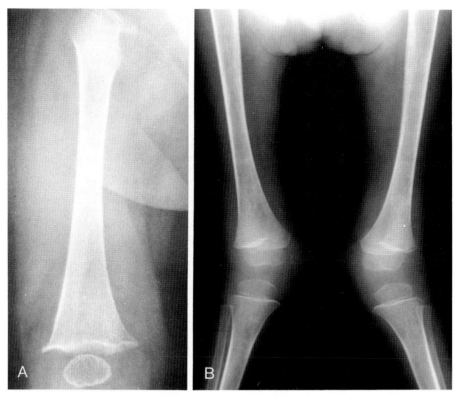

Figure 4.2. Diminished bone density: osteoporosis. A. Scurvy. Note generalized demineralization, but residual, thin white cortices. **B.** Neurogenic problem with knock-knees and diffusely demineralized bones with thin, distinct, white cortices.

(Fig. 4.2*A*) and certain bony dysplasias, the most common of which is osteogenesis imperfecta (see Fig. 4.9). However, it is also seen with Turner syndrome (2), progeria, Ehlers-Danlos syndrome, homocystinuria, and phenylketonuria. Excess loss of bone matrix after normal deposition occurs when osteoclastic activity surpasses osteoblastic activity and bone atrophy results. Most often this is seen with nonuse or immobilization, either acute or chronic (Fig. 4.2*B*), but also it is common with hyperemia associated with infections, inflammation, vasculitides (collagen vascular diseases), and trauma. On a focal basis, it occurs with Sudeck atrophy and localized arteriovenous fistulae.

Osteoporosis due to matrix loss also is seen with idiopathic hypocalcemia, Cushing syndrome (8), hyperthyroidism, steroid therapy, some cases of sarcoidosis, and in the condition known as juvenile osteoporosis (5, 6). The latter condition is of unknown etiology, but can result in profound transient osteoporosis of the entire skeleton. Compression fractures of the vertebra are common, and the condition tends to occur in later childhood and early adolescence.

With immobilization of an extremity or of the whole body, normal stresses on bone are removed and osteoblastic activity is depressed. With continued osteoclastic activity, bone atrophy and osteoporosis result; i.e., old bone is not replaced by new bone, and slowly, bone loss and demineralization occur. Roentgenographically, this is manifested by thinning of the trabeculae and cortices and, with time, disappearance of the smaller trabeculae and increased prominence of the larger ones. Eventually, the bone assumes a very glassy appearance, with thin, white trabeculae and cortices that stand out in prominent relief (Fig. 4.2). Overall, the trabecular and cortical pattern of mineralization becomes rather delicate. The same phenomenon occurs with hyperemia and also in the early stages of bone marrow hypercellularity or impregnation. Hypercellularity usually occurs with chronic anemias (10), leukemia, lymphoma, metastatic disease, and mastocytosis (17), while foreign material impregnation is seen with the various storage diseases. In all of these conditions, increased intraosseous pressure due to the hypercellularity or impregnation results in atrophy of the primary trabeculae. As a result, the number of trabeculae is decreased and the secondary trabeculae stand out in relief. In many of these patients, variable widening of the bones may be seen, especially in the metaphyseal regions.

In osteomalacia, with no matrix or osteoid loss,

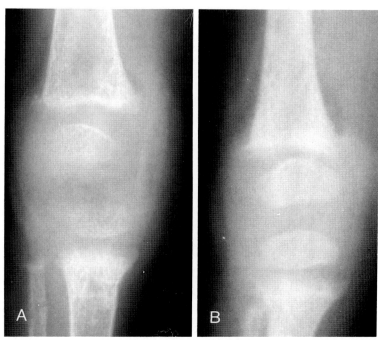

Figure 4.3. Osteomalacia. A. Rickets. Note indistinctness of the cortex and trabeculae. Also note typical rachitic changes in the metaphyses of this infant with rickets. Osteomalacia is characteristic of rickets. **B.** Similar changes in hyperparathyroidism.

the trabeculae and cortex do not become thinned, only demineralized. The result is a coarse, indistinct, fuzzy pattern of demineralization (Fig. 4.3), quite different from the delicate, sharp-appearing pattern seen with osteoporosis. Thereafter, as the changes advance, the cortex becomes so poorly defined that it virtually disappears. A more or less complete list of conditions producing osteomalacia is presented in Table 4.2, but the most common are rickets and hyperparathyroidism. Hyperparathyroidism usually is secondary and seen with renal osteodystrophy, for primary hyperparathyroidism is rare in childhood. Most of the other conditions listed in Table 4.2 would be expected to produce osteomalacia and the fact that they are a part of the list is no surprise, but a comment regarding Jansen metaphyseal dysostosis, gangliosidosis, and mucolipidosis II is in order. Although unrelated to hyperparathyroidism, for some unknown reason these diseases produce changes indistinguishable from it in infancy.

Finally, it should be noted that osteoporosis and osteomalacia can occur together, and then the findings of both are intertwined. Actually, the problem is not uncommon, and the reason for this is that in many of the conditions producing severe osteomalacia, the illness is so severe that the patient becomes bedridden. This then leads to disuse (immobilization) osteoporosis, superimposed on changes of osteomalacia.

REFERENCES

1. Boechat MI, Gormley LS, O'Laughlin BJ: Thickened cortical bones in congenital neutropenia. *Pediatr Radiol* 17:124–126, 1987.
2. Brown DM, Jowsey J, Bradford DS: Osteoporosis in ovarian dysgenesis. *J Pediatr* 84:816–820, 1974.
3. Caffey J: Congenital stenosis of medullary spaces in tubular bones and calvaria in two proportionate dwarfs—mother and son: coupled with transitory hypocalcemic tetany. *AJR* 100:1, 1967.
4. Cremin BJ: Sclerostenosis in children. *Pediatr Radiol* 8:173–177, 1979.
5. Houang MTW, Brenton DP, Renton P, Shaw DG: Idiopathic juvenile osteoporosis. *Skeletal Radiol* 3:17–23, 1978.
6. Jowsey J, Johnson KA: Juvenile osteoporosis: bone findings in seven patients. *J Pediatr* 81:511–517, 1972.
7. Kenny FM, Linarelli L: Dwarfism and cortical thickening of tubular bones: transient hypocalcemia in a mother and son. *Am J Dis Child* 111:201, 1966.
8. McArthur RG, Cloutier MD, Hayles AB, Sprague RG: Cushing's disease in children: findings in 13 cases. *Mayo Clin Proc* 47:318–326, 1972.
9. Mehls O, Willich E, Beduhn D, Schuler HW, Krempien B, Ritz E: Roentgenological findings in the skeleton of dialyzed children. *Pediatr Radiol* 1:183–190, 1973.
10. Moseley JE: Skeletal changes in the anemias. *Semin Roentgenol* 9:169–184, 1974.
11. Robinow M, Silverman FN, Smith HD: A newly recognized dwarfing syndrome. *Am J Dis Child* 117:645–649, 1969.
12. Ivastava KK, Bhattacharya AK, Galatius-Jensen F, Tamaela LA, Borgstein A, Kozlowski K: Pycnodysostosis: report of four cases. *Australas Radiol* 22:70–78, 1978.

13. Swischuk LE: *Radiology of the Newborn and Young Infant.* 3d ed. Baltimore: Williams & Wilkins, 1989: 708.
14. Tebbi K, Zarkowsky HS, Siegel BA, McAlister WH: Childhood myelofibrosis and osteosclerosis without myeloid metaplasia [Abstract]. *Radiology* 114:246, 1975.
15. Weston M, Duffy P: Osteosclerosis in sarcoidosis. *Australas Radiol* 19:191–193, 1975.
16. Wolpowitz A, Matisonn A: A comparative study of pycnodysostosis, cleidocranial dysostosis, osteopetrosis and acro-osteolysis [Abstract]. *Radiology* 113:758, 1974.
17. Wooten WB, de Sants LA, Finkelstein JB: Case report 61—diagnosis: systematic mastocytosis. *Skeletal Radiol* 3:53–55, 1978.

Long Bone Tubulation Abnormalities

With tubulation abnormalities of the long bones one can encounter undertubulated (short, squat) or overtubulated (long, thin) bones. Short, squat bones can be classified as follows: (a) squat bones with metaphyseal flaring, (b) squat bones with excessive metaphyseal flaring (dumbbell configuration), (c) short bones with minimal or no metaphyseal flaring, and (d) bones where middle segment (radius, ulna, tibia-fibula) shortening predominates. With long, thin bones it is not practical to subclassify the findings because the bones tend to appear much the same from condition to condition.

UNDERTUBULATION: SHORT, SQUAT BONES (TABLE 4.3)

Undertubulation of long bones can occur on a focal basis and usually is secondary to injury, infection, or congenital hypoplasia. The problems here are self-evident, and usually the bones are also deformed to one degree or another. Generalized shortening of the bones occurs primarily with bony dysplasias, dwarfing syndromes, and some metabolic conditions, and is the focus of this section.

In terms of bony dysplasias, the one best known to produce short, squat bones is achondroplasia (Fig. 4.4A), a form of dwarfism serving as a prototype for other chondrodystrophies. In addition to the short long bones, the ribs are short, the iliac wings square and hypoplastic, the acetabular angles flat, the calvarial base underdeveloped and constricted, the vertebra small and cuboid, and the spinal canal itself narrower than normal. At the same time, the foramen magnum is smaller than normal, which may lead to obstructive hydrocephalus. Hypochondroplasia probably is related to achondroplasia, but the bone changes are much less pronounced (7, 10). Changes similar to those seen with achondroplasia

Table 4.3
Undertubulation: Short, Squat Bones

Achondroplasia[a] Storage diseases[b,c]	Common
Metaphyseal dysostosis[a] Pseudoachondroplasia[a] Madelung deformity[e] Hypochondroplasia[a] Vitamin D-resistant rickets-type B[c] Neonatal dwarfs[a] Chondrodystrophy with immune deficiency[a]	Moderately common
Rhizomelic punctate epiphyseal dysplasia[a] Diastrophic dwarfism[a,e] Hypophosphatasia[a] Metatropic dwarfism[d] Kniest syndrome[d] Dyggve-Melchior-Clausen[d] Camptomelic dwarfism[b,e] Larsen syndrome[b,e] Weissenbacher-Zweymuller syndrome[a]	Rare

[a] Flared metaphyses.
[b] Hypoplastic ends.
[c] No metaphyseal flaring.
[d] Dumbbell-shaped bones.
[e] Middle segment predominance.

occur with asphyxiating thoracic dystrophy, the Ellis-van Creveld syndrome, and diastrophic dwarfism. However, the pelvis is usually a little different in these latter entities in that it is somewhat more square and more irregular along the acetabular roof (Fig. 4.105A). In addition, in asphyxiating thoracic dystrophy long bone shortening is minimal and there is no metaphyseal flaring. Shortening of the long bones occurs in the Ellis-van Creveld syndrome and, in addition, carpal fusion and polydactyly are hallmarks of the condition. With diastrophic dwarfism the long bones are short, but there is excessive shortening of the middle segment bones of the extremities. In addition, the ends may be hypoplastic and frequently a Madelung deformity is present. The hallmarks of the condition, however, are severe clubbed feet and scoliosis. Hyperextensibility of the thumb, the "hitchhiker's" thumb, is also characteristic. In addition, the various metaphyseal dysostoses if severe enough (see Fig. 4.69) can produce impaired linear growth, resulting in short, squat bones with metaphyseal flaring. These conditions are discussed elsewhere, and while they do produce short bones in some cases, the characteristic irregularity of the metaphysis is the key to proper diagnosis.

In the neonatal period, a number of dwarfs who tend to resemble severely afflicted achondroplasts can be encountered (11). Most have definite features which distinguish them from true achondroplasts,

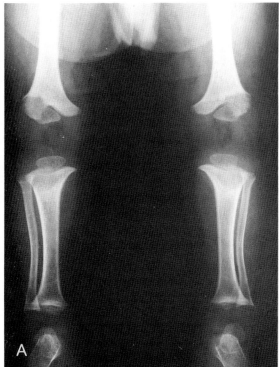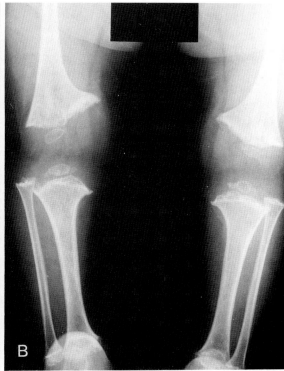

Figure 4.4. Short, broad bones (undertubulation). A. Typical short, broad bones in **achondroplasia. B. Pseudoachondroplasia.** Note overall similar appearance to achondroplasia, but also note that epiphyseal involvement is more marked. In less severe cases, the bones are not as broad, but still quite short.

but a complete review of these is beyond the scope of this book. On the other hand, one might at least be familiar with some of their names and key differentiating features: achondrogenesis types I and II—spine in general and lower spine especially is unossified; thanatophoric dwarfism—looks like severe achondroplasia but has flat vertebra; short rib polydactyly dwarfism—Majewski and Saldino-Noonan types—very short bones and flat vertebra; hypophosphatasia (11)—looks like achondrogenesis; metatropic dwarfism—dumbbell-shaped long bones present; the Kniest (15) and Dyggve-Melchior-Clausen syndromes—resemble metatropic dwarfs; and severe rhizomelic (recessive) punctate epiphyseal dysplasia—stippled epiphyses and severe contractures. In general, all of these dwarfs demonstrate markedly short bones which often are very squat and show pronounced metaphyseal cupping, with or without actual flaring. Many also show small thoraces and short, cupped ribs. They are shown in Figure 4.5.

Short, squat bones also are seen in the condition known as pseudoachondroplasia. Certain features in these children may at first suggest achondroplasia, but the problem is not so much poor enchondral bone formation as epiphyseal maldevelopment. The changes vary in severity and it is in the more severe cases that the findings can be confused with achondroplasia. If one examines the epiphyses closely, however, one will note that they are markedly or predominantly involved (Fig. 4.4B), whereas in achondroplasia, epiphyseal changes are minimal.

There are two forms of pseudoachondroplasia: multiple epiphyseal and spondyloepiphyseal types. In the latter type, severe platyspondyly exists, whereas in the former it does not. In either case, however, along with marked epiphyseal underdevelopment, there is concomitant metaphyseal growth impairment. As a result, metaphyseal flaring and long bone shortening occur, and for this reason achondroplasia is misdiagnosed: hence the term "pseudoachondroplasia." In some conditions in which the long bones are short, metaphyseal flaring is so pronounced that a **dumbbell appearance of the bones results.** Only a few conditions produce such a degree of change and, for the most part, consist of metatropic dwarfism (Fig. 4.6), the Kniest syndrome, the Dyggve-Melchior-Clausen syndrome (24), and the more severe cases of pseudoachondroplasia.

Another variation of short, squat bones with metaphyseal widening is seen with certain chondrodysplasias associated with some immunodeficiency syndromes. These include adenosine deaminase

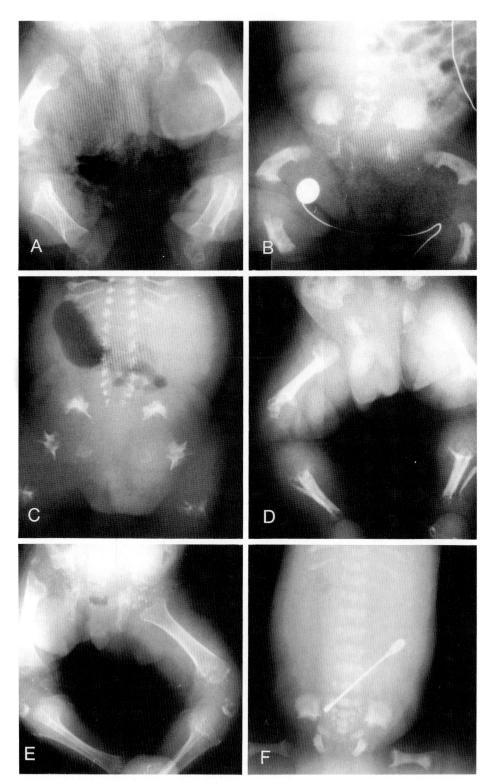

Figure 4.5. Neonatal dwarfs. A. Achondroplasia: homozygous type. Note the extremely short long bones with deeply cupped ends. **B. Thanatophoric dwarf.** Changes resemble those of severe achondroplasia. **C. Achondrogenesis.** Extremely short long bones with deeply cupped ends. Note that the vertebral bodies are underossified and the ribs very short. **D. Hypophosphatasia.** Note short bones and deeply cupped meta-physes. The metaphyses, however, are very irregular. (Courtesy of C. Stuart Houston, M.D.) **E. Punctate epiphyseal dysplasia; rhizomelic type.** Note the extremely short extremities with flexion contractures and marked stippling of the epiphyses and patellae. **F. Short rib-polydactyly syndrome.** Note the short long bones with deeply cupped metaphyses.

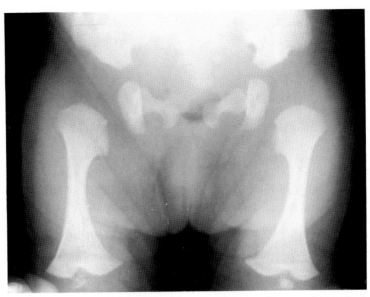

Figure 4.6. Dumbbell long bones. Note the short, squat femurs with very wide metaphyses constituting a dumbbell appearance. Metatropic dwarfism.

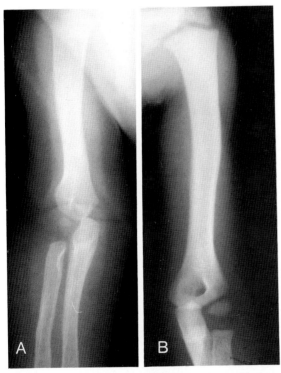

Figure 4.7.   Short, squat humeri. A. Note short, wide humerus in mucopolysaccharidosis. **B.** Similar appearing humerus in vitamin D-resistant hypophosphatemic rickets type B.

deficiency with chondro-osseous dysplasia (3), Schwachman-Diamond syndrome (18, 23, 28) associated with neutropenia and pancreatic insufficiency, and McKusick-type metaphyseal dysostosis also associated with neutropenia and pancreatic insufficiency (4, 13). Another group of patients demonstra-

ting short, squat bones but without metaphyseal flaring are those with vitamin D-resistant rickets, type B (27) and the various storage diseases, including the more penetrant mucopolysaccaridoses and lipidoses,ie, Hunter, Hurler, Marateaux-Lemay, gangliosidosis, and mucolipidosis I and II (Fig. 4.7).

Conditions where **middle segment** (mesomelic) shortening predominates are not particularly common, but include mesomelic dwarfism (Nievergelt and Langer [14] types), dyschondrosteosis or Madelung deformity (upper extremity predominance), the Ellis-van Creveld syndrome (26), the Robinow-Silverman-Smith syndrome (21), diastrophic dwarfism, and the ulnofibular dysplasia syndromes of Rhinehardt and Pfeiffer. In many of these conditions, the bones, in addition to being short, also are curved or bent (Fig. 4.8). This occurs primarily with mesomelic dwarfism, the ulnofibular dysplasia syndromes, diastrophic dwarfism, and dyschondrosteosis, or Madelung deformity. In the latter condition there is also posterior dislocation of the ulna. In mesomelic dwarfism and the ulnofibular dysplasia syndromes, the involved bones also often are severely hypoplastic (Fig. 4.8D).

Middle segment shortening also is seen in the camptomelic dwarfism and Larsen syndromes, and in many of these cases the ends of the long bones also are somewhat hypoplastic and underdeveloped. Such hypoplasia often is most pronounced around the elbow, and in Larsen syndrome multiple joint dislocations coexist.

Bone shortening on an **isolated basis** most often occurs after trauma or infection of a bone (i.e., bat-

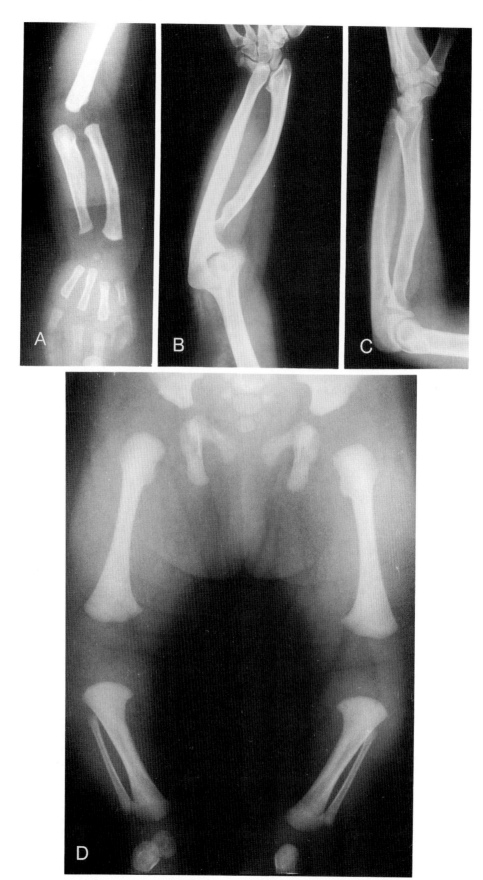

Figure 4.8. Middle segment shortening. A. Markedly shortened and bowed radius and ulna in middle segment dwarfism. **B.** Typical short radius and ulna in Madelung deformity or dyschondrosteosis. **C.** Lateral view showing increased carpal angle, and typical posterior dislocation of the ulna. **D.** Short tibia and hypoplastic fibula in ulnofibular dysplasia.

tered child syndrome, osteomyelitis, radiation, septicemia with small vessel thrombosis, and vitamin A intoxication [20]).

OVERTUBULATION: LONG, THIN BONES (TABLE 4.4)

The major causes of long, thin bones are atrophy and congenital bony dysplasia. The commonest, of

Table 4.4
Overtubulation: Thin, Gracile Bones

Neurologic-neuromuscular disease	Commonest
Osteogenesis imperfecta Arthrogryposis syndromes	Moderately common
Marfan syndrome Homocystinuria	Relatively rare
Cockayne syndrome Winchester syndrome Progeria Kenny-Caffey[a] Marfan contractural arachnodactyly Stickler syndrome Hallermann-Streiff syndrome Seckel bird-headed dwarf	Rare

[a]Medullary stenosis syndrome. Thin bones but thick, sclerotic cortex.

course, is atrophy, which most often is secondary to the chronic disuse seen with a large number of neurologic or neuromuscular diseases (Fig. 4.9A), including the heterogeneous arthrogryposis multiplex congenita group. However, it also can be seen with long-standing debilitating arthritic disease (usually rheumatoid arthritis) and in the debilitating storage disease known as Winchester syndrome (29). In this latter condition, rheumatoid-like findings are seen.

Bony dysplasias leading to long, thin bones include osteogenesis imperfecta (Fig. 4.9B), Cockayne syndrome, progeria, Marfan syndrome (1), Marfan contractural arachnodactyly (6, 12, 16) (Fig. 4.9C), homocystinuria (1, 17, 19, 22), Seckel bird-headed dwarfism, Kenny-Caffey or medullary stenosis syndrome (2, 5) (often associated with hypocalcemia and seizures), and the Stickler, Hallermann-Streiff, and Werdnig-Hoffman syndromes. Osteogenesis imperfecta, of course, is the most common of these conditions, and bone thinning is believed to result from impaired diaphyseal bone formation. In the Kenny-Caffey syndrome, in addition to the bones being thin, the cortices are very thick and sclerotic. Although in all of these conditions the long bones are thin and appear long, when they are truly long the best possibilities are Marfan syndrome, Marfan's contractural arachnodactyly, and homocystinuria.

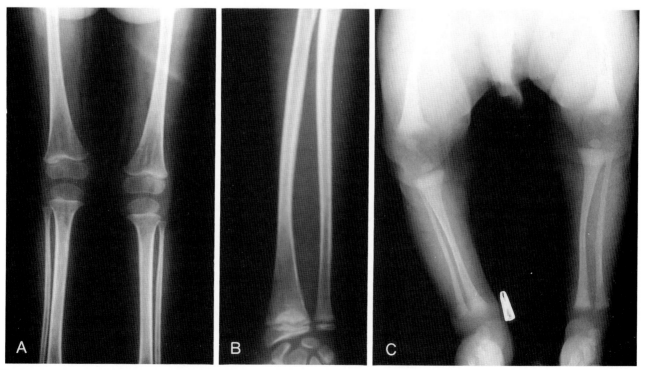

Figure 4.9. Long, thin bones (overtubulation). A. Typical long thin bones in patient with long-standing neurologic disease. **B.** Long, thin forearm bones in osteogenesis imperfecta tarda. **C.** Long, thin bones in infant with Marfan contractural arachnodactyly.

REFERENCES

1. Brenton DP, Dow CJ, James JIP, Hay RL, Wynne-Davies R: Homocystinuria and Marfan's syndrome: a comparison. *J Bone Joint Surg* 54:277–298, 1972.
2. Caffey J: Congenital stenosis of medullary spaces in tubular bones and calvaria in two proportionate dwarfs—mother and son: coupled with transitory hypocalcemic tetany. *Am J Roentgenol Radium Ther Nucl Med* 100:1–11, 1967.
3. Cederbaum SD, Kaitila I, Rimoin DL, Steihm ER: The chondro-osseous dysplasia of adenosine deaminase deficiency with severe combined immunodeficiency. *J Pediatr* 89:737–742, 1976.
4. Chakravarti VS, Borns P, Lobell J, Douglas SD: Chondro-osseous dysplasia in severe combined immunodeficiency due to adenosine deaminase deficiency: chondroosseous dysplasia in ADA deficiency SCID. *Pediatr Radiol* 21:447–448, 1991.
5. Frech RS, McAlister WH: Medullary stenosis of the tubular bones associated with hypocalcemic convulsions and short stature. *Radiology* 91:457–461, 1968.
6. Gruber MA, Graham TP Jr, Engle E, Smith C: Marfan's syndrome with contractural arachnodactyly and severe mitral regurgitation in a premature infant. *J Pediatr* 93:80–82, 1978.
7. Hall BD, Spranger J: Hypochondroplasia: clinical and radiological aspects in 39 cases. *Radiology* 133:95–100, 1979.
8. Haller JO, Berdon WE, Robinow M, Slovis TL, Baker DH, Johnson DF: The Weissenbacher-Zweymuller syndrome of micrognathia and rhizomelic chondrodysplasia at birth with subsequent normal growth. *Am J Roentgenol Radium Ther Nucl Med* 125:936, 1975.
9. Hecht F, Beals RK: "New" syndrome of congenital contractural arachnodactyly originally described by Marfan in 1896. *Pediatrics* 49:574–579, 1972.
10. Heselson NG, Cremin BJ, Beighton P: The radiographic manifestations of hypochondroplasia. *Clin Radiol* 30:79–85, 1979.
11. Houston CS, Awen CF, Kent HP: Fatal neonatal dwarfism. *J Can Assoc Radiol* 23:45–61, 1972.
12. Ho N, Khoo T: Congenital contractural arachnodactyly. *Am J Dis Child* 133:639–640, 1979.
13. Kultursay N, Tanelli B, Cavusoglu A: Pseudoachondroplasia with immune deficiency. *Pediatr Radiol* 18:505–508, 1988.
14. Langer LO: Mesomelic dwarfism of the hypoplastic ulna, fibula, mandible type. *Radiology* 89:654–660, 1967.
15. Lachman RS, Rimoin DL, Hollister DW, Dorst JP, Siggers DC, McAlister W, Kaufman RL, Langer LO: The Kniest syndrome. *AJR* 123:805–814, 1975.
16. MacLeod PM, Fraser FC: Congenital contractural arachnodactyly: an inheritable disorder of connective tissue distinct from Marfan's syndrome. *Am J Dis Child* 126:810–812, 1973.
17. McCarthy JMI, Carey MC: Bone changes in homocystinuria. *Clin Radiol* 19:128, 1968.
18. McLennan TW, Steinbach HL: Schwachman's syndrome: the broad spectrum of bony abnormalities. *Radiology* 112:167–173, 1974.
19. Morreels CL Jr, Fletcher BD, Weilbaecher RG, Dorst JP: The roentgenographic features of homocystinuria. *Radiology* 90:1150-1158, 1968.
20. Pease CN: Focal retardation and arrest of growth of bones due to vitamin A intoxication. *JAMA* 182:980–985, 1962.
21. Robinow M, Silverman FN, Smith HD: A newly recognized dwarfing syndrome. *Am J Dis Child* 117:645–649, 1969.
22. Schedewie H, Willich E, Grobe H, Schmidt H, Muller KM: Skeletal findings in homocystinuria: a collaborative study. *Pediatr Radiol* 1:12–23, 1973.
23. Schwachman H, Diamond LK, Oski FK: The syndrome of pancreatic insufficiency and bone marrow dysfunction. *J Pediatr* 65:645–663, 1974.
24. Schorr S, Legum C, Ochshorn M, Hirsch M, Moses S, Lasch EE, El-masri M: The Dyggve-Melchior-Clausen syndrome. *AJR* 128:107–113, 1977.
25. Spranger J, Maroteaux P, der Kaloustian VM: The Dyggve-Melchior-Clausen syndrome. *Radiology* 114:415–421, 1975.
26. Stokes NJ, Sheat JH: Chondroectodermal dysplasia (Ellis-van Creveld syndrome): case report. *Australas Radiol* 15:259–263, 1971.
27. Swischuk LE, Hayden CK Jr: Rickets: a roentgenographic scheme for diagnosis. *Pediatr Radiol* 8:203–208, 1979.
28. Taybi H, Mitchell AD, Friedman GD: Metaphyseal dysostosis and the associated syndrome of pancreatic insufficiency and blood disorders. *Radiology* 93A:563–571, 1969.
29. Winchester P, Grossman H, Lim WN, Danes BS: A new acid mucopolysaccharidosis with skeletal deformities simulating rheumatoid arthritis. *AJR* 106:128–136, 1969.

BALLOONED BONES

Ballooned bones are characterized by very wide shafts and thin cortices. As listed in Table 4.5, conditions producing ballooned bones generally consist of medullary cavity expansile processes and subperiosteal bleeding problems, but in addition a few bony dysplasias also may be encountered. The medul-

Table 4.5
Diffusely Ballooned Bones (Osteoectasia)

Generalized		
Severe anemia	}	Common
Familial hypophosphatemia Mastocytosis Craniodiaphyseal dysplasia	}	Rare
Asymmetric or localized		
Fracture with subperiosteal bleeding[a] Battered child syndrome[a] Hemophilia[a] Neurogenic fracture[a]	}	Common
Fibrous dysplasia	}	Moderately common
Scurvy[a] Neurofibromatosis[a]	}	Rare

[a] Subperiosteal bleed.

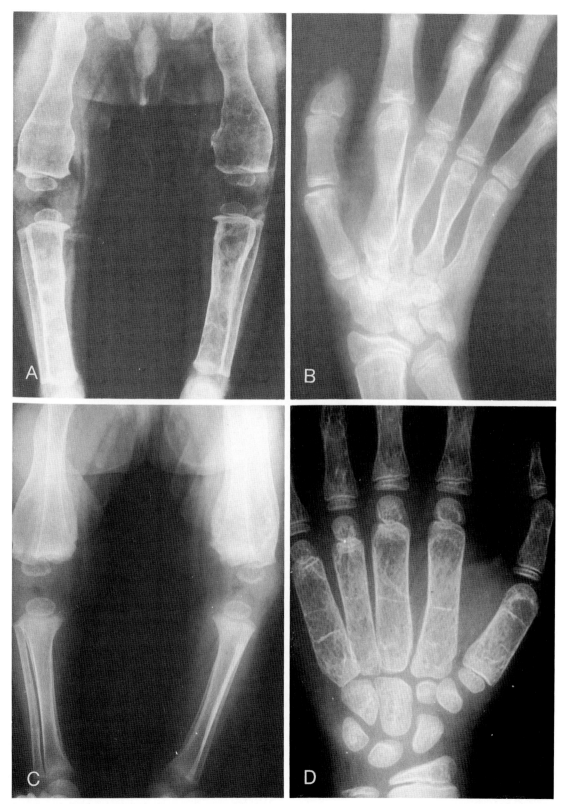

Figure 4.10. Balloned bones. A. Typical expansion and ballooning due to bone marrow infiltration. This patient had mastocytosis. **B.** Generalized ballooning of the metaphyses, especially of the small bones in the hands in the otopalatodigital syndrome. **C.** Pseudoballooning due to subperiosteal bleeding in scurvy. **D.**

Ballooned bones in Cooley's anemia secondary to marrow hyperplasia. (Part **A** reproduced with permission from Wooten WB, DeSantos LA, Finkelstein JB: Case Report 61. *Skeletal Radiol* 3:53–55, 1978.

lary expansile processes include familial hyperphosphatemia (1), mastocytosis (early stages) (2, 3), and severe anemias (especially Cooley's anemia). With anemias and mastocytosis, ballooning results from marrow hypercellularity (Fig. 4.10A and D), whereas in familial hyperphosphatemia it is the result of altered tubulation secondary to bone hypermetabolism and overgrowth. In terms of bony dysplasias, the one most commonly producing wide bones with thin cortices is craniometaphyseal dysplasia (Fig. 4.10B). In this condition the long bones and the bones of the hands and feet tend to be somewhat ballooned, while the remainder of the skeleton, especially the thorax and calvarium, undergo extensive hyperostosis resembling that seen with van Buchem disease.

Apparent ballooning of bones occurs in the healing stages of massive periosteal bleeding such as occurs with pathologic fractures in patients with scurvy (Fig. 4.10C) or neurologic disease, and with the epiphyseal-metaphyseal fractures encountered in the battered child syndrome. Similar subperiosteal bleeding is seen with neurofibromatosis (loose periosteal attachment) and blood dyscrasias such as hemophilia. In all of these cases the outwardly displaced periosteal lining, as it deposits new bone, produces a wavy, undulating ballooned appearance of the long bones.

REFERENCES

1. Iancu TC, Almagor G, Friedman E, Hardoff R, Front D: Chronic familial hyperphosphatasemia. *Radiology* 129:669–676, 1978.
2. Lucaya J, Perez-Candela V, Aso C, Calvo J: Mastocytosis with skeletal and gastrointestinal involvement in infancy: two case reports and review of the literature. *Radiology* 131:363–366, 1979.
3. Wooten WB, de Santos LA, Finkelstein JB: Case report 61—diagnosis: systemic mastocytosis. *Skeletal Radiol* 3:53–55, 1978.

BOWED BONES

Bowed bones can occur on a generalized or focal basis (Table 4.6). Focally bowed bones usually result from injury or infection, whereas generalized bowing usually occurs with (a) bony dysplasias or syndromes where inherent disturbances of bone growth result in bowing, and (b) metabolic diseases where bones bow because they are osteomalacic and soft.

GENERALIZED BOWING

Generalized bowing resulting from metabolic disease (leading to osteomalacia) occurs in rickets, hyperparathyroidism, hypophosphatasia, and hyper-

Table 4.6
Bowed Bones

Generalized bowing	
Rickets }	Common
Osteogenesis imperfecta[a] Madelung deformity[b] Neonatal dwarfs Hyperparathyroidism }	Moderately common
Diastrophic dwarfism[c] Camptomelic dwarfism[c] Larsen syndrome[c] Neonatal Ellis-van Creveld syndrome[c] Parastremmatic dwarfism Hypophosphatasia Hyperphosphatemia }	Rare
Localized bowing	
Plastic bending fracture Normal Bowed legs[d] }	Common
Posttrauma or osteomyelitis Neurofibromatosis (tibia-fibula) Fractures in softened bones }	Moderately common
Tibial kyphosis w/ or w/o absent fibula }	Relatively rare

[a] Especially congenita form with fracture.
[b] Dyschondrosteosis.
[c] Symmetric middle segment dwarfism predominates.
[d] See Table 4.7.

phosphatemia. Rickets, of course, is most common, and in all of these conditions, because of weight bearing, bowing is most pronounced in the lower extremities. However, bowing also can occur in the upper extremities (Fig. 4.11A). Weight bearing is not the problem in the bony dysplasias, such as achondroplasia, hypochondroplasia, a large variety of neonatal dwarfs (8, 10, 11), Ellis-van Creveld syndrome, camptomelic dwarfism, Larsen syndrome, pseudo-achondroplasia (multiple epiphyseal dysplasia and spondyloepiphyseal dysplasia types), diastrophic dwarfism, the mucopolysaccharidoses, the mucolipidoses, and parastremmatic dwarfism. In camptomelic dwarfism (Fig. 4.11 B) and Larsen syndrome, in addition to bowing, the long bones usually are underdeveloped, and varying degrees of hypoplasia frequently are best seen around the elbow. Larsen syndrome also is characterized by multiple joint dislocations, and while in any of these conditions bowing is rather nonspecific, it still is an important part of their diagnosis. Bowing also occurs in osteogenesis imperfecta (Fig. 4.11C) and often is most pronounced in the congenita form (Fig. 4.11D).

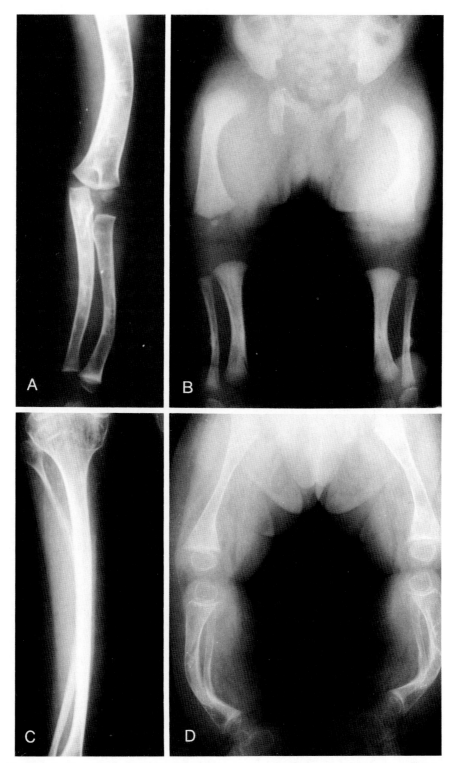

Figure 4.11.   Bowed bones. A. Typical bowing of the bones of the upper extremity in rickets. **B.** Bowing of the shortened bones of the lower extremity in camptomelic dwarfism. Also note exos- toses on the fibula. **C.** Bowing of the bones in osteogenesis imperfecta tarda. **D.** Bowing of thin bones in osteogenesis imperfecta congenita.

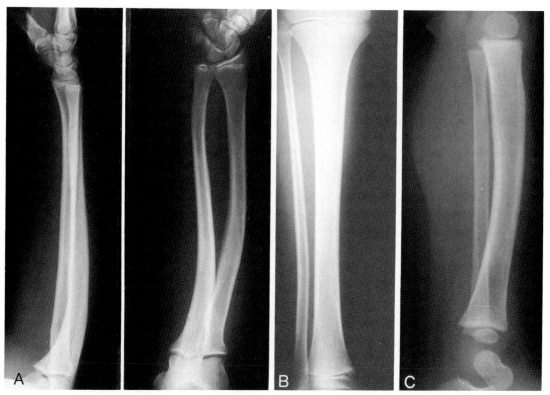

Figure 4.12. Normal bowing of bones. A. Typical bowing of the radius and ulna on both frontal and lateral views. **B.** Typical inward bowing of the fibula on frontal view. **C.** Typical bowing of the tibia on lateral view.

In some conditions, although bowing is generalized it is most noticeable in the middle segments of the upper or lower extremities (i.e., radius and ulna, tibia and fibula). Classically, in the upper extremities such bowing occurs with Madelung deformity, or "dyschondrosteosis" (6). The typical distal ulnar subluxation, increased carpal angle, tilting of the radial epiphysis, and bowing of the radius and ulna confirm the diagnosis (see Fig. 4.8B and C). Middle-segment bowing also occurs in mesomelic dwarfism and the ulnofibular dysplasia syndromes of Reinhardt and Pfeiffer (see Fig. 4.8D).

All of the foregoing abnormalities must be differentiated from normal curvatures of bones. For the most part, these involve the radius, ulna, fibula, and tibia. The typical normal curved shapes of these bones are shown in Figure 4.12.

FOCAL BOWING

Focal, asymmetric bowing of one or two bones most commonly is secondary to trauma and is seen with the so-called "plastic" bending, or bowing, fractures of childhood (1, 2, 5). With minimal injuries, the bowing deformity will be missed unless the other extremity is examined at the same time (Fig. 4.13). Actually, these fractures are a variation of the well-known greenstick fracture and can be considered the **"greenest of greenstick fractures."** Most often, they occur in the bones of the forearm, but they also can be seen in the fibula and clavicle. Rarely, they are seen in the other long bones (3).

Bending, or plastic, fractures usually heal with persistent deformity, and many years are required for remodeling to occur. Indeed, complete remodeling may never occur, and in addition, periosteal new bone deposition, in the healing phase, rarely is seen. Isotope bone scans, however, will be positive, but once the fracture is appreciated on plain films, there is little reason to obtain them. Perhaps the most important points regarding these fractures are: (a) be aware of their existence, and (b) obtain views of the normal extremity for comparison. Otherwise, even the more obvious of these fractures can be overlooked.

Unilateral or bilateral focal bowing of the extremities also is seen with faulty intrauterine fetal positioning. In the broadest sense, such bowing is due to trauma and actually is a form of the plastic bending fracture. However, these bent bones, unlike those seen with bending fractures in older infants and chil-

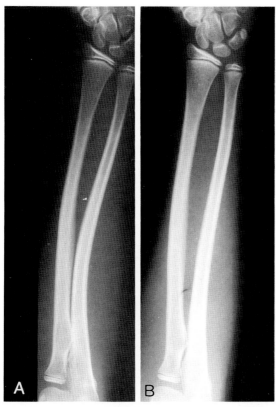

Figure 4.13. Focal bone bowing. A. Note exaggerated, abnormal bowing of the radius and ulna due to a plastic bending fracture. Alone, these findings could be missed, but when compared with the normal side in Part **B,** bowing is more apparent.

dren, tend to correct with time. Other instances where plastic bowing fractures occur include osteogenesis imperfecta and bones softened by metabolic disease such as rickets, hyperparathyroidism, hypophosphatasia, and hyperphosphatemia.

Localized bowing, more pronounced at one end of a long bone, can be seen after epiphyseal injury secondary to trauma, infection, or irradiation (Fig. 4.14). Most often the problem is trauma and, indeed, such bowing is common in the battered child syndrome. Similar epiphyseal-metaphyseal injuries are seen in metabolically weakened bones such as those occurring in rickets, hyperparathyroidism, scurvy, leukemia, and neonatal infections such as syphilis. Indeed, any time the epiphyseal-metaphyseal junction is weakened, epiphyseal-metaphyseal fractures are more prone to occur and bowing deformities can then result.

Congenital pseudoarthrosis is another cause of focal bowing and, although it can occur in almost any long bone, most commonly it occurs in the lower extremity, in the tibia and fibula. In most of these patients, the problem is believed to be just another

manifestation of the generalized mesenchymal defect seen in neurofibromatosis (Fig. 4.15A and B) and, while at first, only bowing and dysplasia are seen, later frank pseudoarthrosis develops (see Fig. 4.28B). Recently, stabilization of the bony fragments with intramedullary nails has proven somewhat successful, but in the past, even with bone grafting, true healing seldom occurred. Very often the end result was amputation of the extremity. For this reason, it is important to differentiate this form of tibiofibular bowing from the more benign form where pseudoarthrosis does not develop (Fig. 4.16). For the most part, this differentiation is accomplished by the fact that, in the latter, curvature of the bones occurs in the opposite direction to that seen with the congenital pseudoarthrosis of neurofibromatosis. In addition, with this type of bowing there is no evidence of bony dysplasia, while with the bowing of neurofibromatosis, the bone in the area of maximal bending is narrower than normal, dysplastic, and associated with virtual obliteration of the medullary canal (Fig. 4.15). The tibia and fibula in the more benign form often are short (Fig. 4.16), and even though pseudoarthrosis does not develop, the extremity usually remains short and bowed, suggesting an inherent

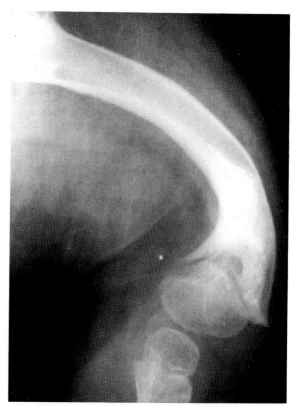

Figure 4.14. Severe bowing after epiphyseal insult. Note marked bowing of this femur secondary to osteomyelitis in the past.

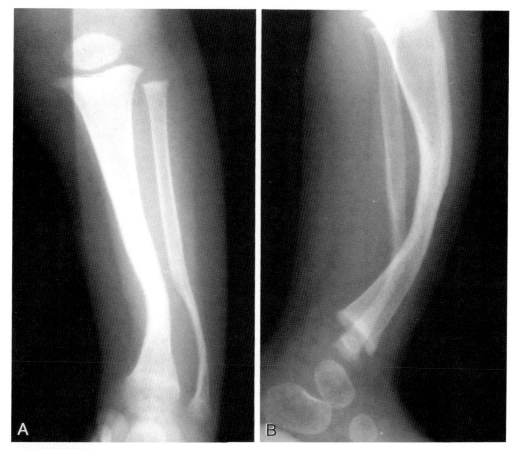

Figure 4.15. Focal bowing: neurofibromatosis-type congenital pseudoarthrosis of lower extremity. A. Typical bowing and dysplasia of the tibia and fibula. **B.** Typical findings on lateral view. Note especially the dysplastic appearance of the thinned bones. Corticomedullary distinction is poor, and eventually a pseudoarthrosis will develop through the area (see Fig. 4.28B).

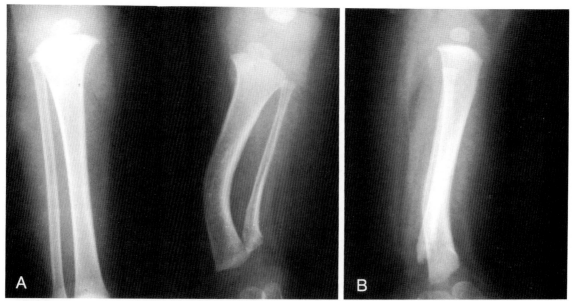

Figure 4.16. Focal bowing: non-neurofibromatosis type. A. Typical frontal view of bowing due to non-neurofibromatosis dysplasia of the left tibia and fibula. Note the difference in appearance from the bending seen in Figure 4.15. **B.** Lateral view demonstrating typical findings, which again are quite different from those seen in Figure 4.15. Shortening, however, is present and may persist.

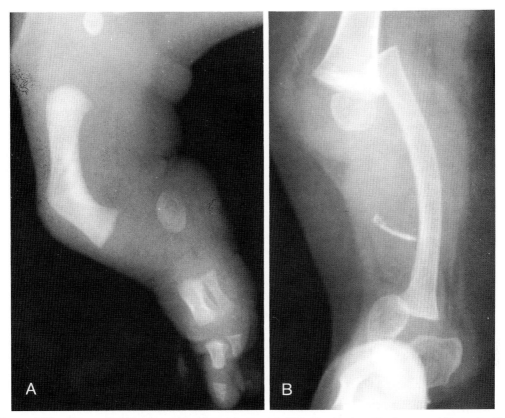

Figure 4.17. Congenital bowing with absent bones. A. Tibial kyphosis, with absence of fibula. **B.** Fibular bowing with absence of tibia.

growth problem. This is quite different from simple positional intrauterine bending, in which the bones are completely normal except for the bending configuration. Most often this is seen in the lower extremities, and eventually the bones become straight.

Bowing of the tibia, on an isolated basis, usually occurs with congenital absence or hypoplasia of the fibula (4, 7), but also can occur with an intact fibula (9). When the fibula is absent, the tibia is quite kyphotic (Fig. 4.17A), and the opposite, that is, absence of the tibia, also can occur (Fig. 4.17B). Other causes of localized bowing of long bones include fibrous dysplasia and juvenile (tertiary) syphilis. Fibrous dysplasia, of course, can involve any bone, but bending tends to involve the weight-bearing bones of the lower extremity. Juvenile syphilis usually involves the tibia, resulting in the "sabre-shin" tibia. It is quite rare in the pediatric age group.

REFERENCES

1. Borden S: Roentgen recognition of acute plastic bowing of the forearm in children. *AJR* 125:524–530, 1975.
2. Borden S: Traumatic bowing of the forearm in children. *J Bone Joint Surg* 56A:611–616, 1974.
3. Cail WS, Keats TE, Sussman MD: Plastic bowing fracture of the femur in a child. *AJR* 130:780–782, 1978.
4. Coventry MB, Johnson EW Jr: Congenital absence of the fibula. *J Bone Joint Surg* 34A:646, 1952.
5. Crowe JW, Swischuk LE: Acute bowing fractures of the forearm in children: a frequently missed injury. *AJR* 128:981–984, 1977.
6. Felman AH, Kirkpatrick JA: Madelung's deformity: observations in 17 patients. *Radiology* 93:1037–1042, 1969.
7. Hootnick D, Boyd NA, Fixsen JA, Lloyd-Roberts GC: The natural history and management of congenital short tibia with dysplasia or absence of the fibula. *J Bone Joint Surg* 59B:267–271, 1977.
8. Houston CS, Awen CF, Kent HP: Fetal neonatal dwarfism. *J Can Assoc Radiol* 23:45–61, 1972.
9. Jones D, Barnes J, Lloyd-Roberts GC: Congenital aplasia and dysplasia of the tibia with intact fibula. *J Bone Joint Surg* 60B:31–39, 1978.
10. Kozlowski K, Butzler HO, Galatius-Jensen F, Tulloch A: Syndromes of congenital bowing of the long bones. *Pediatr Radiol* 7:48, 1978.
11. Thompson W, Oliphant M, Grossman H: Bowed limbs in the neonate; significance and approach to diagnosis. *Pediatr Ann* 5:50–62, 1976.

Twisted or Tortuous Curved Bones

Twisted or tortuous bones are not common and, in the ribs, are referred to as "ribbon-like" bones. This type of rib deformity is seen most often in neurofibromatosis and the basal cell nevus syndrome (see Fig. 4.116). In both instances, the deformity represents a dysplastic aberration of bone growth, and in the basal cell nevus syndrome, vertebral anomalies, a large head, dentigerous cysts in the mandible and maxilla, and cyst-like lesions of the phalanges also are seen (1, 2, 4, 5). Occasionally, isolated congenital rib maldevelopment or postsurgical deformity of a rib or clavicle also can produce a "ribbon-like" deformity of these bones.

Generalized deformity of the skeleton, resulting in tortuous, twisted-appearing bones occurs in the rather rare Melnick-Needles syndrome (3, 6, 7). This generalized progressive bony dysplasia can lead to very bizarre-appearing bones (Fig. 4.18A). Curved, somewhat tortuous bones also can be seen in the otopalatodigital syndrome (Fig. 4.18B), and in Pyle metaphyseal dysostosis. On an isolated basis, a long bone can appear twisted or curved after trauma, surgery, or infection, and also in osteogenesis imperfecta (Fig. 4.18C).

REFERENCES

1. Becker MH, Kopf AW, Lande A: Basal cell nevus syndrome—its roentgenologic significance: review of the literature and report of four cases. *AJR* 99:817, 1967.
2. Dunnick NR, Head GL, Peck GL, Yoder FW: Nevoid basal cell carcinoma syndrome: radiographic manifestations including cystlike lesions of the phalanges. *Radiology* 127:331–334, 1978.
3. Eggli K, Giudici M, Ramer J, Easterbrook J, Madewell J: Melnick-Needles syndrome: four new cases. *Pediatr Radiol* 22:257–261, 1992.
4. Gorlin RJ, Golz R: Multiple nevoid basal cell epithelioma, jaw cysts and bifid rib syndrome. *New Engl J Med* 262:908, 1960.
5. Lile HA, Rogers JF, Gerard B: The basal cell nevus syndrome. *AJR* 103:214, 1968.
6. Melnick JC, Needles CF: An undiagnosed bone dysplasia: a 2 family study of 4 generations and 3 generations. *AJR* 97:39–48, 1966.
7. Moadel E, Byrk D: Melnick-Needles syndrome (osteodysplasia). *Radiology* 123:154, 1977.

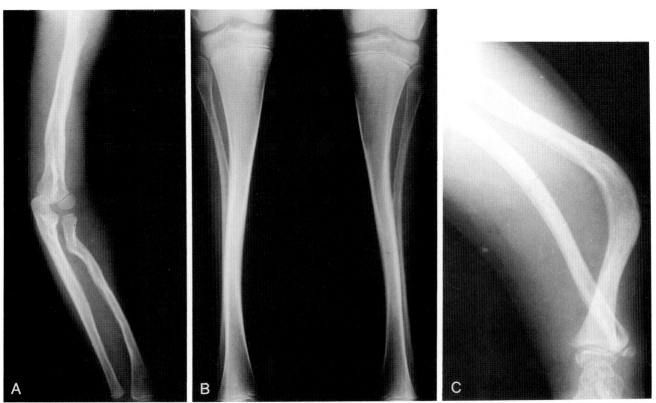

Figure 4.18. Twisted or tortuous bones. A. Typical twisted undulating appearance of long bones in Melnick-Needles syndrome. **B.** Swayed, somewhat "S"-shaped bones of the lower extremity in the otopalatodigital syndrome. **C.** Curved bones in osteogenesis imperfecta. This patient had numerous episodes of fracturing.

Bowed Legs and Knock-Knees

Both bowed legs and knock-knees are common in childhood and, actually, in either case the problem most often is physiologic (1, 4, 7, 8). This is especially true of bow legs, but the deformity, in either case, is due to increased vertical stresses being applied to one or other side of the knee joint. With medial stresses bowed legs result, while with lateral stresses knock-knees occur (6). The effects of these stresses on the metaphyses of the growing bones are shown in Figure 4.19. Bowed legs and knock-knees also occur in certain bony dysplasias and syndromes, and less commonly with any number of epiphyseal plate insults.

The many causes of bowed legs and knock-knees are summarized in Table 4.7, but the commonest cause of bowed legs is the condition known as physiologic tibial torsion. In these infants the lower tibias are twisted forward and medially so that there is intoeing and accommodative bowing of the legs. Most often, the problem is self-limiting and corrects itself by 3 or 4 years of age (4, 7, 8). For this reason, it is considered "physiologic," and hasty "corrective" osteotomies should be avoided (7). In terms of etiology, it is curious that the muscles in these patients almost always are well developed, and that the infants themselves are early walkers (1). It is likely that these factors lead to extra medial stress, which then causes bending of the normal, but yet quite plastic, infantile bones (Fig. 4.20A).

In those patients in whom tibial torsion does not resolve, medial stresses lead to impaction and beaking of the medial tibial metaphysis and growth disturbance of the medial physis. This leads to increased bowing (especially through the upper tibia) and Blount disease (2) (Fig. 4.20B and C). Unlike physiologic bowing, bowing due to Blount disease is persistent or progressive and often requires corrective osteotomy. The condition can be unilateral or bilateral, and in some cases there is diastasis of the contralateral aspect (lateral) of the epiphyseal-metaphyseal junction (3). In other words, while there are compressive, fragmenting forces medially, distracting forces act laterally (i.e., see-saw-like effect).

Table 4.7
Bowed Legs and Knock-Knees

Bowed legs		
Physiologic		
Rickets		
Femoral anteversion	}	Common
Blount disease		
Bone dysplasias[a]		
Epiphyseal injuries		
Hypophosphatasia		
Hyperphosphatemia	}	Relatively rare
Hyperparathyroidism		
Metaphyseal dysostoses		
Knock-knees		
Physiologic	}	Common
Muscular weakness		
Epiphyseal-metaphyseal injuries	}	Relatively rare
Trevor disease		

[a]See Table 4.6.

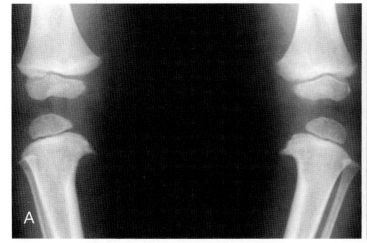
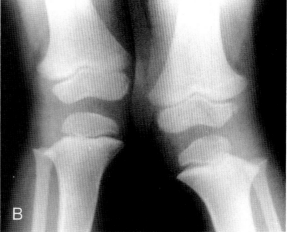
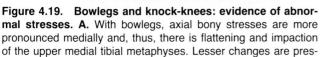

Figure 4.19. Bowlegs and knock-knees: evidence of abnormal stresses. A. With bowlegs, axial bony stresses are more pronounced medially and, thus, there is flattening and impaction of the upper medial tibial metaphyses. Lesser changes are present in the medial femoral metaphyses. **B.** With knock-knees, changes are reversed. Note that there is flattening and impaction of the lateral aspects of the metaphyses, and that in addition there is cupping (impaction) of the fibula.

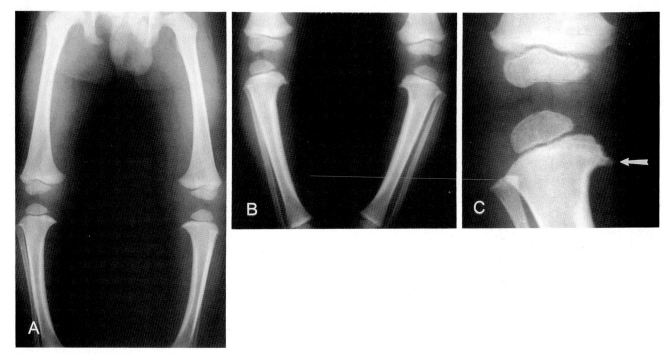

Figure 4.20. Bowed legs. A. Physiologic bowing; except for bowing the bones are normal. **B. Blount disease: young infant.** Note bilateral impaction and fragmentation of the upper medial metaphysis. **C. Blount disease** with typical tibial beaking and fragmentation *(arrow)*.

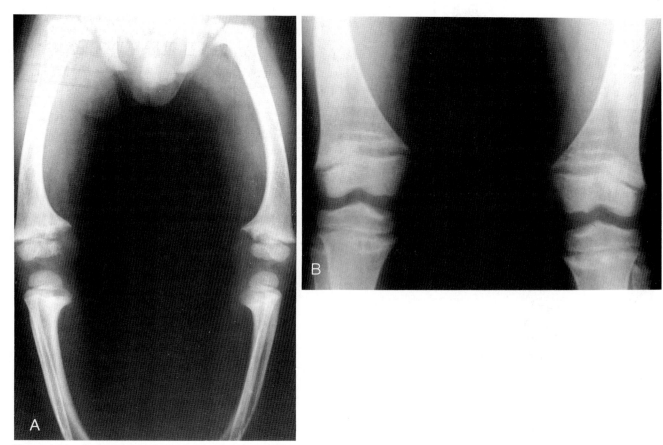

Figure 4.21. Bowed legs. A. Typical bowed legs in hypophosphatemic vitamin D-resistant rickets in young infant. **B. Bowed legs** in older child with hypophosphatemic rickets. Note numerous growth repair lines. This is typical of this form of rickets.

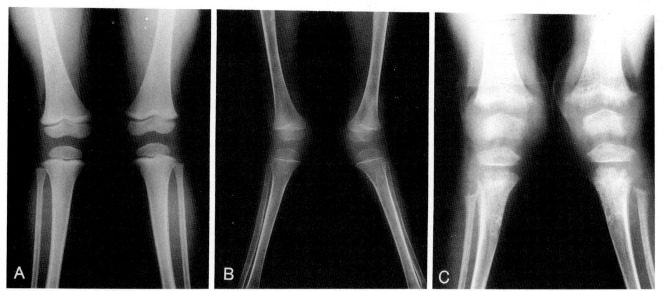

Figure 4.22. Knock-knees. A. Normal knock-knees in 4-yr-old girl. **B.** Severe knock-knees in neurologic disease. Note marked loss of soft tissue bulk. **C.** Knock-knees in advanced rickets. This patient had vitamin D-dependent rickets and was bedridden. If the patient were ambulant, bowing would result.

Blount disease occurs at two different age periods. The first is early in infancy around the time of ambulation and probably is due to the mechanical stresses of strong muscle pull. In this age group, it probably is related to normal, physiologic bowing, which usually resolves spontaneously. A few cases, however, go on to Blount disease. With the second group of patients, the problem is a little different. This group consists of stocky, or overweight, adolescents and, once again, increased compressive force on the medial aspect of the tibia is the most likely underlying etiologic problem (5, 10).

A less common cause of bowed legs is femoral anteversion, or forward and internal rotation of the femur on its neck. This also is a physiologic or normal state in infancy, and as the patient grows older it tends to correct itself. In those cases where correction is incomplete, pathologic femoral anteversion persists. This also occurs in patients with neuromuscular problems such as cerebral palsy, presumably because of the lack of normal weight bearing and associated normal stresses on the bones. Clinically, intoeing similar to that seen with tibial torsion occurs but, roentgenographically, the bow legs are not apparent. To determine whether anteversion is present, CT cross-sectional views of the femoral neck demonstrating its relationship (angle) to the femoral shaft can be utilized.

Bowed legs due to soft bones most often are seen in rickets (9) (Fig. 4.21), but also occur in hyperparathyroidism, hypophosphatasia, and hyperphosphatemia. Inherent bowing of the lower extremities occurs in a variety of bone dysplasias and dwarfing syndromes where there is bowing of the long bones in general (see Table 4.6).

The commonest cause of knock-knees, once again, is physiologic growth variation, occurring at about 3 to 6 years of age (Fig. 4.22A), more commonly in girls (4, 9). As with physiologic bowing, spontaneous correction is the rule. With pathologic knock-knee deformity, the most common underlying problem is muscular weakness due either to neurologic or neuromuscular disease (Fig. 4.22B). Indeed, even in rickets, where bowing is characteristic, if associated hypotonia exists, knock-knee deformity results (9) (Fig. 4.22C). For the same reason (i.e., associated muscle weakness), one can see knock-knees in conditions such as Pyle disease, the storage diseases, nail-patella syndrome, Englemann diaphyseal dysostosis, and severe rheumatoid arthritis. Unilateral knock-knee deformity can be seen with any type of epiphyseal-metaphyseal injury, and Trevor's disease or dysplasia epiphysealis hemimelica.

REFERENCES

1. Bateson EM: Non-rachitis bow leg and knock-knee deformities in young Jamaican children. *Br J Radiol* 39:92–101, 1966.
2. Bateson EM: The relationship between Blount's and bow legs. *Br J Radiol* 41:107–114, 1968.
3. Currarino G, Kirks DR: Lateral widening of epiphyseal plates in knees of children with bowed legs. *AJR* 129:309–312, 1977.
4. Greenberg LE, Swartz AA: Genu varum and genu valgum: another look. *Am J Dis Child* 121:219–221, 1971.

5. Henderson RC: Tibia vara: a complication of adolescent obesity. *J Pediatr* 121:482–486, 1992.

6. Kettlekamp DB, Chao EY: A method for quantitative analysis of medial and lateral compression forces at the knee during standing. *Clin Orthop* 83:202–213, 1972.

7. Shopfner CE, Cramer R, Cramer R: Growth remodelling of long bone osteotomies. *Br J Radiol* 46:512–519, 1973.

8. Shopfner CE, Coin CG: Genu varus and valgus in children. *Radiology* 92:723–732, 1969.

9. Swischuk LE, Hayden CK Jr: Rickets: a roentgenographic scheme for diagnosis. *Pediatr Radiol* 8:203–208, 1979.

10. Thompson GH, Carter JR: Late-onset tibia vara (Blount's disease): current concepts. *Clin Orthop* 255:24–35, 1990.

Coxa Vara and Coxa Valga

Normally, with the legs internally rotated and the toes pointing inward, the femoral neck to femoral shaft angle measures about 130° to 140°. However, if the roentgenogram is obtained with the toes pointing upward or outward, the angle is increased, and an erroneous impression of coxa valga results. Consequently, it is most important that correct positioning of the hips be accomplished, and then if the angle between the neck and shaft is increased, true coxa valga is present, and if it is decreased, coxa vara is present (Table 4.8).

Coxa vara deformities most frequently result from downward bending of the femoral neck in bones that are softer than normal or downward slipping of the femoral capital epiphysis because of a weakened epiphyseal-metaphyseal junction. In other cases, the deformity is due to a growth disturbance as part of a generalized bony dysplasia, and, occasionally, coxa vara occurs because of an actual bony defect in the femoral neck. Such defects usually are congenital (i.e., congenital coxa vara) but sometimes can be acquired after severe infections or epiphyseal-metaphyseal fractures. The latter most often occurs in the battered child syndrome.

In those cases where coxa vara is due to bending of soft bones, the problem usually is some metabolic disease such as rickets, hyperparathyroidism, or hypophosphatasia. Coxa vara deformities secondary to actual downward slipping of the femoral capital epiphysis usually occur in the condition known as idiopathic slipped capital femoral epiphysis (Fig. 4.23A). The etiology of this condition is unknown, but it does tend to occur in more obese adolescents, and is a little more common in boys (6, 7). There also seems to be a genetically inheritable predisposition and, in this regard, it has been noted that often there is skeletal (bone age) immaturity in these patients. This may well be an important factor, for it is quite

Table 4.8
Coxa Vara and Coxa Valga

Coxa vara	
Idiopathic slipped epiphysis Legg-Perthes disease[a] Rickets	Common
Fracture or infection of femoral neck Sickle cell disease, steroid therapy (femoral head necrosis)	Moderately common
Slipped epiphysis (secondary)[b] Radiation therapy[c] Gaucher disease[c] Osteogenesis imperfecta[d] Metatropic dwarfism Storage diseases Congenital coxa vara	Rare

Coxa valga	
Neurologic disease Chronic muscle hypotonia	Common
Turner syndrome Storage diseases	Moderately common
Melnick-Needles syndrome Prader-Willi syndrome Progeria Pyle metaphyseal dysplasia Stickler syndrome	Rare

[a] Healing.
[b] Hyperparathyroidism, hypothyroidism, pseudo- or pseudopseudohypoparathyroidism.
[c] Femoral head necrosis.
[d] Congenita form.

possible that a combination of skeletal immaturity and increased vertical stress (i.e., being overweight) leads to the problem. The disease usually is unilateral, but bilateral disease occurs in approximately 20 to 30% of patients. In these patients, one side tends to slip earlier than the other, and it is uncommon to have simultaneous slipping of both sides.

The coxa vara deformity in such cases is a late manifestation and, thus, before any significant degree of slippage occurs, the findings consist solely of (a) demineralization of the bones of the hip, (b) some soft tissue muscle atrophy, and (c) widening and hyperlucency of the epiphyseal line (see Fig. 4.74C). This latter sign is most important and the one to look for in the early detection of this condition.

Chronic, and occasionally acute, slippage of the proximal femoral epiphysis also can occur with severe rickets, hyperparathyroidism, and hypothyroidism (5). In terms of rickets, renal osteodystrophy usually is the underlying cause (4, 8, 9, 11), but of course, slippage can occur with any form of rickets.

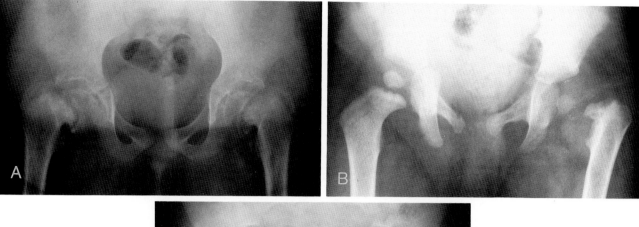

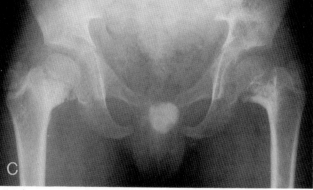

Figure 4.23. Coxa vara. A. Bilateral coxa vara deformity secondary to markedly slipped femoral capital epiphyses. **B.** Congenital coxa vara on the left. Note that there is deficiency of ossification of the femoral neck. The femoral head remains relatively normal. **C.** Bilateral coxa vara deformities in older child with metaphyseal dysostosis.

In rickets and hyperparathyroidism, the cause probably is related to weakened and softened bones, but in hypothyroidism the pathophysiology may be similar to that postulated in idiopathic slippage of the femoral capital epiphysis (i.e., delayed skeletal maturity and overweightness).

Downward displacement of the femoral capital epiphysis also can be seen in the late, healing stages of ischemic necrosis of the femoral head (i.e., Legg-Perthes disease), steroid-induced infarction, infarction with the various collagen vascular diseases, Gaucher disease, radiation therapy (3, 14), and, occasionally, with congenital dislocation of the hip. In patients with dislocating hips, infarction of the femoral head is a complication of prolonged immobilization of the hips in a plaster splint. It does not occur very often.

"Congenital" coxa vara is not particularly common and often is considered to be the most minimal manifestation of the proximal focal femoral deficiency syndrome (2, 12). In this syndrome, when abnormality is severe, the upper end of the femur is phocomelic (see Fig. 4.25B) and the coxa vara deformity so gross that often it escapes observation. In milder cases, variable degrees of bony deficiency of the femoral neck lead to femoral shortening and a coxa vara deformity (Fig. 4.23B). Similar femoral neck defects leading to coxa vara deformity also can be seen with cleidocranial dysostosis, osteogenesis imperfecta, and, on an acquired basis, with trauma or infection. Usually these latter problems occur in infancy, and as far as trauma is concerned, the battered child syndrome probably accounts for most cases.

Other causes of coxa vara include a variety of dysplasias and dwarfing syndromes where intrinsic abnormal growth patterns of the upper femur lead to its presence—i.e., achondroplasia, diastrophic dwarfism, metatropic dwarfism, Kniest syndrome, metaphyseal dysostosis (Fig. 4.23C), multiple epiphyseal dysplasia, Morquio disease, spondyloepiphyseal dysplasia, and pseudo- or pseudopseudohypoparathyroidism (13). However, other more specific findings usually are used for final diagnosis.

As far as **coxa valga** deformities of the upper femur are concerned, the commonest cause is underlying neurologic or neuromuscular disease (10). In these patients, lack of upright posture reduces vertical stresses on the femur and allows the femoral neck to grow in a more vertical direction (Fig.

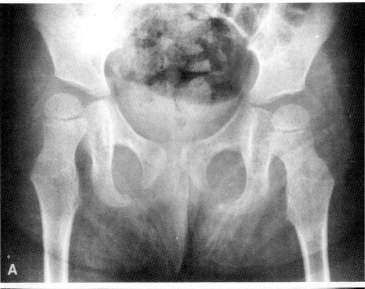

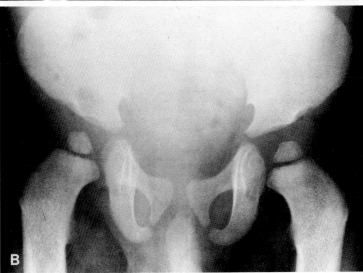

Figure 4.24. Coxa valga. A. Typical coxa valga deformity of the hips in neurologic disease. **B.** Coxa valga deformity in Hurler disease. Also note that the bones are broad, and that the waist of the iliac wing is underdeveloped and narrow.

4.24*A*). In many of these patients, the hips also are subluxated or frankly dislocated. The same problem occurs in a number of syndromes and dysplasias where hypotonia is inherently present (i.e., Turner syndrome, Stickler syndrome (1), the mucopolysaccharidoses (Fig. 4.24*B*), the mucolipidoses, Melnick-Needle syndrome, Prader-Willi syndrome, progeria, pyknodysostosis, and Pyle metaphyseal dysplasia).

REFERENCES

1. Bennett JT, McMurray SW: Stickler syndrome. *J Pediatr Orthop* 10:760–763, 1990.
2. Calhoun JD, Pierret G: Infantile coxa vara. *AJR* 115:561–568, 1972.
3. Chapman JA, Deakin DP, Green JH: Slipped upper femoral epiphysis after radiotherapy. *J Bone Joint Surg* 62B:337–339, 1980.
4. Goldman AG, Lane JM, Salvati E: Slipped capital femoral epiphyses complicating renal osteodystrophy: a report of three cases. *Radiology* 126:333–339, 1978.
5. Hirano T, Stamelos S, Harris V, Dumbovic N: Association of primary hypothyroidism and slipped capital femoral epiphysis. *J Pediatr* 93:262–264, 1978.
6. Kelsey JL: Epidemiology of slipped capital femoral epiphysis. *J Pediatr* 93:262–264, 1978.
7. Kelsey JL, Acheson RM, Keggi KJ: The body build of patients with slipped capital femoral epiphysis. Am J Dis Child 124:276–281, 1972.
8. Kirkwood JR, Ozonoff MB, Steinbach HL: Epiphyseal displacement after metaphyseal fracture in renal osteodystrophy. *Am J Roentgenol Radium Ther Nucl Med* 115:647–654, 1972.
9. Mehls O, Ritz E, Krempien B, Gilli G, Link K, Willich E,

Scharer K: Slipped epiphyses in renal osteodystrophy. *Arch Dis Child* 50:545–554, 1975.

10. Griffiths GJ, Evans KT, Roberts GM, Lloyd KN: The radiology of the hip joints and pelvis in cerebral palsy. *Clin Radiol* 28:187–192, 1977.
11. Nixon JR, Douglas JF: Bilateral slipping of the upper femoral epiphysis in end-stage renal failure. *J Bone Joint Surg* 62B:18–21, 1980.
12. Pavlov H, Goldman AG, Freiberger RH: Infantile coxa vera. *Radiology* 125:631–640, 1980.
13. Steinback HL, Young DA: The roentgen appearance of pseudohypoparathyroidism (PH) and pseudo-pseudohypoparathyroidism (PPH), differentiation from other syndromes associated with short metacarpals, metatarsals, and phalanges. *AJR* 97:49–66, 1966.
14. Wolf EL, Berdon WE, Cassady JR, Baker DH, Freiberger R, Pavlov H: Slipped femoral capital epiphysis as sequela to childhood irradiation for malignant tumors. *Radiology* 125:781–784, 1977.

Cubitus Valgus (Increased Carrying Angle)

Most commonly, this deformity of the elbow results from improperly reduced fractures or growth plate damage to the distal humerus. It also occurs as a basic growth disturbance in Turner syndrome, Noonan syndrome, and the cerebrohepatorenal syndrome.

Clubfeet

There are so many syndromes in which typical clubfoot deformity occurs that it is of questionable value to list all of them. Indeed, seldom does one make the diagnosis in any one of these conditions on the basis of clubfeet alone; the only exception might be diastrophic dwarfism where clubbing is so pronounced that is becomes quite characteristic.

Overall, the commonest causes of typical clubfoot deformity are (a) faulty intrauterine positioning in otherwise normal infants and (b) underlying neurologic or neuromuscular disease. Clubfoot due to faulty positioning also occurs in infants developing in an amniotic fluid-deficient uterus, a phenomenon that occurs most commonly with Potter's syndrome (renal agenesis) but also with prolonged leakage of amniotic fluid from the uterus (2, 3). It also can occur when the fetus develops in an abnormal saccule or portion of a bifed uterus. In all of these cases, direct compression of the fetus by the uterus results in a number of physical deformities, and clubfoot is one of these. The thorax in these patients also is chroni-

cally compressed in utero, and this is believed to inhibit lung growth and result in pulmonary hypoplasia (1).

REFERENCES

1. Blanc WW, Apperson JW, McNally J: Pathology of newborn and of placenta in oligohydramnios. *Bull Sloane Hosp Women* 8:51–64, 1962.
2. Potter EL: Facial characteristics of infants with bilateral renalagenesis. *Am J Obstet Gynecol* 51:885–888, 1946.
3. Stern L, Fletcher BD, Dunbar JS, Levant MN, Fawcett JS: Pneumothorax and pneumomediastinum associated with renal malformations in newborn infants. *AJR* 116:785–791, 1972.

Phocomelias, Hypoplasias, and Aplasias

Phocomelic abnormalities probably are the result of fetal vascular insults and in the past thalidomide embryonopathy often was the cause (3). Currently, however, this is not a problem. In other infants with hypoplastic extremities, the problem is believed to lie with an embryonic peripheral neuropathy (8). The neuropathy probably results from drug or infection-induced (virus?) damage to a primitive sclerotome. In turn, this leads to undergrowth of that portion of the extremity originating from the sclerotome (i.e., radius, ulna, tibia, fibula). Such deformities often are generalized and widespread, but focal hypoplasia of one or more of the long bones also can occur (Fig. 4.25).

Focal hypoplasia of the proximal femur, on a congenital basis, is referred to as the proximal focal femoral deficiency syndrome (5, 7, 10), and in severe cases results in a very short femur with a "pencil-sharpened" or "clubbed" upper femoral end (Fig. 4.25B). In these more severe cases, the femoral head usually also does not develop properly. With lesser degrees of abnormality, the femoral head may develop to nearly normal size, but the upper femur remains hypoplastic and a femoral neck pseudoarthrosis (bony defect in the neck) may prevent normal ambulation. In the mildest form of this abnormality, the femoral neck is short and wide, the epiphyseal line wide and irregular, and although a major neck defect does not exist, a congenital coxa vara deformity is present (see Fig. 4.23B).

Of the sclerotome injury-induced hypoplasias, perhaps one of the best known examples is the "radial ray" syndrome (Table 4.9). In this condition, the radius and first and second digits of the hand are vari-

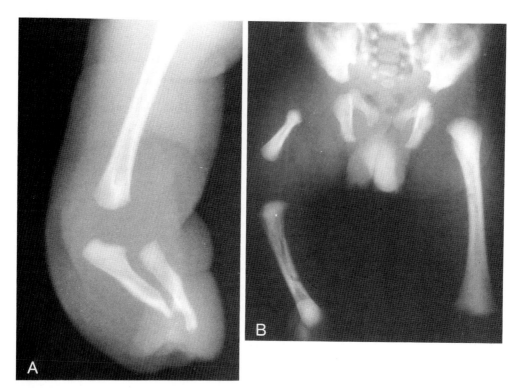

Figure 4.25. Phocomelias and focal hypoplasias. A. Typical phocomelic abnormality of the forearm. **B.** Focal femoral deficiency causing underdevelopment of the right femur and absence of the upper femur and femoral neck. The clubbed end is typical of focal femoral deficiency. In other cases, the end is more pencil sharpened.

Table 4.9
Focal Bony Hypoplasias

Radial ray syndrome 　Holt-Oram syndrome 　Poland syndrome 　Fanconi anemia 　Thrombocytopenia-absent radius 　　syndrome VATER syndrome	Common
Hypoplastic radial head with congenital dislocation Nonspecific focal hypoplasias[a]	Moderately common
Proximal focal femoral deficiency Absent fibula	Relatively rare
Absent tibia Mermaid deformity Thalidomide embryonopathy[b]	Rare

[a]Cause unknown.
[b]Currently not seen.

ably underdeveloped (Fig. 4.26), and, for the most part, these changes occur in VATER syndrome, Holt-Oram syndrome, Poland syndrome, Fanconi anemia, and the thrombocytopenia-absent radius (TAR) syndrome. In the latter, the thumb often is not as hypoplastic as in Fanconi anemia. Poland syndrome is associated with ipsilateral underdevelopment of the pectoralis muscle and chest cage, and in the Holt-Oram syndrome abnormally curved or hooked (handlebar) clavicles can occur (see Fig. 4.99*B*), other congenital bone deformities, and cardiac disease (atrial septal defect, ventricular septal defect, or pulmonary stenosis) coexist.

Isolated hypoplasia of either the tibia or fibula also can occur, and when the fibula is severely hypoplastic or absent a marked bowing deformity of the tibia results (see Fig. 4.17). On the other hand, absence or hypoplasia of the tibia usually is associated with a less bowed fibula and in some cases the fibula may be intact (6). Extensive underdevelopment of the lower extremities and sacrum occurs in the "mermaid," or caudal regression, syndrome. Imperforate anus commonly is associated, and the condition is more common in infants of diabetic mothers. It is believed that the entire deformity results from intrauterine vascular insufficiency of the lower segment of the body (1, 2, 4, 9).

Focal hypoplasia, or underdevelopment, of a bone also can result when severe infection or injury causes impaired epiphyseal-metaphyseal growth. Generalized hypoplasia of the bones occurs in many dwarfing syndromes and, for the most part, these

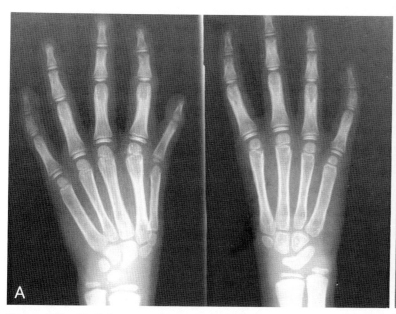

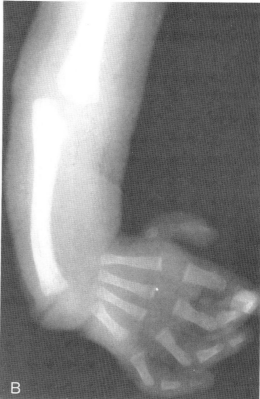

Figure 4.26. Radial ray syndrome. A. Patient with Holt-Oram syndrome demonstrating absence of the thumb on one side, and severe hypoplasia of the thumb on the other. Also note corresponding carpal bone abnormalities. **B.** Another patient with the radial ray syndrome showing absence of the radius and a small, underdeveloped thumb.

have been dealt with in the section dealing with tubulation abnormalities of the long bones.

REFERENCES

1. Assemany SR, Muzzo S, Gardner LI: Syndrome of phocomelic diabetic embryopathy (caudal dysplasia). *Am J Dis Child* 123:489–491, 1972.
2. Becker MH, Szatkowski JA, Bant EE: Case report 75—diagnosis: caudal regression syndrome. *Skeletal Radiol* 3:191–192, 1978.
3. Cuthbert R, Spiers AL: Thalidomide induced malformations: a radiological survey. *Clin Radiol* 14:163, 1963.
4. Duhamel B: From mermaid to anal imperforation: syndrome of caudal regression. *Arch Dis Child* 36:152–155, 1961.
5. Goldman AB, Schneider R, Wilson PD: Proximal focal femoral deficiency. *J Can Assoc Radiol* 29:101–107, 1978.
6. Jones D, Barnes J, Lloyd-Roberts GC: Congenital aplasia and dysplasia of the tibia with intact fibula. *J Bone Joint Surg* 60:31–39, 1978.
7. Levinson ED, Ozonoff MB, Royen PM: Proximal femoral focal deficiency (PFFD). *Radiology* 125:197–204, 1977.
8. McCredie J: Segmental embryonic peripheral neuropathy. *Pediatr Radiol* 3:163–168, 1975.
9. Passarge E, Lenz W: Syndrome of caudal regression in infants of diabetic mothers: observations of further cases. *Pediatrics* 37:672–675, 1966.
10. Schatz SL, Kopits SE: Proximal femoral focal deficiency. *AJR* 131:289–295, 1978.

Ankyloses

Acquired ankylosis is more common than congenital ankylosis and most often the problem is prior joint infection or inflammation (Fig. 4.27A). Ankylosis after trauma is less common. On a congenital basis, ankylosis can occur in isolated form, and often involves the elbow (1) (Fig. 4.27B).

REFERENCE

1. Card RY, Strachman J: Congenital ankylosis of the elbow. *J Pediatr* 46:81–85, 1955.

Synostoses

Synostosis of bones can occur after severe inflammatory periostitis, and the best-known example of this is Caffey infantile cortical hyperostosis. Similar synostoses can occur after extensive bleeding sec-

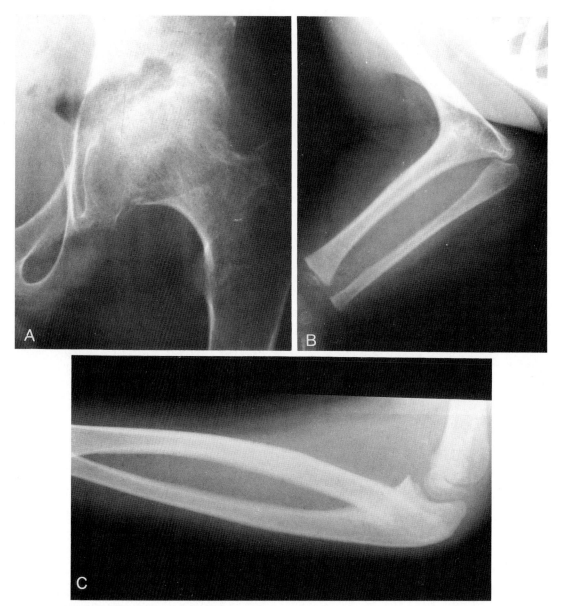

Figure 4.27. Ankyloses and synostoses. A. Ankylosis of hip joint in rheumatoid arthritis. **B.** Congenital ankylosis of the elbow. **C.** Typical appearance of **radioulnar synostosis.** Note associated radial head dislocation.

ondary to trauma, but overall congenital synostoses are more common and tend to occur in a variety of sex chromatin abnormalities. For the most part, these include Klinefelter syndrome and the XXXY syndrome (1). In many of these patients, the synostoses involve the proximal radioulnar area and are associated with congenital radial head dislocation (Fig. 4.27C). Of course, similar synostoses can occur in patients without these syndromes and synostoses also can be seen with the "clover-leaf skull" syndrome (Kleeblattschädel), acrocephalosymphalangism (Pfeiffer type), Ehlers-Danlos syndrome, Holt-Oram syndrome, Nager syndrome, Wolf (4P) syndrome (2), and the mesomelic dwarfism syndrome.

REFERENCES

1. Jancu J: Radioulnar synostosis: a common occurrence in sex chromosomal abnormalities. *Am J Dis Child* 122:10–11, 1971.
2. Katz DS, Smith TH: Wolf syndrome. *Pediatr Radiol* 21:369–372, 1991.

Pseudoarthroses

Pseudoarthroses most commonly occur after nonunion of fractures, either in normal bones or in bones with structural weakness secondary to osteomyelitis, tumor, or cysts (Fig. 4.28A) (Table 4.10). Pseudoarthroses also are encountered in conditions where bone fragility is increased (i.e., osteogenesis imperfecta, osteoporosis, and osteomalacia). On a congenital basis, pseudoarthroses most commonly occur in the clavicle (1, 7, 9) and lower extremity. In the clavicle, most often they are isolated findings but also can be seen with cleidocranial dysostosis. In the lower extremity, the tibia and fibula usually are involved, and the finding most commonly is associated with neurofibromatosis (Fig. 4.28B).

Congenital pseudoarthroses of the clavicle must be differentiated from nonunited clavicular fractures, and this usually is accomplished by noting absence of callus formation, shortening of both remaining portions of the clavicle, and smoothness of the margins of the clavicular defect (Fig. 4.28C). Congenital pseudoarthroses of other bones occurs rarely, but can be seen in the radius and ulna

(2, 3), fibula (4, 10), and upper femur. In the femur, the problem occurs as part of the proximal focal femoral deficiency syndrome (5, 6, 8) (see Fig. 4.23B).

Table 4.10
Pseudoarthroses

Postfracture long bones or clavicle }	Common
Congenital: clavicle Neurofibromatosis: tibia-fibula Postinfection-osteomyelitis[a] Osteogenesis imperfecta-fracture[a] }	Moderately common
Congenital: radius, ulna, fibula Proximal focal femoral deficiency: upper femur Postirradiation[a] }	Rare

[a] Pathologic fracture.

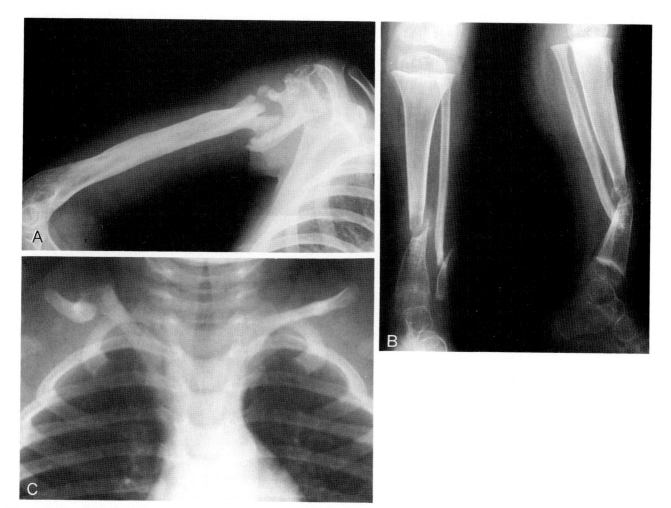

Figure 4.28. Pseudoarthroses. A. Acquired pseudoarthrosis of humerus after pathologic fracture secondary to osteomyelitis. **B.** Typical pseudoarthrosis of tibia and fibula in neurofibromatosis. **C.** Typical congenital pseudoarthrosis of the right clavicle. There are no signs of an old, healing, ununited fracture. The bone ends are smooth and rounded.

REFERENCES

1. Behringer BR, Wilson FC: Congenital pseudoarthrosis of the clavicle. *Am J Dis Child* 123:511–517, 1972.
2. Bell DF: Congenital forearm pseudoarthrosis: report of six cases and review of the literature. *J Pediatr Orthop* 9:438–443, 1989.
3. Cleveland RH, Gilsanz V, Wilkinson RH: Congenital pseudoarthrosis of the radius. *AJR* 130:955–957, 1978.
4. Dooley BJ, Menelaus MB, Paterson DC: Congenital pseudoarthrosis and bowing of the fibula. *J Bone Joint Surg* 56A:739–743, 1974.
5. Goldman AB, Schneider R, Wilson PD: Proximal focal femoral deficiency. *J Can Assoc Radiol* 29:101–107, 1978.
6. Levinson ED, Ozonoff MB, Royen PM: Proximal femoral focal deficiency (PFFD). *Radiology* 125:197–204, 1977.
7. Manashil G, Laufer S: Congenital pseudoarthrosis of the clavicle: report of three cases. *AJR* 132:678–679, 1979.
8. Schatz SL, Kopits SE: Proximal femoral focal deficiency. *AJR* 131:289–295, 1978.
9. Schnall SB, King JD, Marrero G: Congenital pseudoarthrosis of the clavicle: a review of the literature and surgical results of six cases. *J Pediatr Orthop* 8:316–321, 1988.
10. Sprague BL, Brown GA: Congenital pseudoarthrosis of the radius. *J Bone Joint Surg* 56A :191–194, 1974.

Subperiosteal Bone Resorption

Subperiosteal bone resorption (Table 4.11) can occur at multiple sites, and on a practical basis, is almost synonymous with hyperparathyroidism. In children, as in adults, such bone resorption occurs at sites of musculotendinous attachment, but in children, certain areas are more likely to be involved. These include the upper proximal tibia, femoral neck (especially the inner curvature), inner proximal humerus, and distal radius and ulna (Fig. 4.29). Of course, resorption also occurs at other sites and, as in the adult, can be seen at either end of the clavicle (11), the middle phalanges of the hand, terminal tufts of the phalanges (9), and the lamina dura of the teeth. In more severe cases, almost all these sites are positive, but in early cases one of the best places to look for subperiosteal bone resorption in children is along the inner upper tibia (Fig. 4.29A). In addition, in all cases both endosteal and trabecular bone resorption occur (1), but subperiosteal bone resorption receives the most attention. Nonetheless, the other findings should be appreciated because the combination of endosteal, subperiosteal, and trabecular bone resorption produces a rather characteristic picture of an indistinct, fuzzy cortex and coarse trabeculae (Fig. 4.29C and D).

Both primary and secondary forms of hyperparathyroidism can be encountered in children, but the secondary form is much more common. Most often, it is seen with chronic renal disease, and then it is referred to as renal osteodystrophy (1, 2). In these children, both rickets and hyperparathyroidism coexist, but eventually the findings of hyperparathyroidism predominate. Rickets in these patients results from renal tubular dysfunction, and hyperparathyroidism from glomerular dysfunction (i.e., the latter leads to phosphorus retention, overstimulation of the parathyroid glands, and secondary hyperparathyroidism). In kidney disease where only tubular impairment occurs, secondary hyperparathyroidism is not seen. Conditions in which renal osteodystrophy is seen include chronic glomerulonephritis, chronic pyelonephritis, hypoplastic kidneys, kidneys destroyed by hydronephrosis, and bilateral cystic disease of the kidneys.

Secondary hyperparathyroidism also can occur with severe nonrenal rickets, and in these cases it is believed that profound, chronic hypocalcemia leads to rebound, or secondary, hyperparathyroidism (10). Early or mild cases of rickets do not demonstrate this phenomenon, and actually only those forms of rickets capable of producing severe bony change show changes of hyperparathyroidism. For the most part, these include vitamin D deficiency, vitamin D-dependent, and Dilantin-phenobarbital rickets (10).

Another uncommon cause of secondary hyperparathyroidism is pancreatitis. The problem here should not be confused with pancreatitis occurring in patients with primary hyperparathyroidism. There is an increased incidence of pancreatitis in these patients, but pancreatitis-induced hyperparathyroidism can occur in any patient, with any type of pancreatitis. We have seen the findings in one patient with viral pancreatitis in whom features of hyperparathyroidism developed 3 to 4 weeks after the on-

Table 4.11
Subperiosteal Bone Resorption

Hyperparathyroidism Secondary, renal osteodystrophy	Common
Hyperparathyroidism Secondary, severe rickets Focal, with tendon avulsion	Moderately common

Hyperparathyroidism
    Primary
    Secondary, in pancreatitis
    Secondary, in neonate
Focal with subperiosteal hematoma
	Relatively rare

Jansen metaphyseal dysostosis[a] Generalized gangliosidosis[a] Mucolipidoses[a] Lipogranulomatosis[a] Pseudohypohyperparathyroidism	Rare

[a] Present in infancy.

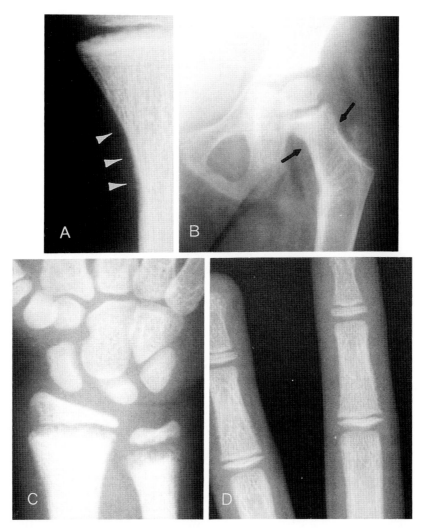

Figure 4.29. Subperiosteal bone resorption: periosteal and endosteal. A. Hyperparathyroidism. Typical subperiosteal resorption along the upper medial tibia *(arrows)*. **B.** Subperiosteal bone resorption around the femoral neck *(arrows)*. **C.** Another patient demonstrating subperiosteal bone resorption around the radius and ulna. **D.** Subperiosteal and endosteal bone resorption in the phalanges.

set of pancreatitis and disappeared as the patient recovered. It is presumed that liberation of lipase in this patient caused binding of calcium, hypocalcemia, and rebound hyperparathyroidism.

Rarely, secondary hyperparathyroidism is seen in association with pseudo- or pseudopseudohypoparathyroidism (8). In these cases, hyperparathyroidism again is believed to result from hypocalcemia, and when the findings of both of these aberrations of bone metabolism are seen together, the term "pseudohypohyperparathyroidism" is applied.

Primary hyperparathyroidism in the pediatric age group is quite uncommon, but both sporadic and familial forms exist (5). Neonates also can be hyperparathyroid as a result of their mothers' hypoparathyroidism (10), and, finally, subperiosteal bone resorption, very similar to that seen with hyperparathyroidism, can occur in a few nonrelated conditions.

It is not known exactly why this occurs, but the findings can mimic those of hyperparathyroidism exactly. For the most part, this occurs in infants with the following conditions: Jansen metaphyseal dysostosis (4), generalized gangliosidosis (3), mucolipidoses (6), and lipogranulomatosis (7).

Focal, or isolated, subperiosteal resorption occurs with adjacent soft tissue inflammation, or tendon avulsions (Fig. 4.30). The latter is more common, and can occur at any tendon insertion site.

REFERENCES

1. Jensen PS, Klinger AS: Early radiographic manifestations of secondary hyperparathyroidism associated with chronic renal disease. *Radiology* 125:645–652, 1977.
2. Mehls O, Ritz E, Krempien B, Willich E, Bommer J, Scharer K: Roentgenological signs of the skeleton of ure-

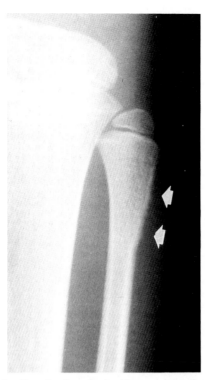

Figure 4.30. Focal subperiosteal bone resorption. Note area of subperiosteal bone resorption *(arrows)* from a chronic avulsion injury in a patient with cerebral palsy.

mic children. An analysis of the anatomical principles underlying the roentgenological changes. *Pediatr Radiol* 1:183–190, 1973.

3. O'Brien JS, Stern BB, Landing BH, O'Brien JK, Donnell GN: Generalized gangliosidosis: another inborn error of ganglioside metabolism. *Am J Dis Child* 109:338–346, 1965.

4. Ozonoff MB: Metaphyseal dysostosis of Jansen. *Radiology* 93:1047–1050, 1969.

5. Sandler LM, Moncrieff MW: Familial hyperparathyroidism. *Arch Dis Child* 55:146–147, 1980.

6. Scott CR, Langunoff D, Trump BF: Familial neurovisceral lipidosis. *J Pediatr* 71:357–366, 1967.

7. Schultz G, Lang EK: Disseminated lipogranulomatosis: early roentgenographic changes. *Radiology* 82:675–678, 1964.

8. Steinback HL, Young DA: The roentgen appearance of hyperparathyroidism (PH) and pseudo-pseudo-hypoparathyroidism (PPH), differentiation from other syndromes associated with short metacarpals, metatarsals, and phalanges. *AJR* 97:49–66, 1966.

9. Sundaram M, Joyce PF, Shields JB, Riaz MA, Sagar S: Terminal phalangeal tufts: earliest site of renal osteodystrophy findings in hemodialysis patients. *AJR* 133:25–29, 1979.

10. Swischuk LE, Hayden CK Jr: Rickets: a roentgenographic scheme for diagnosis. *Pediatr Radiol* 8:203–208, 1979.

11. Teplick JG, Eftekhari F, Haskin ME: Erosion of the sternal ends of the clavicles: a new sign of primary and secondary hyperparathyroidism. *Radiology* 113:323–326, 1974.

Cortical Defects and Erosions

Cortical defects and erosions can result from (a) intrinsic cortical lesions and (b) extrinsic focal erosions or areas of demineralization (Table 4.12).

INTRINSIC CORTICAL LESIONS

The commonest intrinsic cortical lesion producing a localized cortical defect is the benign cortical fibrous defect. These growth disturbances, primarily of long bones, are identified by their very eccentric and completely intracortical location. They occur in the metaphyses: some appear as small cortical cysts, but others are just thin, flat defects (Fig. 4.31). Often they are more readily demonstrable on one view than another (Fig. 4.32) and, of course, the tangential view is the one that best demonstrates their cortical location. When seen en face, a more serious lesion often is erroneously suggested (i.e., osteomyelitis, primary or secondary bone tumor, and bone cyst).

Benign cortical defects often are multiple and tend to be most common in the lower extremities. For the most part, they seem to cluster around the knees and ankles, but they can be seen in other long bones and, occasionally, even in a flat bone. Eventually they heal and become replaced by sclerotic bone (Fig. 4.32C), but in their early stages they are a problem for the unwary. In this regard, it should be noted that benign cortical defects, for the most part, are silent lesions. Usually they are noted when the extremity is being examined for some other reason. It is most important not to misinterpret these benign

Table 4.12
Cortical Defects and Erosions

Benign cortical defect Tendon avulsion injuries	Commonest

Focal subperiosteal bone resorption[a]
Metaphyseal bone destruction with
   Lymphoma, leukemia
   Metastatic disease
   Infection, infarction, congenital
     syphilis
Juxta-articular erosion with rheumatoid arthritis
	Moderately common

Adjacent soft tissue tumors Humeral notch (Gaucher disease)	Relatively rare

[a]See Table 4.11.

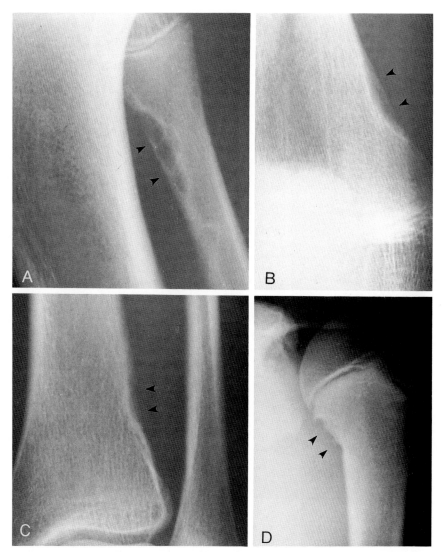

Figure 4.31. Benign cortical defects. A. Rather large, multi-loculated benign cortical defect *(arrows)*. This type of defect could qualify for the related lesion, a nonossifying fibroma. **B.** Smaller, somewhat cystic-appearing benign cortical defect *(arrow)*. **C.** Small, almost invisible benign cortical defect *(arrow)*. **D.** Lobulated benign cortical defect in upper humerus *(arrow)*.

cortical defects for some more serious lesion, and the major step in avoiding such a misinterpretation is knowing what they look like and where they are likely to be seen. They are related to the larger, but still generally eccentric, cortical lesion known as the nonossifying fibroma (see Fig. 4.139A).

Another lesion that may mimic a benign cortical defect is the condition referred to as cortical osteofibrous dysplasia of long bones (1, 12). In the tibia this lesion may have the appearance of a solitary adamantinoma, but more often it presents with multiple lytic lesions which closely resemble benign cortical defects or some cases of low-grade histiocytosis-X (Fig. 4.33). For the most part, these fibrous lesions are benign and tend to heal on their own.

EXTRINSIC FOCAL CORTICAL EROSIONS

Such erosions can result from adjacent soft tissue masses, tendon avulsion injuries, or focal, subperiosteal bone resorption. Erosions by **adjacent soft tissue masses** usually are smooth edged, but are uncommon. For the most part, these masses include tumors such as neurofibroma, fibroma, lipoma, and hemangioma. The malignant counterparts of these tumors (generally quite rare) may give the edge of the defect a moth-eaten and irregular appearance.

Focal cortical erosions produced by **tendon avulsion injuries** are the most common cause of an extrinsic cortical defect or erosion. Of course, if the avulsed piece of bone is visible there is no problem

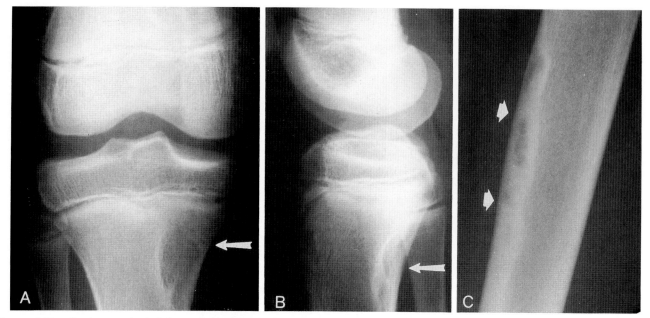

Figure 4.32. Benign cortical defects. A. Typical appearance on frontal view *(arrow)*. **B.** On lateral view, note eccentric cortical location *(arrow)*. **C.** Another patient demonstrating a sclerotic, healing benign cortical defect *(arrow)*.

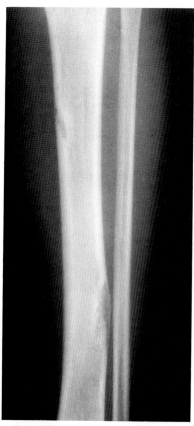

Figure 4.33. Osteofibrous dysplasia. Note cortical, cystic lesions mimicking benign cortical defects or fibrous dysplasia.

with the diagnosis, but unfortunately in some cases no avulsed fragment of bone is seen (see Fig. 4.30). Initially, there is soft tissue change only, but with subsequent inflammation, bone resorption at the site of avulsion occurs. These injuries can occur anywhere a tendon inserts onto a bone, but they are most common in the lower extremity around the hip and knee. In the hip they tend to occur over the superior crest of the iliac wing, just above the edge of the acetabulum along the anterior inferior iliac spine, just above this area in the region of the anterior superior iliac spine, around either trochanter, and along the lower edge of the ischium (6, 13, 14). At most of these sites, in most cases, an avulsed piece of bone is visible from the onset, but in other cases, especially along the lower edge of the ischium, this may not occur. Indeed, all that usually is present in the early stages is slight fuzziness of the cortex (Fig. 4.34) **and the finding is so subtle that most often it is missed.** On the other hand, when it is seen it tends to be misinterpreted as a more serious lesion such as a malignant bone tumor or an area of osteomyelitis. This pitfall can be avoided if the characteristic site of this avulsion injury is remembered.

In the healing phase of an avulsion injury, as new bone is deposited the finding may even more closely resemble a bone tumor (Fig. 4.35). Indeed, it is at this stage of the evolution of the lesion that one must maintain confidence in one's original diagnosis. Bone biopsy must be avoided because there is a tendency to misinterpret the histologic findings as those of a malignant bone tumor. In addition, there is no point in obtaining an isotope bone scan, because although it is positive it does not differentiate between trauma, tumor, or infection. Realistically, then, once one identifies the lesion on plain films, the diagnosis must be made from the plain films (14).

In the knee, a similar cortical erosion occurs with avulsion of the adductor magnus muscle tendon as it inserts into the medial supracondylar ridge of the fe-

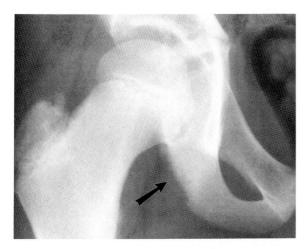

Figure 4.34. Cortical defect: tendon avulsion. Indistinct but typical cortical defect due to tendon avulsion along the ischium *(arrow)*. This patient had hip pain (see healing in Fig. 4.35*A*).

mur (Fig. 4.36). This lesion usually is asymptomatic, and most cases are discovered incidentally when the knee is being investigated for some other reason. In spite of this fact and the fact that numerous documentations of this avulsion injury are available (2, 4, 5, 9, 11, 15), it still is commonly misdiagnosed as a bone tumor. In the past these lesions have been referred to as cortical desmoids, but most likely they represent nothing more than healing cortical avulsions (3, 5). All of these points notwithstanding, when the lesion is encountered it is difficult not to entertain thoughts of lesions such as periosteal sarcoma. A helpful clinical observation is that pain usually is not present over the area, and radiographically there is no evidence of an associated soft tissue mass.

Occasionally, as has been mentioned earlier, avulsion-induced erosions similar to those described in the pelvis and knee are seen in other bones. Such injuries can occur around the upper inner tibial metaphysis or at the deltoid insertion on the humerus. None of these sites, however, are as common as those outlined around the hip and knee.

Focal cortical bone loss secondary to subperiosteal bone resorption is seen with hyperparathyroidism and conditions mimicking hyperparathyroidism. For the most part, these have been discussed in the preceding section and are noted in Table 4.11. In addition, however, juxtacortical erosions occur with rheumatoid arthritis (7) and can be mimicked by certain highly aggressive metaphyseal destructive lesions. In such cases, the cortex is destroyed from within,

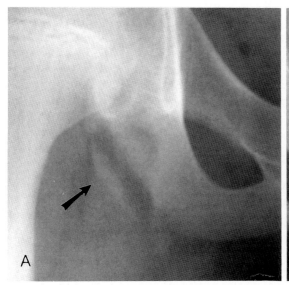
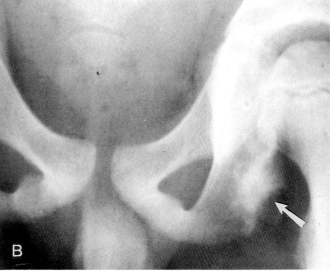

Figure 4.35. Healed ischial avulsions. A. Note new bone deposition during healing of an ischial avulsion *(arrow)*. Same patient as in Figure 4.34. **B.** Another patient with tumor-like healing of an ischial avulsion *(arrow)*.

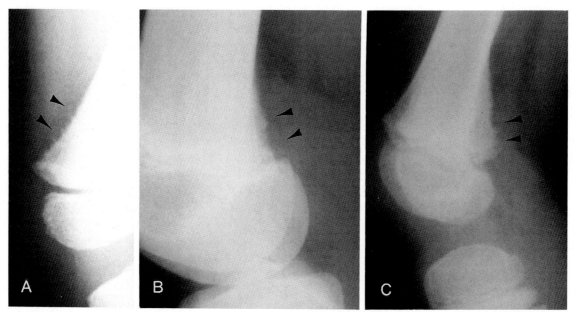

Figure 4.36. Cortical defect-distal femoral irregularity. A. Typical appearance of medial condylar irregularity due to tendon avulsion *(arrows)*. **B.** Lateral view demonstrating similar findings in another patient *(arrows)*. **C.** Another patient with similar findings *(arrows)*.

but the radiograph may suggest that an extrinsic cortical erosive notch is present. Conditions in which this can occur include leukemia (Fig. 4.37*A* and *B*), lymphoma, metastatic disease, the trophic (destructive) bone changes produced by congenital lues (10), and bone infarction. With congenital lues the upper tibial defect is referred to as Wimberger sign (Fig. 4.37*C*). Erosion of the upper medial humerus also is seen with Gaucher disease (8), and smooth notching of the upper humerus is seen in the storage diseases (Fig. 4.37*D*).

REFERENCES

1. Adler C-P: Case report 587. *Skeletal Radiol* 19:55–58, 1990.
2. Barnes GR Jr, Gwinn JL: Distal irregularities of the femur stimulating malignancy. *AJR* 122:180–185, 1974.
3. Barower AC, Culver JE Jr, Keats TE: Histologic nature of cortical irregularity of medial posterior distal femoral metaphysis in children. *Radiology* 99:389, 1971.
4. Bufkin WJ: The avulsion cortical irregularity. *AJR* 112:477–492, 1971.
5. Dunham WK, Marcus NW, Enneking WF, Haun C: Developmental defects of the distal femoral metaphysis. *J Bone Joint Surg* 62A:801–806, 1980.
6. Ellis RE, Green AG: Ischial epiphysiolysis. *Radiology* 87:646–648, 1966.
7. Goel KM, Rawson SP, Shanks RA: Radiological assessment of fifty patients with juvenile rheumatoid arthritis: correlation with clinical and laboratory abnormalities. *Pediatr Radiol* 2:51–60, 1974.
8. Li JKW, Birch PD, Davies AM: Proximal humeral defects in Gaucher's disease. *Br J Radiol* 61:579–583, 1988.
9. Prentice ID: Variations on the fibrous cortical defect. *Clin Radiol* 25:531–533, 1974.
10. Rasool MN, Govender S: the skeletal manifestations of congenital syphilis: a review of 197 cases. *J Bone Joint Surg* 71B:752–755, 1989.
11. Simon H: Medial distal metaphyseal femoral irregularity in children. *Radiology* 90:258–260, 1968.
12. Sweet DE, Vinh TN and Devaney K: Cortical osteofibrous dysplasia of long bone and its relationship to adamantinoma. *Am J Surg Path* 16:282–290, 1992.
13. Slayton CA: Ischial epiphysiolysis. *AJR* 76:1161–1162, 1956.
14. Swischuk LE, John SD, Phillips WA, Shetty B: Early findings in chronic hip problems in childhood. *Contemp Diagn Radiol* in press, 1994.
15. Young, DW, Nogrady MB, Dunbar JS, Wiglesworth FW: Benign cortical irregularities in the distal femur of children. *J Can Assoc Radiol* 23:107–115, 1972.

Cortical Bumps

Focal cortical bumps are most commonly encountered with buckle, or torus, fractures of the long bones. These bumps occur in the metaphyses, where the cortex is weakest. Generally, the normal metaphyseal margins are smoothly curving, and when one sees any type of buckle, kink, or bump, one should suspect a fracture (Fig. 4.38*A*). In more subtle cases, these bumps will be missed unless comparative views of the other extremity are obtained. Other causes of cortical bumps include old healed fractures

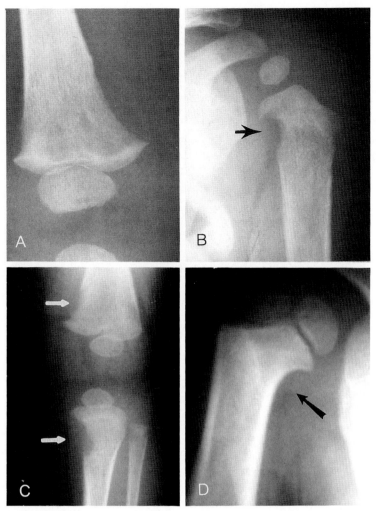

Figure 4.37. Notch-like cortical erosions. A. Leukemia. Note cortical erosions in distal femur. Although destruction is occurring from within, the cortical erosions suggest an extrinsic process. **B.** Similar changes in the humerus *(arrow)*. **C.** Cortical erosion in upper tibia and distal femur *(arrow)* in congenital syphilis (Wimberger sign). **D.** Notching of humerus *(arrow)* in Hurler disease.

(Fig. 4.38*B*) and small sessile osteochondromas and enchondromas (Fig. 4.38*C*).

Cortical Thickening

The commonest cause of localized cortical thickening is a healed fracture or osteomyelitis. It can also be seen after healing of any type of bone lesion that first destroys or expands the cortex. Localized cortical thickening also is seen in osteoid osteoma and with prolonged periosteal new bone deposition for any reason. Thickening of the cortex also occurs in hyperphosphatemia, a condition in which hypermetabolism of the bone leads to thick, coarsely trabeculated cortices. Thick, dense cortices also are seen in thin bones in the Kenny-Caffey syndrome.

Osteolysis

Osteolysis, in general, is an uncommon problem, but three basic types have been identified: (a) massive osteolysis (Gorham disease); (b) essential (carpal-tarsal) osteolysis; and (c) acro-osteolysis. None are particularly common in childhood, and, of the three, acro-osteolysis probably is most common. Massive osteolysis is quite rare and also is known as vanishing, or disappearing, bone disease (1, 3, 7–9, 11). The basic problem in this condition is an underlying hemangioma or, more often, lymphangioma, leading to virtual dissolution of bone. The process can cross joint spaces, generally is progressive, and usually involves the flat bones, including the ribs

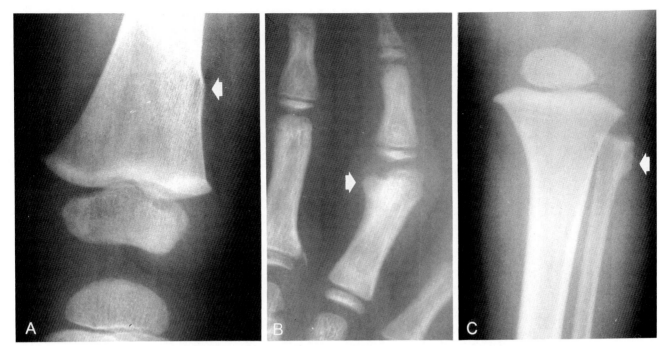

Figure 4.38. Cortical bumps. A. Typical cortical bump due to buckle or torus fracture of the distal femur *(arrow)*. Compare with the smoothly curved normal cortex on the other side. **B.** Cortical bump due to old epiphyseal-metaphyseal fracture *(arrow)*. **C.** Cortical bump due to sessile osteochondroma *(arrow)* in 1-year-old child. This patient came from a family with multiple osteochondromas, and this is about as early as these lesions are seen.

(Fig. 4.39). Essential, carpal-tarsal osteolysis is a progressive, slow, bone resorbing disease affecting the carpal and tarsal bones primarily. It also can involve the metacarpals, metatarsals, and bones around the elbow (4). Basically, two types have been identified: a hereditary autosomal dominant form and a nonfamilial type associated with a fatal nephropathy (2, 5, 6, 10, 12–17). The most likely underlying problem is a vasculitis leading to both bone and cartilage destruction. Similar destruction can be seen with rheumatoid arthritis and the mucopolysaccharidosis known as the Winchester syndrome (18). Bone lysis also occurs with neuropathic joints such as is seen with syphilis, leprosy, syringomyelia, and scleroderma (4).

Acro-osteolysis refers to resorption of the terminal phalanges of the hands and feet, but often the finding is more pronounced in the hands. It is likely that in many cases a vasculitis leads to progressive bone resorption and the condition, along with other causes of phalangeal resorption, is dealt with later with terminal phalangeal resorption (Fig. 4.79).

REFERENCES

1. Abrahams J, Ganick D, Gilbert E, Wolfson J: Massive osteolysis in an infant. *AJR* 135:1084–1086, 1980.

2. Counahan R, Simmons MJ, Charlwood GJ: Multifocal osteolysis with nephropathy. *Arch Dis Child* 51:717–719, 1976.

3. Edeiken J, Hodes PJ: *Roentgen Diagnosis of Diseases of Bone.* 2d ed. Baltimore: Williams & Wilkins, 1973:58, 214, 928.

4. Erickson CM, Hirschberger M, Sticker GB: Carpaltarsal osteolysis. *J Pediatr* 93:779–782, 1978.

5. Gilula LA, Bliznak J, Staple TW: Idiopathic nonfamilial acro-osteolysis with cortical defects and mandibular ramus osteolysis. *Radiology* 121:63–68, 1976.

6. Gluck J, Miller JJ III: Familial osteolysis of the carpal and tarsal bones. *J Pediatr* 81:506–510, 1972.

7. Heyden G, Kindblom LG, Nielsen JM: Disappearing bone disease: a clinical and histological study. *J Bone Joint Surg* 59A:57–61, 1977.

8. Hejgaard N, Olsen PR: Massive Gorham osteolysis of the right hemipelvis complicated by chylothorax: report of a case in a 9-year-old boy successfully treated by pleurodesis. *J Pediatr Orthop* 7:96–99, 1987.

9. Joseph J, Bartal E: Disappearing bone disease: a case report and review of the literature. *J Pediatr Orthop* 7:584–588, 1987.

10. Kohler E, Babbitt D, Huizenga B, Good TA: Hereditary osteolysis: a clinical, radiological and chemical study. *Radiology* 108:99–105, 1973.

11. Kozlowski K, Bacha L, Brachimi L, Massen R: Multicentric/massive idiopathic osteolysis in a 17-year-old girl. *Pediatr Radiol* 21:48–51, 1990.

12. Kozlowski K, Barylak A, Eftekhari F, Pasyk K: Acro-osteolysis: problems of diagnosis-report of four cases. *Pediatr Radiol* 8:79–86, 1979.

13. Lemaitre L, Remy J, Smith M, Nuyts JP, Cousin J, Far-

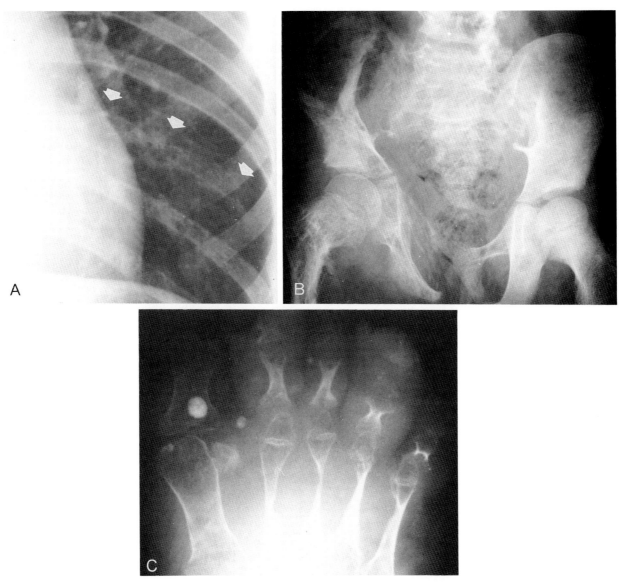

Figure 4.39. Osteolysis. A. Note complete absence of the rib on the left *(arrow)* in this patient with disappearing bone disease secondary to lymphangioma of the bone. **B.** Extensive lysis of the pelvic bones and right femur in a patient with extensive soft tissue hemangiomas. **C.** Another patient with extensive lysis due to hemangioma. Note characteristic phleboliths.

ine MO, Debeugny P: Carpal and tarsal osteolysis. *Pediatr Radiol* 13:219–226, 1983.

14. MacPherson RI, Walker RD, Kinwall MH: Essential osteolysis with nephropathy. *J Can Assoc Radiol* 24:98–100, 1973.

15. Tyler T, Rosenbaum H: Idiopathic multicentric osteolysis. *AJR* 126:23–32, 1976.

16. Torg JS, Steel HH: Essential osteolysis with nephropathy: a review of the literature and case report of an unusual syndrome. *J Bone Joint Surg* 50A:1629–1634, 1968.

17. Torg JS, DiGeorge AM, Kirkpatrick JA, Trujillo MM: Hereditary multicentric osteolysis with recessive transmission: a new syndrome. *J Pediatr* 75:243–246, 1969.

18. Winchester P, Grossman H, Lim WN, Danes BS: A new acid mucopolysaccharidosis with skeletal deformities simulating rheumatoid arthritis. *AJR* 106:121–128, 1969.

Focal Bony Sclerosis

The commonest cause of focal bony sclerosis in childhood is a healing stress fracture (Table 4.13). Most commonly these fractures occur in the upper tibia, and the sclerosis is seen as they heal. At this stage, there also usually is associated periosteal new bone deposition (Fig. 4.40A). In addition to the upper tibia, stress fractures also occur in the femoral neck, the fibula, and in the second metatarsal "march" fractures. Stress fractures in the upper extrem-

Table 4.13
Focal Bony Sclerosis

Stress fracture (healing)	}	Common
Healed cortical defect, nonossifying fibroma		
Fibrous dysplasia		
Bone infarct		Moderately common
Healed histiocytosis-X		
Osteoid osteoma		
Idiopathic, bone island		
Ewing sarcoma (solitary)		
Meningioma (skull)		Relatively rare
Foreign body reaction		
Osteoma		
Osteogenic sarcoma (multiple)		
Tuberous sclerosis		
Healing mastocytosis		Rare
Osteoblastic metastases		

ities or ribs are uncommon except in very active children or those with underlying metabolic bone disease.

Other causes of focal bony sclerosis are not particularly common but perhaps the next group of conditions to be considered includes idiopathic focal sclerosis (4), bone infarction, healed benign cortical defect or nonossifying fibroma, and healed histiocytosis-X. Idiopathic sclerosis occasionally is identified in entirely asymptomatic individuals (Fig. 4.40B). The cause of such areas of sclerosis is not known, but they may represent burned-out osteoid osteomas. Once an osteoid osteoma has burned itself out, sclerosis may remain with no residual symptoms. Small, "bone islands" (2, 5) are not particularly common in children (Fig. 4.40C) and are of no particular consequence.

Bone infarcts causing sclerosis occur, for the most part, in older children with sickle cell disease (Fig. 4.40D) (8), and the findings are no different from those seen in adulthood. They consist of irregular areas of medullary sclerosis that eventually become more generalized and, at the same time, associated with irregular endosteal thickening. Healing in osteomyelitis (Fig. 4.41A), benign cortical defects (Fig. 4.41D), nonossifying fibromas (Fig. 4.41B and C), and histiocytosis-X also can produce nonspecific sclerotic areas in the bone. With nonossifying fibromas and benign cortical defects (these probably are related lesions), the eccentric, cortical location of the healed, sclerotic area is a clue to the etiology (Fig. 4.41D). Osteoid osteoma, a benign bone tumor with

an aberrant, radiolucent nidus of osteoid tissue in the center (Fig. 4.41B) and reactive bony sclerosis around it (Fig. 4.41B and C), is moderately common in childhood (1, 7). It is associated with pain that worsens at night and characteristically is relieved by aspirin. The clinical findings are not always classic, however, and, as noted earlier, some osteoid osteomas seem to "burn-out" and become quiescent (Fig. 4.40B). In addition, when osteoid osteomas are located in the spine or pelvis, they may be difficult to detect radiographically. In such cases, isotope bone scans are quite useful in detecting the more occult of these lesions (6, 10). Some cases of osteoid osteoma are difficult to differentiate from a stress fracture, but when the central radiolucent nidus is demonstrated (Fig. 4.41B), the diagnosis is more or less assured. The radiolucent nidus often is more readily demonstrable with conventional CT.

Other, less common causes of focal bony sclerosis include Ewing sarcoma (single or multiple), osteogenic sarcoma, fibrous dysplasia (usually skull), meningioma (skull), foreign body reaction, osteoma, healing mastocytosis, tuberous sclerosis, and osteoblastic metastases. The latter, of course, are quite uncommon in childhood. As far as osteogenic sarcoma is concerned, when it is multicentric (3, 9), multiple areas of focal sclerosis can be seen throughout the skeleton. This form of the tumor, however, is quite rare. In tuberous sclerosis, patches of dense bone frequently are seen in the flat bones and skull.

REFERENCES

1. Black JA, Levick RK, Sharrard WJW: Osteoid osteoma and benign osteoblastoma in childhood. *Arch Dis Child* 54:459–465, 1979.
2. Blank N, Lieber A: The significance of growing bone islands. *Radiology* 85:508–511, 1965.
3. Cremin BJ, Heselson NG, Webber BL: The multiple sclerotic osteogenic sarcoma of early childhood. *Br J Radiol* 49:416–419, 1976.
4. Freedman S, Taber P, Alter A: Benign osteoblastic lesion in the scapula of a child. *Am J Dis Child* 123:236–237, 1972.
5. Kim SK, Barry WF: Bone islands. *Radiology* 90:77–78, 1968.
6. Omojola MF, Cockshott WP, Beatty EG: Osteoid osteoma: an evaluation of diagnostic modalities. *Clin Radiol* 32:199–204, 1981.
7. Orlowski JP, Mercer RD: Osteoid osteoma in children and young adults. *Pediatrics* 59:526–532, 1977.
8. Rowe CW, Haggard ME: Bone infarcts in sickle cell anemia. *Radiology* 68:661–667, 1957.
9. Singleton EB, Rosenberg HS, Dodd GD, Dolan PA: Sclerosing osteogenic sarcomatosis. *Am J Roentgenol Ther Nucl Med* 88:483–490, 1962.
10. Winter PF, Johnson PM, Hilal SK, Feldman F: Scinti-

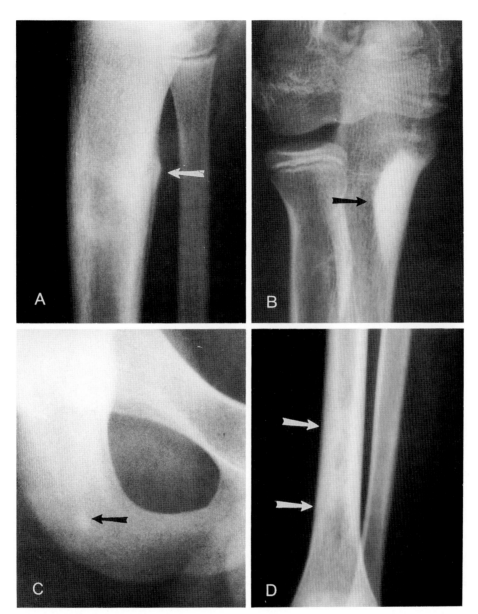

Figure 4.40. Focal bony sclerosis. A. Typical sclerosis due to upper tibial stress fracture *(arrow)*. Also note periosteal new bone. **B.** Idiopathic sclerosis in ulna *(arrow)*. Possible quiescent osteoid osteoma. **C.** Bone island *(arrow)* in pubic bone. **D.** Bony sclerosis secondary to bone infarction *(arrows)* in sickle cell disease.

graphic detection of osteoid osteoma. *Radiology* 122:177–178, 1977.

Bone Sequestrum

For the most part, when a bone sequestrum is seen, the problem is osteomyelitis and the sequestrum may be small or large. Typically, it appears sclerotic (Fig. 4.42), and occasionally a similar finding can be seen with bone infarction in sickle cell disease or Gaucher disease (the latter usually occurs in older children). A bone sequestrum also has been noted in cases of fibrous dysplasia (1). Bone sequestra in the calvarium also can be caused by histiocytosis-X.

REFERENCE

1. Pratt AD, Felson B, Wiot JF, Paige M: Sequestrum formation in fibrous dysplasia. *Am J Roentgenol Radium Ther Nucl Med* 106:162–165, 1969.

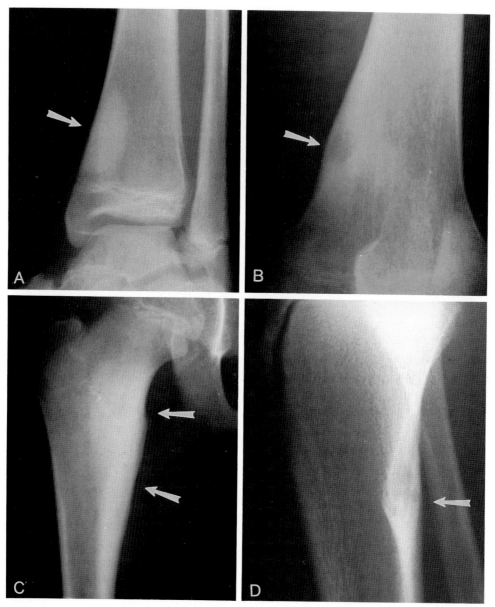

Figure 4.41. Focal bony sclerosis. A. Focal bony sclerosis in healing, low-grade osteomyelitis *(arrow)*. **B.** Osteoid osteoma. Note characteristic focal sclerosis and central radiolucent nidus *(arrow)*. **C.** Another osteoid osteoma along the inner aspect of upper femur *(arrows)*. **D.** Eccentric location identifies this healing, sclerotic nonossifying fibroma or benign cortical defect *(arrow)*. For partial healing of a benign cortical defect see Figure 4.32C.

Bone-within-Bone Appearance

With this finding, a miniature bone (more or less) of the involved bone seems to be present within itself. Most commonly, this is seen in the spine as a normal variation in newborn infants. It is especially common in premature infants and is believed to result from retarded enchondral bone formation secondary to nonspecific perinatal insults to the infant.

Within a few days or weeks, normal bone growth resumes and the old ghosts of the bone are buried into the substance of the newly grown bone (Fig. 4.43A). This phenomenon can be exaggerated in infants with stresses greater than those from birth alone (i.e., sepsis, hyaline membrane disease, gastrointestinal problems, etc.), and occasionally can be seen in other bones (Fig. 4.43B). Apart from this, the bone-within-bone appearance in children is very uncommon, and almost always occurs in osteopetrosis (Fig. 4.43C).

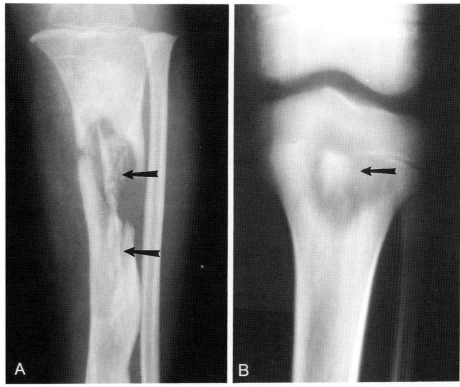

Figure 4.42. Bone sequestrum. A. Note the dense, bone sequestrum *(arrow)* in this patient with treated osteomyelitis. **B.** Another patient with a dense, sclerotic sequestrum *(arrow)*, secondary to osteomyelitis.

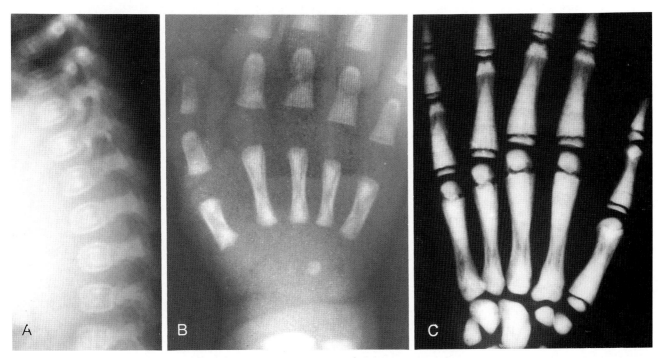

Figure 4.43. Bone in bone appearance. A. Typical bone in bone appearance in vertebra due to trophic disturbances in a premature infant. The radiolucent rings correspond to the radiolucent trophic or stress lines seen in long bones (see Fig. 4.61). **B.** Another infant with bone in bone appearance of the small bones of the hands. **C.** Bone in bone appearance in osteopetrosis. (Part **B** courtesy of Marvin Kogut, M.D., New Orleans.)

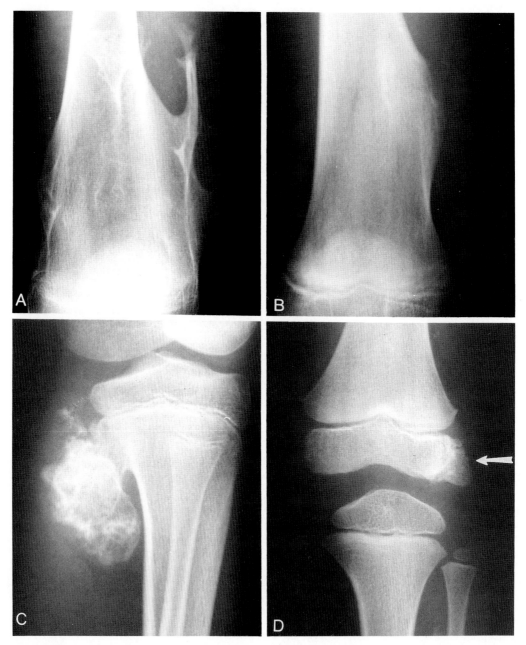

Figure 4.44. Exostoses. A. Typical elongated osteochondroma. **B.** Sessile osteochondroma. **C.** Osteochondroma with irregular edge due to trauma. Note, however, that there is no associated soft tissue mass. **D.** Osteochondroma of epiphysis *(arrow).* This is a case of epiphyseal dysplasia hemimelica or Trevor disease.

Exostoses

Exostoses are bony or cartilaginous outgrowths from long or flat bones, and although most are primary tumors, others occur secondary to traumatic avulsions or myositis ossificans (Table 4.14). The commonest of the primary tumoral outgrowths is the osteochondroma, a benign bone tumor with a cartilaginous cap that behaves like the epiphyseal plate of a growing long bone. Because of this latter feature, osteochondromas grow until the patient's epiphyses fuse, and then growth stops. Morphologically, osteochondromas can be sessile or pedunculated and, when pedunculated, point away from the joint (Fig. 4.44A). Sessile osteochondromas do not demonstrate this phenomenon and, because of their flat and often ragged appearance, are a greater problem in terms of diagnosis (Fig. 4.44B). To be sure, there is a distinct tendency for the uninitiated to as-

Table 4.14
Exostoses

Osteochondroma Calcaneal spurs: normal neonate Healed avulsion injuries Pronounced medial tibial metaphyseal beaks in conditions with bowed legs	} Common

Costoclavicular ligament exostosis-
   midclavicle
Tuberous sclerosis
Myositis ossificans progressiva
Multiple enchondromatosis[a]
Supracondylar spur: humerus
Camptomelic dwarfism: calcaneal
   spur
	} Relatively rare

Fong lesion Epiphyseal osteochondroma[b] Hypertrophic degenerative spurs Iliac spur with tethered cord	} Rare

[a] Ollier disease.
[b] Trevor disease.

sign them a more serious diagnosis such as a malignant tumor or malignant degeneration of the osteochondroma.

Osteochondromas can be single or multiple, and the multiple form is familial (9, 14). Single osteochondromas, however, are much more common, and although they can occur almost anywhere, most occur in the long bones of the lower extremities. Often they lie in close proximity to the joints, and thus can interfere with joint function. This problem is especially prevalent in the multiple exostosis syndrome.

Clinically, osteochondromas produce a variety of palpable lumps and bumps, joint deformities if paraarticular, and, when traumatized, pain. They also may interfere with tendon function and result in friction tendonitis. When growth is complete, the edge of the exostosis is relatively smooth, but when inflammatory or traumatic changes supervene, raggedness of the periphery again may erroneously suggest malignant degeneration (Fig. 4.44C). In fact, malignant degeneration is extremely uncommon in solitary osteochondromas, and overall probably occurs in less than 1% of cases. With multiple familial exostoses, the incidence of malignancy often is quoted as being as high as 5 to 10%, but most likely is considerably lower. When exostoses occur in the ribs, they can produce local bulges of the chest wall, and when posterior, can erode into the vertebral column and cause cord compression (6, 13).

Multiple osteochondromatosis should not be confused with multiple endochondromatosis or Ollier disease. In Ollier disease, the cartilaginous tumor is of central origin, but in some cases the lesions may resemble sessile osteochondromas (see Fig. 4.147). Another point to note in differentiating the two conditions is the fact that the tumors tend to be unilateral in Ollier disease, whereas symmetry is the rule in multiple osteochondromatosis. A peculiar form of osteochondroma is that which occurs with **epiphyseal dysplasia hemimelica, or Trevor disease** (4). This condition tends to occur in the lower extremities (knee, ankle), but also can be seen in the arms (shoulder, wrist). Deformity and interference with joint motion are common, and the whole problem arises because of a sessile epiphyseal osteochondroma (Fig. 4.44D).

In the elbow one occasionally can encounter an exostosis referred to as a **supracondylar spur.** This vestigial structure is located anteromedially on the distal humerus and points toward the elbow (Fig. 4.45A). For the most part, the spur is of no consequence (1), but occasionally it can be fractured or cause traction on the median nerve. **Bony spurs off the iliac wings** (2, 8, 11, 15, 16) are seen in hereditary osteo-onychodysplasia and are termed **Fong lesions** (2) (Fig. 4.45B). This syndrome also is known as the nail-patella syndrome (3), because the nails are hypoplastic and the patellae absent. Another spine-like outgrowth from the iliac bone just adjacent to the greater sciatic notch is associated with sciatic nerve compression, a tethered cord, and a sacral lipoma (5, 7, 12). Calcaneal spurs are relatively uncommon in infants and children, either on a primary basis (10) or as acquired lesions secondary to diseases such as rheumatoid arthritis. Small **calcaneal spurs** have been seen in the neonate in camptomelic dwarfism and also can occur normally (Fig. 4.45C). Another normal exostosis, occasionally seen in children, is that which occurs along the midclavicle just at the insertion of the costoclavicular ligament (Fig. 4.44D).

Bony exostoses also occur with healed avulsion injuries, degenerative joint disease, and myositis ossificans. The latter can be posttraumatic (Fig. 4.45E), posthemorrhagic in hemophilia, or part of the syndrome known as myositis ossificans progressiva (Fig. 4.45F). This latter condition is progressively debilitating, but not very common and of unknown etiology. It is characterized by generalized ligament calcification which often is especially marked in the paraspinal ligaments. Hypertrophic, degenerative exostoses, or spurs, are rare in children, but occasionally can be seen in the foot. At this site they occur most often on the superior aspects of the talus and navicular bone (at the joint) and result from chronic hyperflexion injuries. Elsewhere, degenerative spurs are less common, but can occur with long-standing abnormalities of gait or extremity motion. For example, in little leaguer's elbow, exostoses can develop around the medial epicondyle, and in patients with a short leg and/or chronic limp, similar exostoses can be seen along the inferior aspect of the sacroiliac joints. Exostoses resulting from healed avulsion injuries can occur anywhere a muscle attaches onto a bone, but most commonly are seen along the lower aspect of the ischium (Fig. 4.45E).

REFERENCES

1. Barnard LB, McCoy SM: The suprocondyloid process of the humerus. *J Bone Joint Surg* 28:845–850, 1946.
2. Fong EE: Iliac horns (symmetrical bilateral central posterior iliac processes): case report. *Radiology* 47:517–518, 1946.
3. Guidera KJ, Scatterwhite Y, Ogden JA, Pugh L, Ganey T: Nail patella syndrome: a review of 44 orthopaedic patients. *J Pediatr Orthop* 11:737–742, 1991.
4. Keret D, Spatz DK, Caro PA, Mason DE: Dysplasia epiphysealis hemimelica: diagnosis and treatment. *J Pediatr Orthop* 12:365–372, 1992.
5. Lester PD, McAllister WH: Congenital iliac anomaly with sciatic palsy. *Radiology* 96:397–399, 1970.
6. Madigan R, Worrall T, McClain EJ: Cervical cord compression in hereditary multiple exostosis. *J Bone Joint Surg* 56A:401–404, 1974.
7. McAlister WH, Siegel MJ, Shackelford GD: A congenital iliac anomaly often associated with sacral lipoma and ipsilateral lower extremity weakness. *Skeletal Radiol* 3:161–166, 1978.
8. Palacios E: Hereditary osteo-onychodysplasia: the nail-patella syndrome. *AJR* 101:842–850, 1967.
9. Pazzaglia UE, Pedrotti L, Beluffi G, Monafo V, Savasta S: Radiographic findings in hereditary multiple exostoses and a new theory of the pathogenesis of exostoses. *Pediatr Radiol* 20:594–597, 1990.
10. Robinson HM: Symmetrical reversed plantar calcaneal spurs in children. *Radiology* 119:187–188, 1976.
11. Taybi H: *Radiology of Syndromes.* Chicago: Year Book Medical Publishers, 1975:199.
12. Theander G: Malformation of the iliac bone associated with intraspinal abnormalities. *Pediatr Radiol* 3:235–239, 1975.

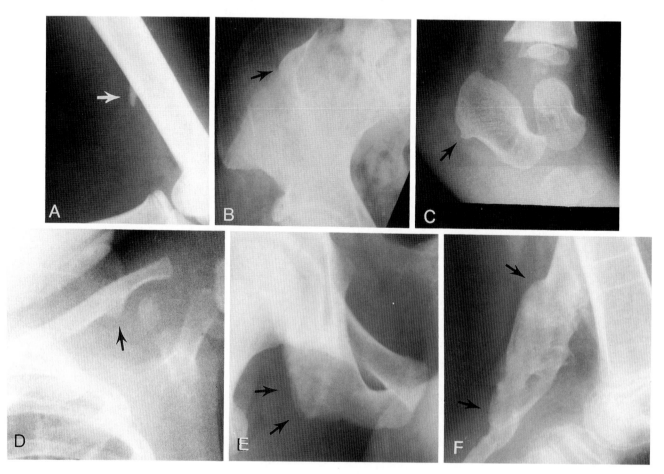

Figure 4.45. Exostoses and spurs. A. Typical supracondylar spur *(arrow)*. **B.** Iliac wing spur (horn) in nail-patella syndrome. The spur *(arrow)* is referred to as the Fong lesion. **C.** Normal calcaneal spur in infant *(arrow)*. **D.** Normal exostosis of clavicle at site of costoclavicular ligament insertion *(arrow)*. **E.** Acquired exostosis due to ischial avulsion injury *(arrow)*. **F.** Acquired exostosis in progressive myositis ossificans *(arrow)*.

13. Twersky J, Kassner EG, Tenner MS, Camera A: Vertebral and costal osteochondromas causing spinal cord compression. *AJR* 124:124–128, 1975.
14. Vinstein AL, Franken EA Jr: Hereditary multiple exostoses. *AJR* 112:405–407, 1971.
15. Williams HJ, Hoyer JR: Radiographic diagnosis of osteoonychodysostosis in infancy. *Radiology* 109:151–154, 1973.
16. Zimmerman C: Iliac horns: a pathognomonic roentgen sign of familial oncho-osteodysplasia. *AJR* 86:478–483, 1961.

Epiphyseal-Metaphyseal Abnormalities

STIPPLED EPIPHYSES

Epiphyses that are stippled (Table 4.15) have a characteristic dense, almost punctate, pattern of ossification (Fig. 4.46) and should be differentiated from epiphyses that are fragmented. The commonest condition in which stippling occurs is punctate epiphyseal dysplasia, also known as chondrodystrophia calcificans congenita, or Conradi disease (6, 9, 10,

Table 4.15
Stippled Epiphyses

Punctate epiphyseal dysplasia[a]	}	Common
Warfarin embryonopathy Fetal alcohol syndrome	}	Moderately common
Cerebrocostomandibular syndrome Smith-Lemli-Opitz syndrome	}	Rare

[a] All forms.

14). Similar findings can be seen in Zellweger cerebrohepatorenal syndrome (1, 4, 12), Warfarin embryonopathy (2, 7, 11, 13), fetal alcohol syndrome (8), cerebrocostomandibular syndrome (3), and Smith-Lemli-Opitz syndrome (5). In all of these conditions, stippling also can be seen in the carpal and tarsal bones (actually quite common), the vertebral synchondroses, and at the cartilaginous junctions of the flat bones of the pelvis (i.e., triradiate cartilage). Indeed, in some cases the findings can be more striking at these sites than at the epiphyses. Two forms of punctate epiphyseal dysplasia exist: a recessive, rhizomelic form in which neonatal death is common, and another milder, more common form that usually progresses to nothing more serious than deformed epiphyses in later life.

REFERENCES

1. Bartoletti S, Armfield SL III, Lesema-Medina J: The cerebrohepatorenal (Zellweger's syndrome): report of four cases. *Radiology* 127:741–745, 1978.
2. Becker MH, Genieser NB, Finegold M, Miranda D, Spackman T: Chondrodysplasia punctata: is maternal Warfarin therapy a factor? *Am J Dis Child* 129:356–359, 1975.
3. Burton EM, Oestreich AE: Cerebrocostomandibular syndrome with stippled epiphysis and cystic fibrosis. *Pediatr Radiol* 18:365–367, 1988.
4. Danks DM, Tippett P, Adams C, Campbell P: Cerebrohepatorenal syndrome of Zellweger. *J Pediatr* 86:382–387, 1975.
5. Herman TE, Seigel MJ, Lee BCP, Dowton SB: Smith-Lemli-Opitz syndrome Type II: report of a case with additional radiographic findings. *Pediatr Radiol* 23:37–40, 1993.
6. Heselson NG, Cremin BJ, Beighton P: Lethal chondrodysplasia punctata. *Clin Radiol* 29:679–684, 1978.

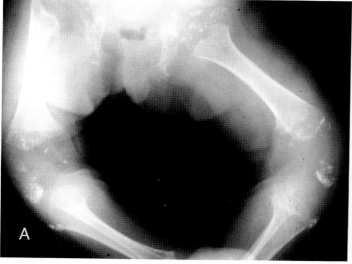
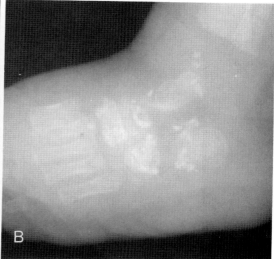

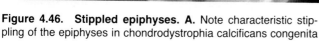

Figure 4.46. Stippled epiphyses. A. Note characteristic stippling of the epiphyses in chondrodystrophia calcificans congenita (punctate epiphyseal dysplasia). **B.** Similar stippling of tarsal bones.

7. Johnson JF: Case report: Coumadin embryonopathy. *Skeletal Radiol* 3:244–246, 1979.
8. Leicher-Duber A, Schumacher R, Spranger J: Stippled epiphyses in fetal alcohol syndrome. *Pediatr Radiol* 20:369–370, 1990.
9. LeMarec B, Passarge E, Dellenbach P, Kerisit J, Signargout J, Ferrang B, Senecal J: Lethal neonatal forms of chondroectodermal dysplasia with five case reports. *Ann Radiol* 16:19–26, 1973.
10. Mason RC, Kozlowski K: Chondrodysplasis punctata: a report of 10 cases. *Radiology* 109:145–150, 1973.
11. Pauli RM, Madden JD, Kranzler KJ, Culpepper W, Port R: Warfarin therapy initiated during pregnancy and phenotypic chondrodysplasis punctata. *J Pediatr* 88:506–508, 1976.
12. Poznanski AK, Nosanchuk J, Baublis J, Holt J: The cerebrohepatorenal syndrome (CHRS): Zellweger's syndrome. *AJR* 109:313–322, 1970.
13. Shaul WL, Emergy H, Hall JG: Chondrodysplasia punctata and maternal Warfarin use during pregnancy. *Am J Dis Child* 129:360–362, 1975.
14. Sheffield LJ, Danks DM, Mayne V, Hutchinson LA: Chondrodysplasia punctata: 23 cases of a mild and relatively common variety. *J Pediatr* 89:916–923, 1976.

FRAGMENTED OR IRREGULAR EPIPHYSES (TABLE 4.16)

Epiphyseal fragmentation or extreme irregularity can occur because of (a) a primary epiphyseal growth disturbance or (b) some insult to the epiphysis. The former is more common and may be normal or pathologic. Normal epiphyseal irregularity is common and most often is seen in the distal femoral epiphysis of infants and young children (Fig. 4.47A). So common is this finding that one would expect to see it in other epiphyses on a regular basis, but this is not the case. Occasionally, one can see normal fragmentation of the capitellum and, even less often, the femoral head, but normal fragmentation of other epiphyses is rare. "Normal" fragmentation of the femoral head constitutes Meyer dysplasia (14), a condition that may be difficult to differentiate from aseptic necrosis (Fig. 4.47B). The changes in Meyer dysplasia may be unilateral or bilateral, but most often are bilateral and may persist for years. Slowly, however, the fragments become larger and unite to form a single, normal ossification center.

Syndromes or diseases in which epiphyseal irregularity or fragmentation occurs as a primary growth disturbance include multiple epiphyseal dysplasia (Fig. 4.47C), spondyloepiphyseal dysplasia, Morquio disease (16) (storage disease that looks like spondyloepiphyseal dysplasia), Dyggve-Melchior-Clausen syndrome (resembles spondyloepiphyseal dysplasia and Morquio disease), and the trichorhinophalangeal syndrome (primarily femoral head involvement). Fragmentation of the epiphyses also occurs in hypo-

Table 4.16
Irregular or Fragmented Epiphyses

Normal: distal femur, capitellum Legg-Perthes disease	Common
Aseptic necrosis[a] Rheumatoid arthritis Hemophilic arthritis	Moderately common

Multiple epiphyseal dysplasia
Spondyloepiphyseal dysplasia
Aseptic necrosis
  Collagen vascular disease
  Congenital hip treatment
  Gaucher disease
  After hip surgery
  After septic hip
  Hip trauma
Hypothyroidism[b]
Frostbite of feet and hands
Osteomyelitis of epiphysis
Pigmented villonodular synovitis
	Relatively rare

Morquio disease
Epiphyseal dysplasia hemimelica:
  Trevor disease
Thiemann disease[c]
Tricho-rhino-phalangeal syndrome:
  femoral head
Dyggve-Melchior-Clausen syndrome
Meyer dysplasia (hips)
Winchester syndrome
Zellweger syndrome
	Rare

[a] Sickle cell disease, steroid therapy.
[b] Epiphyseal dysgenesis.
[c] Hand.

thyroidism and is referred to as epiphyseal dysgenesis (Fig. 4.47D and E). The finding clears with therapy. When multiple epiphyseal dysplasia is seen in infancy, it usually takes the form of punctate epiphyseal dysplasia. In such cases, there is premature and abnormal calcification of the epiphysis in characteristically stippled or punctate fashion (see Fig. 4.46).

As far as some insult leading to epiphyseal irregularity, the commonest problem is ischemic, aseptic necrosis, or Legg-Perthes disease of the femoral head (20, 22). This condition, basically of unknown etiology, but generally believed to result from disruption of the blood supply to the growing femoral head (22), usually has onset with hip pain and limp. In the early stages, because the ossified nucleus of the femoral head stops growing, it becomes noticeably smaller than normal (19). At the same time, the femoral head becomes sclerotic (necrotic and impacted) and then fragmented (Fig. 4.48A). Fragmentation results from irregular resorption of the necrotic head,

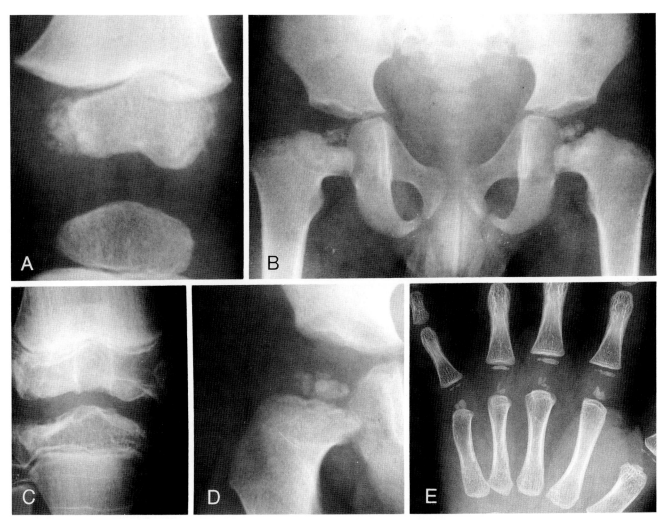

Figure 4.47. Irregular epiphyses. A. Normal irregularity of distal femoral epiphysis in young child. **B.** Bilateral irregular, small, underdeveloped femoral capital epiphyses in asymptomatic patient with Meyer dysplasia. Also note changes in metaphyses. **C.** Scalloped, irregular epiphyses in multiple epiphyseal dysplasia. **D.** Irregular femoral capital epiphysis in hypothyroidism. **E.** Numerous small, fragmented epiphyses and apophyses of the small bones of the hand in another patient with hypothyroidism.

and eventually it is all resorbed. The ossified nucleus of the femoral head then reossifies and continues to grow. Unless the head is contained within the acetabular roof, however, the new femoral head deforms and becomes large (coxa magna) and flat (coxa plana). At the same time, the femoral neck becomes shortened and a coxa vara deformity of the upper femur develops. Legg-Perthes disease is most commonly unilateral.

Avascular necrosis of the femoral head also occurs with other conditions producing ischemia. Roentgenographically, the findings are indistinguishable from Legg-Perthes disease except that bilateral involvement is more common. These conditions include steroid therapy (4), sickle cell disease (9, 12, 15), the collagen vascular diseases (1, 10), Gaucher disease, and a few cases of avascular necrosis as a complica-

tion of closed reduction of congenital hip dislocation (7, 17), surgical hip nailing, hip fracture (displaced femoral head), osteomyelitis of the femoral capital epiphysis, septic arthritis or osteomyelitis of the hip (11), and irradiation therapy to the hip. Of all these, the most common are sickle cell disease and steroid therapy. Avascular necrosis of the other epiphyses is rather uncommon, but occasionally can be seen with steroid therapy (Fig. 4.48B), sepsis with disseminated intravascular coagulation (6, 18), trauma, or frostbite (3, 20). The latter occurs mostly in the hands and feet. In the distal femur, avascular necrosis should be differentiated from normal irregularity of the lateral femoral condyle (see Fig. 4.59C). An unusual cause of a sclerotic, fragmented epiphysis in the hands is Thiemann disease (5), a condition presumed, but not universally accepted, as being a rare

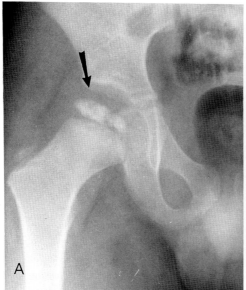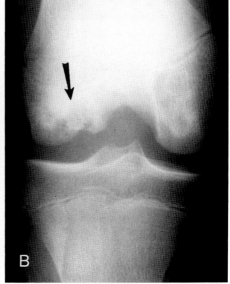

Figure 4.48. Irregular epiphyses. A. Typical, slightly small, sclerotic, and fragmented epiphysis *(arrow)* of advanced Legg-Perthes disease. **B.** Irregular, distal femoral condyle *(arrow)* due to ischemic necrosis in patient on steroid therapy for chronic renal disease.

form of primary aseptic necrosis of the epiphysis of the small bones of the hand.

Rounding out the causes of epiphyseal irregularity are rheumatoid arthritis (8, 13), Winchester syndrome (storage disease which resembles rheumatoid arthritis) (21), other joint inflammations, and epiphyseal dysplasia hemimelica (2, 11). With epiphyseal dysplasia hemimelica, also known as Trevor disease (2), the problem is an osteochondroma of the epiphysis, and most often the changes are seen around knee or ankle (see Fig. 4.44D). However, the disease also can be seen in the upper extremity.

REFERENCES

1. Bergstein JM, Wiens C, Fish AJ, Vernier RL, Michael A: Avascular necrosis of bone in systemic lupus erythematosus. *J Pediatr* 85:31–35, 1974.
2. Carlson DH, Wilkinson RH: Variability of unilateral epiphyseal dysplasia (Dysplasia epiphysealis hemimelic). *Radiology* 133:369–373, 1979.
3. Carrera GF, Kozin F, Flaherty L, McCarty DJ: Radiographic changes in the hands following childhood frostbite injury. *Skeletal Radiol* 16:33–37, 1971.
4. Cole WG, Neal BW: Corticosteroids and avascular necrosis of the femoral head in childhood. *Aust Paediatr J* 11:243–246, 1975.
5. Cullen JC: Thiemann's disease. *J Bone Joint Surg* 52B:532–534, 1970.
6. Fernandez F, Peuyo I, Jimenez JR, Vigil E, Guzman A: Epiphysiometaphyseal changes in children after severe meningococcic sepsis. *AJR* 136:1236–1238, 1981.
7. Gage JR, Winter RB: Avascular necrosis of the capital femoral epiphysis as a complication of closed reduction of congenital dislocation of the hip: a critical review of 20 years' experience at Gillette Children's Hospital. *J Bone Joint Surg* 54A:373–388, 1972.
8. Goel KM, Rawson SP, Shanks RA: Radiological assessment of fifty patients with juvenile rheumatoid arthritis: correlation with clinical and laboratory abnormalities. *Pediatr Radiol* 2:51–60, 1974.
9. Hill MC, Oh KS, Bowerman JW, Siegelman SS, James AE Jr: Abnormal epiphyses in the sickling disorders. *AJR* 124:34–43, 1975.
10. Hurley RM, Steinberg RH, Patriquin H, Drummond KN: Avascular necrosis of the femoral head in childhood systemic lupus erythematosus. *Can Med Assoc J* 111:781–784, 1974.
11. Keret D, Spatz DK, Caro PA, Mason DE: Dysplasia epiphysealis hemimelica: diagnosis and treatment. *J Pediatr Orthop* 12:365–372, 1992.
12. Lee REJ, Golding JSR, Sergeant GR: The radiologic features of avascular necrosis of the femoral head in homozygous sickle cell disease. *Clin Radiol* 32:205–214, 1981.
13. Martel W, Holt JF, Cassidy JT: Roentgenologic manifestations of juvenile rheumatoid arthritis. *AJR* 88:400–423, 1962.
14. Meyer J: Dysplasia epiphysealis capitis femoris. *Acta Orthop Scand* 34:183–197, 1964.
15. Milner PF, Kraus AP, Sebes JI, Sleeper LA, Kukes KA, Embury SH, Bellevue R, Koshy M, Moohr JW, Smith J: Sickle cell disease as a cause of osteonecrosis of the femoral head. *N Engl J Med* 325:1476–1481, 1991.
16. Norman LE, Pischnotte WO: Morquio's disease. *Am J Dis Child* 124:719–722, 1972.
17. Salter RB, Kostuik J, Dallas S: Avascular necrosis of femoral head as a complication of treatment for congenital dislocation of hip in young children: a clinical and experimental investigation. *Can J Surg* 12:44–61, 1969.
18. Santos E, Boavida JE, Barroso A, Seabra J, da Mota HC: Late osteoarticular lesions following meningococcemia with disseminated intravascular coagulation. *Pediatr Radiol* 19:199–202, 1989.

19. Stansberry, SD, Swischuk LE, Barr LL: Legg-Perthes disease: incidence of subchondral fracture. *Appl. Radiol.* 19:30–33, 1990.

20. Wensl JE, Burke EC, Bianco AJ Jr: Epiphyseal destruction from frostbite of the hands. *Am J Dis Child* 114:668–670, 1967.

21. Winchester P, Grossman H, Lim WN, Danes BS: A new acid mucopolysaccharidosis with skeletal deformities simulating rheumatoid arthritis. *Am J Roentgenol Radium Ther Nucl Med* 106:128, 1969.

22. Wynne-Davies R, Gormley J: The etiology of Perthes disease. *J Bone Joint Surg* 60B:6–14, 1978.

IRREGULAR OR FRAGMENTED APOPHYSES (TABLE 4.17)

Apophyses are not true epiphyses, but in many regards function in the same fashion. They are growth centers, but unlike epiphyses, they generally do not have articular surfaces. Overall, they normally tend to be more fragmented and sclerotic than epiphyses, and most commonly occur at sites of tendon insertion in the feet, shoulder, and elbow (Fig. 4.49). The findings should not be misinterpreted as those of avascular necrosis or comminuted fracture. The most common source of such misinterpretation occurs with the

Table 4.17
Irregular—Fragmented Apophyses

Normal Hands, feet Distal humerus Calcaneus Scapula Osgood-Schlatter disease: tibial tubercle	Common
Hypothyroidism Trisomy-21: feet	Relatively rare

apophysis of the calcaneus. Usually, because of chronic heel pain, aseptic necrosis of the calcaneal apophysis is considered to be the cause (i.e., Siever disease) (Fig. 4.49*D*). In fact, Siever disease, as a bone disease, probably does not exist. Indeed, with normal weight bearing the calcaneal apophysis should be dense and sclerotic (2). The problem in patients with heel pain most often is chronic subclinical traumatic tendonitis/bursitis. Irregular, dense apophyses also occur in the scapula, primarily over the coracoid and acromial processes (Fig. 4.49*B*).

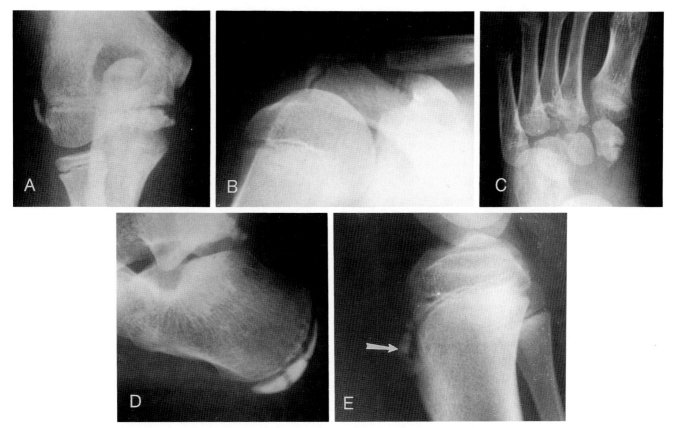

Figure 4.49. Irregular and sclerotic apophyses. A. Normal irregular apophyses and capitellar epiphysis around the elbow. **B.** Normal irregular apophyses around the shoulder. **C.** Normal irregular apophyses of metatarsals. **D.** Normal sclerotic, irregular calcaneal apophysis. **E.** Markedly irregular tibial tubercle in Osgood-Schlatter disease *(arrow)*.

The tibial tubercle, that is, the apophysis of the upper tibia, normally is not fragmented or particularly irregular, but with chronic avulsion of the inserting infrapatellar tendon, irregularity and sclerosis frequently develop. The condition then is known as Osgood-Schlatter disease (1, 3, 4), and is quite common in the active youngster. In the acute phase, it is associated with soft tissue swelling, obliteration of the infrapatellar fat pad, and focal pain over the tibial tubercle. Fragmentation may be minimal, but with healing and repeated avulsions, fragmentation and hypertrophic bone formation can become quite profound (Fig. 4.49E). Irregularity of the apophyses, in general, also occurs in hypothyroidism and trisomy 21, and, once again, in both conditions the changes are most pronounced in the feet (see Fig. 4.47E).

REFERENCES

1. Cohen B, Wilkinson RW: The Osgood-Schlatter lesion: a radiological and histological study. *Am J Surg* 95:731, 1958.
2. Shopfner CE, Coin CG: Effect of weight-bearing on the appearance and development of the secondary calcaneal epiphysis. *Radiology* 86:201–206, 1966.
3. Willner P: Osgood-Schlatter's disease: etiology and treatment. *Clin Orthop* 62:178–179, 1969.
4. Woolfrey BF, Chandler EF: Manifestations of Osgood-Schlatter's disease in later teen age and early adulthood. *J Bone Joint Surg* 42A:327–332, 1960.

IVORY EPIPHYSES

Ivory epiphyses are of normal size and shape, but are very dense (Fig. 4.50). Most often, they occur in the hands and feet, and of the two, occurrence in the hands is more common. In this regard, the distal phalanges most often are involved, and the individuals in whom this is seen usually have been considered normal (2). However, many of these children are examined for short stature, and even though a cause for this problem is not always determined, whether these children are completely normal is debatable. In this regard, ivory epiphyses frequently occur in patients with hypopituitarism, and on a practical basis, **one probably sees more ivory epiphyses in a child of short stature and delayed growth than in a perfectly normal child.** It may be that the ivory epiphysis simply reflects slow bone metabolism with impaired turnover of calcium.

When multiple ivory epiphyses are seen in the proximal phalanges, there is a better chance that some syndrome is present, and then one might consider conditions such as multiple epiphyseal dysplasia, Cockayne syndrome (bone age also usually ad-

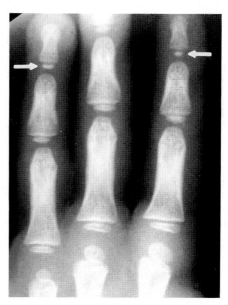

Figure 4.50. Ivory epiphysis. Typical appearance of ivory epiphyses of a number of the small bones of the hands *(arrows)*. This patient had growth retardation of undetermined etiology.

vanced), the trichorhinophalangeal syndrome, Coffin syndrome, Stickler syndrome, Seckel bird-headed dwarfism, and, rarely, Thiemann disease (1). In the latter condition, aseptic necrosis of the epiphysis of the small bones of the hands is believed to be the problem. Dense epiphyses also can occur in any conditions where the bones generally are dense.

REFERENCES

1. Cullen JC: Thiemann disease. *J Bone Joint Surg* 52B:532–534, 1970.
2. Kuhns LR, Poznanski AK, Harper HAS, Garn SM: Ivory epiphyses and the hands. *Radiology* 109:643–648, 1973.

LARGE EPIPHYSES (TABLE 4.18)

Generalized enlargement of all of the epiphyses occurs with many chondrodystrophic dwarfing syndromes in which the long bones are short, the metaphyses are widened, and the epiphyses are enlarged (see Table 4.3). By the same token, epiphyses are disproportionately large in conditions leading to thin bony shafts (e.g., osteogenesis imperfecta, neurologic-neuromuscular disease), but in neither case are the large epiphyses used as a specific diagnostic feature of the conditions. An exception occurs with the rare condition known as megaepiphyseal dwarfism (3). When a large epiphysis is used for diagnostic purposes, it is focal and most often is secondary to chronic joint infection or inflammation. The hyperemia so produced results in epiphyseal overgrowth

Table 4.18
Large—Overgrown Epiphyses

Rheumatoid arthritis[a,b]	
Hemophilic arthritis[a,b]	
Healed Legg-Perthes disease: coxa plana-magna	Common
Chondrodystrophies with short bones and flared metaphyses[c]	
Tuberculous and fungal arthritis[a,b]	Moderately common
Pyogenic arthritis: chronic	
Winchester syndrome[a]	
Epiphyseal dysplasia hemimelica[b]	Rare
Fibrous dysplasia of epiphysis	
Megaepiphyseal dwarfism	

[a] Epiphysis often large and glassy.
[b] Unilateral enlargement usually.
[c] See Table 4.25.

and osteoporosis, and because of this the epiphysis becomes **large, glassy, and coarsely trabeculated** (Fig. 4.51). The most common causes of such epiphyseal enlargement are rheumatoid arthritis (2) and hemophilic arthropathy, but epiphyseal enlargement also occurs in tuberculous arthritis, fungal arthritis, and the rheumatoid arthritis mimicking storage disease known as Winchester syndrome (4, 7). In hemophilic arthropathy, there also is widening of the in-

tercondylar notch of the distal femur (Fig. 4.51B), and although this configuration is near-pathognomonic of the condition, such widening also has been documented with tuberculous arthritis (5). It does not occur with rheumatoid arthritis.

Enlargement of an epiphysis also can occur with lingering, low-grade pyogenic arthritis, but generally this is uncommon. Most often, with pyogenic arthritis, the infection is of short duration and rapid onset, and the epiphysis is more likely to be destroyed than overgrown. In those few, chronic cases where enlargement occurs, it is slight, and the glassy effect does not usually develop.

An enlarged, but flattened, epiphysis is seen in healed Legg-Perthes disease (i.e., coxa plana, coxa magna), and irregular enlargement of an epiphysis, especially of the lower extremity, can be seen with epiphyseal dysplasia hemimelica (1). In this condition, the problem actually is an osteochondroma of the epiphysis, and epiphyseal enlargement usually is eccentric (see Fig. 4.44D). Fibrous dysplasia leading to a large epiphysis also has been recorded (6), but is very rare.

REFERENCES

1. Carlson DH, Wilkinson RH: Variability of unilateral epiphyseal dysplasia (dysplasia epiphysealis hemimelica). *Radiology* 133:369–373, 1979.

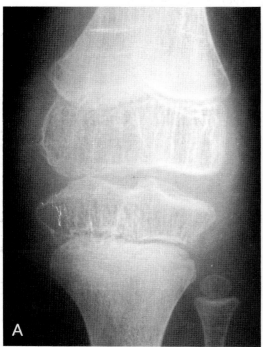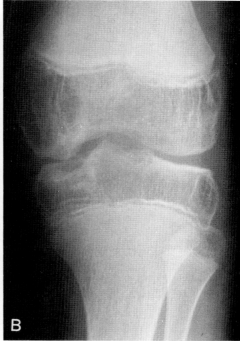

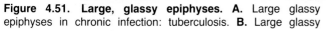

Figure 4.51. Large, glassy epiphyses. A. Large glassy epiphyses in chronic infection: tuberculosis. **B.** Large glassy epiphyses in patient with hemophilia. Also note characteristic widening of the intercondylar notch.

2. Goel KM, Rawson SP, Shanks RA: Radiological assessment of fifty patients with juvenile rheumatoid arthritis: correlation with clinical and laboratory abnormalities. *Pediatr Radiol* 2:51–60, 1974.
3. Gorlin RJ, Alper R, Longer L: Megaepiphyseal dwarfism. *J Pediatr* 83:633–637, 1973.
4. Hollister DW, Rimoin DL, Lachman RS, Cohen AH, Reed WB, Estin GW: The Winchester syndrome: a nonlysosomal connective tissue disease. *J Pediatr* 84:701–709, 1974.
5. Nixon SP: Tuberculosis synovitis with widening of the intercondylar notch of the distal femur. *Br J Radiol* 42:703–704, 1969.
6. Nixon GW, Condon VR: Epiphyseal involvement in polyostotic fibrous dysplasia: a report of two cases. *Radiology* 106:167–170, 1973.
7. Winchester P, Grossman H, Lim WN, Danes BS: A new acid mucopoly-saccharidosis with skeletal deformities simulating rheumatoid arthritis. *AJR* 106:128–136, 1969.

LARGE MEDIAL FEMORAL CONDYLE

In these conditions, the medial condyle of the distal femoral epiphysis is overly prominent and is associated with variable depression of the underlying tibial plateau. For the most part, this finding is seen in the following conditions: Turner syndrome, Prader-Willi syndrome, Cornelia de Lange syndrome, dyschondrosteosis (Fig. 4.52). Prominence of the medial femoral condyle also occurs in most of the chondrodystrophic dwarfs, producing short, bowed bones, but in these conditions it is not of much value for specific diagnosis. Other features of these conditions are more important.

SMALL EPIPHYSES (TABLE 4.19)

Small epiphyses can occur on a generalized or focal basis. On a generalized basis, small epiphyses can be seen with any condition where bone age is delayed, but smallness of the epiphysis is not important in the diagnosis of these conditions. On the other hand, there are certain diseases where small epiphyses are used for specific diagnosis, and these include multiple epiphyseal dysplasia, spondyloepiphyseal dysplasia, Morquio disease (a storage disease that looks like spondyloepiphyseal dysplasia), and hypothyroidism. In both hypothyroidism and the epiphyseal dysplasias, in addition to the epiphyses being small, they are fragmented and irregular (see Fig. 4.47C–E) and, with the epiphyseal dysplasias, frequently sclerotic.

On a focal basis, a small epiphysis results from some insult to the epiphysis or because the extremity on that side is not being used. The latter can occur in any neurologic, neuromuscular, or arthritic disease that leads to disuse of an extremity, and one of the best examples of this phenomenon is congenital dislocation (developmental dysplasia) of the hip. In this condition, the femoral head remains small as long as the hip is located out of the acetabulum (Fig. 4.53A). If, however, early therapy is instituted and the femoral head is relocated under the acetabular roof, head size catches up with that of the normal side. Smallness of an epiphysis, secondary to its de-

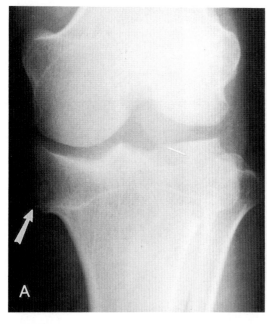
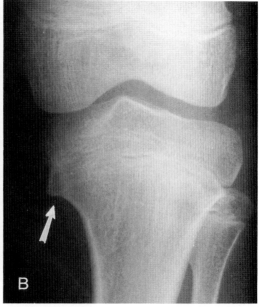

Figure 4.52. Prominent medial femoral condyles. A. Typical prominence of the medial femoral condyle in Turner syndrome. **B.** Similar prominence of the medial femoral condyle in dyschon- drostosis. Also note associated flattening of the upper medial, tibial metaphysis and the small exostosis *(arrow).*

struction or resorption by inflammation, infection, or infarction is self-evident, and in terms of infarction, the most common situation is that of the ischemically necrotic femoral head of Legg-Perthes disease (Fig. 4.53*B* and *C*). To be sure, smallness of the femoral capital epiphysis is one of the earliest findings of this condition (1, 2), and reflects cessation of growth of the ossified nucleus of the femoral head. However, even though the ossified nucleus becomes small and then fragments, the cartilage cap remains relatively intact, and later, in long-standing cases, the femoral head reconstitutes and remodels to become flattened, large, and deformed (i.e., coxa magna and coxa plana). If, however, therapy is instituted early and the femoral head is relocated under the acetabular roof, it retains a more normal, round configuration.

Occasionally, a solitary, normal femoral capital

Table 4.19
Small Epiphyses

Generalized		
Delayed bone age: any cause	}	Common

Hypothyroidism
Dysplasia
    Multiple epiphyseal
    Spondyloepiphyseal
	}	Moderately common

Morquio disease	}	Relatively rare
Unilateral		
Early Legg-Perthes disease Congenital dislocating hip: developmental hip dysplasia	}	Common
Postinfection, injury, etc. Normal[a]	}	Moderately common

[a]Minimal asymmetry; usually hips.

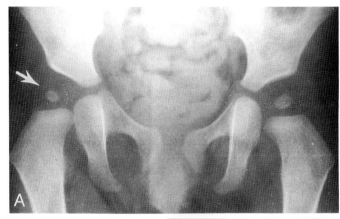

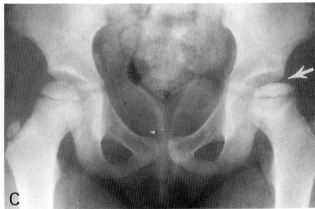

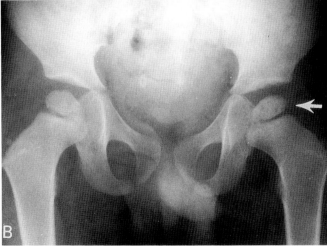

Figure 4.53.   Small, nonfragmented epiphyses. A. Congenital hip dislocation. Note small proximal femoral epiphysis on the right *(arrow).* Also note that the acetabular roof is more slanted and less cupped than normal, and that the hip is laterally displaced. **B.** Small, sclerotic epiphysis *on the left (arrow)* in patient with early Legg-Perthes disease. **C.** Another patient with later stage Legg-Perthes disease demonstrating more smallness of the femoral head *on the left (arrow).* Also note slight lateral subluxation of the hip. Later, the femoral head undergoes fragmentation (see Fig. 4.48*A*).

epiphysis may be small, but usually the difference from the other side is minimal. In such cases, if there is question as to whether the epiphysis is small and normal, or small and ischemically necrotic, one can utilize nuclear scintigraphy or MR scanning to determine whether the head is ischemic and necrotic.

REFERENCES

1. Caffey J: The early roentgenographic changes in essential coxa plana: their significance in pathogenesis. *AJR* 102:620–634, 1968.
2. Stansberry SD, Swischuk LE, Barr LL: Legg-Perthes disease: Incidence of the subchondral fracture. *Appl Radiol* 19:30–33, 1990.

CONE-SHAPED EPIPHYSES (TABLE 4.20)

Cone-shaped epiphyses have a cone-like projection into the center of the metaphysis and most commonly occur in the hands and feet. They can be seen in normal individuals (1, 5), especially in the feet (Fig. 4.54*A*) and occasionally in the knee (Fig. 4.54*B*). On a pathologic basis, coned epiphyses occur in a number of syndromes and the best known such association is with the tricho-rhino-phalangeal syndrome of Giedion (2–4, 6) (Fig. 4.54*C*). Similar coning occurs in the lesser known conorenal syndrome, a condition associated with chronic renal disease in the form of familial nephronophthisis (3, 9). Other conditions in which cone-shaped epiphyses are seen include achondroplasia (see Fig. 4.4*A*), acrodysostosis, Ellis-van Creveld syndrome, cleidocranial dysostosis, osteopetrosis, orodigitofacial syndrome, otopalatodigital syndrome, the acrocephalosyndactyly syndromes, asphyxiating thoracic dystrophy, nonspecific brachydactyly (Fig. 4.54*D*), Marchesani syndrome, Ruvalcaba syndrome, osteopetrosis, multiple and spondyloepiphyseal dysplasia, metaphyseal dysostosis, Seckel bird-headed dwarfism, pseudo- or pseudopseudohypoparathyroidism (10), and multiple osteochondromatosis. In the latter condition, the cone deformity often occurs laterally, whereas in most of the other conditions the cone is central.

On an acquired basis, a cone-shaped epiphysis can develop secondary to any type of epiphyseal-metaphyseal injury or insult (see Fig. 4.14). The specific epiphyseal-metaphyseal injury may be simple trauma, pathologic epiphyseal-metaphyseal fracture, osteomyelitis, bone infarction (i.e., sickle cell disease), sepsis with disseminated intravascular coagulation, radiation injury, frostbite, hypophosphatasia (knees), or chronic vitamin A intoxication (7). In some of these conditions, the resulting cone-shaped deformity is quite pronounced and deep.

REFERENCES

1. de Iturriza JR, Tanner JM: Cone-shaped epiphyses and other minor anomalies in the hands of normal British children. *J Pediatr* 75:265–272, 1969.
2. Giedion A: Cone-shaped epiphyses of the hands and their diagnostic value: the tricho-rhino-phalangeal syndrome. *Ann Radiol* 10:322–329, 1967.
3. Giedion A: Phalangeal cone shaped epiphysis of the hands (PhCSEH) and chronic renal disease: the conorenal syndromes. *Pediatr Radiol* 8:32-38, 1979.
4. Gorlin RJ, Cohen MM Jr, Wolfson J: Trichorhinophalangeal syndrome. *Am J Dis Child* 118:595–599, 1969.
5. Hertzog KP, Garn SM, Church SF: Cone-shaped epiphyses in the hand: population frequencies, anatomic distribution and developmental stages. *Invest Radiol* 3:433–441, 1968.
6. Kozlowski K, Blaim A, Malolepsky E: Tricho-rhino-phalangeal syndrome. *Australas Radiol* 16:411–416, 1972.
7. Pease CN: Focal retardation and arrestment of growth of bones due to vitamin A intoxication. *JAMA* 182:980–985, 1962.
8. Poznanski AK: Diagnostic clues in the growing ends of bones. *J Can Assoc Radiol* 29:7–21, 1978.
9. Saldino RM, Mainzer F: Cone-shaped epiphyses (CSE) in

Table 4.20
Cone-shaped Epiphyses

Normal[a]	}	Common
Trauma Infection Achondroplasia	}	Moderately common
Bone infarction Sickle cell disease Frostbite: hands and feet Multiple osteochondromatosis Metaphyseal dysostosis-dysplasia Metaphyseal and spondyloepiphyseal dysplasia Cleidocranial dysostosis Acrocephalosyndactyly syndrome Asphyxiating thoracic dystrophy Osteopetrosis Pseudo- or pseudopseudohyperparathyroidism	}	Relatively rare
Tricho-rhino-phalangeal syndrome Vitamin A intoxication: chronic Acrodysostosis Ellis-van Creveld syndrome Nonspecific brachydactyly Marchesani syndrome Seckel bird-headed dwarf Oro-facial-digital syndrome Oto-palato-digital syndrome Ruvalcaba syndrome Conorenal syndrome Radiation injury Hypophosphatasia	}	Rare

[a]Especially feet.

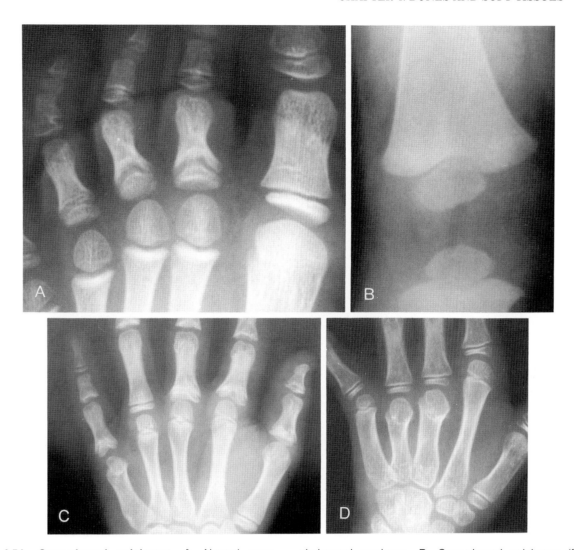

Figure 4.54. Cone-shaped epiphyses. A. Normal cone-shaped epiphyses in feet. **B.** Normal cone-shaped epiphyses in knee of infant. **C.** Typical cone-shaped epiphyses in tricho-rhino-phalangeal syndrome. **D.** Cone-shaped epiphyses (fused in metacarpals) in nonspecific brachydactyly.

siblings with hereditary renal disease and retinitis pigmentosa. *Radiology* 98:39–46, 1971.
10. Steinback HL, Young DA: The roentgen appearance of pseudohypoparathyroidism (PH) and pseudo-pseudohypoparathyroidism (PPH), differentiation from other syndromes associated with short metacarpals, metatarsals, and phalanges. *AJR* 97:49–66, 1966.

INDISTINCT EPIPHYSEAL MARGINS (TABLE 4.21)

Normally the epiphysis has a readily visualized and intact margin around its periphery. When calcification is less than normal, however, the edge of the epiphysis becomes indistinct. Most often, this occurs with conditions producing osteomalacia, that is, rickets and hyperparathyroidism (Fig. 4.55A). However, it also occurs with hypophosphatasia, hypothyroidism (Fig. 4.55B), and, in infancy, in conditions that mimic hyperparathyroidism (i.e., Jansen metaphyseal dysostosis, generalized gangliosidosis, and mucolipidosis II).

RINGED EPIPHYSES (TABLE 4.21)

The commonest cause of a ringed epiphysis is severe, chronic osteoporosis, because, while the center of the epiphysis becomes increasingly radiolucent, the relatively less demineralized cortex remains thin and dense. This can be seen with any cause of osteoporosis, but is most common in neurologic or neuromuscular disease with disuse atrophy (Fig. 4.56A). The finding also is seen in osteogenesis imperfecta, and when seen in scurvy (rare these days), is referred to as the Wimberger ring (Fig. 4.56B).

Less delicate and often very dense rings are seen in the healing phase of any condition that first leads to an indistinct epiphyseal margin. In such conditions, including rickets, hyperparathyroidism, renal

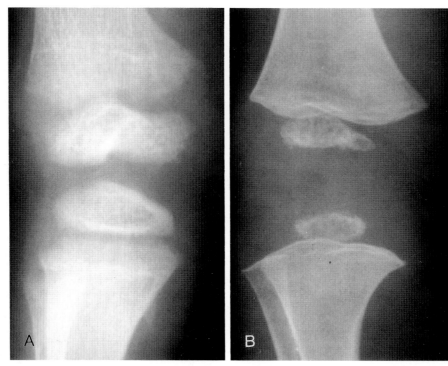

Figure 4.55. Indistinct epiphyseal edges. A. Indistinct epiphyses in rickets. Note generalized osteomalacia. **B. Indis-** tinct epiphyseal edges in hypothyroidism (epiphyseal dysgenesis).

osteodystrophy, and hypothyroidism, the problem is similar to that seen with transverse metaphyseal bands. In other words, when an insult to enchondral bone growth occurs, the edge of the epiphysis be-

comes indistinct, and then, with recovery, the cortex reconstitutes and a white ring is formed.

RAGGED EPIPHYSES

This epiphyseal configuration usually is normal, and most often is seen in the distal femur of infants and young children (Fig. 4.57). It also occasionally can be seen in the hip and in the proximal tibia. In older children, raggedness can be seen with rheumatoid arthritis (1). Ragged epiphyses also are seen with other chronic arthritides and the Winchester syndrome (storage disease that resembles rheumatoid arthritis).

REFERENCE

1. Martel W, Holt J, Cassidy J: Roentgenographic manifestations of juvenile rheumatoid arthritis. *AJR* 88:400–423, 1962.

DEFECTS OF THE EPIPHYSES (TABLE 4.22)

Perhaps the most important point to note with an epiphyseal defect is whether it is associated with joint fluid. The reason for this is that, when fluid is present, infection or trauma almost surely also is present. If the defect is due to an acute avulsion (e.g., cruciate ligament avulsion), the fluid is blood, and because the avulsed fragment is seen, there is no

Table 4.21
Indistinct and Ringed Epiphyses

Indistinct epiphyseal margins		
Rickets	}	Common
Hyperparathyroidism[a]		
Hypothyroidism	}	Moderately common
Hyperparathyroidism[b]		
Jansen metaphyseal dysostosis	}	Relatively rare
Mucolipidosis II		
Gangliosidosis		
Ringed epiphysis		
Severe chronic osteoporosis[c]	}	Commmon
Healing rickets	}	Moderately common
Healing hypothyroidism	}	Relatively rare
Osteogenesis imperfecta		
Scurvy[d]	}	Rare

[a] Secondary.
[b] Primary.
[c] See Table 4.2 for causes.
[d] Wimberger ring.

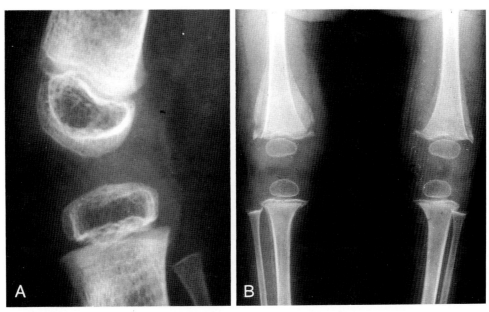

Figure 4.56. Ringed epiphyses. A. Marked disuse osteoporosis causing ringed epiphysis in patient with neurologic disease. **B.** Ringed epiphyses in scurvy. Note other characteristic changes in the metaphyses including the white line of scurvy, the scurvy zone (radiolucent band), corner fracturing, and subperiosteal bleeding with new bone deposition.

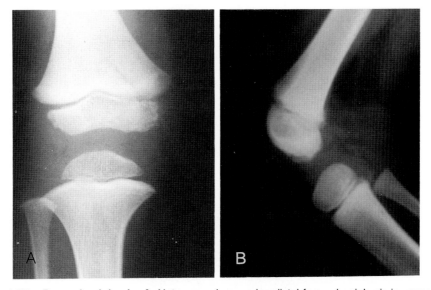

Figure 4.57. Ragged epiphysis. A. Note ragged appearing distal femoral epiphysis in young infant. **B.** Lateral view shows same changes.

problem with the diagnosis. When the problem is infection, chronic synovial hypertrophy is the cause of the defect. Almost invariably in such cases, the problem is tuberculous (Fig. 4.58A) or rheumatoid arthritis (1–3, 6, 8, 9), but occasionally it is due to acute or subacute osteomyelitis (4, 10) (Fig. 4.58B). In the distal femoral epiphysis, normal fibrous defects should not be confused with those due to infection (Fig. 4.58C), and in the hip, the normal defect of the fovea centralis can mimic a pathologic defect (Fig. 4.58D).

In the knee, another common epiphyseal defect is that seen with osteochondritis dissecans (5, 7). The condition may be asymptomatic, and usually there is no significant joint fluid accumulation. Characteristically, the defect involves the medial femoral condyle, is somewhat anterior in position, and is associated with an avulsed bone fragment (Fig. 4.59A). It is especially well delineated with MRI (Fig. 4.59B). A normal defect (Fig. 4.59C), not to be confused with that of osteochondritis dissecans, can occur in either femoral condyle. In such cases, its more posterior lo-

Table 4.22
Epiphyseal Defects

Fovea centralis: normal femoral head defect Osteochondritis dissecans: distal femur Avulsion injuries: anterior tibial spine, knee	Common
Normal femoral condyle defects Rheumatoid arthritis Osteochondritis dissecans: other bones Hemophilic arthritis	Moderately common
Tuberculous arthritis Fungal arthritis Other chronic arthritis Osteomyelitis of epiphysis	Relatively rare
Histiocytosis-X Synovial tumors Fibrous defects	Rare

cation is the clue to proper diagnosis. Osteochondritis dissecans can occur at other sites (i.e., capitellum, patella, talus) (Fig. 4.59D and E). However, it is by far most common in the distal femur. Other causes of epiphyseal defects include histiocytosis-X and, rarely, a synovial tumor.

REFERENCES

1. Cassidy JT, Brody GL, Martel W: Mono-articular juvenile rheumatoid arthritis. *J Pediatr* 70:867–875, 1967.
2. Cremin BJ, Fisher MB, Levinsohn MB: Multiple bone tuberculosis in the young. *Br J Radiol* 43:638–645, 1970.
3. Edeiken J, Hodes PJ: *Roentgen Diagnosis of Diseases of Bone.* 2d ed. Baltimore: Williams & Wilkins, 1973; 2:664, 733.
4. Green NE, Beauchamp RD, Griffin PP: Primary subacute epiphyseal osteomyelitis. *J Bone Joint Surg* 63A: 107–114, 1981.
5. Green WT, Banks HH: Osteochondritis dissecans in children. *J Bone Joint Surg* 35A:26–47, 1953.

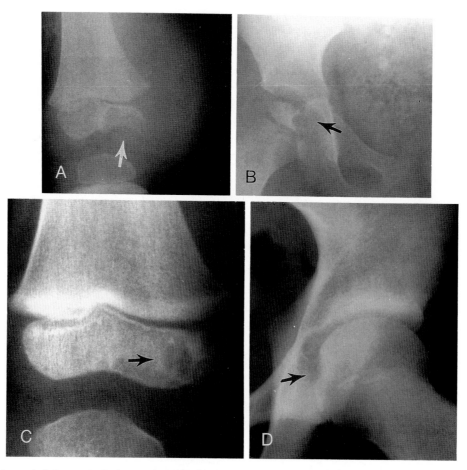

Figure 4.58. Epiphyseal defects. A. Defect *(arrow)* of distal femoral epiphysis due to tuberculous arthritis. **B.** Epiphyseal defect *(arrow)* of proximal femoral epiphysis due to subacute pyogenic osteomyelitis *(arrow)*. **C.** Normal, fibrous defect in distal femoral epiphysis *(arrow)*. **D.** Normal defect in femoral capital epiphysis *(arrow)* due to fovea centralis.

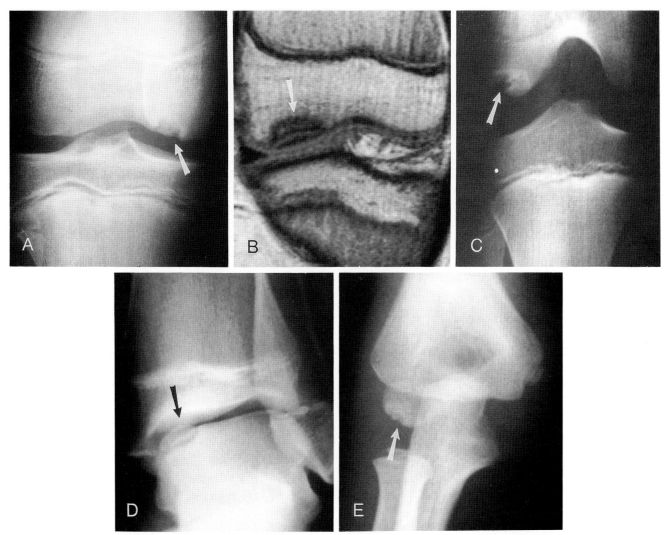

Figure 4.59. A. Epiphyseal defect-osteochondritis dissecans. Note typical defect in medial femoral condyle *(arrow)*. **B.** MRI in another patient shows a typical defect *(arrow)* of osteo-chondritis dissecans. **C.** Normal defect in medial condyle *(arrow)*. **D.** Osteochondritis dissecans of talus *(arrow)*. **E.** Subtle osteochondritis dissecans *(arrow)* of capitellum.

6. Martel W, Holt J, Cassidy J: Roentgenographic manifestations of juvenile rheumatoid arthritis. *AJR* 88:400–423, 1962.
7. Milgram JW: Radiological and pathological manifestations of osteochondritis dissecans of the distal femur: a study of 50 cases. *Radiology* 125:305–311, 1978.
8. Phemister DB: Changes in the articular surfaces in tuberculosis and in pyogenic infections of joints. *AJR* 12:1–14, 1924.
9. Phemister DB, Hatcher CH: Correlation of pathological and roentgenological findings in diagnosis of tuberculosis arthritis. *AJR* 29:736–752, 1933.
10. Rosenbaum DM, Blumhagen JD: Acute epiphyseal osteomyelitis in children. *Radiology* 156:89–92, 1985.

EPIPHYSEAL CLEFTS

Epiphyseal clefts are normal variations in the epiphysis that most commonly occur in the great toe (Fig. 4.60A). They can occur in other epiphyses (1), but are most problematic in the great toe, where often they are misinterpreted for similar clefts caused by fracturing of the epiphysis (Fig. 4.60B). This problem does not arise as often at other sites, because clefts at other sites usually represent epiphyseal fractures.

REFERENCE

1. Harrison RB, Keats TE: Epiphyseal clefts. *Skeletal Radiol* 5:23–27, 1980.

INTRAEPIPHYSEAL GAS

Gas within the epiphysis almost exclusively occurs with aseptic necrosis of the proximal femoral

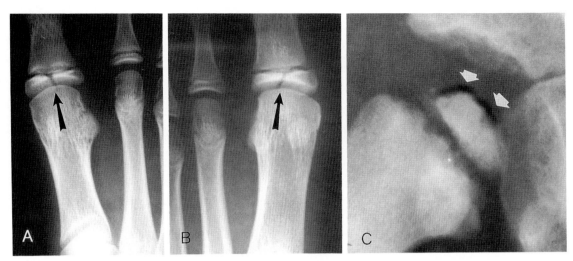

Figure 4.60. Epiphyseal clefts. A. Normal epiphyseal cleft (bipartite epiphysis) of great toe *(arrow).* **B.** Defect of epiphysis due to fracture *(arrow).* **C. Intraepiphyseal gas.** Characteristic intraepiphyseal gas *(arrow)* in Legg-Perthes disease.

epiphysis, i.e., Legg-Perthes disease (1). It has, however, been described with osteochondritis of the capitellum (2), and at either site is quite characteristic (Fig. 4.60C). The phenomenon of gas in the epiphysis is not unlike that which occurs with the so-called "vacuum joint" (see Fig. 4.122C). Intraepiphyseal gas is seen only with traction on a joint, and perhaps this is why it is most commonly recorded in the hip. In the hip, standard roentgenographic examination consists of anteroposterior and frogleg views. On the frogleg view, there is a certain amount of traction applied to the joint, and it may be that this is why intraepiphyseal gas appears so commonly on this study. The reason the gas accumulates in the epiphysis is that there is a subchondral fracture present, and because of this the fractured fragment can separate from the main portion of the head. The negative pressures then are transmitted intraepiphyseally, and intraepiphyseal gas results.

REFERENCES

1. Caffey J: The early roentgenographic changes in essential coxa plana: their significance in pathogenesis. *AJR* 103:620–634, 1968.
2. Jacobs P: Intra-epiphyseal gas in osteochondritis of capitellum. *Clin Radiol* 21:318–319, 1970.

Metaphyseal Abnormalities

TRANSVERSE METAPHYSEAL BANDS (TABLE 4.23)

These bands can be radiolucent or radiodense and, actually, most often both coexist. Radiolucent bands generally reflect episodes of poor enchondral bone formation and dense bands develop in the ensuing recovery phase. Often the dense bands are referred to as growth arrest or Parks's lines (4, 5, 9), even though the term "arrest" is somewhat of a misnomer. **More accurately, the dense lines are recovery lines,** for they result from the rapid deposition of new bone after the insult causing poor bone growth is gone.

The foregoing combination of radiolucent and radiodense transverse metaphyseal bands is rather nonspecific, but at the same time, quite common (Fig. 4.61). The reason is that these lines can result from almost any form of insult to the growing body—i.e., severe infections or fractures and chronic relapsing diseases such as asthma, diabetes, cystic fibrosis, osteopetrosis, treated malignancies (chemotherapy, radiation therapy), rheumatoid arthritis (8), and the battered child-deprivational dwarf syndromes (6). These bands also occur in the neonate as a result of the "normal" insults sustained during birth and the immediate postnatal period (especially in premature infants) and, pathologically, in perinatal infections such as rubella, cytomegalovirus, herpes, toxoplasmosis, and syphilis (1, 2, 11, 12). These lines even can develop before birth as a result of maternal infections or fetal insults such as intestinal perforation (14). In addition, the lines occur with healing rickets and treated hypothyroidism.

As noted earlier, these transverse bands frequently are multiple and the alternating radiolucent-opaque sequence is clearly visible (Fig. 4.61A–D). However, if one obtains a roentgenogram during the first, or only, episode of impaired enchondral bone formation, then one will see only a single transverse radiolucent band such as occurs after a fracture (Fig. 4.61E). Similar and more ominous bands

Table 4.23
Transverse Metaphyseal Bands

Alternating radiolucent and radio-opaque	
Severe illness, trauma[a]	
Battered child syndrome, deprivational dwarf[b]	Common
Healing rickets[a]	
Healing neonatal infections[a]	
Chronic diseases[b]	Moderately common
Chemotherapy[b]	
Osteopetrosis[b]	
Prenatal stress[a]	Rare
Solitary radiolucent band (no opaque band)	
Severe illness, trauma	
Leukemia, lymphoma[c]	
Metastatic disease[c]	Common
Prematurity[a]	
Trauma: fracture	
Neonatal infections (especially syphilis)[c]	Moderately common
Scurvy[c]	Rare
Hypermagnesemia	
Solitary radiodense band	
Normal, physiologic	Common
Chronic lead intoxication	Moderately common
Other heavy metal or chemical intoxication	
Radiation injury by bone-seeking isotopes	
Idiopathic hypercalcemia	Relatively rare
Hypervitaminosis D	
Hypothyroidism: treated	
Biphosphonate therapy	

[a] Single line usually.
[b] Multiple lines.
[c] Fracture (pathologic) may occur.

also can be seen with more serious problems such as leukemia (Fig. 4.61*F*), lymphoma, metastatic disease, and, in the distant past, scurvy. **In leukemia the transverse radiolucent line is referred to as the "leukemia line," whereas in scurvy it is termed the scurvy zone.** The thin white line just distal to the radiolucent line in scurvy is called the scurvy line. In most of these pathologic states, the bone through the radiolucent zone also is weakened, and pathologic fractures through the area are common (Fig. 4.62). Indeed, grossly disorganized epiphyseal-metaphyseal areas often result (see Fig. 4.73).

Radiodense bands, in the absence of preceding radiolucent lines, also occur in both normal and abnormal patients. Overall, however, the commonest cause of such a line is overexuberant calcification of the zone of provisional calcification in normal children. This commonly is seen in children exposed to extended periods of sunlight, especially after the winter months. Indeed, in some of these cases the line is so dense that chronic lead intoxication is suggested (Fig. 4.63*A*). A similar phenomenon can occur with vitamin D intoxication and hypercalcemia, but certainly both are far less common and, of course, also are pathologic.

Other pathologic radiodense lines occur with chronic lead poisoning (Fig. 4.63*B*) (7), and in some cases the lines are multiple. When they are multiple, they can be associated with a modeling error of the metaphysis leading to splaying or an Erlenmeyer flask deformity (see Fig. 4.70*B*) (10). The deformity and dense bands occur together only with chronic lead intoxication, and although some lead is deposited in the region of the white lines, most of the increase in whiteness is due to excess deposition of calcium in thicker and more numerous trabeculae (10). Similar lines can be seen in bismuth, arsenic, phosphorus, fluoride, mercury, lithium, and radium poisoning. They also have been noted in biophosphonate therapy (13) and hypermagnesemia (3). In most of these cases, the problem is impaired osteoclastic activity with the production of thicker and more numerous bony trabeculae.

REFERENCES

1. Coblentz DR, Cimini R, Mikity VG, Rosen R: Roentgenographic diagnosis of congenital syphilis in the newborn. *JAMA* 212:1061–1064, 1970.
2. Cremin BJ, Fisher RM: The lesions of congenital syphilis. *Br J Radiol* 43:333–341, 1970.
3. Cumming WA, Thomas VJ: Case report—hypermagnesemia: a cause of abnormal metaphyses in the neonate. *AJR* 152:1071–1072, 1989.
4. Follis RH Jr, Park EA: Some observations on bone growth, with particular respect to zones and transverse lines of increased density in the metaphysis. *AJR* 68:709–724, 1952.
5. Garn SM, Silverman FN, Hertzog KP, Robmann CG: Lines and bands of increased density: their implication to growth and development. *Med Radiogr Photogr* 44:58–88, 1968.
6. Hernandez RJ, Poznanski AK, Hopwood NJ, Kelch RP: Incidence of growth lines in psychosocial dwarfs and idiopathic hypopituitarism. *AJR* 131:477–479, 1978.
7. Leone AJ Jr: On lead lines. *AJR* 103:165–167, 1968.
8. Martel W, Holt JF, Cassidy JT: Roentgenologic manifestations of juvenile rheumatoid arthritis. *AJR* 88:400–423, 1962.
9. Park EA: The imprinting of nutritional disturbances on growing bone. *Pediatrics* 33(suppl, Pt 2):815, 1964.

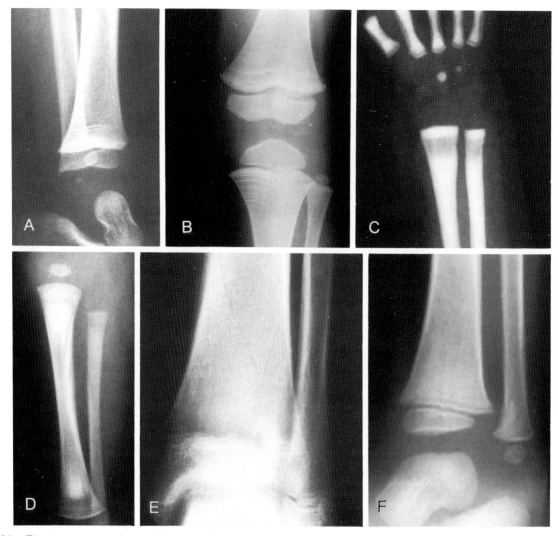

Figure 4.61. Transverse metaphyseal lines. A. Repeated alternating radiolucent and radio-opaque lines in patient with asthma. **B.** Numerous transverse lines in deprivational dwarfism. **C.** Broad radiolucent and dense bands in osteopetrosis. **D.** Broad, nonspecific radiolucent bands in patient with arthrogryposis. **E.** Broad radiolucent metaphyseal band in patient with fracture of tibia. **F.** Transverse radiolucent band in distal tibia in leukemia.

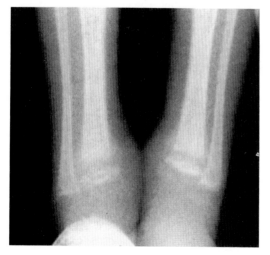

Figure 4.62. Trophic lines with pathologic fracture. Note pathologic fractures through wide trophic lines in this premature infant.

10. Pease CN, Newton GB: Metaphyseal dysplasia due to lead poisoning. *Radiology* 79:233–240, 1962.
11. Rabinowitz JG, Wolf BS, Greenberg EI, Rausen AR: Osseous changes in rubella embryopathy (congenital rubella syndrome). *Radiology* 85:494–499, 1965.
12. Rudolph AJ, Singleton EB, Rosenberg HS, Singer DB, Phillips CA: Osseous manifestations of congenital rubella syndrome. *Am J Dis Child* 110:428–433, 1965.
13. vanPersijn van Meerten EL, Kroon HM, Papapoulos SE: Epi- and metaphyseal changes in children caused by administration of biophosphonates. *Radiology* 184:249–254, 1992.
14. Wolfson JJ, Engel RR: Anticipating meconium peritonitis from metaphyseal bands. *Radiology* 92:1055–1060, 1969.

DENSE VERTICAL METAPHYSEAL LINES

These lines are not particularly common but, on an isolated basis, can be seen after any type of epiphyseal injury. In such cases, the finding probably

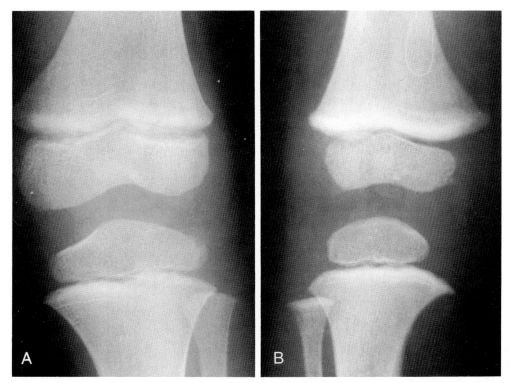

Figure 4.63. Transverse white metaphyseal bands. A. Normal, dense zones of provisional calcification. **B.** Dense white lines in chronic lead intoxication.

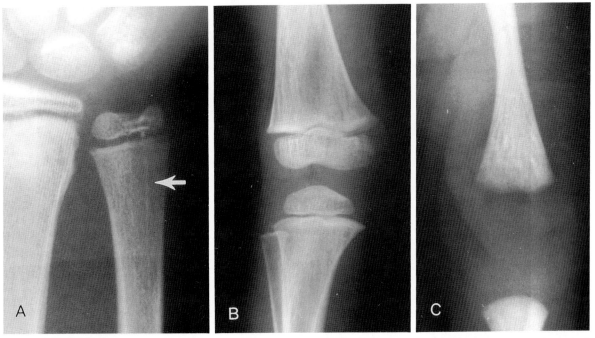

Figure 4.64. Vertical metaphyseal lines. A. Note normal, vertical metaphyseal line *(arrow)* associated with a normal epiphyseal line spicule. **B.** Vertical metaphyseal lines in osteopathia stri-ata. **C.** Vertical, somewhat coarse, metaphyseal lines in congenital rubella. Note also that the bones are dense, a common feature of this infection.

results from a focally induced aberration of metaphyseal growth that causes a streak of thickened trabecular bone to extend into the metaphysis. Occasionally, this also is seen on an entirely normal basis (Fig. 4.64*A*).

When numerous vertical lines are seen in the metaphyses, one should think of the rare condition known as osteopathia striata (Fig. 4.64*B*). Usually an innocuous problem, in some instances it can be associated with hearing difficulties, cranial nerve dysfunction, frontal bossing, a depressed nasal bridge, apparent hypertelorism, and thickening and sclerosis of the skull and facial bones (1). Vertical metaphyseal lines, although less distinct, also are seen in congenital infections such as rubella (Fig. 4.64C). The finding is much less common with cytomegalic inclusion disease and lues. The appearance of the vertical striations in the metaphyses of these latter conditions has led to the term **"celery stalk metaphysis."** A less delicate form of celery stalk metaphysis can be seen with hypophosphatasia and the occasional case of metaphyseal dysostosis.

REFERENCE

1. Paling MR, Hyde I, Dennis NR: Osteopathia striata with sclerosis and thickening of the skull. *Br J Radiol* 54:344–348, 1981.

SPOTTED METAPHYSES

Basically, there is only one condition that produces this finding, and in childhood it is not particularly common. It is termed "osteopathia condensans dissemenata," or osteopoikilosis, and usually is asymptomatic (1–3). The dense areas in the metaphyses are small islands of compact bone, and also can be seen in the epiphyses, the tarsal and carpal bones (Fig. 4.65), and the flat bones of the pelvis. Osteopoikilosis can be seen in association with melorheostosis and pachydermoperiostosis (2, 3) as well.

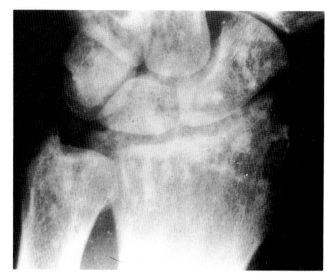

Figure 4.65. Spotted metaphyses. Note dense bone islands in the metaphyses and carpal bones of this young adult with osteopoikilosis.

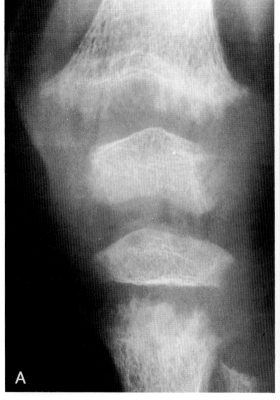

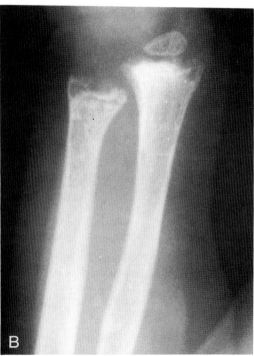

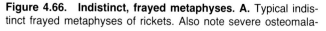

Figure 4.66. Indistinct, frayed metaphyses. A. Typical indistinct frayed metaphyses of rickets. Also note severe osteomalacia and indistinctness of the epiphyseal margins. **B.** Indistinct, somewhat frayed metaphyses in hypophosphatasia.

REFERENCES

1. Archer MC, Fox KW: Osteopoikilosis: report of two new cases. *Radiology* 47:279–283, 1946.
2. Green AE, Ellswood WH, Collins JR: Melorheostosis and osteopoikilosis. *AJR* 87:1096–1111, 1962.
3. Holly LE: Osteopoikilosis: a five year study. *AJR* 36:512–517, 1936.

INDISTINCT-FRAYED METAPHYSES

Indistinctness, with fraying of the metaphysis, is due to poor calcification of the zone of provisional calcification. For the most part, this occurs in conditions producing osteomalacia (see Table 4.2), and certainly the most common of these is rickets (Fig. 4.66A). It also occurs in hypophosphatasia (Fig. 4.66B), in a few cases of metaphyseal dysostosis, in severe hyperparathyroidism, and in oxalosis (1).

REFERENCE

1. Schnitzler CM, Kok JA, Jacobs DWC, Thomson PD, Milne FJ, Mesquita JM, King PC, Fabian VA: Skeletal manifestations of primary oxalosis. *Pediatr Nephrol* 5:193–199, 1991.

CRINKLED, DENSE METAPHYSEAL EDGE

Normally, the edge of the metaphysis is smooth and demarcated by a variably sclerotic line, the zone of provisional calcification. In some instances, however, metaphyseal growth is so disturbed that the edge of the metaphysis becomes very irregular or crinkled, and unusually dense. Most commonly, this occurs with healing epiphyseal-metaphyseal fractures, either overt or subclinical (2) (Fig. 4.67A), but in more florid form occurs in conditions such as metaphyseal dysostosis (1) (Fig. 4.67B), hypophosphatasia, pseudoachondroplasia (spondylo-epiphyseal and multiple types), and healing congenital infections (Fig. 4.67C and D).

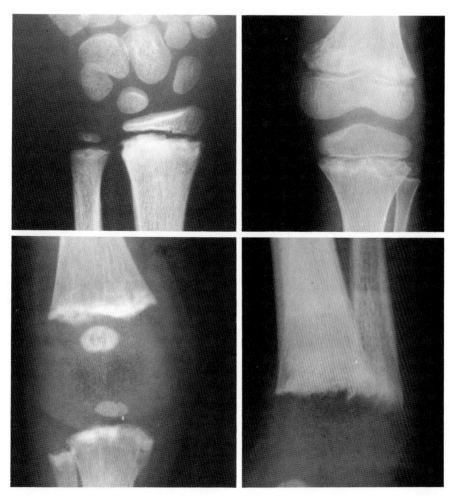

Figure 4.67. **Crinkled dense metaphyses. A.** Typical, irregular and sclerotic (crinkled) metaphysis in healing epiphyseal-metaphyseal fracture. **B.** Crinkled metaphyses in metaphyseal dysostosis. **C.** Crinkled, dense metaphyses in rubella infection of infancy. **D.** Crinkled, irregular metaphyses in congenital syphilis.

REFERENCES

1. Kleinman PK: Case report: Schmid-like metaphyseal chondrodysplasia simulating child abuse. *AJR* 156:576–578, 1991.
2. Roy S, Caine D, Singer KM: Stress changes of the distal radial epiphysis in young gymnasts: a report of twenty-one cases and a review of the literature. *Am J Sports Med* 13:301–308, 1985.

METAPHYSEAL BEAKS (TABLE 4.24)

Metaphyseal beaks may be solid or fragmented, and most commonly occur as corner fractures in epiphyseal injuries, where they become more pronounced as healing occurs (Fig. 4.68A and B). Such beaking usually is focal and asymmetric, but when it occurs in the battered child syndrome, may be more widespread and even reasonably symmetric. Similar beaking resulting from trauma also is seen in the neonate delivered by breech presentation and with pathologic fractures occurring in neurologic disease with bone atrophy, scurvy (beaks are termed Pelkan spurs [see Fig. 4.56B]), hyperparathyroidism, rickets, metabolic bone disease in premature infants, hypophosphatasia (4), Menkes syndrome, leukemia, lymphoma, metastatic disease, osteomyelitis, and congenital syphilis, CMV, and rubella.

The next most common cause of metaphyseal beaking is that which occurs as a normal variation

(3) along the upper medial tibia and distal femur (Fig. 4.68C). In other cases, tibial torsion, leading to so-called "physiologic" bowing of the legs, can lead to more pronounced, but similar beaking of the tibia and femur. There is a distinct tendency for this phe-

Metaphyseal Beaking

Normal (knees) in bowed legs
  Other causes of bowed legs[a]
Epiphyseal metaphyseal fractures in
  normal bones and battered child
  syndrome
Blount disease
	Common

Epiphyseal metaphyseal fractures in
  Breech delivery
  Rickets
  Hyperparathyroidism
  Neurologic disease
  Leukemia, lymphoma
  Metastatic disease
  Osteomyelitis
  Congenital infections
  Metabolic bone disease (premature)
	Moderately common

Menkes kinky hair syndrome Scurvy (Pelkan spurs) Hypophosphatasia Desbuquois syndrome	Rare

[a]See Table 4.7.

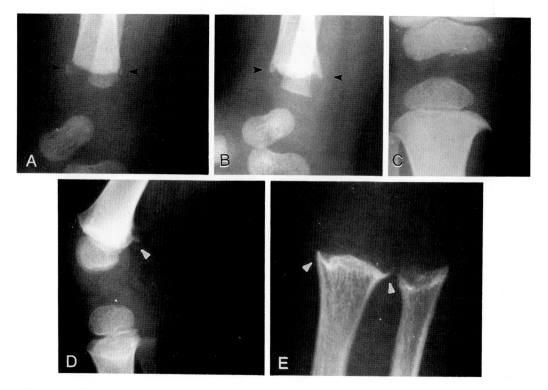

Figure 4.68. Metaphyseal beaking. A. Typical corner fractures with epiphyseal-metaphyseal injury *(arrow).* **B.** Later on with healing, metaphyseal beaks are seen *(arrow).* **C.** Normal upper tibial metaphyseal beaking. **D.** Oblique view showing normal but rather worrisome distal femoral beaking *(arrow).* **E.** Beaking, associated with cupping in spondyloepiphyseal dysplasia *(arrow).*

nomenon to occur in sturdy infants, with more muscle bulk and early ambulation. In more advanced cases, the beaking of the distal femur can be especially worrisome on oblique views (Fig. 4.68D). Going one step further, when the tibial beak is large and fragmented, the condition then is known as Blount disease (see Fig. 4.17B) (1, 2). Unlike physiologic bowing and beaking of the young infant, Blount disease is a true pathologic state requiring treatment, but the entire complex just discussed represents a spectrum of change. Beaking around the knees also occurs with other causes of bowed legs, i.e. rickets, various chondrodystrophies, and metaphyseal dysplasias. With the latter other bones also show beaking (Fig. 4.62E).

REFERENCES

1. Bateson EM: The relationship between Blount's disease and bowlegs. *Br J Radiol* 41:107, 1968.
2. Golding JSR, Bateson EM, McNeil-Smith JDG: Infantile tibia vara (Blount's disease or osteochondrosis deformans tibiae). In: Rang M, ed. *The Growth Plate and Its Disorders*. Baltimore: Williams & Wilkins, 1969:109–119.
3. Kleinman PK, Belanger PL, Karellas A, Spevak MR: Pictorial essay: normal metaphyseal radiologic variants not to be confused with findings of infant abuse. *AJR* 156:781–783, 1991.
4. Oestreich AE, Bofinger MK: Prominent transverse (Bowdler) bone spurs as a diagnostic clue in a case of neonatal hypophosphatasia without metaphyseal irregularity. *Pediatr Radiol* 19:341–342, 1989.

METAPHYSEAL FLARING, WIDENING, AND CUPPING (TABLE 4.25)

Very often, both flaring and cupping are seen together and, indeed, it is difficult to have cupping without flaring, but not the opposite. These changes occur as (a) inherent bone growth disturbances with some bony dysplasias or syndromes and (b) acquired growth disturbances associated with epiphyseal-metaphyseal injury or metabolic bone disease leading to impaired epiphyseal-metaphyseal growth transfer with resultant tubulation abnormality. With injury, the changes often are asymmetric and localized to one joint, whereas with the other conditions they usually are generalized. In all instances, the problem is failure of proper long bone tubulation, causing failure of the metaphyses to decrease in diameter as they become incorporated into the diaphyses.

Inherent flaring and cupping of the metaphyses occurs in a large number of chondrodystrophies and bone dysplasias—i.e., achondroplasia (Fig. 4.69A), hypochondroplasia, pseudoachondroplasia (Fig. 4.63B), thanatophoric dwarfism, metatropic dwarfism, Kniest syndrome, Ellis-van Creveld syndrome, meso-

Table 4.25
Metaphyseal Flaring, Widening, and Cupping

Metaphyseal flaring and cupping[a]	
Rickets	} Common
Epiphyseal-metaphyseal injury Achondroplasia Metaphyseal dysostosis	} Moderately common
Hypochondroplasia Pseudoachondroplasia Thanatophoric dwarfism Hypophosphatasia Immunologic diseases Bone infarction	} Relatively rare
Metatropic dwarfism Kniest syndrome Ellis-van Creveld syndrome Mesomelic dwarfism Short rib-polydactyly syndromes Diastrophic dwarfism Stippled epiphyses congenita Hypophosphatasia Spondylometaphyseal dysplasia Taybi-Lindner syndrome Osteodysplasia: Melnick-Needles Hypervitaminosis A Scurvy Phenylketonuria Weissenbacher-Zweymuller syndrome Achondrogenesis Trichorhinophalangeal syndrome	} Rare
Metaphyseal widening without cupping[b]	
Chronic anemias: sickle cell, Cooley	} Common
Pyle disease Oto-palato-digital syndrome Other craniometaphyseal dysostoses Gaucher disease	} Relatively rare
Chronic lead intoxication Mastocytosis Weaver syndrome	} Rare

[a] Also affects anterior rib ends.

melic dwarfism, the short rib-polydactyly syndromes, diastrophic dwarfism, punctate epiphyseal dysplasia congenita, the various metaphyseal dysostoses (Fig. 4.63C) (5), hypophosphatasia (Fig. 4.63E), spondylometaphyseal dysplasia (Kozlowski type), the Taybi-Lindner syndrome, osteodysplasia or the Melnick-Needles syndrome, Weissenbacher-Zweymuller syndrome, phenylketonuria and a variety of immune deficiency syndromes such as the metaphyseal

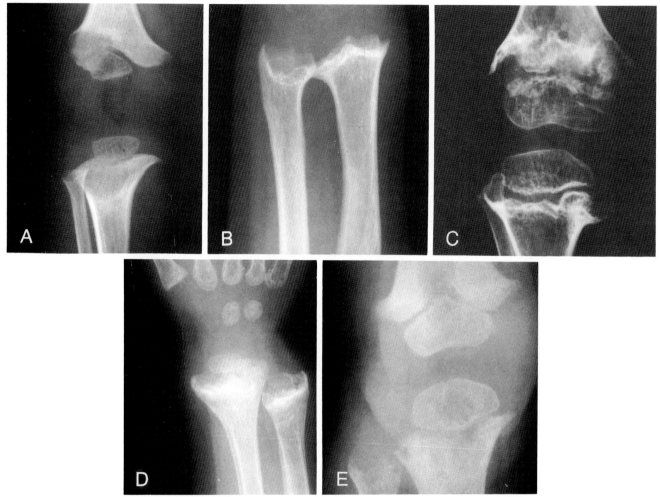

Figure 4.69. Metaphyseal splaying and cupping. A. Metaphyseal splaying and cupping in achondroplasia with ball and socket epiphysis. **B.** Rather marked cupping in pseudoachondroplasia. Note well-defined zone of provisional calcification, but delayed epiphyseal development. **C.** Marked cupping in metaphyseal dysostosis. Also note severe irregularity of the epiphyseal-metaphyseal junction (dense, crinkled metaphyseal edge).

D. Marked cupping in healing rickets. Cupping in rickets often is more pronounced during the healing phase. Also note periosteal new bone formation. **E.** Hypophosphatasia. Note cupping of the fibula *(arrow)*. Cupping was less marked in the other bones. Note, however, a deep ball-and-socket epiphyseal-metaphyseal junction in the femur.

dysostosis-thymolymphopenia syndrome, the Schwachman-Diamond syndrome, and McKusick metaphyseal dysostosis associated with neutropenia and pancreatic insufficiency (1, 4, 6, 9, 12, 14, 15).

The best known cause of acquired metaphyseal flaring and cupping is rickets, and when combined with indistinctness of the epiphyseal-metaphyseal junction (i.e., loss of zone of provisional calcification), is quite characteristic. Often cupping is more readily detectable when healing ensues (Fig. 4.69D). Acquired flaring and cupping also can be seen after epiphyseal-metaphyseal injury due to trauma (3), infection, radiation therapy, bone infarction (2), hypervitaminosis A, and scurvy (usually after pathologic fracturing). In many of these conditions, cupping is very deep so that the epiphysis becomes buried in

the metaphysis and a **ball and socket metaphysis** results (Fig. 4.69E). Actually, the deformity also can be described as a cone-shaped epiphysis. This phenomenon probably is more common with acquired cupping, but also can be seen in some chondrodystrophies and hypophosphatasia.

METAPHYSEAL WIDENING WITHOUT CUPPING (TABLE 4.25)

Metaphyseal widening without cupping occurs most commonly with bone marrow hypercellularity problems and the storage diseases. As far as bone marrow hypercellularity is concerned, the problem arises almost exclusively in Cooley anemia and mas-

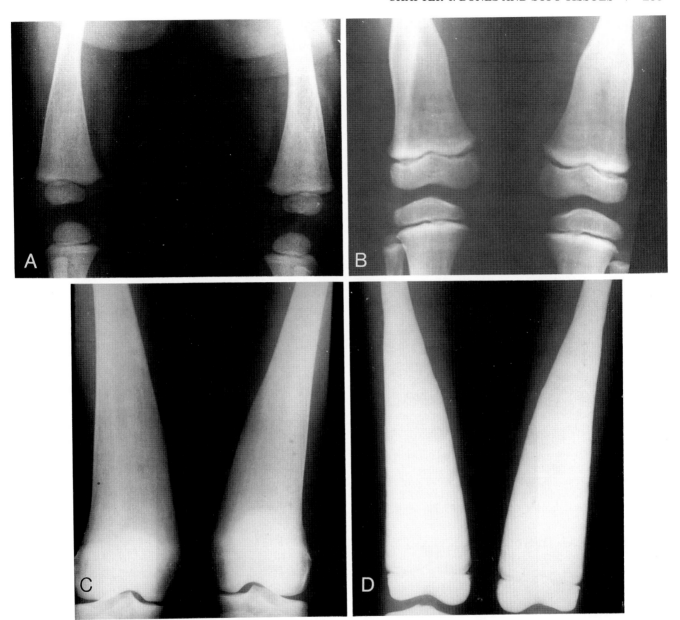

Figure 4.70. Metaphyseal widening without cupping. A. Minimal widening of the metaphyses of the femurs in a young child with sickle cell disease. **B.** Marked widening in chronic lead intoxication. Note faint radio-opaque transverse lines. **C.** Marked metaphyseal widening in older patient with Gaucher disease. **D.** Pronounced widening of the metaphyses and extreme increase in bone density in osteopetrosis.

tocytosis. Occasionally, it can be seen in sickle cell disease (Fig. 4.70A), and with the storage diseases the most common offender is Gaucher disease (Fig. 4.70C) (8, 10). Occasionally, however, similar widening can be seen with Niemann-Pick disease and, very rarely, with histiocytosis-X.

Metaphyseal widening also occurs in chronic lead intoxication (11) and, here, lead lines provide a clue to its etiology (Fig. 4.70B). Similar widening of the metaphysis, but without the lead lines, is seen in Pyle craniometaphyseal dysostosis, the otopalatodigital syndrome (7), and other craniometaphyseal dysplasias. Metaphyseal widening also is seen in osteopetrosis (Fig. 4.70D) and the Weaver syndrome (12). In most of these conditions, when widening is pronounced, the term **"Erlenmeyer flask deformity"** often is used.

REFERENCES

1. Alexander WJ, Dunbar JS: Unusual bone changes in thymic alymphoplasia. *Ann Radiol* 11:389–394, 1968.
2. Bohrer SP: Growth disturbances of the distal femur following sickle cell bone infarcts and/or osteomyelitis. *Clin Radiol* 25:221–235, 1974.

3. Caffey J: Traumatic cupping of the metaphyses of growing bones. *AJR* 108:451–460, 1970.
4. Cederbaum SD, Kaitila I, Rimoin DL, Steihm ER: The chondro-osseous dysplasia of adenosine deaminase deficiency with severe combined immunodeficiency. *J Pediatr* 89:737–742, 1976.
5. Daeschner CW, Singleton EB, Hill LL, Dodge WF: Metaphyseal dysostosis. *J Pediatr* 57:844–854, 1960.
6. Felman K, Kozlowski K, Senger A: Unusual bone changes in exocrine pancreas insufficiency with cyclic neutropenia. *Acta Radiol* 12:428–432, 1972.
7. Gendall PW, Kozlowski K: Otopalatodigital syndrome Type II: report of two related cases. *Pediatr Radiol* 22:267–269, 1992.
8. Meyers H, Cremin B, Beighton P, Sacks S: Chronic Gaucher's disease: radiological finding in 17 South African cases. *Br J Radiol* 48:465–469, 1975.
9. McLennan TW, Steinbach HL: Schwachman's syndrome: the broad spectrum of bony abnormalities. *Radiology* 112:167–173, 1974.
10. Pastakia B, Brower AC, Chang VH, Barranger JA: Skeletal manifestations of Gaucher's disease. *Semin Roentgenol* 21:264–274, 1986.
11. Pease CN, Newton GG: Metaphyseal dysplasia due to lead poisoning in children. *Radiology* 79:233–240, 1962.
12. Ramos-Arroyo MA, Weaver DD, Banks ER: Weaver syndrome: a case without early overgrowth and review of the literature. *Pediatrics* 88:1106–1111, 1991.
13. Say B, Tinaztepe B, Tinaztepe K, Kiran O: Thymic dysplasia associated with dyschondroplasia in an infant. *Am J Dis Child* 123:240–244, 1972.
14. Schwachman H, Diamond LK, Oski FA, Kwaw K: The syndrome of pancreatic insufficiency and bone marrow dysfunction. *J Pediatr* 65:645–663, 1964.
15. Taybi H, Mitchell AD, Friedman GD: Metaphyseal dysostosis and the associated syndrome of pancreatic insufficiency and blood disorders. *Radiology* 93:563–571, 1969.

METAPHYSEAL DESTRUCTION (TABLE 4.26)

Although bone destruction is the same wherever it occurs, many times with generalized diseases, bone destruction localized to the metaphyses provides the first clue to the diagnosis. For this reason, it is of some merit to consider metaphyseal destruction alone, and in this regard the patterns of destruction encountered include (a) mottled destruction, (b) homogeneous destruction, and (c) focal, cyst-like or scalloped destruction.

MOTTLED DESTRUCTION

Mottled, irregular, or permeative destruction usually belies a serious problem and, indeed, underlying malignancy usually is the cause. Associated permeative destruction of the cortex commonly occurs and, overall, one's first diagnostic considerations should be leukemia, lymphoma, or metastatic disease (Fig. 4.71A). In the early stages, the findings may be difficult to differentiate from simple coarse trabecular

Table 4.26
Metaphyseal Destruction

Mottled destruction	
Leukemia, lymphoma	
Metastatic disease	Common
Osteomyelitis	
Primary malignant bone tumors	Moderately common
Homogeneous destruction: no mottling	
Osteomyelitis	
Congenital syphilis[a]	Common
Bone infarction: sickle cell	
Histiocytosis-X	
Leukemia, lymphoma	Moderately common
Metastatic disease	
Primary malignant bone tumors	
Scurvy[a]	Relatively rare
Intantile fibromatosis	
Focal cyst-like destruction	
Osteomyelitis	
Histiocytosis-X	Common
Benign cortical defect: en face	
Small bone cysts	
Leukemia[a]	
Lymphoma	Moderately common
Metastatic disease	
Primary benign bone tumor	Relatively rare

[a]Often through trophic lines.

demineralization, but with advancing disease, the destructive pattern becomes more obvious. Mottled destruction tends not to occur with infection or infarction but, of course, commonly occurs with primary malignant bone tumors such as fibrosarcoma, osteosarcoma, chondrosarcoma, and Ewing tumor.

Metaphyseal destruction that is more homogeneous can occur with all the conditions producing mottled destruction (Fig. 4.71C), but also is common with osteomyelitis (Fig. 4.71B). It can also be seen with bone infarction (usually in sickle cell disease), histiocytosis-X, scurvy (Fig. 4.71F), or bone necrosis secondary to trophic (ischemic) bone disturbances associated with intrauterine infections, but primarily with syphilis (2, 3). In most cases of syphilis and scurvy, destruction occurs across the entire metaphysis (Fig. 4.71E and F), but in other cases of syphilis large scooped out metaphyseal areas are seen. These most commonly occur in the upper, medial tibia, where they are known as Wimberger sign (Fig. 4.71D). Similar lesions also can be seen in infants with osteomyelitis, bone infarction (usually sickle

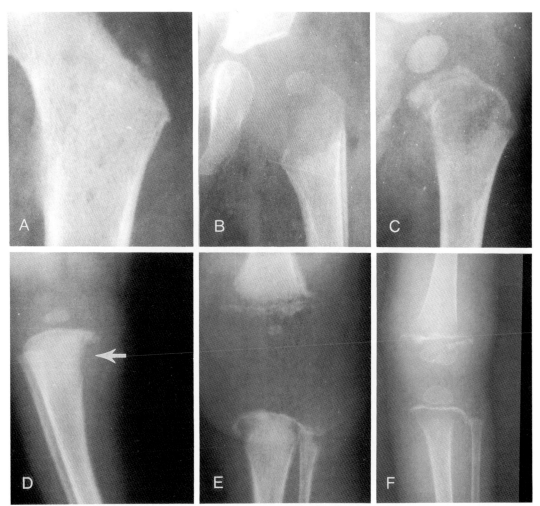

Figure 4.71. Metaphyseal destruction. A. Typical, mottled destruction characteristic of malignancy. This patient had metastatic neuroblastoma. **B.** Diffuse, homogeneous destruction of upper femur, more characteristic of infection, infarction, etc. This patient had atypical tuberculosis of the bone and hip joint. Note periosteal new bone deposition. **C.** Homogeneous destruction, with pathologic fracture through upper femur *(arrow)* in patient with leukemia. **D.** Metaphyseal destruction (Wimberger sign) in syphilis. **E.** Metaphyseal destruction through trophic lines of syphilis. **F.** Similar changes in patient with scurvy. For additional metaphyseal destruction producing metaphyseal notching see Figure 4.37.

cell disease), lymphoma, leukemia, metastatic disease, and in the condition known as infantile fibromatosis (1, 4–6). Indeed, the lesions in this condition often are virtually indistinguishable from those of congenital syphilis. The cause of the condition is unknown, but both bony and systemic varieties exist. If only bone involvement occurs, the prognosis is good, but if widespread visceral involvement is present, the prognosis is poor. In all of these cases, pathologic fractures through the destroyed metaphysis commonly occur.

The commonest cause of **focal, cyst-like destruction** within a metaphysis is osteomyelitis (Fig. 4.72*A*). Many times, a variably sclerotic margin of osteoblastic reaction is seen around the area of destruction (Fig. 4.72*B*). The degree of sclerosis depends on the chronicity of the lesion, and the lesion itself is referred to as a Brodie abscess. Focal, cyst-like destructive lesions without any significant sclerosis are characteristic of histiocytosis-X, and occasionally a small, benign bone tumor such as a hemangioma, fibroma, chondroma, or chondromyxoid fibroma can be encountered.

Small bone cysts usually pose no problem in diagnosis because their thin, well-defined margin and markedly radiolucent interior are characteristic. However, the benign cortical defect, when seen en face, can mimic a focal, cystic, intramedullary lytic lesion and cause problems in diagnosis. It is only when the eccentric nature of this lesion is appreciated that its true identity is established (Fig. 4.72*C* and *D*).

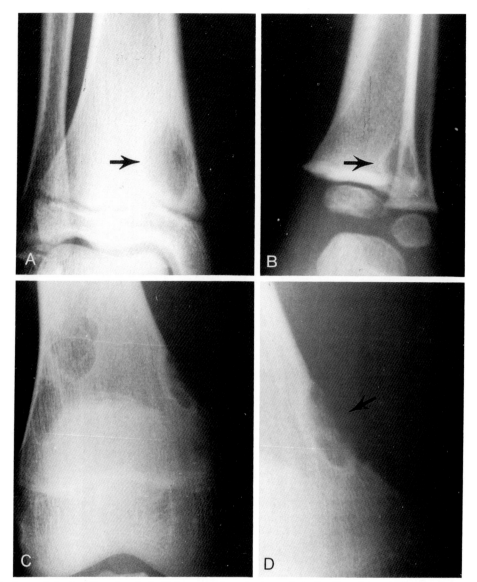

Figure 4.72. Metaphyseal destruction-focal. A. Note area of homogeneous destruction *(arrow)* in distal tibia. There is no marginal sclerosis. This patient had osteomyelitis. **B.** Another patient with osteomyelitis showing slight sclerosis around an area of me-taphyseal destruction *(arrow)*. A cyst-like appearance is mimicked, but note that the lesion extends into the epiphyseal plate. **C.** Typical benign cortical defects in distal femur. **D.** The eccentric cortical location of one of them *(arrow)* is diagnostic.

REFERENCES

1. Baer JW, Radkowski MA: Congenital multiple fibromatosis: a case report with review of the world literature. *AJR* 118:200–205, 1973.
2. Coblentz DR, Cimini R, Mikity VG, Rosen R: Roentgenographic diagnosis of congenital syphilis in the newborn. *JAMA* 212:1061–1064, 1970.
3. Cremin BJ, Fisher RM: The lesions of congenital syphilis. *Br J Radiol* 43:333–341, 1970.
4. Familusi JB, Nottidge VA, Anita AU, Attah EB: Congenital generalized fibromatosis. *Am J Dis Child* 130:1215–1217, 1976.
5. Morettin LB, Mueller E, Schreiber M: Generalized hamartosis (congenital generalized fibromatosis). *AJR* 114:722–734, 1972.
6. Plaschkes J: Congenital fibromatosis: localized and generalized forms. *J Pediatr Surg* 9:95–101, 1074.

GROSSLY DISORGANIZED EPIPHYSEAL-METAPHYSEAL AREAS (TABLE 4.27)

When one encounters grossly disorganized epiphyseal-metaphyseal areas, almost always an epiphyseal-metaphyseal fracture is present. In such cases, excessive motion and bleeding at the fracture site lead to fragmentation, hypercallosis, and marked periosteal new bone deposition. The phenomenon is common in the battered child syndrome and

Table 4.27
Grossly Disorganized Epiphyseal Metaphyseal Junctions

Battered child syndrome Fractures in neurologic or neuromus- cular disease	} Common

Fractures in weakened bone
  Osteomyelitis
  Infarction
  Neonatal infections
  Metastatic disease
  Rickets
  Hyperparathyroidism
	} Moderately common

Congenital insensitivity to pain
Other sensory neuropathies
  Diabetes mellitus
  Syringomyelia
  Lues
  Amyotrophic lateral sclerosis
	} Rare

in patients with underlying neurologic or neuromuscular disease (3, 4), because, in either case, excessive postinjury motion is common (Fig. 4.73A–C). In neurogenic patients, even with passive flexion and extension, such fractures are commonly induced. Other grossly disorganized epiphyseal-metaphyseal fractures are associated with sensory neuropathies such as occurs in chronic diabetes mellitus, syringomyelia, peripheral nerve injury (Fig. 4.73D), tertiary syphilis, amyotrophic lateral sclerosis, and congenital insensitivity to pain (1, 2, 5). All of these conditions are relatively rare in children.

Gross disorganization of the epiphyseal-metaphyseal regions secondary to fractures also occurs in pathologically diseased bones weakened by severe bone infection (especially osteomyelitis in neonates and infants), bone infarction (usually sickle cell disease in infancy), neonatal infections with trophic

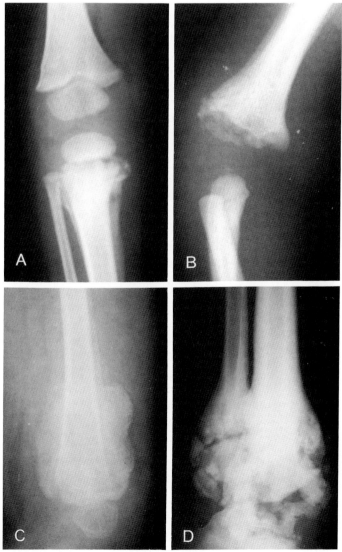

Figure 4.73. Grossly disorganized epiphyseal-metaphyseal areas. A. Moderately disorganized upper tibial epiphyseal-metaphyseal area secondary to healing fracture in battered child syndrome. **B.** Extensive disorganization of the distal humerus in an infant with fractures in the battered child syndrome. **C.** Hypercallosis in neurogenic fracture. Note atrophy of muscle and abundance of fat. Also note that the bones are osteoporotic and thin. **D.** Severe disorganization-Charcot joint secondary to peripheral nerve injury.

disturbances (i.e., syphilis, rubella, CMV), widespread metastatic disease, scurvy, rickets, and hyperparathyroidism (see Fig. 4.71*E* and *F*).

REFERENCES

1. Dehen H, Willer JC, Boureau F, Cambier J: Congenital insensitivity to pain, and endogenous morphine-like substances. *Lancet* 2:293–294, 1977.
2. Drummond RP, Rose GK: A twenty-one-year review of a case of congenital indifference to pain. *J Bone Joint Surg* 57B:241–243, 1975.
3. Gyepes MT, Newbern DH, Neuhauser EBD: Metaphyseal and physeal injuries in children with spina bifida and meningo-myeloceles. *AJR* 95:168–177, 1965.
4. Siegelman SS, Heimann WG, Manin MC: Congenital indifference to pain. *AJR* 97:242, 1966.
5. Silverman FN, Gilden JJ: Congenital insensitivity to pain: a neurologic syndrome with bizarre skeletal lesions. *Radiology* 72:176, 1959.
6. Vardy PA, Greenberg LW, Kachel C, Falewski de Leon G: Congenital insensitivity to pain with anhidrosis. *Am J Dis Child* 133:1153, 1979.

Epiphyseal Line Abnormalities

WIDENED EPIPHYSEAL LINE (TABLE 4.28)

Abnormal widening of the epiphyseal line (physis) generally is due to (a) traumatic separation of the epiphysis from the metaphysis or (b) impaired enchondral bone formation at the epiphyseal-metaphyseal junction. With the latter, the findings tend to be generalized, whereas with the former they are localized. As far as defective enchondral bone formation is concerned, the commonest cause is some form of rickets (Fig. 4.74*A*), including renal osteo-

Table 4.28
Widened Epiphyseal Line

Epiphyseal metaphyseal fractures: normal bones	Commonest
Epiphyseal metaphyseal fractures: pathologic bones Rickets: any type Hyperparathyroidism: secondary in renal osteodystrophy	Moderately common
Hyperparathyroidism: primary Metaphyseal dysostosis	Relatively rare
Hypophosphatasia Jansen metaphyseal dysostosis[a] Gangliosidosis[a] Mucolipidosis II[a]	Rare

[a] Mimics hyperparathyroidism in infancy.

dystrophy. In addition to widening of the epiphyseal line in such cases, the edges of the metaphyses and epiphyses also are indistinct. Similar findings occur with hyperparathyroidism, hypophosphatasia, and conditions mimicking hyperparathyroidism in infancy (i.e., Jansen metaphyseal dysostosis, gangliosidosis, and mucolipidosis II). In the more chronic forms of hypophosphatasia and in the other metaphyseal dysostoses, although the epiphyseal line may be widened, the edges of the epiphysis and metaphysis are less fuzzy or frayed. Indeed, in metaphyseal dysostosis, the edges may be white and undulating or crinkled (see Fig. 4.67*B*).

Separation of the epiphysis from the metaphysis, secondary to trauma, most commonly occurs in normal bones (Fig. 4.74*B*), but it also occurs in structurally weakened bones with metaphyseal bone dissolution (e.g., scurvy, rickets, leukemia, lymphoma, metastatic disease, hyperparathyroidism). In any of these conditions, shearing forces applied across the weakened epiphyseal-metaphyseal junction are the cause of the separations. In such cases, when the epiphysis is markedly displaced, or when there are associated corner fractures of the metaphysis, the fact that an epiphyseal fracture has occurred is not difficult to detect. However, when these associated findings are not present, widening of the epiphyseal line may be the only clue to the presence of the fracture (Fig. 4.74*B*). Indeed, this is a common situation in the pediatric age group, and it is under such circumstances that examination of the normal side for comparison is extremely important.

Chronic, posttraumatic widening of the epiphyseal line most commonly is seen as one of the earliest findings in idiopathic slipped capital femoral epiphysis of adolescence. This condition, of unknown etiology but common in overweight adolescents (slightly more so in boys), begins with insidious onset of pain, which then lasts for weeks or months. Often the first roentgenographic findings consist of little more than increased radiolucency and slight widening of the epiphyseal line (Fig. 4.74*C*).

Finally, before leaving the topic of the widened epiphyseal line, it should be noted that in many perfectly normal children the line may appear unduly wide to the uninitiated examiner. This is especially prone to occur in the wrist, and many times only comparative views finally convince one that the finding is normal.

EPIPHYSEAL LINE SPICULES

Most commonly, epiphyseal line spicules are seen in perfectly normal children (Fig. 4.75). They probably represent lingering fingers of calcified cartilage

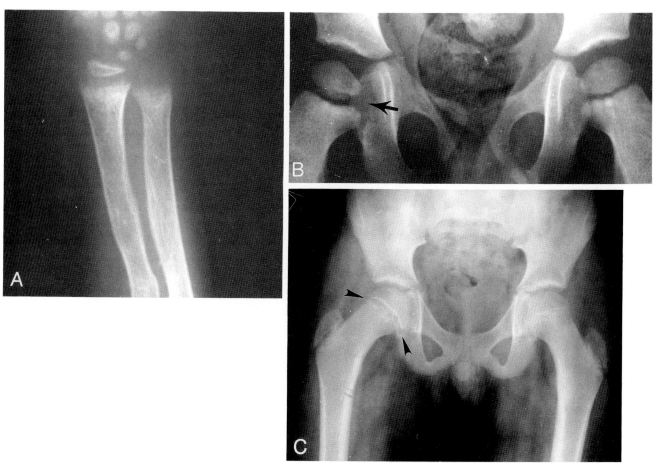

Figure 4.74. Widened epiphyseal line. A. Widening of the epiphyseal line in rickets. Also note fraying of the metaphysis. **B.** Widened epiphyseal line *(arrow)* secondary to epiphyseal-metaphyseal fracture. Compare with the normal left side. **C.** Widening of the epiphyseal line *on the right (arrow)* secondary to slipped capital femoral epiphysis.

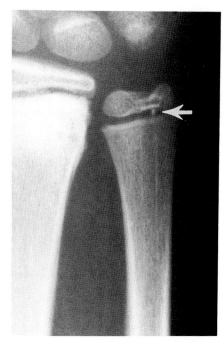

Figure 4.75. Epiphyseal line spicules. Note spicule *(arrow)* in the epiphyseal line of the ulna. This patient was normal.

that have no particular clinical significance. However, they also have been described with phenylketonuria, homocystinuria, and other aminoacidurias (1–5). In addition, they also can be seen in some cases of healing rickets. In all cases, these spicules, as growth progresses, can be incorporated into the metaphysis as short, vertical dense lines (see Fig. 4.65A). In phenylketonuria, it has been demonstrated that these spicules do not occur in adequately treated children (6).

REFERENCES

1. Feinberg SB, Fisch RO: Roentgenologic findings in growing long bones in phenylketonuria. *Radiology* 78:394–397, 1962.
2. Feinberg SB, Fisch RO: Bone changes in untreated neonatal phenylketonuric patients, a new roentgenographic observation and interpretation. *J Pediatr* 81:540–543, 1972.
3. Fisch RO, Craven HJ, Feinberg SB: Growth and bone characteristics of phenylketonurics: comparative analysis of treated and untreated phenylketonuric children. *Am J Dis Child* 112:3–10, 1966.

4. Holt JF, Allen RJ: Radiologic signs in the primary amino-acidurias. *Ann Radiol* 10:317–321, 1967.
5. Morreels CL: The roentgenographic features of homocystinuria. *Radiology* 90:1150–1153, 1968.
6. Woodring JH, Rosenbaum HD: Bone changes in phenylketonuria reassessed. *AJR* 137:241–243, 1981.

The Hands and Feet

There are so many findings, both normal and abnormal, in the hands and feet that one can be overwhelmed with details. By the same token, not all are of equal importance, and thus this section deals with those findings utilized most often in sorting out the various diseases, syndromes, and dysplasias. Generally, changes in the hands are more important than those in the feet, and foot changes are alluded to only if they are diagnostically specific. If they are similar to those in the hands, no specific mention is made.

TERMINAL PHALANGES

Before analyzing terminal phalangeal changes, it should be noted that there is considerable difference in appearance of these bones from one normal person to another. Some terminal phalanges are tapered, while others are more clubbed, and differentiation between normal and abnormal may be difficult. However, a few of the changes are specific enough to allow them to be utilized in the differential diagnosis of certain conditions.

Clubbing of Terminal Phalanges

Clubbing of the digits is a soft tissue phenomenon and usually is more readily detectable clinically than roentgenographically. However, in some cases there is enough widening of the terminal tufts of the distal phalanges to allow roentgenographic identification. Clinical clubbing occurs with chronic cyanotic congenital heart disease, chronic gastrointestinal disease, chronic respiratory disease, intrathoracic tumors such as mesothelioma, and in the condition known as pachydermoperiostitis. The latter condition is familial and is associated with idiopathic periosteal new bone deposition and calvarial defects. Clubbing also occurs in acromegaly, but in childhood, gigantism is the counterpart of the problem, and clubbing is not a significant feature.

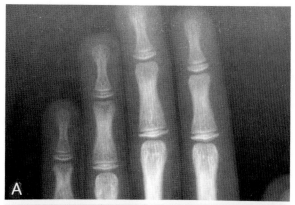

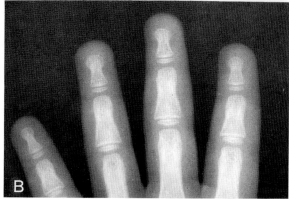

Figure 4.76. Drumstick terminal phalanges. A. Typical drumstick-shaped terminal phalanges in Turner syndrome. **B.** Another patient with suspected Turner syndrome and squat, drumstick terminal phalanges.

Drumstick Terminal Phalanges

Drumstick terminal phalanges result any time the shaft of the phalanx is disproportionately thinned in comparison to the tuft (Fig. 4.76). Clearly, the problem can be in the tuft or the shaft and, furthermore, to complicate the problem, some degree of drumsticking is present in normal individuals. However, true drumstick terminal phalanges have been identified in Turner syndrome, trisomy-21, the cri-du-chat syndrome, Coffin syndrome, and the cardiomelic or Holt-Oram syndrome (1–5). One must hasten to add, however, that not every case of these syndromes demonstrates drumstick terminal phalanges.

REFERENCES

1. Coffin GS, Siris E, Wegienka LC: Mental retardation with osteocartilaginous anomalies. *Am J Dis Child* 112:205, 1066.
2. Kosowicz J: The roentgen appearance of the hand and wrist in gonadal dysgenesis. *AJR* 93:354–361, 1965.
3. Necic S, Grant DB: Diagnostic value of hand x-rays in Turner's syndrome. *Acta Paediatr Scand* 67:309–313, 1978.

4. Poznanski AK: *The Hand in Radiologic Diagnosis.* Philadelphia: WB Saunders, 1974:228.
5. Procopis PG, Turner B: Mental retardation, abnormal fingers and skeletal anomalies: Coffin's syndrome. *Am J Dis Child* 214:258–261, 1972.

Hypoplastic Terminal Phalanges

Hypoplastic terminal phalanges should be differentiated from destroyed or eroded terminal phalanges. The latter are dealt with in the next section, and in this section only those terminal phalanges that are inherently underdeveloped, or hypoplastic, are considered. Such phalanges may appear spindle-shaped or frankly truncated, but, again, variation is common. Truncated phalanges are common in the normal foot (Fig. 4.77), but in the hand, when a hypoplastic terminal phalanx is encountered, some pathologic condition should be considered. For the most part, these include any number of conditions associated with hypoplastic fingernails: trisomy 18, trisomy 13, Aarskog syndrome, cleidocranial dysostosis (Fig. 4.78A and B), asphyxiating thoracic dystrophy, Dilantin embryonopathy (2, 7) (Fig. 4.78C and D), fetal alcohol syndrome, Ellis-van Creveld syndrome, otopalatodigital syndrome, scalp defect and hand anomaly syndrome (1), pseudo- and pseudopseudohypoparathyroidism, Marshall-Smith syndrome (3), Larsen syndrome, Coffin-Siris syndrome (1, 6), Turner syndrome (2–5), and all of the conditions producing a spade hand (see Fig. 4.86). In some cases of terminal phalangeal underdevelopment, the epiphysis is overgrown and equals the size of the hypoplastic phalanx. In such cases, hyperphalangism erroneously is suggested (7) (Fig. 4.78D).

REFERENCES

1. Barr M Jr, Poznanski AK, Schmickel RD: Digital hypoplasia and anticonvulsants during gestation: a teratogenic syndrome? *J Pediatr* 84:254–256, 1974.
2. Coffin GS, Siris E, Wegienka LC: Mental retardation with osteocartilaginous anomalies. *Am J Dis Child* 112:205, 1966.
3. Eich GF, Silver MM, Weksberg R, Daneman A, Costa T: Marshall-Smith syndrome: new radiographic, clinical, and pathologic observations. *Radiology* 181:183–188, 1991.
4. Kosowicz J: The roentgen appearance of the hand and wrist in gonadal dysgenesis. *AJR* 93:354–361, 1965.
5. Necic S, Grand DB: Diagnostic value of hand x-rays in Turner's syndrome. *Acta Paediatr Scand* 67:309–313, 1978.
6. Procopis PG, Turner B: Mental retardation, abnormal fingers and skeletal anomalies: Coffin's syndrome. *Am J Dis Child* 214:258–261, 1972.
7. Wood BP, Young LW: Pseudohyperphalangism in fetal Dilantin. *Radiology* 131:371–372, 1979.

Distal Phalangeal Resorption or Destruction

The most common cause of resorption of the terminal tufts of the distal phalanges is hyperparathyroidism and, in childhood, secondary hyperparathyroidism, or renal osteodystrophy, is much more common than primary hyperparathyroidism. Nonetheless, in either situation resorption of the terminal phalanges is rather characteristic (Fig. 4.79). Other acquired causes of terminal phalangeal resorption or destruc-

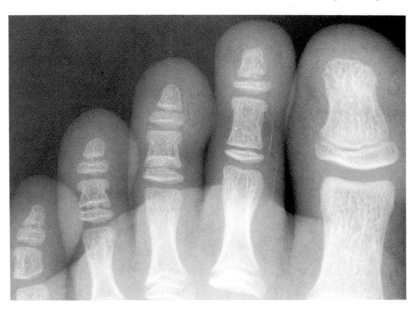

Figure 4.77. Hypoplastic terminal phalanges. A. Normal, small terminal phalanges in foot.

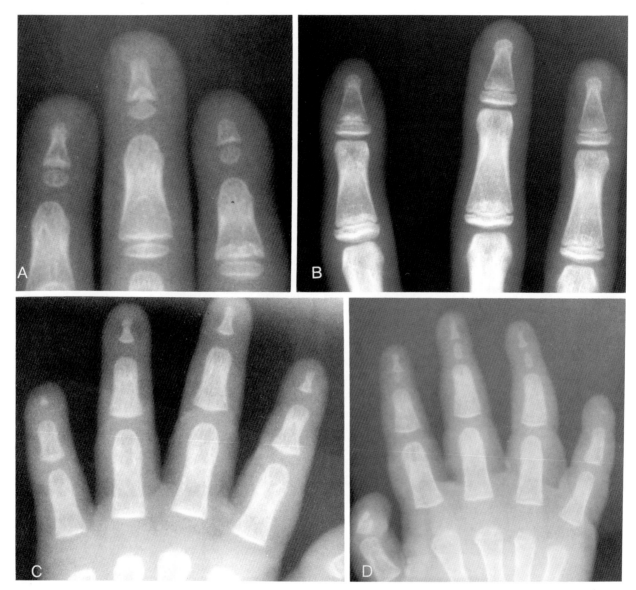

Figure 4.78. Hypoplastic terminal phalanges. A. Small hypoplastic terminal phalanges in young child with cleidocranial dysostosis. Also note slightly cone-shaped epiphysis. **B.** Older child with cleidocranial dysostosis showing thin, tapered distal phalanges. **C.** Infant with Dilantin embryonopathy and small hypoplastic terminal phalanges. **D.** Another child with Dilantin embryonopathy showing small, hypoplastic terminal phalanges and so-called **"pseudohyperphalangealism."**

tion include frostbite, thermal injury, syringomyelia, trauma, infection, leprosy (6), psoriasis, the hyperuricemia (fingerbiting) syndrome of Lesch-Nyhan (1), and polyvinyl chloride toxicity (2). In almost all of these conditions, except for hyperparathyroidism, the problem probably results from a vasculitis or vascular spasm leading to ischemic bone necrosis. Indeed, even in congenital causes of distal phalangeal resorption, the same problem likely is present, and with regard to these syndromes, one should consider the following: idiopathic acro-osteolysis (2), progeria, pyknodysostosis, osteopetrosis (5), Ehler-Danlos syndrome (3), pseudoxanthoma elasticum, Rothmund

syndrome (4), congenital insensitivity to pain (congenital sensory neuropathy), and epidermolysis bullosa. Distal phalangeal resorption also can occur, on an isolated basis, with osteomyelitis of the distal phalanx, and on a more generalized basis, in patients with burn injury and contractures (with or without associated osteomyelitis).

REFERENCES

1. Becker MH, Wallin JK: Congenital hyperuricosuria: associated radiologic features. *Radiol Clin North Am* 6:239–243, 1968.

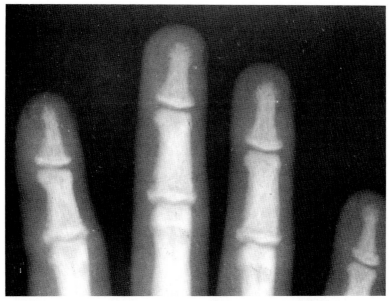

Figure 4.79. Distal phalangeal resorption. Note resorption of terminal phalanges in advanced secondary hyperparathyroidism.

2. Brown DM, Bradford DS, Gorlin RJ, Desnick RJ, Langer LO Jr, Jowsey J, Sauk JJ Jr: The acro-osteolysis syndrome: morphologic and biochemical studies. *J Pediatr* 88:573–575, 1976.
3. Mabille JP, Castera D, Chapuis JL, Lambert D, Chapelon M: A case of Ehlers-Danlos syndrome with acroosteolysis. *Ann Radiol* 15:781–786, 1972.
4. Maurer RM, Langford OL: Rothmund's syndrome: a cause of resorption of phalangeal tufts and dystrophic calcification. *Radiology* 89:706–708, 1967.
5. Moss A, Mainzer F: Osteopetrosis: an unusual cause of terminal-tuft erosion. *Radiology* 97:631–632, 1970.
6. Newman H, Casey B, DuBois JJ, Gallagher T: Roentgen features of leprosy in children. *AJR* 114:402–410, 1972.

MIDDLE AND PROXIMAL PHALANGES

Except for the middle phalanx of the fifth digit, middle or proximal phalangeal hypoplasia is relatively uncommon. Middle phalangeal hypoplasia is seen with certain primary brachydactyly syndromes. Hypoplasia of the middle phalanx of the fifth digit is dealt with later (see Fig. 4.85*B*). Middle, or proximal, phalangeal underdevelopment can be acquired after osteomyelitis, bone infarction, trauma, or septic arthritis. On a congenital basis, generalized shortening of the middle phalanges often is associated with hypoplasia of the distal phalanges and can be seen in the following syndromes: acrocephalosyndactyly (Apert syndrome), Poland syndrome, and trichorhino-phalangeal syndrome (see Fig. 4.54*C*). There are no specific syndromes where the proximal phalanges are shortened on an isolated basis.

Metacarpals and Metatarsals

For the most part, metacarpal and metatarsal problems center around shortening of one or more of these bones. Overly long metacarpals and metatarsals, however, also can be seen, and usually occur as part of an underlying syndrome such as Marfan syndrome or homocystinuria. In such cases, they are not selectively used for diagnosis.

Shortening of the first metacarpal and metatarsal is dealt with later (see Fig. 4.84), as are other abnormalities of the thumb and great toe. In this section, shortening of the other metacarpals and metatarsals is considered, and generally what can be said for the metacarpals is true of the metatarsals.

Short Metacarpals and Metatarsals

It is helpful to consider the third, fourth, and fifth metacarpals as a unit, even though in any given case only one of these may be shortened. The reason for this is that many syndromes cause shortening of these bones as a unit. When only the fourth and fifth metacarpals appear shortened, however, it is important to determine whether one's observations are true. This is important because in some cases perfectly normal metacarpals appear shortened. To de-

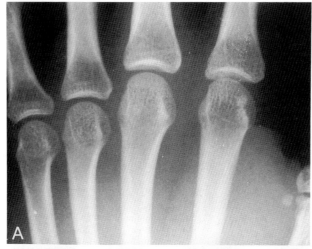

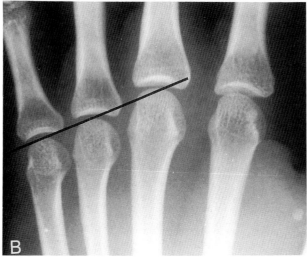

Figure 4.80. Positive, metacarpal sign. A. Note shortening of the fourth and fifth metacarpals. **B.** Metacarpal line drawn across the heads of the fourth and fifth metacarpals intersects head of the third metacarpal.

termine whether the fourth and fifth metacarpals are truly shortened one can apply the "metacarpal line." Originally developed for assessing metacarpal shortening in Turner syndrome (2, 5), the line is drawn along the heads of the fourth and fifth metacarpals and then where it intersects the third metacarpal is noted. When the sign is positive, the line intersects the head of the third metacarpal (Fig. 4.80), when borderline it just grazes the head, and when normal it misses the head. Always apply this line before making a final judgment.

Perhaps the two conditions best known for producing shortening of the third through fifth metacarpals are the just-mentioned Turner syndrome (3, 4) and pseudo- or pseudopseudohypoparathyroidism (Fig. 4.81A and B) (5, 6). In addition to these conditions, the metacarpals or metatarsals can be shortened on an isolated basis (Fig. 4.81C) and with the following syndromes: basal cell nevus syndrome, Beckwith-Wiedemann syndrome, Biedmon syndrome, Larsen syndrome, multiple exostoses syndrome, the various epiphyseal dysplasias, and the tricho-rhino-phalangeal syndrome. In any of these conditions, only the fifth metacarpal may be shortened. Other conditions in which only the fifth metacarpal is shortened include the cri-du-chat syndrome and Russell-Silver dwarfism (congenital hemiatrophy). Finally, it should be noted that short fourth and fifth metacarpals of no consequence at all occur in approximately 10% of normal individuals (1).

REFERENCES

1. Bloom RA: The metacarpal sign. *Br J Radiol* 43:133–135, 1970.
2. Finby N, Archibald RM: Skeletal abnormalities associated with gonadal dysgenesis. *AJR* 89:1222–1235, 1963.
3. Kosowicz J: The roentgen appearance of the hand and wrist in gonadal dysgenesis. *AJR* 93:354–361, 1965.
4. Necic S, Grant DB: Diagnostic value of hand x-rays in Turner's syndrome. *Acta Paediatr Scand* 67:309–312, 1978.
5. Poznanski AK, Werder EA, Giedion A: The pattern of shortening of the bones of the hand in PHP and PPHP: a comparison with brachydactyly E, Turner syndrome, and acrodysostosis. *Radiology* 123:707–718, 1977.
6. Steinback HL, Young DA: The roentgen appearance of pseudohypoparathyroidism (PH) and pseudo-pseudo hypoparathyroidism (PPH): differentiation from other syndromes associated with short metacarpals, metatarsals and phalanges. *AJR* 97:49–66, 1966.

The Thumb and Great Toe

SHORT, BROAD THUMB OR GREAT TOE

Shortening of the first digit often is more evident clinically than radiographically, and perhaps the most striking radiologic findings are seen in the Rubenstein-Taybi (mental retardation and broad thumbs) and acrocephalosyndactyly syndromes (Fig. 4.82A–C). In both of these conditions, the thumbs and great toes also may be duplicated. Other conditions demonstrating broad thumbs and great toes, but not usually duplicated, include the otopalato-digital syndrome (Fig. 4.82D), the frontodigital syndrome, the hand-foot-uterus syndrome, Robinow syndrome, Weaver-Smith syndrome, progressive myositis ossificans (Fig. 4.82E), diastrophic dwarfism, Larsen syndrome, and pleonostenosis. The thumb also is short and broad when there is isolated hypoplasia of the distal phalanx of the thumb. This particular deformity has no diagnostic specificity, and

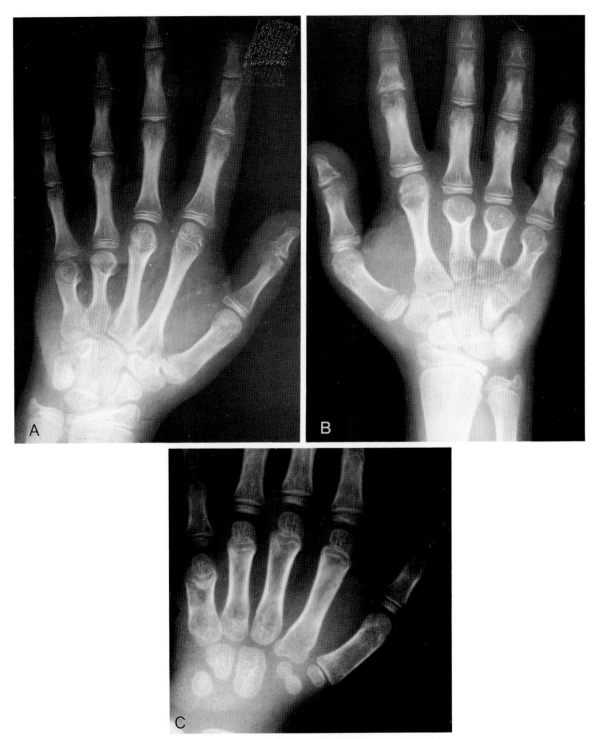

Figure 4.81. Short metacarpals. A. Typical short fourth and fifth metacarpals in Turner syndrome. Also note carpal fusion and drumstick terminal phalanges. **B.** Similar shortening of the third, fourth, and fifth metacarpals in pseudohypoparathyroidism. Note that all of the small bones of the hands are shortened. **C.** Isolated, incidental shortening of the fifth metacarpal *(arrow)* in normal child.

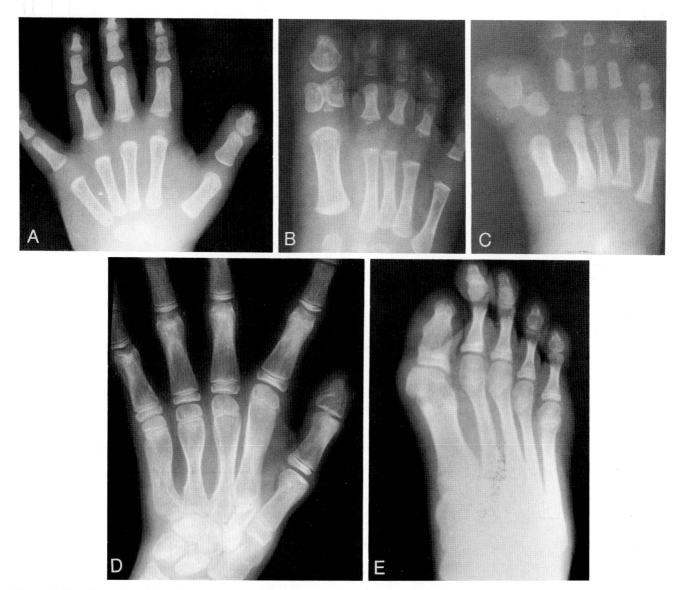

Figure 4.82. Short broad thumbs and toes. A. Broad thumb in Rubenstein-Taybi syndrome. **B.** Broad, bifid great toe in same patient. **C.** Short broad toe in acrocephalosyndactyly. Note other anomalies including symphalangism and hypoplasia of the pha-langes. **D.** Broad thumb in otopalatodigital syndrome. Note other characteristic changes. **E.** Short, somewhat broad great toe, with fusion of the phalanges, in progressive myositis ossificans.

usually occurs as an isolated finding in otherwise normal individuals.

HYPOPLASTIC, THIN THUMB

Conditions producing a hypoplastic but thin thumb include the Holt-Oram syndrome (see Fig. 4.26), Fanconi anemia, the thrombocytopenia-absent radius syndrome (thumb only minimally hypoplastic or normal), trisomy-18, Cornelia de Lange syndrome, Smith-Lemli-Opitz syndrome, and any of the conditions leading to a triphalangeal thumb (see next section).

TRIPHALANGEAL THUMB

In this deformity, the thumb has an extra phalanx and appears more like the other digits. Rarely, it can occur as a normal variation, and in any case may be associated with duplication of the thumb or absence of the contralateral thumb. As far as syndromes are concerned, triphalangeal thumbs can occur in the Blackfan-Diamond congenital anemia syndrome (2, 3), Holt-Oram syndrome (Fig. 4.83), trisomy-13–15 (rarely), Poland (absent pectoralis muscle) syndrome, VATER (vertebral defects, anal anomalies, tracheo-esophageal fistula with esophageal atresia, and radial and renal anomalies) association, Werner mesomelic dysplasia (1), Juberg-Hayward syndrome, thalidomide embryonopathy (4), and Dilantin embryonopathy.

REFERENCES

1. Hall CM: Werner's mesomelic dysplasia and ventricular septal defect and Hirschsprung's disease. *Pediatr Radiol* 10:247–249, 1981.

2. Jones B, Thompson H: Triphalangeal thumbs associated with hypoplastic anemia. *Pediatrics* 52:609–612, 1973.
3. Murphy S, Lubin B: Triphalangeal thumbs and congenital erythroid hypoplasia: report of a case with unusual features. *J Pediatr* 81:987–989, 1972.
4. Poznanski AK, Garn SM, Holt JF: The thumb in the congenital malformation syndromes. *Radiology* 100:115–129, 1971.

Hypoplastic First Metacarpal or Metatarsal

A hypoplastic first metacarpal or metatarsal can be seen as an isolated anomaly, but more often is indicative of some syndrome (1). Perhaps the best known conditions resulting in shortening of the first metacarpal are those constituting the "radial ray" syndromes (hypoplastic radius and thumb). For the most part, these include Fanconi anemia, Holt-Oram syndrome (see Fig. 4.26), and the thrombocytopenia-absent radius syndrome. In the latter, however, changes in the thumb usually are minimal or virtually nonexistent. Hypoplasia of the first metacarpal also occurs with syndromes exhibiting a triphalangeal thumb (see previous section). Other syndromes in which the first metacarpal or metatarsal is shortened or hypoplastic include Juberg-Hayward syndrome, Cornelia de Lange syndrome, progressive myositis ossificans (Fig. 4.84A), trisomy-18 (Fig. 4.84B), hand-foot-uterus syndrome, diastrophic dwarfism, the VATER syndrome, and all of the conditions marked by short, broad thumbs and toes.

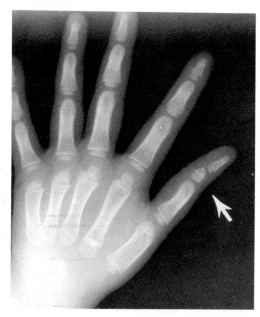

Figure 4.83. Triphalangeal thumb. Typical triphalangeal thumb *(arrow)* in Holt-Oram syndrome.

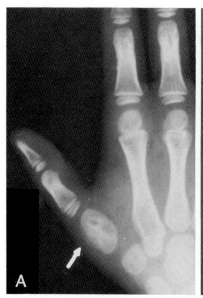
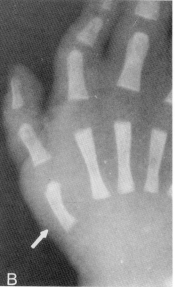

Figure 4.84. Short, hypoplastic first metacarpal or metatarsal. A. Note short metacarpal in progressive myositis ossificans *(arrow)*. **B.** Short metacarpal *(arrow)* with slight shortening of the phalanges of the thumb in trisomy-18 *(arrow)*. For a thin, hypoplastic metacarpal in Fanconi anemia, see Figure 4.26.

REFERENCE

1. Poznanski AK, Garn SM, Hold JF: The thumb in the congenital malformation syndromes. *Radiology* 100:115–129, 1971.

Fifth Digit Abnormalities

For the most part, abnormalities of the **fifth digit involve the hand,** and are incurving deformities, i.e., clinodactyly and Kirner deformity. Clinodactyly of the fifth digit is associated with hypoplasia of the middle phalanx (Fig. 4.85*B* and *C*), while Kirner deformity is isolated to the terminal phalanx. Some believe it to be a form of epiphyseal dysplasia (1, 3, 5). The condition usually is bilateral and occurs as an isolated finding (Fig. 4.85*A*). However, it can be seen with some frequency in the Cornelia de Lange and Russell-Silver syndromes. The findings are rather typical but often misinterpreted as posttraumatic or infectious changes.

Ordinary clinodactyly of the fifth digit (4) is seen in so many conditions that its diagnostic value is diminished (Table 4.29). In addition, on an isolated basis it can be seen in some normal individuals (1, 2).

REFERENCES

1. Blank E, Girdany BR: Symmetric bowling of the terminal phalanges of the fifth fingers in a family (Kirner's deformity). *AJR* 93:367–373, 1965.

Table 4.29
Clinodactyly Fifth Digit

More common conditions	Less common conditions
Normal	**Syndromes**
Sporadic	Aarskog syndrome
Syndromes	Bloom syndrome
Acrocephalosyndactyly	Cerebrohepatorenal syndrome
Camptomelic dwarfism	Cri-du-chat syndrome
Cornelia de Lange syndrome	Hand-foot syndrome
	Nievergelt syndrome
Fanconi anemia	Oculodentodigital syndrome
Goltz syndrome	Oculodento-osseous dysplasia
Holt-Oram syndrome	Orofaciodigital syndrome I and II
Klinefelter syndrome	
Laurence-Moon-Biedl-Bardet syndrome	Popliteal pterygium syndrome
	Rieger syndrome
Marfan syndrome	Senior syndrome
Myositis ossificans progressiva	Seckel bird-headed syndrome
	Thrombocytopenia absent radius syndrome
Noonan syndrome	
Oto-palato-digital syndrome	Tricho-rhino-phalangeal syndrome
Poland syndrome	
Russell-Silver syndrome	Penta X (XXXXX) syndrome
Trisomy-18	Wolf syndrome: 4p syndrome
Trisomy-21	XXXY syndrome
Trisomy-13	Whistling face syndrome

2. Greulich WW: A comparison of the dysplastic middle phalanx of the fifth finger in mentally normal Caucasians, Mongoloids, and Negroes with that of individuals of the racial groups who have Down's syndrome. *AJR* 118:259–281, 1973.

3. Kaufmann HJ, Taillard WF: Bilateral incurving of the ter-

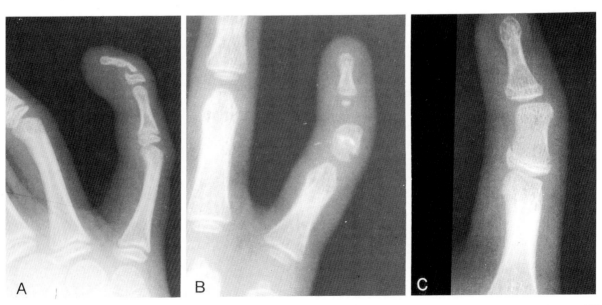

Figure 4.85. Curved fifth digit. A. Typical configuration of Kirner deformity. Note that the terminal phalanx of the fifth digit appears dysplastic. **B.** Curved fifth digit with hypoplastic middle phalanx in trisomy-21. **C.** Normal individual with curved fifth digit and hypoplastic middle phalanx.

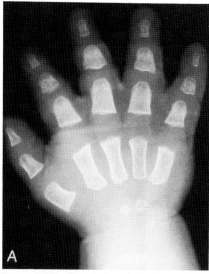 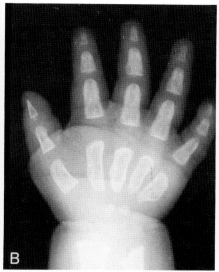 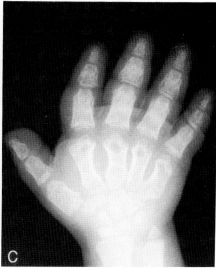

Figure 4.86. Spade hand. A. Typical spade hand of achondroplasia. **B.** Spade hand in Hurler disease. Note bullet-shaped, proximally tapered metacarpals. **C.** Spade hand in acrodysostosis.

minal phalanges of the fifth fingers: an isolated lesion of the epiphyseal plate. *AJR* 86:490, 1961.
4. Laporte G: Clinodactyly. *Ann Radiol* 23:60–68, 1980.
5. Staheli LT, Clawson DK, Capps JH: Bilateral curving of terminal phalanges of little fingers: report of two cases. *J Bone Joint Surg* 48A:1171–1176, 1966.

Other Hand and Foot Deformities

SPADE HAND

The spade hand is quite square and results from shortening of all of the bones of the hand. There are a fair number of conditions in which such a hand occurs, but the largest group consists of the chondrodystrophies: i.e., achondroplasia (Fig. 4.86*A*), pseudoachondroplasia (multiple epiphyseal and spondyloepiphyseal types), hypochondroplasia (mild changes), thanatophoric dwarfism, achondrogenesis, the storage diseases, the short rib-polydactyly syndromes, metatropic dwarfism, Kniest syndrome, diastrophic dwarfism, peripheral dysostosis or acrodysostosis (Fig 4.86*C*) (1, 2, 4), asphyxiating thoracic dystrophy (minimal changes), pleonosteosis, and metaphyseal dysostosis (more severe in Jansen type). In the storage diseases, in addition to the hands being spade-like, the metacarpals are proximally tapered and bullet-shaped (Fig. 4.86*B*).

A spade hand also can occur in osteogenesis imperfecta (due to multiple fractures in the congenita form), punctate epiphyseal dysplasia, Ruvalcaba syndrome (3), Taybi-Lindner syndrome, and the oto-palato-digital syndrome.

Table 4.30
Camptodactyly

More common conditions	Less common conditions
Holt-Oram syndrome	Isolated phalangeal hypoplasia or absence
Arthrogryposis congenita	Oro-facio-digital syndromes I and II
Poland syndrome	Aarskog syndrome
Trisomy-18	Cerebrohepatorenal or Zellweger syndrome
Acquired	Goltz syndrome
Burns	Marfan contractural arachnodactyly
Infections	Osteo-onychodysplasia
Fractures	Popliteal pterygium syndrome
Contractures	Tricho-rhino-phalangeal syndrome
	Camptodactyly-ankylosis-pulmonary hypoplasia syndrome

REFERENCES

1. Arkless R, Graham CB: An unusual case of brachydactyly: peripheral dysostosis? Pseudo-pseudo-hypoparathyroidism? Cone epiphyses? *AJR* 99:724–735, 1967.
2. Robinow M, Pfeiffer RA, Gorlin RJ, McKusick VA, Renuart AW, Johnson GF, Summitt RL: Acrodysostosis. *Am J Dis Child* 121:195–203, 1971.
3. Ruvalcaba RHA, Reichert A, Smith DE: A new familial syndrome with osseous dysplasia and mental deficiency. *J Pediatr* 79:450–455, 1971.
4. Singleton EB, Daeschner CW, Teng CT: Peripheral dysostosis. *AJR* 84:499–505, 1960.

CAMPTODACTYLY

The term "camptodactyly" designates a flexion deformity of one or more of the digits, and the findings

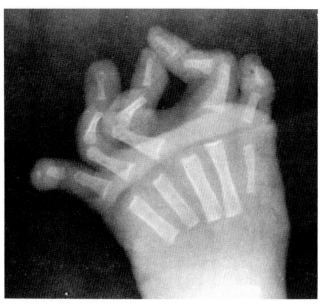

Figure 4.87. Camptodactyly. Note bent fingers in trisomy-18. Also note hypoplastic thumb and first metacarpal.

usually are more striking in the hand than in the foot. Bending occurs primarily at the proximal interphalangeal joints, and one or more fingers may be involved. Clinical detection is easier than roentgenographic detection, for the findings may be difficult to differentiate from faulty positioning of the fingers. Camptodactyly occurs in a large number of syndromes, but only the more common ones are listed in Table 4.30. Usually, the first one that comes to mind is trisomy-18 (Fig. 4.87). It also should be noted that flexion deformities of the digits can be acquired secondary to burns, infections, and fractures.

SYNDACTYLY AND POLYDACTYLY

Syndactyly can involve either the soft tissues alone or both the bones and soft tissues (Fig. 4.88A). In addition, it can occur as an isolated finding or as a feature of certain syndromes (Table 4.31). In a few cases, the metacarpals also can be fused, while in others polydactyly or duplication of the middle digits occurs.

Polydactyly can involve the outer or inner aspect of the hand (Fig. 4.88B). When it involves the ulnar side, it is termed "postaxial"; on the radial side, it is called "preaxial" polydactyly. Polydactyly often is associated with syndactyly, and both can occur on an isolated sporadic basis. However, polydactyly also occurs with a number of syndromes and is useful in defining these syndromes (Table 4.32).

SYMPHALANGISM

In this condition there is fusion of the phalanges in the same digit. Most often, the condition is seen as an isolated abnormality in the hands or feet. Because the condition is believed to have existed in John Talbot, the first Earl of Shrewsbury, the finding often is referred to as the mark of Shrewsbury. It is inherited as a mendelian dominant trait, and most often the proximal interphalangeal joints of the fingers (Fig. 4.88C) and distal interphalangeal joints of the toes are affected (1–7). However, involvement of the distal interphalangeal joints of the hands also can occur. Other anomalies may be seen in some patients, and the condition has been reported in association with carpal and tarsal coalition (2, 3). It also occurs in diastrophic dwarfism, isolated brachydactyly, popliteal pterygium syndrome, and some cases of the acrocephalosyndactyly syndrome (4).

REFERENCES

1. Daniel GH: A case of hereditary anarthrosis of the index finger, with associated abnormalities in the proportions of the fingers. *Ann Eugen* 7:281–296, 1936.
2. Elkington SG, Huntsman RG: The Talbot fingers: a study in symphalangism. *Br Med J* 1:407–411, 1967.
3. Geelhoed G, Neel JV, Davidson RT: Symphalangism and tarsal coalitions—a hereditary syndrome: a report on two families. *J Bone Joint Surg* 51B:278–298, 1969.
4. Harle TS, Stevenson JR: Hereditary symphalangism associated with carpal and tarsal fusions. *Radiology* 89:91–94, 1967.
5. Strasburger AK, Hawkins MR, Eldridge R, Hargrave RL, McKusick VA: Symphalangism: genetic and clinical aspects. *Johns Hopkins Med J* 117:108–127, 1965.
6. Walker G: Remarkable cases of hereditary anchyloses, or absence of various phalangeal joints. *Johns Hopkins Med J* 12:129–133, 1901.
7. Wildervanck LS, Goedhard G, Meijer S: Proximal symphalangism of fingers associated with fusion of os tibiale externum in an European-Indonesian-Chinese family. *Acta Genet* 17:166–177, 1967.

ABSENT OR AMPUTATED DIGITS

Acquired conditions such as trauma, burns, and infection most commonly cause amputation of the digits. Less common acquired causes include advanced psoriasis and frostbite. Congenital amputation also occurs and is seen in the aglossia-adactyly, Cornelia de Lange, Möbius, and thalidomide embryonopathy syndromes. Amputation of the digits also can occur with amniotic (Streeter) bands (Fig. 4.89A).

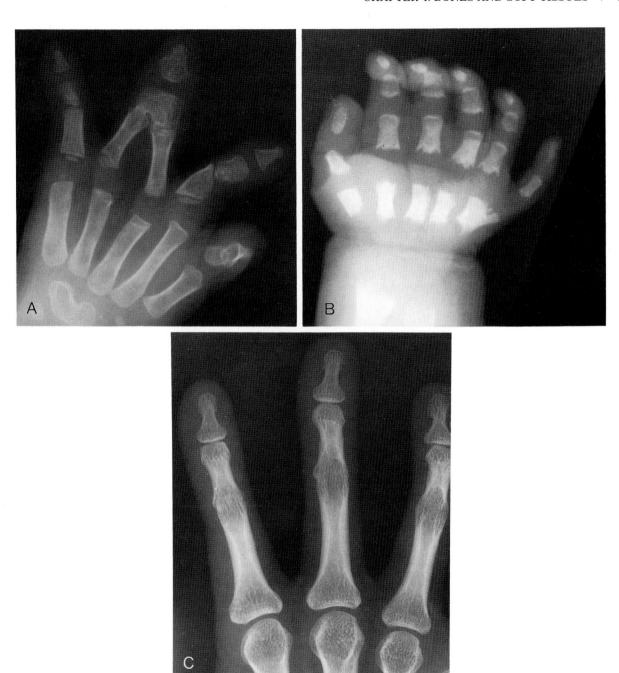

Figure 4.88. Syndactyly and polydactyly. A. Note typical syndactyly and peripheral hypoplasia in Apert syndrome. Also note carpal bone fusion. **B.** Short-rib polydactyly syndrome of Saldino-Noonan. **C. Symphalangism.** Note fusion of the proximal intraphalangeal joints.

Absence of the middle digits of the hands can be seen with the "claw hand" deformity (Fig. 4.89*B*). This deformity often is seen with anomalies of the face, such as cleft lip and palate, mandibulofacial dysostosis, or congenital deafness. Absence of the digits on one or the other side of the hand is termed either the **"radial" or "ulnar ray" syndrome.** The radial ray syndrome is more common, and often the thumb bears the brunt of the hypoplasia. Conditions demonstrating the radial ray syndrome include Klippel-Feil deformity, ectodermal dysplasia, Fanconi anemia, Holt-Oram syndrome, thrombocytopenia-absent radius syndrome (thumb usually well developed but radius absent), thalidomide embryonopathy, VATER syndrome, and trisomy-18. Conditions associated with the ulnar ray syndrome (i.e., fourth and fifth digits) include the Cornelia de Lange syndrome, Nievergelt and Pfeiffer ulnofibular dysplasias, Wegner syndrome, and Weyer oligodactyly.

Table 4.31
Syndactyly

More common conditions	Less common conditions
Acrocephalosyndactyly[a]	**Isolated**
Cornelia de Lange syndrome	Sporadic
Fanconi anemia	**Syndromes**
Holt-Oram syndrome	Aarskog syndrome
Thrombocytopenia absent radius syndrome	Aglossia-adactyly syndrome
Trisomy-13	Bloom syndrome
Trisomy-18	Carpenter syndrome
Syndromes with polydactyly[b]	Punctate epiphyseal dysplasia: Conradi syndrome
	Goltz syndrome
	Laurence-Moon-Biedl syndrome
	Möbius syndrome
	Nager syndrome
	Mesomelic dwarfism
	Otopalatodigital syndrome
	Popliteal pterygium syndrome
	Robinow-Silverman syndrome
	Rothmund-Thomson syndrome
	Rubinstein-Taybi syndrome
	Smith-Lemi-Opitz syndrome
	Tricho-rhino-phalangeal syndrome

[a]Including Apert.
[b]See Table 4.32.

Table 4.32
Polydactyly

More common conditions	Less common conditions
Acrocephalosyndactyly[a]	**Isolated**
Blackfan-Diamond anemia[a]	Sporadic
Dubowitz syndrome[a]	**Syndromes**
Fanconi anemia[a]	Acro-pectoro-vertebral dysplasia[a]
Holt-Oram syndrome[a]	Asphyxiating thoracic dystrophy[b]
Rubinstein-Taybi syndrome[b]	Biedmond syndrome[b]
VATER syndrome[a]	Bloom syndrome[a]
	Ellis-van Creveld syndrome[a]
	Goltz syndrome[b]
	Grieg syndrome[b]
	Hereditary hydrometrocolpos[b]: McKusick-Kaufman syndrome
	Kaufman-McKusick syndrome[b]
	Mohr syndrome[a,b]
	Möbius syndrome
	Myositis ossificans progressiva
	Nager syndrome[a]
	Oro-facio-digital syndrome
	Poland syndrome[a]
	Short-rib polydactyly syndrome[a,b]
	Smith-Lemli-Opitz syndrome[b]
	Trisomy-13
	Werner mesomelic dysplasia[a]
	Weyer syndrome[b]

[a]Preaxial (radial side).
[b]Postaxial (ulnar side).

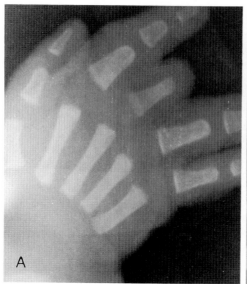
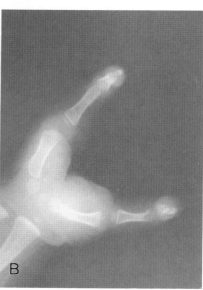

Figure 4.89. Amputated digits. A. Note amputation of middle digit due to amniotic band syndrome. **B.** Absent middle digits in claw hand deformity.

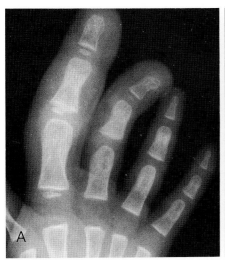
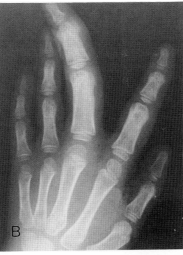
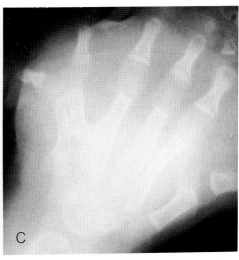

Figure 4.90. Gigantism. A. Note enlargement of the second and third digits in this patient with neurofibromatosis. **B.** Digital gigantism in Proteus syndrome. **C.** Gigantism in macrodystrophia lipomatosa congenita.

MACRODACTYLY

Enlargement of one or more of the digits (Fig. 4.90) is not common, and most often is associated with a hemangiomatous or lymphangiomatous tumor of the hand or foot, neurofibromatosis, macrodystrophia lipomatosa congenita (1), or the Proteus syndrome (2–4).

REFERENCES

1. Baruchin AM, Herold ZH, Shmueli G, and Lupo L: Macrodystrophia lipomatosa of the foot. *J Pediatr Surg* 23:192–194, 1988.
2. Demetriades D, Hager J, Nikolaides N, Malamitsi-Puchner A, Bartsocas CS: Proteus syndrome—musculoskeletal manifestations and management: a report of two cases. *J Pediatr Orthop* 12:106–113, 1992.
3. Strickler S: Musculoskeletal manifestations of proteus syndrome: report of two cases with literature review. *J Pediatr Orthop* 12:667–674, 1992.
4. Wiedemann HR, Burgio GR, Aldenhoff P, Kunze J, Kaufmann HJ, Schirg E: The proteus syndrome. *Eur J Pediatr* 140:5, 1983.

DACTYLITIS

Dactylitis infers an infection or inflammation of the fingers (Table 4.33). As far as infection is concerned, perhaps the most common cause of dactylitis is osteomyelitis in certain immune deficiency syndromes and tuberculosis (spina ventosa). Many times the findings in the bones consist of destruction, sclerosis with healing, and generalized expansion of the bone (Fig. 4.91A). Similar findings can be seen with bone infarction (hand-foot syndrome of sickle cell

Table 4.33
Dactylitis

Infection: osteomyelitis Infarction: hand-foot syndrome	Common
Frostbite	Relatively rare

Radiation injury
Microgeodic syndrome
Tumor mimicking dactylitis
  Ewing sarcoma
  Hemangioma
  Metastatic neuroblastoma
	Rare

disease) (1) (Fig. 4.91B), frostbite (3), radiation necrosis, and, rarely, tumors such as Ewing sarcoma, hemangiomas, and metastatic neuroblastoma. With Ewing sarcoma and metastatic neuroblastoma, spiculated new bone formation may accompany the changes. Changes resembling dactylitis are seen in the rare phalangeal microgeodic syndrome of infancy (2).

REFERENCES

1. Bennett OM: Salmonella osteomyelitis and the hand-foot syndrome in sickle cell disease. *J Pediatr Orthop* 12:534–538, 1992.
2. Maroteaux P: Cinq observations d'une affection microgeodique des phalanges du nourrisson d'etiologie inconnue. *Ann Radiol* 13:229, 1970.
3. Sweet EM, Smith MGH: Winter fingers: bone infarction in Scottish children as a manifestation of cold injury. *Ann Radiol* 22:71–75, 1979.

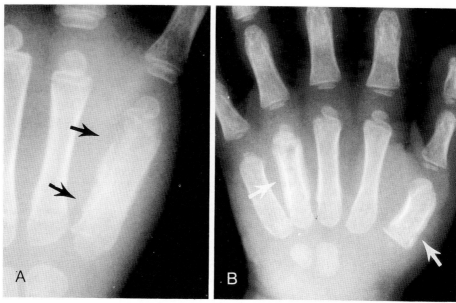

Figure 4.91. Dactylitis. A. Coccidiomycosis of metacarpal *(arrows).* **B.** Hand-foot syndrome causing dactylitis in sickle cell disease. Note bone destruction and periosteal reaction on the first and fourth metacarpals *(arrows).*

Carpal and Tarsal Abnormalities

DECREASED (MORE ACUTE) CARPAL ANGLE

The carpal angle is the angle formed by the lines drawn tangentially to the lunate, scaphoid, and triquetral bones. Normally, the angle measures somewhere between 125° and 140° (1). When it is decreased (i.e., more acute), especially in more severe cases, there is associated slanting of the distal radial and ulnar articulating surfaces (Fig. 4.92). The most common condition associated with a decreased carpal angle is Turner syndrome (1–3), but other conditions where it can be decreased include dyschondrosteosis (Madelung deformity), Morquio disease, multiple osteochondromatosis, Hurler syndrome (1), and other storage diseases with more severe bony changes (Fig. 4.92). When angulation is profound, often there is an erosion of the upper medial aspect of the radius (Fig. 4.92B). This erosion probably is the result of herniation of the synovial lining of the wrist joint.

REFERENCES

1. Harper HAS, Poznanski AK, Garn SM: The carpal angle in American populations. *Invest Radiol* 9:217–221, 1974.
2. Kosowicz J: The roentgen appearance of the hand and wrist in gonadal dysgenesis. *AJR* 93:354–361, 1965.
3. Necic S, Grant DB: Diagnostic value of hand x-rays in Turner's syndrome. *Acta Paediatr Scand* 67:309–312, 1978.

CARPAL-TARSAL COALITION

The carpal bones probably undergo fusion more often than the tarsal bones, and the phenomenon can occur on an isolated basis in normal patients or as a part of certain syndromes. On an isolated basis (most common), carpal coalition is more common among black individuals (1, 2, 4) and, in this regard, fusion is most common between the triquetral and the lunate bones (Fig. 4.93A). However, numerous other combinations can occur both in the hand and foot (Fig. 4.93B). In the foot, isolated coalition between the talus and calcaneus (Fig. 4.93C) is not uncommon and may be associated with pes planus. It is best demonstrated with CT scanning (Fig. 4.93D).

In syndromes, coalition patterns may be more bizarre, and in the foot they are likely to involve mainly the cuneiforms and the metatarsals (3). Syndromes in which fusion occurs are outlined in Table 4.34, but the one that first comes to mind is the Ellis-van Creveld syndrome. Acquired carpal or tarsal fusion can be seen after trauma, inflammation, or infection. In terms of inflammation, the best known cause is rheumatoid arthritis (Fig. 4.93E).

REFERENCES

1. Cockshott WP: Carpal fusions. *AJR* 89:1260–1271, 1963.
2. Cope JR: Carpal coalition. *Clin Radiol* 25:261–266, 1974.
3. Poznanski AK: Foot manifestations of the congenital malformation syndromes. *Semin Roentgenol* 5:354–366, 1970.
4. Poznanski AK, Holt FF: The carpals in congenital malformation syndromes. *AJR* 112:443–459, 1971.

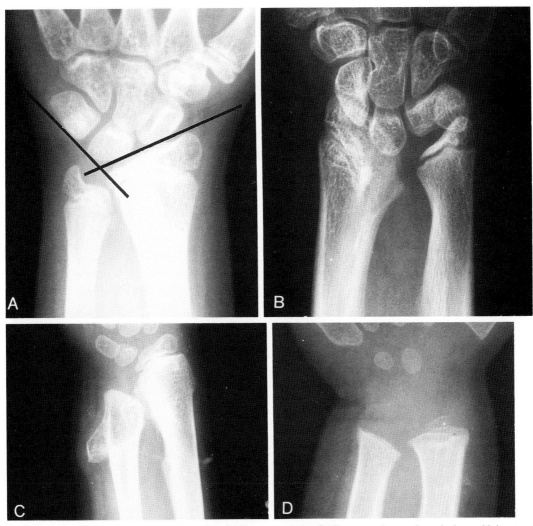

Figure 4.92. Decreased (more acute) carpal angle. A. Decreased carpal angle in Turner syndrome. Carpal angle (lines) measures approximately 112°. **B.** Decreased carpal angle and associated distal radial and ulnar deformities in dyschondros- teosis. **C.** Decreased carpal angle in multiple exostosis. **D.** Decreased carpal angle and associated slanting of distal radius and ulna in Hurler disease.

SCALLOPED CARPAL-TARSAL BONES

Scalloping deformities of the carpal or tarsal bones most commonly occur with multiple epiphyseal dysplasia (Fig. 4.94A), but similar findings can be seen with neurofibromatosis (Fig. 4.94B), adjacent soft tissue hemangiomas or lymphangiomas, and neurotrophic diseases such as tertiary syphilis, syringomyelia, and diabetic neuropathy. Most of these latter conditions tend to occur in adults, but occasionally they are encountered in children. Focal, solitary scallopings are seen with adjacent tumors (Fig. 4.94C) and after infection, trauma, or bone necrosis. Scalloped tarsal and carpal bones also occur in rheumatoid arthritis (synovial erosion) (Fig. 4.94D), Winchester syndrome (a storage disease mimicking rheumatoid arthritis), and pigmented villinodular

synovitis. In all of these conditions, scalloping is due to synovial hypertrophy.

FRAGMENTED OR IRREGULAR CARPAL-TARSAL BONES

Irregular development suggesting fragmentation of the tarsal, but not the carpal, bones is common in normal individuals. Indeed, in such cases aseptic necrosis often is erroneously suggested (Fig. 4.95A and B). Such normal fragmentation can occur in any of the tarsals but tends to involve the cuneiforms and navicular more than the others. Fragmentation due to avascular necrosis most commonly occurs in the tarsal navicular and is known as Köhler disease (Fig. 4.95C) (1). Clinically, pain is present and soft tissue swelling is demonstrable roentgenographi-

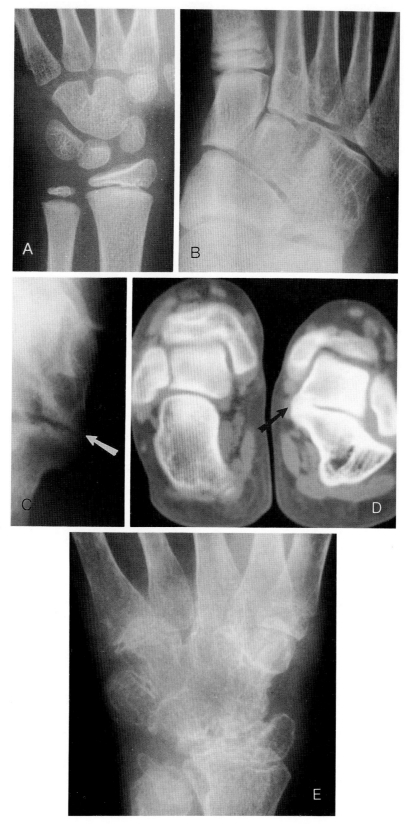

Figure 4.93. Carpal-tarsal coalitions. A. Incidental carpal coalition. **B.** Multiple coalitions of the tarsal bones in a foot. **C.** Talocalcaneal coalition *(arrow).* **D.** CT scan shows the coalition *(arrow)* more clearly. **E.** Postinflammatory coalition in rheumatoid arthritis.

Table 4.34
Carpal-Tarsal Coalition

More common conditions	Less common conditions
Idiopathic, isolated	Diastrophic dwarfism
Ellis-van Creveld syndrome	Hand-foot-uterus syndrome
Holt-Oram syndrome	Kniest syndrome
Acrocephalosyndactyly	Nievergelt mesomelic dwarfism
Arthrogryposis congenita	Otopalato-digital syndrome
Turner syndrome	Frontometaphyseal dysplasia
Dyschondrosteosis: Madelung deformity	Stickler syndrome
Acquired	
Trauma	
Inflammation, infection	

cally over the involved bone. This is a useful point in differentiating normally irregular navicular bones from those undergoing avascular necrosis (2). This point is of more than just passing interest, for the normal navicular bone not uncommonly is irregular and sclerotic. In the hand, the carpal navicular can undergo posttraumatic avascular necrosis and become irregularly sclerotic, but in children this is not common.

The tarsal and carpal bones also are irregular and sclerotic in multiple epiphyseal dysplasia, punctate epiphyseal dysplasia (stippling and fragmentation), spondyloepiphyseal dysplasia (Fig. 4.95*D*), Morquio disease (resembles spondyloepiphyseal dysplasia), rheumatoid arthritis, Winchester syndrome (storage

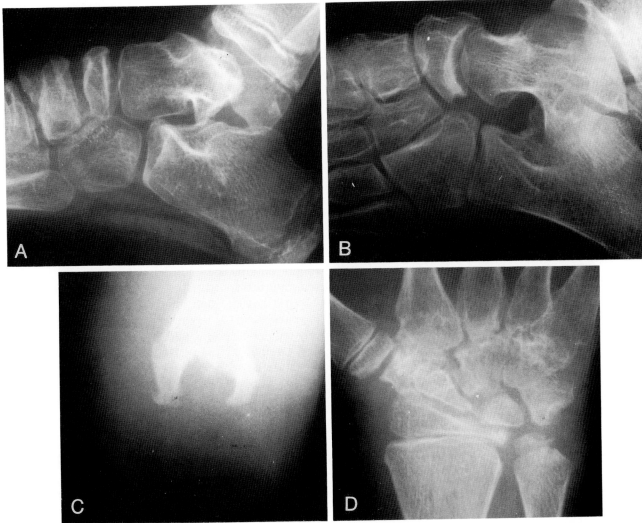

Figure 4.94. Scalloped carpal-tarsal bones. A. Excessive scalloping of the tarsal bones in epiphyseal dysplasia. **B.** Similar scalloping in neurofibromatosis. **C.** Scalloping of calcaneus by neurofibroma. **D.** Scalloped, small, and irregular carpal bones in rheumatoid arthritis.

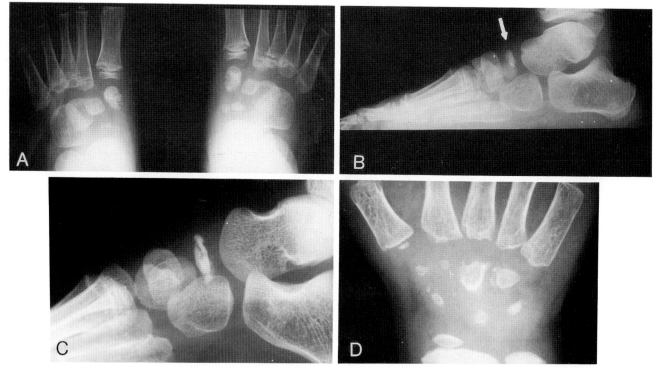

Figure 4.95. Fragmented, irregular carpal and tarsal bones. A. Normal, irregular navicular, and cuneiform bones. **B.** Irregular, small navicular bone *(arrow)*, in normal patient. **C.** Small, irregu-lar and sclerotic navicular bone in Köhler disease. Pain was present in this patient. **D.** Irregular, fragmented, carpal bones in spondyloepiphyseal dysplasia.

disease mimicking rheumatoid arthritis), and after trauma or infection.

REFERENCES

1. Waught W: The ossification and vascularization of the tarsal-navicular and a relation to Kohler's disease. *J Bone Joint Surg* 40B:765, 1958.
2. Weston WJ: Kohler's disease of the tarsal scaphoid. *Australas Radiol* 22:332–337, 1978.

BIPARTITE TARSAL OR CARPAL BONES

Occasionally, one of these bones will be bipartite on a congenital basis. This is especially true in early childhood, before bone formation is complete. A bipartite calcaneus is seen in Larsen syndrome, and an acquired bipartite carpal or tarsal navicular can occur after avascular necrosis.

VERTICAL TALUS

A vertical talus is seen in flat foot deformities, either idiopathic or associated with neurologic or neuromuscular disease (Fig. 4.96). It also is seen with pes calcaneovalgus, a foot deformity commonly present in trisomy-18.

Abnormalities of the Flat Bones
PATELLA

Perhaps the most problematic finding encountered in the patella is **normal irregularity or pseudofragmentation during its development (Fig. 4.97A).** Indeed, when the patella begins to ossify (3–5 years of age), it rather routinely appears fragmented and sclerotic, and, thereafter, an almost endless number of fragmentation configurations can be encountered. A bipartite patella, with two separate ossification centers, also is common, and very often is bilateral. The upper outer quadrant of the patella usually is involved, and the anomaly is best seen on frontal view (Fig. 4.97*B*). A tripartite patella is much less common.

Irregularity of the inferior pole of the patella usually denotes a chronic tendon avulsion injury or Sinding-Larsen-Johansson disease (Fig. 4.97*C*). It is the counterpart of Osgood-Schlatter disease of the tibial tubercle, and in addition to its occurrence in normal, active children, it also commonly is seen in spastic cerebral palsy (5, 7). It should not be confused

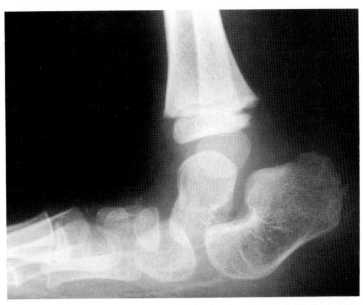

Figure 4.96. Vertical talus. Typical vertical talus in neurogenic flatfoot deformity.

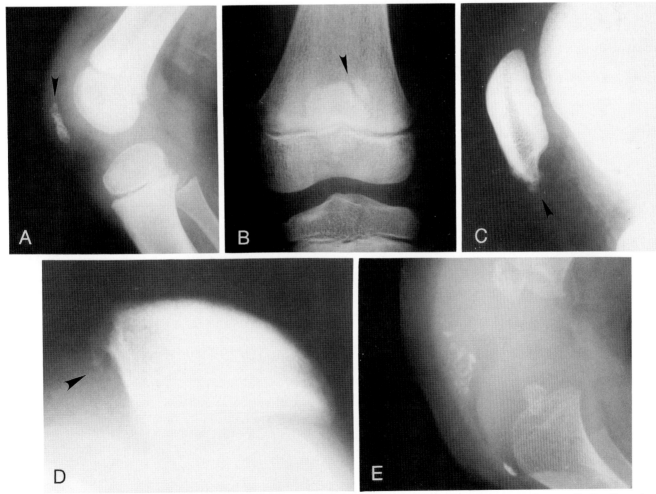

Figure 4.97. Patellar abnormalities. A. Normal, irregular patella of young child *(arrow)*. **B.** Typical fragment of bipartite patella *(arrow)*. **C.** Slight fragmentation of inferior patellar pole *(arrow)* in Sinding-Larsen-Johansson disease. **D.** Small, avulsed medial fragment *(arrow)*, with acute patellar dislocation. **E.** Typical stippled patella in punctate epiphyseal dysplasia.

with normal ossification irregularities of the patella involving the inferior pole (Fig. 4.98).

Dislocation of the Patella

Dislocation of the patella can be acute or chronic, but chronic patellar dislocation is more common. With acute dislocation, by the time roentgenograms are obtained the patella usually reduces to normal position. However, on skyline views with 30°, 60°, and 90° knee flexion, one may see an avulsed fragment of bone medially (Fig. 4.97D). With chronic dislocation, the 30°, 60°, 90° knee flexion (skyline) views are most important. With these views, patellar dislocation can be demonstrated, and in many cases an associated defect on the medial undersurface of the patella is seen. The defect results from the patella riding over the lateral condyle as it dislocates. Chronically dislocating patellae most often occur as isolated abnormalities, but also can be seen in acrocephalosyndactyly (especially Carpenter syndrome), multiple epiphyseal dysplasia, and the Rubinstein-Taybi, Stickler (hereditary arthro-ophthalmopathy), and Larsen syndromes. **Absence or hypoplasia of the patella** occurs in the nail-patella (hereditary osteo-onychodysplasia) syndrome, neurofibromatosis, diastrophic dwarfism, the popliteal pterygium syndrome, bird-headed dwarfism, and on a familial basis in otherwise normal individuals (1, 2).

Defects and Lytic Lesions

Defects and lytic lesions of the patella are not nearly as common as they are in the long bones, but they do occur. Usually they are presumed to be fibrous or cartilaginous in origin (4), but occasionally they can be due to chronic osteomyelitis, histiocytosis-X, or osteochondritis dissecans. Defects produced by other benign tumors and cysts of the patella are relatively rare. Occasionally, one can encounter irregularity along the posterior surface of the patella. Although probably normal, one is never sure that the finding is not due to old osteochondritis dissecans.

Fuzzy, Indistinct Patella

A fuzzy, indistinct patella can be seen with osteomyelitis and any cause of osteomalacia. **Massive destruction of the patella** due to tumors such as Ewing sarcoma, leukemia, metastatic disease, lymphangioma, and hemangioma is rare.

Miscellaneous Abnormalities of the Patella

Punctate patellar calcifications occur in the same conditions as do stippled epiphyses (i.e., punctate epiphyseal dysplasia (Fig. 4.97E), the cerebrohepatorenal, or Zellweger, syndrome, and Warfarin embryonopathy). **Enlargement of the patella** can occur with a number of chronic arthritides, but primarily is seen with rheumatoid arthritis, hemophilic arthropathy, and tuberculous arthritis. Much as with the epiphyses, the patellae in these conditions not only become large, but osteoporotic and glassy as well. In addition, it has been noted that in hemophilia the patella remains rather long, but in rheumatoid arthritis it is short and squat, almost cuboid (3). **Patella alta** denotes a patellar position higher than normal, and the abnormality can be confirmed by specific measurements on lateral view (6). However, in most cases one can make a subjective judgement alone, and the problem occurs in some cases of chronic dislocation (6), spastic cerebral palsy, and on an isolated idiopathic basis.

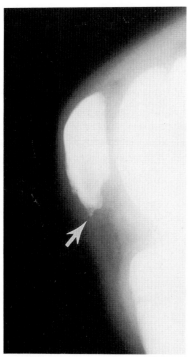

Figure 4.98. Normal inferior patellar pole irregularity. Irregularity of the lower patellar pole *(arrow)* resembles an avulsion injury.

REFERENCES

1. Berhang AM, Levine SA: Familial absence of the patella. *J Bone and Joint Surg* 55:1088, 1973.

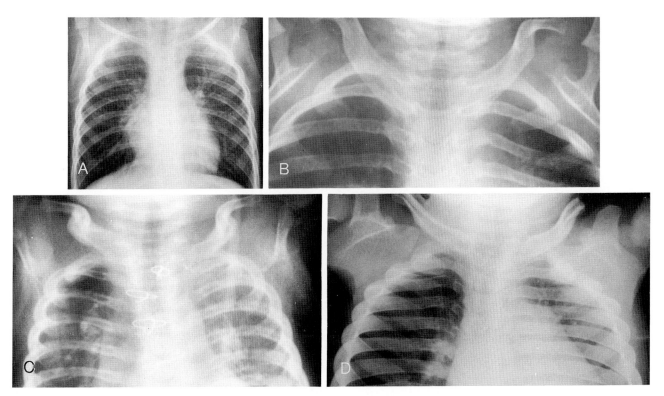

Figure 4.99. Hypoplasia of clavicle. A. Thin clavicles in trisomy-18. **B.** Hypoplastic, somewhat squat and handlebar-shaped clavicles in Holt-Oram syndrome. **C.** Pseudo-handlebar appearance in normal infant due to positioning with upwardly stretched arms. **D.** Short, squat, deformed clavicles in Hurler syndrome.

2. Braun H-St: Familial aplasia or hypoplasia of the patella. *Clin Genet* 13:350, 1978.
3. Chlosta EM, Kuhns LR, Holt JF: The "patellar ratio" in hemophilia and juvenile rheumatoid arthritis. *Radiology* 116:137–138, 1975.
4. Haswell DM, Berne AS, Graham CB: The dorsal defect of the patella. *Pediatr Radiol* 4:238–242, 1976.
5. Kaye JJ, Freiberger RH: Fragmentation of the lower pole of the patella and spastic lower extremities. *Radiology* 101:97, 1971.
6. Lancourt JE, Cristini JA: Patella alta and patella infera. Their etiological role in patellar dislocation, chondromalacia, and apophysitis of the tibial tubercle. *J Bone Joint Surg* 57:1112–1115, 1975.
7. Rosenthal RK, Levine DB: Fragmentation of the distal pole of the patella in spastic cerebral palsy. *J Bone Joint Surg* 59:934–939, 1977.

CLAVICLE

Clavicular **hypoplasia** is not uncommon and occurs with cleidocranial dysostosis, pyknodysostosis, focal dermal hypoplasia (Goltz syndrome), Larsen syndrome, Holt-Oram syndrome, progeria, and trisomy-13 and -18. In the latter three conditions, hypoplasia manifests primarily in **thinness of the clavicle** (Fig. 4.99A), a configuration also commonly seen on a normal basis in premature infants. In Holt-

Oram syndrome, the hypoplastic clavicles often are somewhat squat and **handlebar** in appearance (Fig. 4.99B). The configuration also can be seen in diastrophic dwarfism, camptomelic dwarfism, thrombocytopenia-absent radius syndrome, trisomy-18 (1), and also as a normal variation due to hyperextension of the arms (Fig. 4.99C).

In cleidocranial dysostosis, the clavicle can be hypoplastic, completely absent (Fig. 4.100A), or defective in any of the thirds from which its ossification centers are derived (Fig. 4.100B). When the defect is central, it should be differentiated from that seen with congenital pseudoarthrosis of the clavicle (Fig. 4.100C), a finding usually seen as an isolated phenomenon. In some cases of congenital pseudoarthrosis, the findings are suggestive of an ununited fracture, but in most cases, smoothness and bulbous ends of the remaining portions of the clavicle provide a clue to proper diagnosis.

Short, squat clavicles occur in any of the conditions leading to short, squat tubular bones (see Table 4.3), or conditions with splayed metaphyses (see Table 4.25), but the clavicles may be exceptionally short in the storage diseases (see Fig. 4.99D). As far as **defects of the clavicle** are concerned, most occur

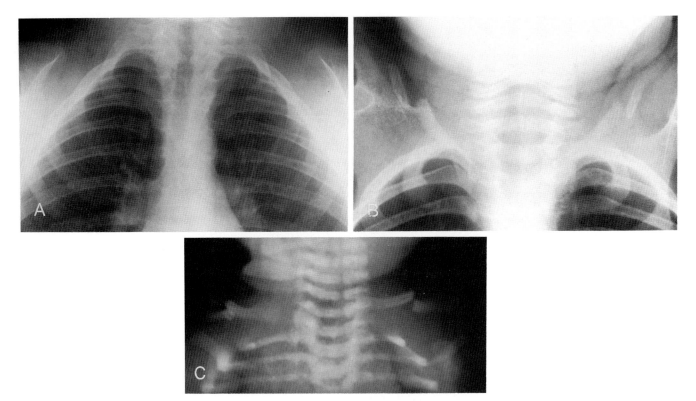

Figure 4.100. Absent and defective clavicles. A. Absent clavicles: cleidocranial dysostosis. **B.** Hypoplastic, defective clavicles in cleidocranial dysostosis. **C.** Bilateral congenital pseudoarthroses of the clavicles. Note smooth, bulbous ends of the clavicular fragments.

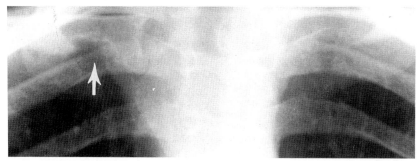

Figure 4.101. Rhomboid fossa. Note typical, normal notch on undersurface of medial aspect of the clavicle *(arrow)*.

after trauma and infection. Overall, however, the normal rhomboid fossa is the most common cause of a clavicular defect. Characteristically, it is located along the lower edge of the medial aspect of the clavicle (Fig. 4.101). **Erosion of the distal end of the clavicle** occurs primarily with hyperparathyroidism (Fig. 4.102A), rheumatoid arthritis, rickets, osteomyelitis, and after trauma. In the healing phase of trauma, the distal end of the clavicle can become quite bulbous and flared, and indeed the finding can be diagnostic in the battered child syndrome (Fig. 4.102B) (2). Other conditions in which distal clavicular erosion occurs include progeria, pyknodysostosis, scleroderma, gout, and the storage diseases.

Destruction, with **narrowing of the acromioclavicular joint,** occurs primarily with pyogenic infections, but also can be seen with rheumatoid arthritis and traumatic dislocation. **Defects and lytic lesions** of the clavicle have the same causes as do those of long bones, and **pseudoarthrosis** of the clavicle has been discussed earlier (see Fig. 4.28). In review, most commonly it is seen on a congenital, anomalous basis and thereafter with nonunited fractures.

REFERENCES

1. Igual M, Giedion A: The lateral clavicle hook: its objective measurement and its diagnostic value in Holt-Oram syn-

drome, diastrophic dwarfism, thrombocytopenia-absent radius syndrome and trisomy 8. *Ann Radiol* 22:136–141, 1979.

2. Kogutt MS, Swischuk LE, Fagan CJ: Patterns of injury and significance of uncommon fractures in the battered child syndrome. *AJR* 121:143–149, 1974.

SCAPULA

Enlargement of the scapula occurs with Caffey infantile cortical hyperostosis, histiocytosis-X, chronic osteomyelitis, metastases and primary tu-

mors such as Ewing sarcoma, malignant fibrous histiocytoma, hemangioma, lymphangioma, and aneurysmal bone cysts (1). Scapular involvement in Caffey disease may be the only lesion present in some infants, and clinically is associated with swelling and redness over the area. Roentgenographically, the enlarged scapula often initially shows fuzzy margins, but thereafter, with periosteal new bone deposition, increased sclerosis is seen around the edges (Fig. 4.103*A*). Generally, Caffey disease does not occur after the age of 5 months and, conse-

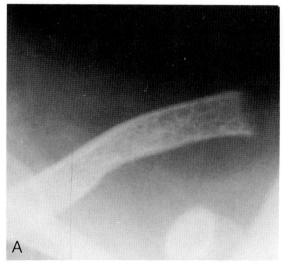

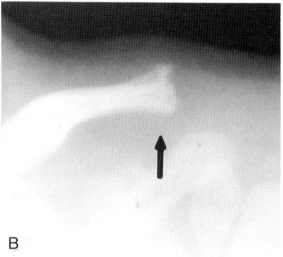

Figure 4.102. Distal clavicular erosion and flaring. A. Note typical erosion and slight cupping of clavicle in hyperparathyroid-ism, secondary to renal osteodystrophy. **B.** Irregular, flared distal clavicle due to fracture in battered child syndrome.

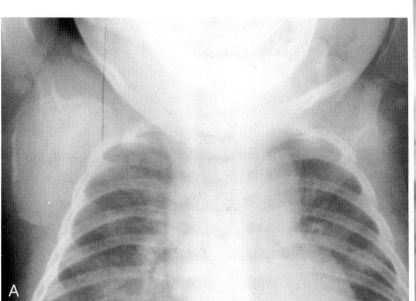

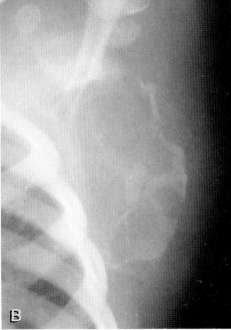

Figure 4.103. Scapular enlargement. A. Note slightly ballooned right scapula with sclerotic edges in healing Caffey disease. **B.** Markedly ballooned, destroyed scapula in histiocytosis-X.

quently, if one sees a similar appearance in an older infant one should consider histiocytosis-X (Fig. 4.103*B*). In addition, currently, Caffey disease is quite rare.

Focal **destruction** has the same etiologies as it does in long bones, but **massive destruction of the scapula** deserves special attention. Such destruction can occur with acute osteomyelitis, metastatic disease, Ewing sarcoma, leukemia, and lymphoma. In terms of lymphoma, malignant fibrous histiocytoma (reticulum cell sarcoma) often is the offender. **Bubbly expansion of the scapula** most often occurs with healing histiocytosis-X, but also can be seen with chronic osteomyelitis, lymphangiomas and hemangiomas, fibrous dysplasia, and aneurysmal bone cyst (1). Solitary cystic lesions of the scapula have the same etiology as do they in any bone in the body, and the problem has been dealt with elsewhere (see Fig. 4.145).

Smallness of the scapula occurs with many of the chondrodystrophies and dwarfing syndromes seen in infancy, but for the most part there is little specificity to the configuration. The only exception might be the small scapula with a **shallow glenoid fossa** commonly seen in the storage diseases (Fig. 4.104**A**). A **small glenoid fossa** also can be seen in the thrombocytopenia-absent radius syndrome and as the result of chronic dislocation of the shoulder (usually neurologic disease). It also can be seen with

simple hypoplasia of the scapula and with Sprengle deformity, a condition where the scapula is rotated and fixed in an abnormally high position (Fig. 4.104*B*). The findings are rather characteristic and often associated with the Klippel-Feil syndrome (fusion-segmentation anomalies of the cervical spine). In some cases, an anomalous bone between the spine and scapula is seen, the "omo-vertebral" bone.

Indistinctness of the scapular edges is seen with severe osteomalacia, and for the most part occurs with rickets and hyperparathyroidism (usually secondary in renal osteodystrophy). In some of these cases, the scapula is so soft that the bottom end becomes bent outward. Irregularity of the acromion process occurs with trauma and, in infants, is virtually pathognomonic of the battered child syndrome (2).

REFERENCES

1. Hope JW, Gould RJ: Scapular lesions in childhood. *AJR* 88:496–502, 1962.
2. Kogutt MS, Swischuk WE, Fagan CJ: Patterns of injury and significance of uncommon fractures in the battered child syndrome. *AJR* 121:143–149, 1974.

PELVIS

There are a number of findings in the pelvis that are useful in the differential diagnosis of various

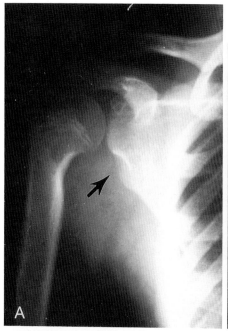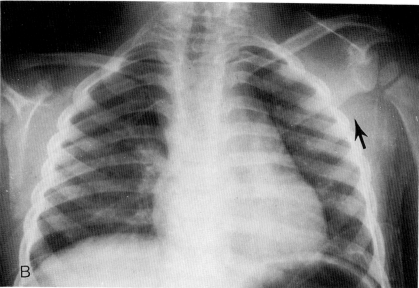

Figure 4.104. **A. Shallow, hypoplastic glenoid fossa** *(arrow)* in Hurler disease. The scapula also is hypoplastic. Also note notch in upper humerus. **B. Sprengel deformity.** Note typical upwardly rotated left scapula *(arrow)*.

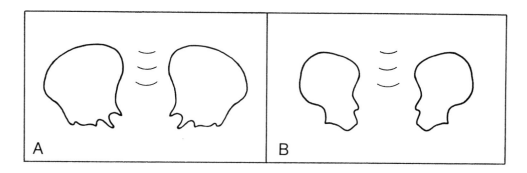

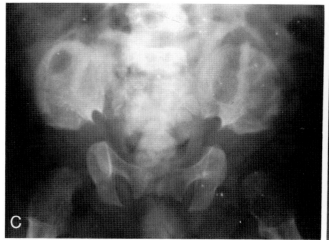
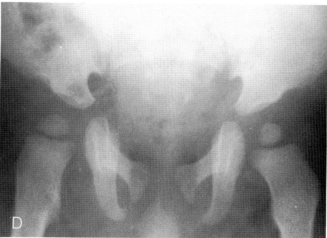

Figure 4.105. Pelvis: squared iliac wings. A. In the **type A pelvis,** the iliac wings are markedly underdeveloped, very square, and show considerable irregularity of the acetabular roofs. **B.** In the **type B pelvis,** changes are less pronounced and the iliac wings are less square and more tapered. **C.** Typical **type A pelvis** in achondroplasia. **D.** Typical **type B pelvis** in Hurler disease.

syndromes and dysplasias, but one of the more common is the small, **squared iliac wing.** In these cases, the iliac wings are smaller than normal, appear rotated outwardly, and are associated with flat acetabular roofs or angles (5). Basically, two types can be identified, arbitrarily designated as types A and B (Fig. 4.105). **In type A,** the iliac wings are more hypoplastic and outwardly rotated. They also appear more square, have deep sciatic notches, and have a crinkled or irregular acetabular roof. All of these changes tend to become less pronounced as the patient grows older. **In the type B wing,** there is less hypoplasia and a more normal appearance of the sciatic notch and acetabular roof. The inferior portion of the iliac wing still is hypoplastic, but more tapered in appearance than square (Fig. 4.105B). A list of conditions producing these iliac wing deformities is presented in Table 4.35.

Narrowing of the lower iliac wing similar to that seen in the type B pelvic configuration also can be seen with the Melnick-Needles syndrome. It also oc-

curs with chronic hip dislocation (i.e., idiopathic or with the trisomy-18 and Larsen syndromes). Narrowing is enhanced by the development of a pseudo-acetabulum above the normal acetabulum (Fig. 4.106). In addition to these causes, narrowing of the waist of the iliac wing can occur with bone-deforming conditions such as neurofibromatosis and hemangiomas or lymphangiomas in the area (see Fig. 4.39B).

Flat or Steep Acetabular Angles

Flat acetabular angles occur in most of the chondrodystrophies demonstrating the type A pelvis and square iliac wing (see Table 4.35). Otherwise, flat acetabular angles are due to outwardly flared iliac wings and are characteristic of trisomy 21 (Fig. 4.107A). Steep acetabular angles are due to inward turning of the iliac wings, are characteristic of trisomy-18 (Fig. 4.107C), and also occur with congenital hip dislocation (Fig. 4.107B).

Table 4.35
Small Squared and Flared Iliac Wings—Decreased Acetabular Angle

Type A
Achondroplasia
Achondrogenesis
Asphyxiating thoracic dystrophy
Ellis-van Creveld syndrome
Short rib-polydactyly syndromes
Metatropic dwarfism
Kniest syndrome
Spondyloepiphyseal dysplasia congenita
Punctate epiphyseal dysplasia: rhizomelic form
Thanatophoric dwarfism
Morquio disease
Severe metaphyseal dysostoses
Dyggve-Melchior-Clausen syndrome
Immune deficiency syndromes

Type B
Trisomy-21: Down syndrome
Mucopolysaccharidoses: except Morquio
Mucolipidoses
Other storage diseases
Cleidocranial dysostosis
Cockayne syndrome
Acrocephalosyndactyly
Aminopterin-induced syndrome
Arthrogryposis
Cornelia de Lange syndrome
Hypophosphatasia
Popliteal pterygium syndrome
Osteo-onchodysplasia
Prune-belly syndrome
Rubinstein-Taybi syndrome
Bladder extrophy
Sacral agenesis
Trisomy-13, -18
Metaphyseal dysostoses: mild cases
Osteogenesis imperfecta
Weissenbacher-Zweymuller syndrome
Larsen syndrome
Congenital dislocating hip
Melnick-Needles syndrome

Delayed or Defective Ossification of the Pubic Bones

This type of ossification is not uncommon in normal premature infants, but, on a pathologic basis, occurs in certain syndromes (2, 3). For example, the pubic bones are underossified in most of the neonatal and infantile chondrodystrophies, but the finding is not utilized for specific diagnosis. On the other hand, it is a specific finding in cleidocranial dysostosis (Fig. 4.108A). It also is used as an adjunctive finding in punctate epiphyseal dysplasia, spondyloepiphyseal dysplasia congenita (Fig. 4.108B), Wolf (chromosome 4p) syndrome, and the Taybi-Lindner syndrome. In all of these conditions, because the pubic bones are unossified, the **interpubic distance is increased.** Other conditions where the distance is increased, but not necessarily associated with hypoplastic pubic bones, include extrophy of the bladder, cryptophthalmia syndrome, prune-belly syndrome, Sjögren-Larsson syndrome, Goltz syndrome, epispadias, and occasionally hypospadias. Separation of the pubic bones also can be seen with diastasis recti and has been noted in patients demonstrating anorectal, genital, and urinary tract abnormalities (3). Acquired widening of the pubic symphysis is seen after trauma, osteomyelitis, and, rarely, with destructive tumors.

Protusio Acetabuli

Protusio acetabuli is uncommon in the pediatric age group, but can be seen with Turner syndrome, osteogenesis imperfecta, Still's disease (juvenile rheumatoid arthritis), and renal osteodystrophy (Fig. 4.109).

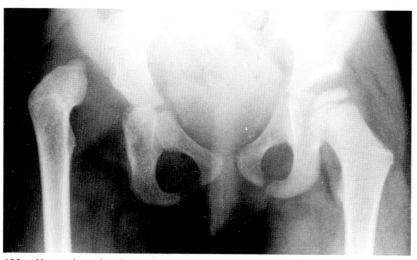

Figure 4.106. **Narrowing of waist or lower part of iliac bone.** Narrowed iliac waist *(arrow)* in chronic congenital hip dislocation with pseudoacetabulum formation.

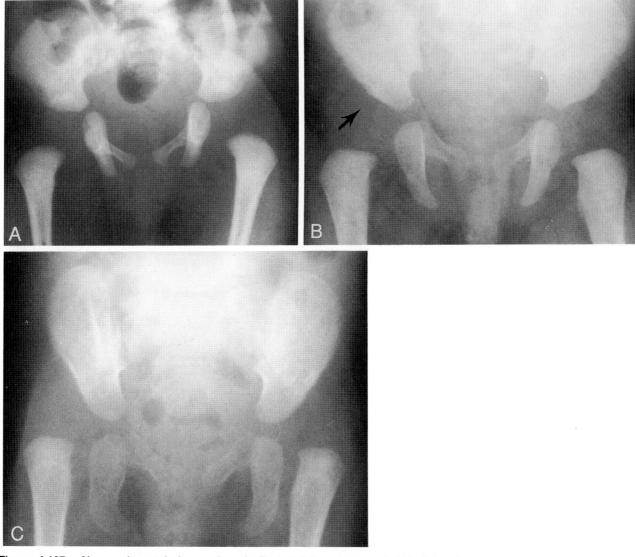

Figure 4.107. Abnormal acetabular angles. A. Typical flat acetabular roof in trisomy-21. Also note flat acetabular roofs in achondroplasia in Figure 4.105C. **B.** Increased acetabular slope in congenital hip dislocation on the right *(arrow)*. **C.** Note bilateral increased acetabular slope in trisomy-18. Both hips also are dislocated.

Miscellaneous Abnormalities

Exostoses from the iliac wing (Fong lesion) have been dealt with elsewhere (see Fig. 4.45B). **Complete destruction of the pelvic bones** occurs in the same conditions as with any bone (e.g., acute osteomyelitis, malignant sarcomas, metastatic disease, hemangioma, lymphangioma), and cysts, bony tumors, and osteomyelitis appear much the same as they do in other bones of the body.

Abnormal Configurations of the Sacroiliac Joints

These abnormal configurations are not particularly common, and apart from a variety of congenital articulation disturbances between the sacrum and iliac bone, consist primarily of **abnormal widening of the sacroiliac joint.** In many cases, there is associated sclerosis of the joint edges, and the commonest causes of this configuration are trauma (Fig. 4.110A), infection, or inflammation. Infection can be pyogenic (Fig. 4.110B) or tuberculous, whereas inflammation usually is due to rheumatoid arthritis. Widening secondary to acute trauma is self-evident but, on a chronic basis, can be seen in the child with a longstanding limp. In such children, the findings are the result of chronic stresses sustained by the joint as a result of the limp. In most of these conditions, the findings are difficult to distinguish from one another, and when osteomyelitis is suspected, bone scanning should be utilized (1, 4, 6). However,

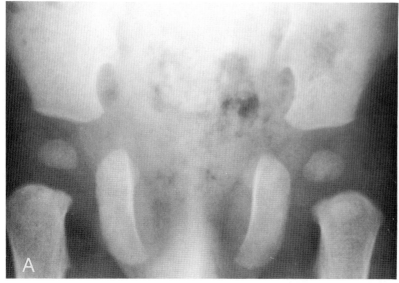
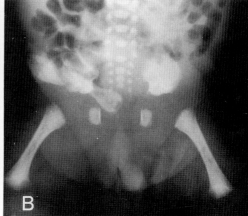

Figure 4.108. Delayed or defective ossification of pubic bones. A. Virtual absence of pubic rami in cleidocranial dys- ostosis. **B.** Hypoplastic pubic rami in spondyloepiphyseal dyspla- sia congenita.

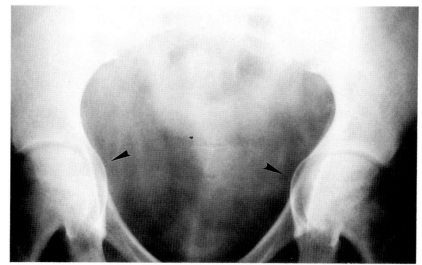

Figure 4.109. Protusio acetabuli. Note inward bulging of medial acetabular margins *(arrow)* in long- standing renal osteodystrophy.

the bone scan will not necessarily confirm that osteo- myelitis is the problem, for it is a nonspecific screen- ing modality and also is positive after trauma and conditions such as rheumatoid arthritis. Computed tomography also is very useful for detecting subtle sacroiliac joint widening (Fig. 4.110C).

REFERENCES

1. Ailsby RL, Stheli LT: Pyogenic infections of the sacroiliac joint in children: radioisotope bone scanning as a diagnos- tic tool. *Clin Orthop* 100:96–100, 1974.

2. Cortina H, Vallcanera A, Andres V, Gracia A, Aparici R, Mari A: The non-ossified pubis. *Pediatr Radiol* 8:87–92, 1979.

3. Muecke EC, Currarino G: Congenital widening of the pubic symphysis. *AJR* 103:179–185, 1968.

4. Schaad UB, McCracken GH Jr, Nelson JD: Pyogenic ar- thritis of the sacroiliac joint in pediatric patients. *Pediat- rics* 66:375–379, 1980.

5. Taybi H, Kane P: Small acetabular and iliac angles and associated diseases. *Radiol Clin North Am* 6:215–221, 1968.

6. Trauner DA, Connor JD: Radioactive scanning in diagnosis of acute sacroiliac osteomyelitis. *J Pediatr* 87:751–753, 1975.

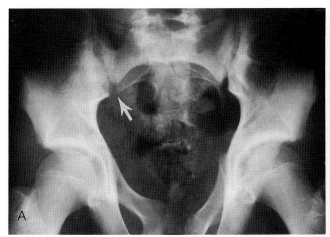

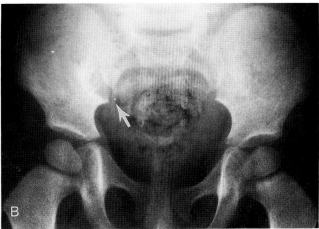

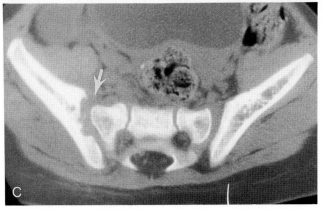

Figure 4.110. Sacroiliac joint abnormalities. A. Widening of the sacroiliac joint *(arrow)* in pelvic trauma. **B.** Widened, indis- tinct joint in acute pyogenic infection *(arrow).* **C.** CT demonstra- ting wide, irregular sacroiliac joint *(arrow)* secondary to infection.

STERNUM

Hypersegmentation of the sternum occurs in the trisomy-21, and **undersegmentation** in the trisomy-18 syndrome (Fig. 4.111*A* and *B*). Undersegmenta- tion also occurs in camptomelic dwarfism, Noonan syndrome, and the Brachmann-de Lange syndrome and, in all of these conditions, often is associated with hypoplasia and premature fusion of the ster- num. A **pectus carinatum** deformity (Fig. 4.112*A* and *B*) may result, and also can be seen in congenital heart disease, especially the chronic cyanotic variety (2–6). Pectus carinatum also can occur as an isolated finding, but on an isolated basis **pectus excavatum** is more common (Fig. 4.112*C* and *D*). A pectus exca- vatum deformity of the chest also occurs any time the bones are softened (e.g., osteomalacia, newborn with respiratory distress) and after trauma with a flail chest.

Retrosternal thickening of the soft tissues most commonly is due to some disease process in the ster- num, such as tumor, extramedulary hematopoiesis, osteomyelitis, or trauma, and often the soft tissue thickening is localized or undulating. However, it also can appear as a more uniform retrosternal arc. The latter configuration also can be seen with pleu- ral fluid accumulations and the hypogenetic right lung syndrome (see Fig. 1.15*D*). A rare cause of lo- calized thickening of the retrosternal soft tissues, just behind the manubrium, is posterior dislocation of the medial end of the clavicle. A congenital **bifid sternum** can occur as an incidental anomaly or with ectopia cordis (1), and lytic and destructive lesions of the sternum have the same differential diagnosis as they do with other bones of the skeleton.

REFERENCES

1. Chang CH, Davis WC: Congenital bifid sternum with par- tial ectopia cordis. *AJR* 86:513–516, 1961.
2. Currarino G, Silverman FN: Premature obliteration of the sternal sutures and pigeon-breast deformity. *Radiology* 70:532–540, 1958.
3. Fischer KC, White RI, Jordan CE, Dorst JP, Neill CA: Sternal abnormalities in patients with congenital heart disease. *AJR* 119:530–538, 1973.
4. Gabrielsen TO, Ladyman GH: Early closure of the sternal

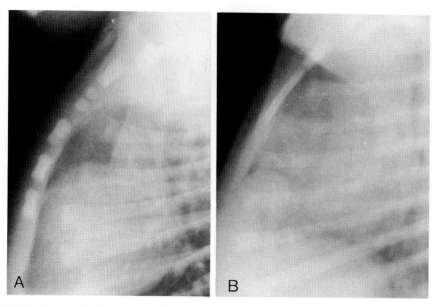

Figure 4.111. Segmentation abnormalities of sternum. A. Note hypersegmentation of sternum in trisomy-21. **B.** Undersegmentation of sternum in trisomy-18.

sutures and congenital heart disease. *AJR* 89:975–983, 1963.
5. Kim OH, Gooding CA: Delayed sternal ossification in infants with congenital heart disease. *Pediatr Radiol* 10:219–223, 1981.
6. Lees RF, Caldicott WJH: Sternal anomalies and congenital heart disease. *AJR* 124:423–427, 1975.

RIBS

Abnormalities of rib shape consist of under- or overtubulation, cupped or straight anterior rib ends, rib notching, twisted ribs, and rib defects (Table 4.36). Other abnormalities also occur, but basically these are no different from those that occur in other bones of the body (e.g., destructive lesions, fractures, demineralization, periosteal new bone).

Overtubulation of the ribs leads to **thin ribs,** while undertubulation causes **short, broad ribs.** Basically, the same conditions producing these abnormalities in the long bones and clavicles also produce them in the ribs, and most are documented in Tables 4.3 and 4.4. However, thin ribs are most pronounced in premature infants, trisomy 18, progeria, and osteogenesis imperfecta. **Wide, paddle-shaped ribs** constitute a specific type of rib widening where there is a short and narrow posterior, juxtaspinal segment, and then broadening out of the rib to produce a paddle shape. Almost exclusively, this configuration occurs in the storage diseases (Fig. 4.113), but not all of the conditions in this group of diseases produce the same degree of change and, actually, the most profound changes are seen in Hurler disease,

Hunter disease, mucopolysaccharidosis IV (Marateaux-Lamy), mucolipidosis II (I cell disease), and generalized gangliosidosis.

Cupping or Straightening of the Ribs

Cupping (Fig. 4.114) is comparable to splaying of the metaphyses of the long bones, and the causes of both are very similar (see Table 4.25). Traumatic cupping resulting from healing costochondral injuries (Fig. 4.114C) is nearly pathognomonic of the battered child syndrome in infants (3). **Undue straightening of the anterior rib ends** (Fig. 4.114D) occurs when bone growth is impaired, and most often is seen with hypothyroidism, osteopetrosis, and the storage diseases (mucopolysaccharidoses, mucolipidoses, and gangliosidosis). Usually, normal anterior rib ends show slight cupping, but in these conditions they appear rather straight.

Rib Notching

This is not overly common in childhood but, when seen, most often is due to coarctation of the aorta (1, 2, 9). Notches in this condition occur on the inferior surface of the ribs (most often, fourth through eighth ribs) and usually are seen in the older child (Fig. 4.115A). Even then, however, only about one half of the cases of coarctation of the aorta demonstrate the finding. The next most common cause of rib notching is normal variation, where slight undulations of the

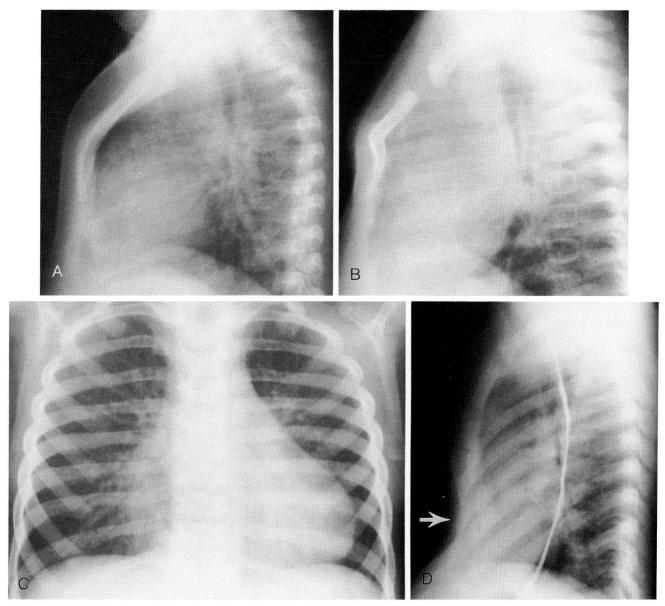

Figure 4.112. Pectus deformity. A. Typical bulging chest of pectus carinatum deformity in patient with congenital heart disease. **B.** Another patient with a pectus carinatum deformity. **C.** Pectus excavatum deformity leading to shift of the mediastinum to the left, downward slanting of the anterior ribs, a more horizontal position of the posterior ribs, and apparent infiltrate along the right cardiac border. **D.** Lateral view showing dipping sternum *(arrow)* characteristic of the pectus excavatum deformity.

inferior rib margins may suggest notching. Most often the finding is very subtle and overlooked. Thereafter, unilateral notching can be seen with Blalock-Taussig shunts for tetralogy of Fallot or other similar congenital heart lesions. In these patients, because the subclavian artery is anastomosed to the hypoplastic pulmonary artery, arterial flow to the involved extremity is diminished, and over the years collateral circulation and rib notching develop. Notching or undulation of the lower rib margins also can occur with neurofibromatosis, Melnick-Needles osteodysplasia, from collateral circulation in long-standing pulmonary valve atresia or pulmonary trunk agenesis (i.e., the old, "persistent" truncus arteriosis type IV), superior vena caval obstruction, arteriovenous fistula of the chest wall, intercostal nerve tumors, intercostal arteritis, and poliomyelitis. All of these, however, are rare in childhood and, thus on a practical basis, when rib notching is seen in a child, it either is normal, associated with coarctation of the aorta, or secondary to a Blalock-Taussig shunt.

Table 4.36
Rib Abnormalities

Anterior rib cupping[a]

Anterior rib straightening	
Hypothyroidism	
Osteopetrosis	} Common
Storage diseases	
Rib notching	
Coarctation of aorta	} Common
Postoperative Blalock-Taussig shunt	} Moderately common
Normal	
Neurofibromatosis	} Relatively rare
Melnick-Needles osteodysplasia	
Collaterals with pulmonary valve atresia	
Superior vena cava obstruction	
Arteriovenous fistula of the chest wall	} Rare
Intercostal nerve tumors	
Intercostal arteritis	
Poliomyelitis	

[a]Same as metaphyseal cupping (see Table 4.25).

Rib Defects

Rib defects are not particularly common in children, but can be seen after infection, surgery, or fracture. On a congenital basis, they occur in the cerebro-costo-mandibular syndrome (10), and the finding is rather pathognomonic (Fig. 4.115B). Associated smallness of the mandible in this condition has caused most to consider it a variation of the Pierre-Robin syndrome (5, 8).

Twisted Ribs

Twisted ribs can be seen with neurofibromatosis (Fig. 4.116A and B), the basal cell nevus syndrome, Melnick-Needles osteodysplasia (6) (Fig. 4.116C), spondylothoracic dysplasia (4, 7), congenital hypoplasia with synostosis, and after thoracotomy. In most of these conditions, the ribs also are thinned, but in neurofibromatosis, they can be wide and ribbon-like (Fig. 4.116B).

Destructive Lesions

These lesions have the same differential diagnosis as they do in long and other flat bones, but massive destruction usually occurs with osteomyelitis, histiocytosis-X (Fig. 4.117A), Ewing sarcoma (Fig. 4.117B and C), metastatic disease, leukemia, lymphoma, and hemangioma or lymphangioma. In the latter, very often the bone is totally dissolved (i.e., vanishing bone disease [see Fig. 4.39]). With Ewing sarcoma and histiocytosis-X, the destroyed rib also may be expanded (Fig. 4.117A and C).

Lumpy Target Lesions

Lumpy, target lesions of the ribs are seen with healing rib fractures (Fig. 4.117D). The finding re-

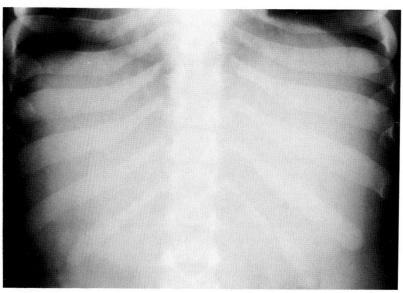

Figure 4.113. **Wide paddle-shaped ribs** characteristic of Hurler disease. Note marked narrowing posteriorly and considerable broadening laterally.

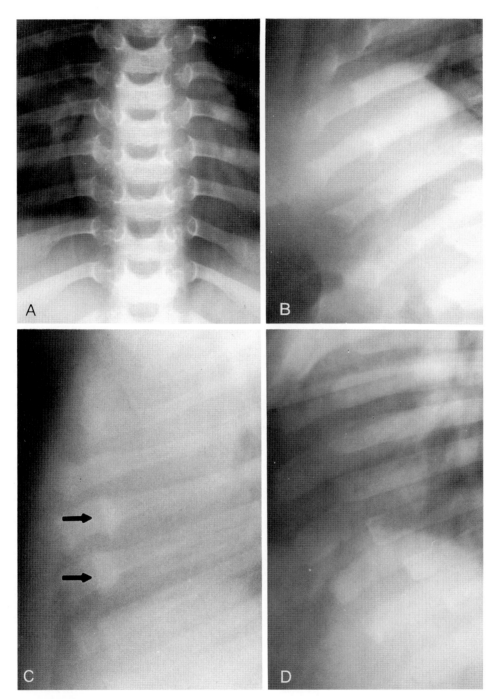

Figure 4.114. Cupping of the ribs. A. Cupping of the ribs in spondyloepiphyseal dysplasia. **B.** Same patient showing anterior cupping. **C.** Cupping of two ribs *(arrows)* in costochondral injury in battered child syndrome. **D. Undue straightening of anterior rib ends** in Hurler disease.

sults from callus formation, and also can be seen with rib infarction in sickle cell disease and with healing after destruction secondary to infection or tumor. As far as fractures are concerned, most often they are sustained in the battered child syndrome.

REFERENCES

1. Babbitt DP, Cassidy GE, Godard JE: Rib notching in aortic coarctation during infancy and early childhood. *Radiology* 110:169–171, 1974.
2. Gooding CA, Glickman MG, Suydam MJ: Fate of rib notching after correction of aortic coarctation. *Am J Roentgenol Radium Ther Nucl Med* 106:21–23, 1969.

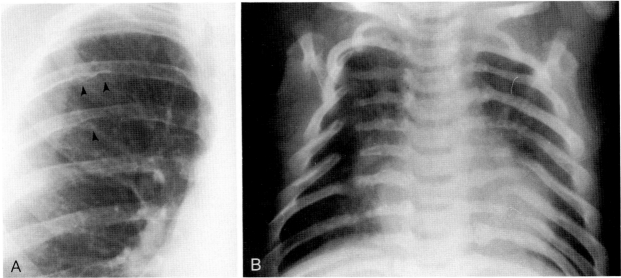

Figure 4.115. **A.** Rib notching. Typical rib notching *(arrows)* in coarctation of the aorta. **B. Rib defects.** Typical extensive rib defects in cerebrocostomandibular syndrome. (Reproduced with permission from Williams HJ, Sane SM: Cerebro-costo-mandibular syndrome: long-term follow-up of a patient and review of the literature. *AJR* 126:1223–1228, 1976).

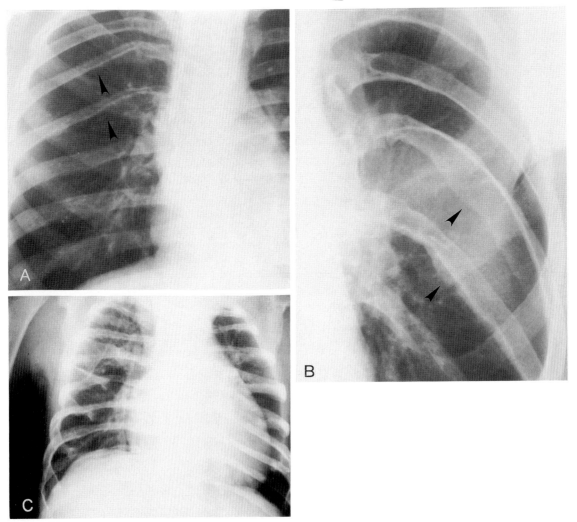

Figure 4.116. **Twisted ribs. A.** Thin, slightly twisted ribs in neurofibromatosis *(arrows)*. **B.** Twisted, ribbon-like ribs in neurofibromatosis *(arrows)*. **C.** Twisted, thin ribs in Melnick-Needles osteodysplasia.

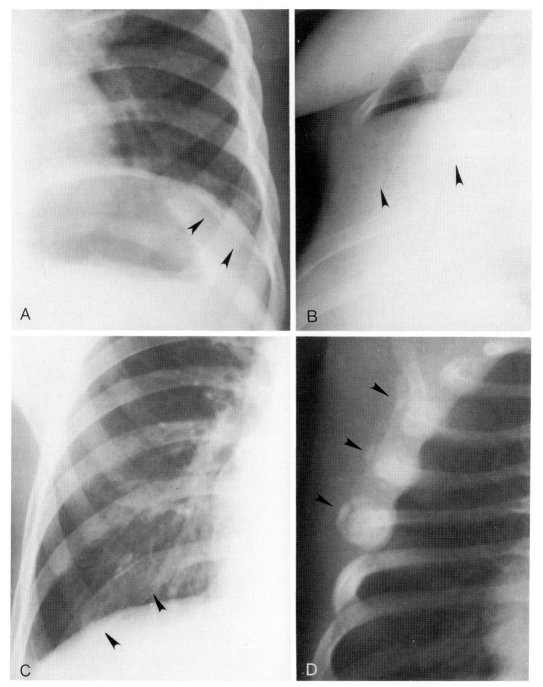

Figure 4.117. Massive destruction of ribs. A. Destruction, with expansion of rib in histiocytosis-X *(arrows).* **B.** Completely destroyed rib in Ewing sarcoma *(arrows).* **C.** Widespread destruction with moderate expansion of a rib in Ewing sarcoma *(arrows).* **D. Lumpy target lesion of rib.** Multiple target lesions *(arrows)* of ribs due to healing rib fractures in the battered child syndrome.

3. Kogutt MS, Swischuk LE, Fagan CJ: Patterns of injury and significance of uncommon fractures in the battered child syndrome. *AJR* 121:143–149, 1974.

4. Kozlowski K: Spondylo-costal dysplasia-severe and moderate types: report of 8 cases. *Australas Radiol* 25:81–90, 1981.

5. Leroy JG, Devos EA, Bulcke LJV, Robbe NS: Cerebro-costo-mandibular syndrome with autosomal dominant inheritance. *J Pediatr* 99:441–443, 1981.

6. Melnick JC, Needles CF: An undiagnosed bone dysplasia: a 2 family study of 4 generations and 3 generations. *AJR* 97:39–48, 1966.

7. Moseley JE, Bonforte RJ: Spondylothoracic dysplasia: a syndrome of congenital anomalies. *AJR* 106:166–169, 1969.

8. Silverman FN, Strefling AM, Stevenson DK, Lazarus J: Cerebro-costo-mandibular syndrome. *J Pediatr* 97:406–416, 1980.

9. Sloan RD, Cooley RN: Coarctation of aorta: roentgenologic aspects of one hundred and twenty-five surgically confirmed cases. *Radiology* 61:701–721, 1953.
10. Williams HJ, Sane SM: Cerebro-costo-mandibular syndrome; long term follow-up of a patient and review of the literature. *AJR* 126:1223–1228, 1976.

Joint Abnormalities

JOINT SPACE WIDENING

Widening of the joint space can occur because of (a) traumatic dislocation, (b) joint laxity, (c) synovial thickening, and (d) joint fluid accumulation (Table 4.37). In the pediatric age group, the latter is most common but occurs almost exclusively in the shoulder and hip (Fig. 4.118A and B). Lateral dislocation of the humerus or femur occurs readily with fluid accumulation in these joints (1), especially in infants and young children; but, in the other joints, the ligaments and capsules are too strong to allow much distraction of the bones. As far as the type of fluid is concerned, no specificity exists because it can be blood, serous effusion, or pus. Traumatic effusions or hemarthroses and pyogenic exudates are most common, however. Indeed, in children, in the absence of trauma, pus (septic arthritis) should be considered the diagnosis until proven otherwise.

Serous effusions are seen with rheumatoid arthritis, the collagen vascular diseases, tuberculous arthritis, and other chronic arthritides. In the hip, one also can add toxic or transient synovitis (3) and Legg-Perthes disease. In Legg-Perthes disease, joint space widening probably is due to a combination of joint fluid accumulation and joint laxity, while in toxic synovitis, the problem is simple joint effusion. In the latter, however, only a few of the more severe cases accumulate enough fluid to develop visible joint widening. Indeed, most cases demonstrate very little in the way of roentgenographic change or systemic reaction. Clinically, the problem is a limp of rather sudden onset, and although viral infection and/or subclinical trauma have been suggested as causes, the etiology remains unknown. Transient synovitis is rare in other joints, but we believe that we have seen it in the shoulder and knee.

Hemarthroses leading to joint space widening most often occur with trauma, but occasionally can be seen with bleeding disorders, vascular synovial tumors, or with chronic inflammation of the synovium. Inflammatory synovial thickening most often occurs with tuberculous arthritis, hemophilic arthropathy, rheumatoid arthritis, Winchester syndrome (storage disease which looks like rheumatoid arthritis), Farber lipogranulomatosis, and pigmented villinodular synovitis. The latter three conditions are quite rare, and in all of the conditions it should be noted that, while synovial thickening first produces joint space widening, eventually it leads to cartilage destruction and joint space narrowing. This phenomenon occurs at different rates in the various conditions, with the slowest being tuberculous and fungal arthritis. Indeed, it may take many months before any significant joint space narrowing is seen, because there are few proteolytic enzymes produced by tuberculosis infections. With rampant pyogenic arthritis, on the other hand, proteolytic enzymes

Table 4.37
Joint Space Widening and Narrowing

Joint space widening[a]	
Pyogenic arthritis: hip, shoulder	
Traumatic effusion or hemarthrosis: hip, shoulder	Common
Toxic (transient) synovitis: usually hip	
Developmental hip dysplasia	
Rheumatoid arthritis	
Traumatic dislocation	
Joint laxity: neurogenic-neuromuscular	Moderately common
Tuberculous arthritis	
Fungal arthritis	
Pigmented villinodular synovitis	
Ligamentum teres rupture: hip	
Retained cartilage fragment: hip	
Synovial tumors	
Winchester syndrome	Relatively rare
Congenital dislocation—other joints	
Farber lipogranulomatosis	
Larsen syndrome	
Desbuquois syndrome	
Joint space narrowing	
Septic arthritis	Common
Rheumatoid arthritis	
Hemophilic arthropathy	
Tuberculous arthritis	Moderately common
Fungal arthritis	
Degenerative arthritis	
Slipped capital femoral epiphysis: postoperative	
Pigmented villinodular synovitis	
Winchester syndrome	Relatively rare
Degenerative arthritis: primary	
Traumatic dislocation	
Farber lipogranulomatosis	

[a] Also use for joint dislocation.

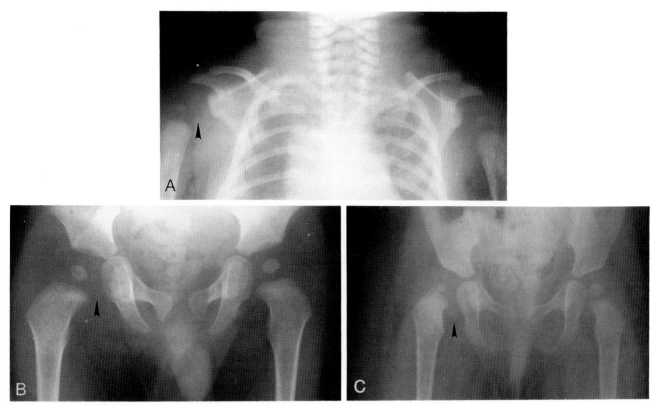

Figure 4.118. Joint space widening. A. Typical widening of the right shoulder joint *(arrows)* in septic arthritis. **B.** Similar widening of right hip joint *(arrows)* in infant with septic arthritis. **C.** Widening of the right hip joint *(arrow)* with congenital dislocation. Note delayed ossification of right femoral head and increased steepness of acetabular roof.

abound and joint cartilage destruction occurs rapidly. Consequently, the joint space may narrow within a few days. With rheumatoid arthritis, one may go for months or years without significant narrowing, and then, after a serious exacerbation, a joint may narrow within weeks.

Traumatic dislocation with widening of the joint space is self-evident and, in such cases, not only is the joint space widened, but the involved bone is so out of position that the diagnosis is relatively obvious. Joint dislocations in children are less common than in adults, because most often an epiphyseal-metaphyseal fracture occurs rather than a joint dislocation. The reason for this is that, in a growing bone, the epiphyseal-metaphyseal junction is a weak area, and forces are dissipated through it before they are exerted on the joint proper. Nonetheless, joint dislocations still can occur, and one of the most peculiar is that which results from rupture of the ligamentum teres in the hip. In such cases, no bony abnormality is seen, but there is a lateral displacement of the femur causing widening of the joint space. In other cases of traumatic dislocation of the hip, a piece of avulsed, unossified cartilage may remain in

the joint. This prevents the joint from reducing, and chronic joint space widening results. The finding should serve as a signal for the presence of the cartilage fragment (2), which can then be detected with CT.

Congenital dislocations occur in any joint, but, again, are most common in the hip (i.e., developmental dysplasias of the hip). In this condition, joint space widening is associated with outward and upward displacement of the femur, dysplasia and underdevelopment of the acetabular roof, increase in its pitch, and loss of its normal cupping (Fig. 4.118C). All of these acetabular changes occur because of the lack of normal femoral head articulation, and are not seen with dislocation due to fluid accumulation. With fluid accumulation, the acetabular roof is normal, and displacement of the femoral head is predominantly in the lateral direction. If it occurs in any other direction, usually it is downward. Joint space widening due to laxity of the muscles and tendons around the joint almost always is the result of underlying neurologic or neuromuscular disease. However, in some cases of septic arthritis, enough destruction of the ligaments and joint capsule occurs

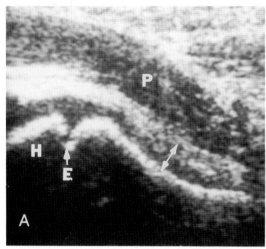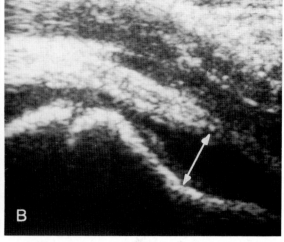

Figure 4.119. Hip joint fluid: ultrasound findings. A. Normal side. Note space between the femoral neck and joint capsule *(arrow).* **B. Abnormal side.** Fluid distends this space *(arrow).* Femoral head *(H)*, epiphyseal line *(E)*, psoas muscle *(P)*.

to cause chronic laxity and joint space widening. In addition, it is seen in conditions such as the Larsen and Desbuquois syndromes where ligament laxity is present.

Joint fluid causing joint widening, especially in the hip, now is best evaluated with ultrasound where widening of the joint space between the femoral head and joint capsule are readily demonstrable (Fig. 4.119).

REFERENCES

1. Hayden CK Jr, Swischuk LE: Paraarticular soft tissue changes in infections and trauma of the lower extremity in children. *AJR* 134:307–311, 1980.
2. Smith GR, Loop JW: Radiologic classification of posterior dislocation of the hip: refinements and pitfalls. *Radiology* 119:569–574, 1976.
3. Neuhauser EBD, Wittenborg MH: Synovitis of the hip in infancy and childhood. *Radiol Clin North Am* 1:13–16, 1963.

JOINT SPACE NARROWING

Joint space narrowing occurs with (a) traumatic joint dislocation and (b) joint cartilage destruction (Table 4.37). In the former, the finding is due to overlap of the dislocated bones, a finding easily demonstrable on a view taken at right angles to the one showing the narrowing. Cartilage destruction causing joint space narrowing occurs with a number of diseases, but most often is seen with septic arthritis (Fig. 4.120A). Thereafter, one should consider rheumatoid arthritis (Fig. 4.120B), hemophilic arthropathy, and tuberculous and fungal arthritis. However,

it should be remembered that joint space narrowing with tuberculosis and fungal infections occurs only after many months, because with tuberculous and fungal infections, proteolytic enzyme activity and subsequent cartilage destruction are minimal. With septic arthritis, on the other hand, proteolytic activity is high and cartilage destruction rapid. The incidence of tuberculous and fungal arthritis varies from one geographic location to another.

Less common causes of joint space narrowing include pigmented villinodular synovitis, Winchester syndrome, primary degenerative arthritis (very rare in children), Farber lipogranulomatosis, Stickler hereditary arthrophthalmopathy, and slipped capital femoral epiphysis. In the latter condition, cartilage destruction and joint space narrowing occur, but usually only after surgical intervention (3). It is not known just why this happens, but it is believed to result from an autoimmune phenomenon. The problem generally is not particularly debilitating and not overly common. Joint space narrowing with degenerative arthritis in children is rare except as it occurs secondarily, as a long-term complication of Legg-Perthes disease, other causes of avascular necrosis, septic arthritis, and trauma.

JOINT HYPER- AND HYPOMOBILITY

These abnormalities are more readily assessed clinically than radiographically, for often there is very little in the way of roentgenographic change. As far as **hypermobility** is concerned, one should consider the following conditions: trisomy-21, Marfan syndrome, Morquio disease, Ehlers-Danlos syn-

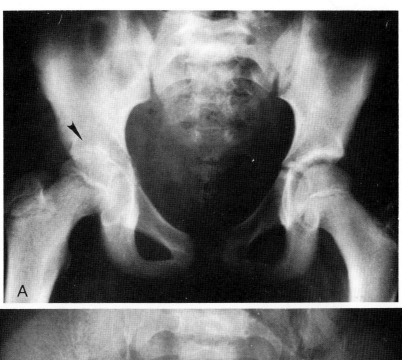

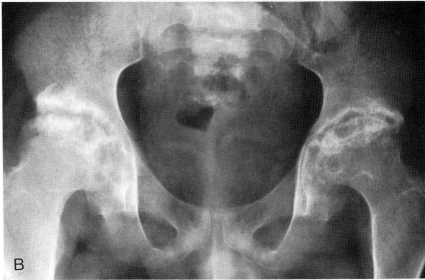

Figure 4.120. Joint space narrowing. A. Narrowing of the right hip joint in staphylococcal septic arthritis *(arrow)*. **B.** Narrowing of both hip joints, with irregularity of the articular surfaces, in rheumatoid arthritis.

drome, Goltz syndrome (focal dermal hypoplasia), hereditary arthro-ophthalmopathy (Stickler syndrome), and the various storage diseases. In terms of joint **hypomobility,** the commonest cause, on a generalized basis, is joint contracture in arthrogryposis multiplex congenita (1) and related syndromes. Contractures also are seen in rheumatoid arthritis, punctate epiphyseal dysplasia (severe recessive form), contractural arachnodactyly, the storage diseases, hereditary arthro-ophthalmopathy (Stickler syndrome), Winchester syndrome, diastrophic dwarfism, metatropic dwarfism, the more severe forms of metaphyseal dysostosis, and diabetes mellitus (2).

In terms of isolated joint **hyper- or hypomobility,** the commonest causes of both are infection and trauma. However, isolated joint hypomobility also can occur with bony exostoses around the joint, congenital radial head dislocation, various congenital and acquired bony synostoses, and Madelung deformity of the wrist, or "dyschondrosteosis."

REFERENCES

1. Beckerman RC, Buchino JJ: Arthrogryposis multiplex congenita as part of an inherited symptom complex: two case reports and a review of the literature. *Pediatrics* 61:417–422, 1978.
2. Grgic A, Rosenbloom AL, Weber FT, Giodano B, Malone

JI, Shuster JJ: Joint contracture-common manifestation of childhood diabetes mellitus. *J Pediatr* 88:584–588, 1976.

3. Urettos BC, Hoffman EB: Chondrolysis in slipped upper femoral epiphysis. *J Bone Joint Surg* 75B:956–961, 1993.

FRANK JOINT DISLOCATION (TABLE 4.38)

The same problems causing joint space widening (i.e., joint fluid, trauma, lax muscles, and loose ligaments) also cause the joint to dislocate. This section deals with frank joint dislocation, however, and trauma, of course, is most common. On a congenital basis, developmental hip dysplasia or congenital dislocation of the hip is the most common problem.

Table 4.38
Frank Joint Dislocation

Traumatic[a] Developmental hip dysplasia[a] Rheumatoid arthritis[a,b] Neurologic-neuromuscular disease[a,b]	Common
Congenital radial head dislocation[a] Madelung deformity[a]	Relatively rare
Larsen syndrome[b] Genu recurvatum[a] Winchester syndrome[a,b] Farber syndrome[b] Werner mesomelic syndrome[b] Stickler syndrome[b]	Rare

[a] Single joint involvement.
[b] Generalized joint involvement.

Next most common is radial head dislocation. Congenital dislocation of the hip is characterized by lateral and upward displacement of the hip, widening of the hip joint, underdevelopment of the femoral head, increased slant to the acetabular roof, and loss of cupping of the acetabular roof (see Fig. 4.118C). With radial head dislocation, proximal radioulnar synostosis commonly is associated, and the radial head is somewhat hypoplastic and bent dorsally (Fig. 4.121A). This type of radial head dislocation can be seen in isolated form or as part of syndromes such as the Cornelia de Lange and Noonan syndromes, and sex chromosome abnormalities. Another peculiar congenital dislocation is posterior dislocation of the proximal tibia on the distal femur or "genu recurvatum" (Fig. 4.121B). Usually the problem results from faulty intrauterine positioning of the legs, but genu recurvatum also occurs in syndromes such as the Larsen and Desbuquois syndromes (5), where generalized joint dislocation is present. Posterior dislocation of the distal ulna occurs in Madelung deformity or dyschondrosteosis (see Fig. 4.8C).

Multiple joint dislocations are seen in conditions where neurologic, neuromuscular, or chronic arthritic disease predisposes the patient to joint laxity or contracture. These include conditions such as rheumatoid arthritis, Winchester syndrome (a storage disease that resembles rheumatoid arthritis), Stickler hereditary arthro-ophthalmopathy, Farber lipogranulomatosis, and Desbuquois (5) and Larsen syndromes. This latter condition is characterized by multiple joint dislocations, severe clubbed feet,

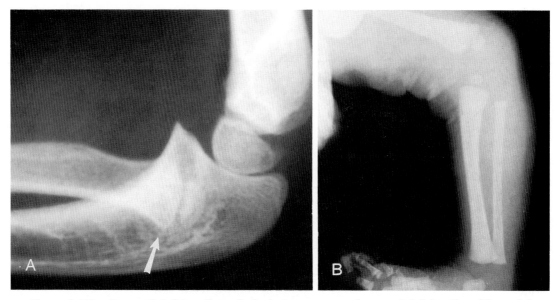

Figure 4.121. Congenital dislocations. A. Typical appearance of congenital dislocation of the radial head *(arrow).* **B.** Genu recurvatum in neonate.

and dwarfism. In addition, shortening of some of the long bones can occur, especially the distal humerus.

JOINT ANKYLOSES

Ankyloses most commonly are acquired and secondary to infection, inflammation (i.e., rheumatoid arthritis), or trauma. Actually, most of these conditions first lead to joint space narrowing (see Table 4.37) but, with time, joint ankylosis occurs. Occasionally, ankyloses are congenital and most often this occurs around the elbow (see Fig. 4.27B).

JOINT CALCIFICATION

Joint calcification can be intra- or periarticular (Table 4.39). **Intraarticular calcification** is rare in children, but occasionally can be seen after trauma or infection. Idiopathic calcifications in the hip joints have been demonstrated in young infants, but in follow-up observations, are believed to have resulted from previous joint taps (7, 8). Problems such as pseudogout, ochronosis, oxalosis, and synovial chondromatosis (2) are all uncommon in children. Every so often, however, one can see a solitary calcification within a joint, usually the knee, in association with osteochondritis dissecans. This also can occur in other joints, (e.g., in the ankle from the talus), but most often, with osteochondritis dissecans, one sees only the cartilaginous defect on the articular surface of the involved bone. Acute trauma, with avulsion of

pieces of an articular surface, also can lead to intraarticular calcification, and most often this occurs with cruciate ligament avulsions in the knee. Calcification of synoviomas is rare in childhood because the tumor itself is rare.

Calcification around a joint or, in other words, **periarticular calcification,** also is rare in children. However, it can be seen after burns (4), pyogenic arthritis (1, 9), rheumatoid arthritis (6), dermatomyositis, other collagen vascular diseases, hyperparathyroidism (10), hypervitaminosis D, hypervitaminosis A (3), tumoral calcinosis, and trauma. In most of these conditions, calcification is nonspecific and sheath-like in its distribution (Fig. 4.122A), but with tumoral calcinosis, the calcifications become large and flocculent (Fig. 4.122B). Some also may show calcium-fluid levels, and a similar phenomenon has been documented with paraarticular calcifications in hyperparathyroidism (10).

REFERENCES

1. Arnold S, Sty JR, Starshak RJ: Periarticular soft tissue calcification and ossification in the septic joint. *Pediatr Radiol* 19:433–434, 1989.
2. Cahuzac JP, Lebarbier P, Germaneau J, Pasque M: Synovial chondromatosis in children: four cases. *Chir Pediatr* 20:89–93, 1979.
3. DiGiovanna JJ, Helfgott RK, Gerber LH, Peck GL: Extraspinal tendon and ligament calcification associated with long-term therapy with etretinate. *N Engl J Med* 315:1177–1182, 1986.
4. Faure C, Viatl C, Gueriot JC: Para-articular calcifications and ossifications in children with burns. *Ann Radiol* 15:733–738, 1972. Abstract: *Radiology* 108:238, 1973.
5. Jequier S, Perreault G, Maroteaux P: Desbuquois syndrome presenting with severe neonatal dwarfism, spondyloepiphyseal dysplasia and advanced carpal bone age. *Pediatr Radiol* 22:440–442, 1992.
6. Martel W, Holt JF, Cassidy JT: Roentgenologic manifestations of juvenile rheumatoid arthritis. *AJR* 88:400–423, 1962.
7. Nahum H, Pissarro B, Sauvegrain J: Calcification of the cartilages of the hip in infants. *Ann Radiol* 11:288–297, 1968.
8. Sauvegrain J, Millet G, Manlot G, Vacher H: Calcifications of the hip in infants and children: new cases and long-term followup. *Pediatr Radiol* 11:29–33, 1981.
9. Shawker TH, Dennis JM: Periarticular calcifications in pyogenic arthritis. *AJR* 113:650–654, 1971.
10. Smith FW, Junor BJR: Peri-articular calcification with fluid levels in secondary hyperparathyroidism. *Br J Radiol* 51:741–742, 1978.

GAS IN THE JOINT

The commonest cause of gas in the joint (Table 4.40) is the "vacuum joint effect" (1). When stress is applied to a normal joint, intraarticular pressures

Table 4.39
Joint Calcification

Intraarticular	
Traumatic avulsion	Common
Osteochondritis dissecans	
Idiopathic: in infants	
Synovial chondromatosis	
Ochronosis	Rare
Oxalosis	
Synovial inflammation	
Synovial tumors	
Periarticular	
Collagen diseases: especially	Common
dermatomyositis	
Trauma	
Infection	
Hypervitaminosis D and A	Relatively rare
Hyperparathyroidism	
Tumoral calcinosis: large, clumpy	

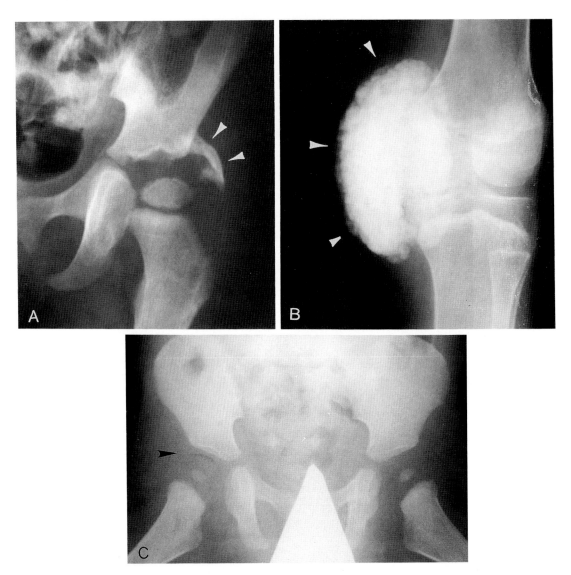

Figure 4.122. Periarticular calcifications. A. Postseptic arthritis calcification around left hip *(arrows)*. **B.** Typical large, bulky calcification *(arrows)* of tumoral calcinosis. **C. Gas in joint.** Typical vacuum joint *(arrow)*. Characteristically, these air configurations are crescentic, but there is debate as to whether the gas is water vapor, nitrogen, or just a vacuum.

become negative and the vacuum joint results (Fig. 4.122C). There is debate as to whether the gas is nitrogen, water vapor, or an actual vacuum. The point is moot, however, for the finding is of no particular consequence, and is seen with greater frequency in patients with flaccid extremities. Intraarticular gas also can be seen after penetrating trauma, postoperatively, after arthrography, and, occasionally, with gas-producing organisms causing infection.

REFERENCE

1. Deffrenne P, Beraud C: Intraarticular vacuum effect. *Ann Radiol* 18:401–406, 1975.

Soft Tissues

HEMIATROPHY AND HEMIHYPERTROPHY

It is important to distinguish between these two abnormalities because, while both give rise to asymmetric limbs, in hemiatrophy the affected limb is smaller than normal, and in hemihypertrophy it is larger. **Hemiatrophy** for the most part occurs with underlying, unilateral neurologic disease, and the problem is more common in the lower extremities. However, hemiatrophy also is seen in the Russell-Silver syndrome (Fig. 4.123A), a condition character-

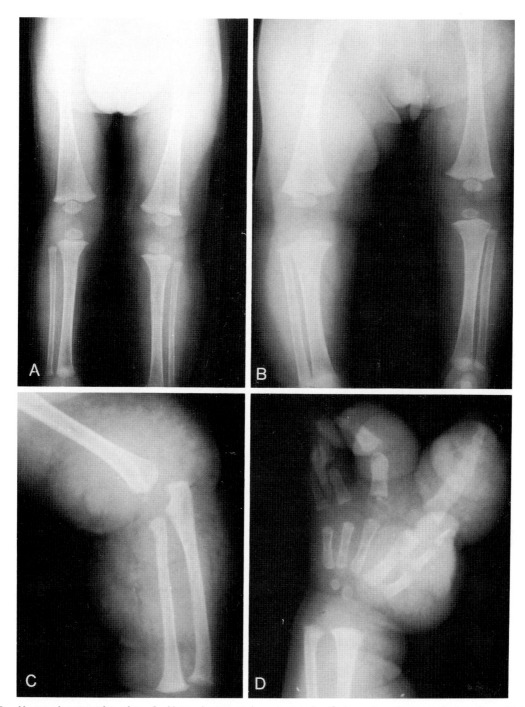

Figure 4.123. Unequal extremity size. A. Note shorter and smaller right lower extremity in Russell-Silver dwarfism. **B.** Note large, slightly longer right lower extremity in congenital hemihy-pertrophy. **C. Lymphangioma and gigantism.** Note typical reticulation of soft tissues and hypertrophy of the soft tissues. **D.** Hand in same patient.

Table 4.40
Gas in Joint

Normal vacuum joint	}	Common
Vacuum joint with hypotonia	}	Moderately common
Penetrating trauma Infection	}	Rare

ized by dwarfism, enlargement of the head, abnormal sexual development, and variable smallness of the extremities on one side of the body (1, 3). In most cases, changes are more pronounced in the lower extremity and the problem is one of congenital growth disturbance rather than neurologic deficit.

Hemihypertrophy usually also is more pronounced in the lower extremities and, although it occurs on a isolated basis (Fig. 4.123B), it also frequently is seen in association with intraabdominal tumors. This is especially true of Wilms tumor of the kidney, but other abdominal tumors also can be encountered. Hemihypertrophy also is seen in the Beckwith-Wiedemann (infantile gigantism) syndrome, and even with benign cystic diseases of the kidney (2). In all of these conditions, the involved extremity is larger than normal both in its bony and soft tissue components. The etiology of this type of hypertrophy is unknown and should not be confused with that due to localized gigantism resulting from soft tissue vascular or lymphatic tumors, or lymphatic obstruction (Fig. 4.123C and D), (discussion in next section).

REFERENCES

1. Moseley JE, Moloshok RE, Freiberger RH: The silver syndrome: congenital asymmetry, short stature, and variations in sexual development. *AJR* 97:74–81, 1966.
2. Pfister RC, Weber AL, Smith EH, Wilkinson RH, May DA: Congenital asymmetry (hemihypertrophy) and abdominal disease: radiological features in 9 cases. *Radiology* 116:685–691, 1975.
3. Silver HK: Asymmetry, short stature and variations in sexual development: a syndrome of congenital malformations. *Am J Dis Child* 107:495–515, 1964.
4. Swischuk LE: *Radiology of the Newborn and Young Infant.* 2d ed. Baltimore: Williams & Wilkins, 1980:730.

ISOLATED EXTREMITY ENLARGEMENT OR GIGANTISM

Perhaps the commonest cause of a locally enlarged extremity is a vascular or lymphangiomatous tumor, or arteriovenous fistula or malformation of the extremity. Hyperemia in these cases causes overgrowth of all of the tissues and, in some cases, the changes are profound (Fig. 4.123C and D). Localized gigantism also can be seen in neurofibromatosis (due to a poorly understood mesenchymal defect), macrodystrophia lipomatosa (1), and the Proteus syndrome. Localized gigantism also can occur with lymphatic obstruction, which can be due to congenital atresia or hypoplasia of the lymphatic channels, or compression of the lymphatics by pelvic tumors, inflammatory masses, or the like. In the tropics, of course, it is also seen with filariasis or "elephantiasis." Hemangiomatous tumors can exist in isolated form or be seen with multiple enchondromatosis (Maffucci syndrome) or multiple hemangioma syndromes such as the Klippel-Trenaunay-Weber syndrome (2).

REFERENCES

1. McCarthy DM, Dorr CA, Mackintosh CE: Unilateral localized gigantism of the extremities with lipomatosis, arthropathy and psoriasis. *J Bone Joint Surg* 51B:348–353, 1969.
2. Tetamy SA, Rogers JG: Macrodactyly, hemihypertrophy, and connective tissue nevi: report of a new syndrome and review of the literature. *J Pediatr* 89:924–928, 1976.

MUSCLE-FAT RATIO ABNORMALITIES

It is relatively easy to define the muscles, subcutaneous fat, and skin of the extremities of infants and children. This being the case, one can determine whether muscle and fat are present in normal proportions, or whether one or the other is lacking or predominates (2, 4). **Four basic categorizations are possible: increased muscle with normal fat, decreased muscle with excess fat, decreased fat with normal muscle, and increased fat with normal muscle (Table 4.41).**

An absolute, abnormal increase in muscle bulk is not that common, but it does occur in pseudohypertrophic muscular dystrophy (Fig. 4.124A), and primary infections of the muscle such as pyomyositis (3). It also can occur on an idiopathic basis in so-called "congenital muscle hypertrophy" (4) and on a focal basis with exercise hypertrophy. Diminution of muscle bulk occurs with a number of neuromuscular diseases including Werdnig-Hoffman disease, amyotonia congenita, poliomyelitis, arthrogryposis multi-

Table 4.41
Muscle-Fat Ratio Abnormalities

Increased muscle—normal fat
  Muscular dystrophy
  Congenital muscular hypertrophy
  Pyomyositis
  Exercise hypertrophy
Decreased muscle—excess fat
  Neurologic disease: multiple causes
  Arthrogryposis multiplex
  Amyotonia congenita
  Werdnig-Hoffman disease
  Muscular dystrophy
  Prolonged muscle paralysis (6–8)
Decreased fat—normal muscle
  Malnutrition, cachexia[a]
  Diencephalic syndrome
  Total lipodystrophy
Increased fat—normal muscle
  Exogenous obesity
  Cushing syndrome
  Laurence-Moon-Biedl syndrome
  Prader-Willi syndrome
  Steroid therapy

[a] In late, severe stages, muscle is also decreased due to protein catabolism.

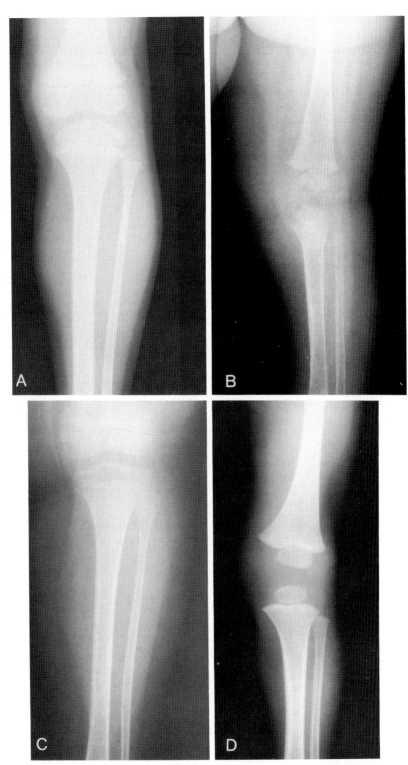

Figure 4.124.   A. Increased muscle, normal fat. Patient with pseudohypertrophic muscular dystrophy. Note bulbous calf. **B. Decreased muscle and increased fat.** Neurologic disease producing thin, wasted muscles and overabundance of subcutaneous fat. **C. Excessive fat, relatively normal muscles.** Note extra fat in Prader-Willi syndrome. **D. Decreased fat, normal or** **increased muscle.** Note homogeneous appearance of soft tissues of legs of this patient with diencephalic syndrome. Virtually no subcutaneous fat is present. All the density is due to muscle. Clinically, the patient appeared very muscular. This is characteristic of the condition.

plex, meningocele, brain damage, and prolonged muscle paralysis with pancuronium bromide (6–8). In all of these cases, there is muscle atrophy and, in many, an associated increase in subcutaneous fat (Fig. 4.124B). Often this increase is only relative, but in some patients it is absolute, for caloric intake is greater than their physical activity requires. Other causes of an absolute increase in subcutaneous fat include exogenous obesity, steroid therapy, Cushing syndrome, Laurence-Moon-Biedl syndrome, and the Prader-Willi syndrome (Fig. 4.124C).

Conditions where subcutaneous fat is diminished include severe undernutrition (2), cachexia, the diencephalic syndrome (5), and total lipodystrophy (1, 9). In the diencephalic syndrome, a brain tumor is located around the anterior third ventricle, and the location of the tumor leads to hypothalamic disturbances causing abnormality of fat metabolism (Fig. 4.124D). In total lipodystrophy, a brain tumor is not present. Decreased fat is self-evident in severe malnutrition, and in very severe cases with protein loss, both fat and muscle decrease.

REFERENCES

1. Fairney A, Lewis G, Cotton D: Total lipodystrophy. *Arch Dis Child* 44:368–372, 1969.
2. Frank J, Klidjian MM, Karran SJ: The radiological assessment of arm muscle and fat stores in normal and malnourished patients. *Clin Radiol* 32:467–470, 1981.
3. Goldberg JS, London WL, Nagel DM: Tropical pyomyositis: a case report and review. *Pediatrics* 63:298–300, 1979.
4. Litt RE, Altman DH: Significance of the muscle cylinder ratio in infancy. *AJR* 100:80–87, 1967.
5. Poznanski AK, Manson G: Radiographic appearance of the soft tissues in the diencephalic syndrome of infancy. *Radiology* 81:101–106, 1963.
6. Rutledge ML, Hawkins EP, Langston C: Skeletal muscle growth failure induced in premature newborn infants by prolonged pancuronium treatment. *J Pediatr* 109:883–886, 1986.
7. Sinha SK, Levene MI: Pancuronium bromide-induced joint contractures in the newborn. *Arch Dis Child* 59:73–75, 1984.
8. Torres CF, Maniscalco WM, Agostenelli T: Muscle weakness and atrophy following prolonged paralysis with pancuronium bromide in neonates. *Ann Neurol* 18:403, 1985.
9. Wesenberg RL, Gwinn JL, Barnes GR Jr: The roentgenographic findings in total lipodystrophy. *AJR* 103:154–164, 1968.

RETICULATED SOFT TISSUES

Normally the interface between fat and muscle is quite sharp, but when soft tissue edema occurs reticulation of the fat is seen (Fig. 4.125). This causes obliteration of the fat-muscle interface and generalized thickening of the soft tissues. Most often, this is

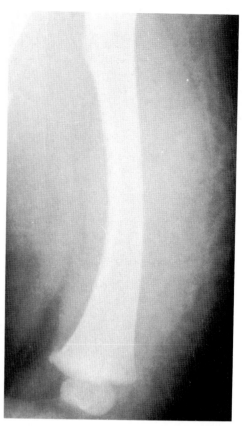

Figure 4.125. Soft tissue reticulation. Note reticulation of soft tissues of the thigh. This is due to edema and was secondary to cellulitis.

seen with infection or trauma, but it also can be seen with soft tissue vascular and lymphatic tumors (see Fig. 4.123C and D).

TENDON WIDTH CHANGES

The tendons of many muscles are relatively easy to visualize in infants, but most often one is dealing with the Achilles tendon in the ankle, and the infra- and suprapatellar tendons around the knee. As far as thickening of any of these tendons is concerned, usually it is due to trauma or inflammation (i.e., tendonitis). In most locations the findings are straightforward (Fig. 4.126A and B), but in the knee, apparent thickening of the suprapatellar tendon can be due to accumulation of fluid (pus, blood, serous effusion) in the immediately adjacent suprapatellar bursa. In such cases, the normally collapsed bursa slowly fills with fluid and distends, and in so doing blends with the quadriceps tendon and causes it to falsely appear thickened (Fig. 4.126C). This is a very valuable finding in identifying knee joint effusions in infants and children (1). Tendon thickening now

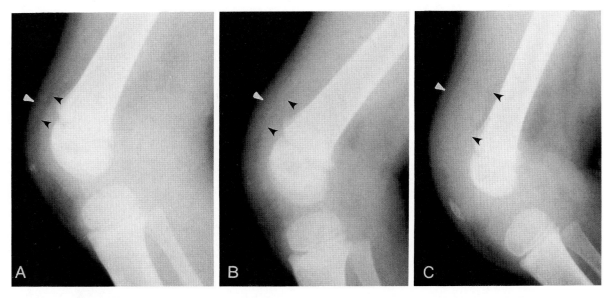

Figure 4.126. Normal and thickened quadriceps tendon. A. Normal quadriceps tendon *(arrows).* **B.** Thickened quadriceps tendon *(arrows)* due to tendonitis. **C.** Marked pseudothickening of quadriceps tendon by massive accumulation of fluid in suprapatellar bursa *(arrows)* in infant with septic arthritis.

also is readily demonstrable with ultrasound, and even with MRI.

REFERENCE

1. Hayden CK Jr, Swischuk LE: Para-articular soft tissue changes in infections and trauma of the lower extremity in children. *AJR* 134:307–311, 1980.

OBLITERATED AND DISPLACED FAT PADS

There are numerous fat pads around the joints of the body and many are used for the detection of joint abnormality. Basically, a fat pad can be displaced or obliterated (Fig. 4.127). Obliteration is due to surrounding edema (any number of causes) and displacement (usually outward) is caused by joint fluid. Fat pads next to bones can be displaced outward by bony masses, pus or edema in osteomyelitis, and hematomas with trauma. All of these assessments are quite important, but their complete discussion is beyond the scope of this book. Therefore, one is referred to a number of articles and books on the subject (1–10).

REFERENCES

1. Bledsoe RC, Izenstark JL: Displacement of fat pads in disease and injury to the elbow. *Radiology* 73:717–724, 1959.
2. Bohrer SP: The fat sign following elbow trauma: its usefulness and reliability in suspecting "invisible" fractures. *Clin Radiol* 21:90–94, 1970.
3. Hayden CK Jr, Swischuk LE: Para-articular soft tissue changes in infections and trauma of the lower extremity in children. *AJR* 134:307–311, 1980.
4. Kohn AM: Soft tissue alteration in elbow trauma. *AJR* 82:867–875, 1959.
5. MacEwen DW: Changes due to trauma in the fat plane overlying the pronator quadratus muscle: a radiologic sign. *Radiology* 82:879–886, 1964.
6. Norell HG: Roentgenologic visualization of the extracapsular fat: its importance in the diagnosis of traumatic injuries to the elbows. *Acta Radiol* 42:205–210, 1954.
7. Rogers SL, MacEwan DW: Changes due to trauma in the fat plane overlying the spinator muscle: a radiologic sign. *Radiology* 92:954–958, 1969.
8. Swischuk LE: *Emergency Radiology of the Acutely Ill or Injured Child.* Ed. 3. Baltimore: Williams & Wilkins, 1993:362–547.
9. Terry DW Jr, Ramin JE: The navicular fat stripe: a useful roentgen feature for evaluating wrist trauma. *AJR* 124:25–28, 1975.
10. Towbin R, Dunbar JS, Clark R: Teardrop sign: plain film recognition of ankle effusion. *AJR* 134:985–990, 1980.

SOFT TISSUE CALCIFICATION AND OPACITIES

Opacities due to **foreign bodies** can assume a variety of sizes and shapes and usually provide no real problem in identification. However, some, such as glass, may or may not be radiopaque. Graphite, in a "lead" pencil, usually is just faintly visible on regular roentgenograms, but most fish spines are not visible.

As far as **soft tissue calcification** is concerned, it can be irregular, formed, or punctate. **Irregular calcifications** occur after deep abscesses, hemato-

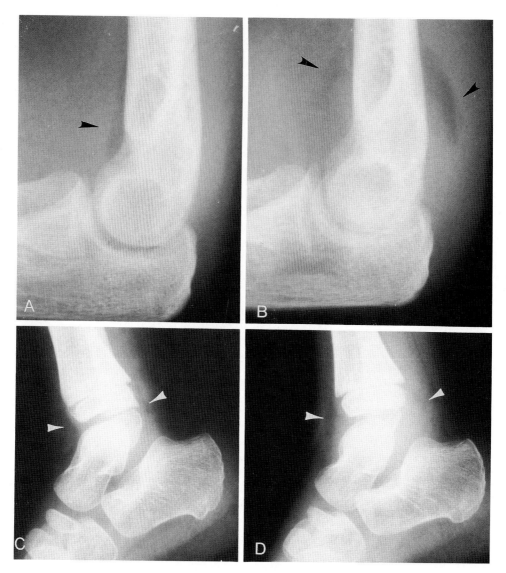

Figure 4.127. Fat pad abnormalities. A. Normal anterior fat pad in elbow *(arrows).* **B.** Displacement of anterior and posterior fat pads *(arrow)* of the elbow by joint fluid. Normally, as in A, the posterior fat pad is not visible. **C.** Normal anterior and posterior ankle fat pads *(arrow).* **D.** Outwardly displaced ankle fat pads *(arrows),* secondary to the presence of joint fluid.

mas, and with collagen vascular disease, namely dermatomyositis (5, 19, 21, 25). Calcification in the collagen vascular diseases usually is subcutaneous and, at an early stage, rather delicate. Later, it can become more extensive and sheath-like (Fig. 4.128A). Irregular subcutaneous calcifications have been noted in the basal cell nevus syndrome (18) as well, and also can occur in the extremities after extravasation of calcium containing injections (1, 11, 14, 15, 20). This latter phenomenon commonly occurs in neonates (Fig. 4.128B). Rather extensive, irregular soft tissue calcification occurs with fat necrosis in infancy (Fig. 4.128C). This condition is of unknown etiology, but some believe that it is related to both hypothermia and trauma (3, 6, 7, 22, 23). Most often, these

calcifications slowly disappear. Irregular calcifications in the soft tissues also can be seen with calcinosis universalis, Ehlers-Danlos syndrome, hyperparathyroidism, hypervitaminosis D, and end-stage renal disease (17).

Formed calcifications usually occur in the muscle in the form of posttraumatic myositis ossificans (Fig. 4.129A and B) and also may be seen after bleeding in hemophilia. In the inherited condition known as progressive myositis ossificans (10), the calcifications tend to be solid and occur around the joints or posterior spinal ligaments (Fig. 4.129C and D). Vascular calcifications are rare in children (8, 16, 24, 26), but when seen, characteristically are tubular, linear, and parallel (Fig. 4.130A). Most often, they are idio-

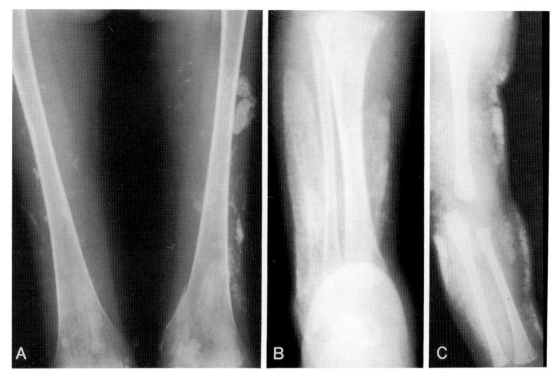

Figure 4.128. Soft tissue calcifications. A. Typical, irregular, almost sheath-like calcifications in collagen vascular disease.
B. Typical calcifications after calcium salt injections in infancy.
C. Typical subcutaneous calcifications of fat necrosis in infancy.

pathic and occur in infancy (2, 26), but they can occur with a variety of idiopathic or iatrogenic hypercalcemic states. A peculiar aortic calcification has been documented by Singleton and Merten in a storage disease problem (21), and we have seen similar calcification in a case of supposed Gaucher disease (see Fig. 1.54A). Punctate calcifications almost invariably are associated with hemangiomatous or lymphangiomatous tumors (Fig. 4.130B), or varices.

The large, flocculent paraarticular calcifications of tumoral calcinosis (4, 9, 12, 13, 27) have been discussed elsewhere (see Fig. 4.122B). In some cases, these calcifications can take the form of milk of calcium and be associated with calcium fluid levels within the lesion (12, 13). Eventually, surgical removal of the calcified soft tissue masses is required, because they interfere with joint function. Tumoral calcinosis tends to occur in families and can be associated with osteomyelitis-like lesions of the long bones. There is no known cause for these lesions, but they are difficult to differentiate from osteomyelitis.

REFERENCES

1. Berger PE, Heidelberger KP, Poznanski AK: Extravasation of calcium gluconate as a cause of soft tissue calcification in infancy. *AJR* 121:109–117, 1974.

2. Bird T: Idiopathic arterial calcification in infancy. *Arch Dis Child* 49:82–89, 1974.

3. Blake HA, Goyette EM, Lyter CS, Swan H: Subcutaneous fat necrosis complicating hypothermia. *J Pediatr* 46:78–80, 1955.

4. Bostrom B: Tumoral calcinosis in an infant. *Am J Dis Child* 135:246–247, 1981.

5. Budin JA, Feldman F: Soft tissue calcifications in systemic lupus erythematosus. *AJR* 124:358–364, 1975.

6. de Vel L, Bolin ZA: Traumatic necrosis of the subcutaneous fat of the newborn infant. *Am J Dis Child* 37:112, 1929.

7. Duhn R, Schoen EJ, Siu M: Subcutaneous fat necrosis with extensive calcification after hypothermia in two newborn infants. *Pediatrics* 41:661–664, 1968.

8. Field MH: Medial calcifications of the arteries of infants. *Arch Pathol* 42:607–618, 1946.

9. Hacihanefioglu U: Tumoral calcinosis: a clinical and pathological study of eleven unreported cases in Turkey. *J Bone Joint Surg* 60A:1131–1135, 1978.

10. Hall CM, Sutcliffe J: Fibrodysplasia ossificans progressiva. *Ann Radiol* 22:119–123, 1979.

11. Harris V, Ramamurthy RS, Pildes RS: Late onset of subcutaneous calcifications after intravenous injections of calcium gluconate. *AJR* 123:845–849, 1975.

12. Hug I, Guncaga J: Tumoral calcinosis with sedimentation sign. *Br J Radiol* 47:734–736, 1974.

13. Kolawole TM, Bohrer SP: Tumoral calcinosis with "fluid levels" in the tumoral masses. *AJR* 120:461–465, 1974.

14. Leape LL: Calcification of the leg after calcium infusion. *J Pediatr Surg* 5:831–833, 1975.

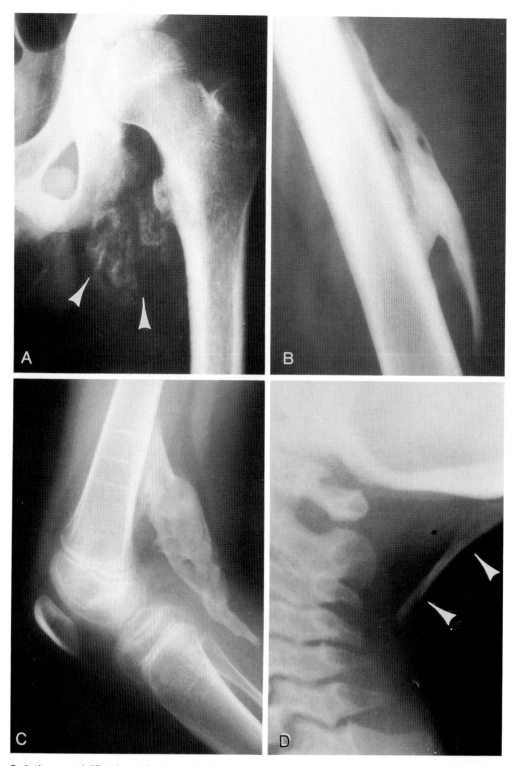

Figure 4.129.   Soft tissue calcifications. A. Irregular calcifications of myositis ossificans due to chronic tendon avulsion in neurogenic patient *(arrows).* **B.** Typical mature, traumatic myositis ossificans. **C.** Similar appearing solid calcifications in myositis ossificans progressiva. **D.** Posterior spinal ligament calcifications *(arrows)* in progressive myositis ossificans.

15. Lee FA, Gwinn JL: Roentgen patterns of extravasation of calcium gluconate in the tissues of the neonate. *J Pediatr* 86:598–601, 1975.
16. Meradjim M, de Villeneuve VH, Huber J, de Bruijn WC,

Pearse RG: Idiopathic infantile arterial calcification in siblings: radiologic diagnosis and successful treatment. *J Pediatr* 92:401–405, 1978.
17. Milliner DS, Zinsmeister AR, Lieberman E, Landing B:

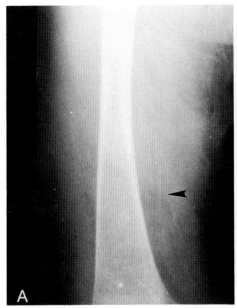

Figure 4.130. Vascular soft tissue calcifications. A. Tubular calcifications of arteries in infancy *(arrow).* (Courtesy of AH Weens, M.D.) **B.** Typical calcified phleboliths in hemangiomatous lesion of lower extremity *(arrow).*

Soft tissue calcification in pediatric patients with end-stage renal disease. *Kidney Int* 38:931–936, 1990.

18. Murphy KJ: Subcutaneous calcification in nevoid basal cell carcinoma syndrome: response to parathyroid hormone and relationship to pseudohypoparathyroidism. *Clin Radiol* 20:287–293, 1969.

19. Ozonoff MB, Flynn FJ Jr: Roentgenologic features of dermatomyositis of childhood. *AJR* 118:206–212, 1973.

20. Ramamurthy RS, Harris V, Pildes RS: Subcutaneous calcium deposition in the neonate associated with intravenous administration of calcium gluconate. *Pediatrics* 55:802–806, 1975.

21. Sewell JR, Liyanage B, Ansell BM: Calcinosis in juvenile dermatomyositis. *Skeletal Radiol* 3:137–143, 1978.

22. Shackelford GD, Barton LL, McAlister WH: Calcified subcutaneous fat necrosis in infancy. *J Can Assoc Radiol* 26:203–207, 1975.

23. Sharlin DN, Koblenzer P: Necrosis of subcutaneous fat with hypercalcemia, a puzzling and multifaceted disease. *Clin Pediatr* 9:290–294, 1970.

24. Singleton EB, Merten DF: An unusual syndrome of widened medullary cavities of the metacarpals and phalanges, aortic calcification and abnormal dentition. *Pediatr Radiol* 1:2–7, 1973.

25. Steiner RM, Glassman L, Schwartz MW, Vanance P: The radiological findings in dermatomyositis of childhood. *Radiology* 111:385–393, 1974.

26. Weens HS, Marin CA: Infantile arteriosclerosis. *Radiology* 67:168–174, 1956.

27. Yaghmai I, Mirbod P: Tumoral calcinosis. *AJR* 111:573–578, 1971.

SOFT TISSUE AIR

Air in the soft tissues can be seen with penetrating injuries, explosions, severe contusion-abrasion injuries (Fig. 4.131A), and gas-forming infections (Fig. 4.131B). Air in the soft tissues of the neck and chest usually is secondary to mediastinal emphysema resulting from pulmonary air-trapping in conditions such as asthma (most often) or with a bronchial foreign body (rather rare). However, it also can be seen with blunt chest trauma and rupture or puncture of the airway (Fig. 4.131C). Vascular air usually is iatrogenic and secondary to vessel catheterization, but also can be seen with penetrating trauma to the heart or great vessels. In infancy, gas commonly is seen in the portal veins with necrotizing enterocolitis. It is secondary to intestinal necrosis and can be seen with other causes of bowel necrosis.

SOFT TISSUE MASSES

Soft tissue masses either are well defined or blend in with the adjacent soft tissues. When well defined, they tend to be benign tumors or cysts, but some malignant tumors can have a surprisingly well-defined margin (Fig. 4.132A). Soft tissue tumors blending with the soft tissues tend to be malignant sarcomas, vascular lesions, or inflammatory masses (Fig. 4.132B). Vascular lesions such as hemangiomas or arteriovenous malformations often show trailing or tortuous vessels (Fig. 4.132C). If these masses are associated with punctate calcifications, they are almost certain to be vascular or lymphangiomatous in origin. Other soft tissue tumors do not calcify very of-

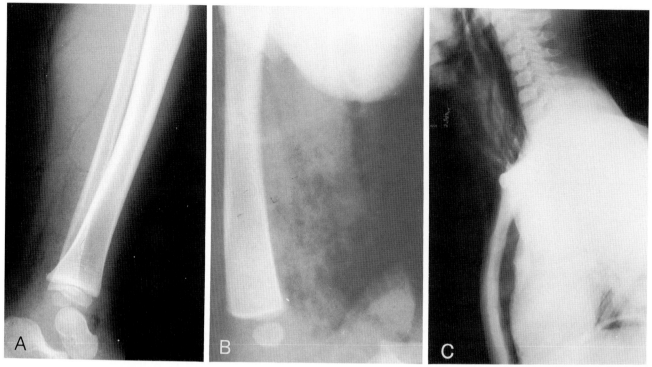

Figure 4.131. Soft tissue gas. A. Note gas around the ankle and in the lymphatics of the calf. This occurred after a severe contusion-abrasion of the lower leg. No open wounds of the skin were present. **B.** Extensive gas secondary to gas-forming infec- tion of the soft tissues. **C.** Extensive subcutaneous and mediasti- nal air after laceration of larynx and trachea secondary to dog bite.

ten, but occasionally one can encounter an "ossifying fibroma" of the soft tissues. Lipomas are not particu- larly common in children, but may produce exagger- ated radiolucency on plain films (Fig. 4.132D) and CT scans. This is more true of benign lipomas, be- cause liposarcomas often do not demonstrate the typ- ical fat density.

Currently, soft tissue masses are best assessed with MRI and ultrasound (1, 2). Clinically, these masses are either inflammatory, soft and/or fluctu- ant, or firm to hard. Ultrasonographically, inflam- matory masses (abscesses) may show fluid (pus) or debris. Soft or fluctuant masses usually are lymph- angiomas, hemangiomas, or lipomas. With ultra- sound, lymphangiomas appear cystic with very little intervening tissue, while hemangiomas are hetero- geneously echogenic, often lobulated, and septated. Venous lakes and feeding and draining vessels also may be seen. Lipomas show a fine, granular homoge- neous echogenicity on ultrasound. With MRI, lymph- angiomas show medium signal on T_1-weighted im- ages and high signal on T_2-weighted images. If bleeding occurs into the lymphangioma, the signal intensity on the T_2-weighted images in those por- tions involved is not as high. Hemangiomas charac- teristically show very high intensity on T_2-weighted

images, especially on second echo images. Lipomas, of course, show high signal on T_1-weighted images and lesser signal on T_2-weighted images. All of the features of these inflammatory, or soft tissue, lesions as seen with ultrasound and MRI enable one to fre- quently make the correct diagnosis. The characteris- tics of firm, solid soft tissue masses are usually non- specific. A variety of these tumors are shown in Figure 4.133.

REFERENCES

1. Cohen MD, DeRosa GP, Kleiman M, Passo M, Cory DA, Smith JA, McKinney l: Magnetic resonance evaluation of disease of the soft tissues in children. *Pediatrics* 79:696– 701, 1987.
2. Glasier CM, Seibert JJ, Williamson SL, Seibert RW, Cor- bitt SL, Rodgers AB, Lange TA: High resolution ultra- sound characterization of soft tissue masses in children. *Pediatr Radiol* 17:233–237, 1987.

PERIOSTEAL NEW BONE DEPOSITION

Periosteal new bone is deposited in reaction to any type of periosteal irritation, and can assume **one of the following configurations: (a) layered (single**

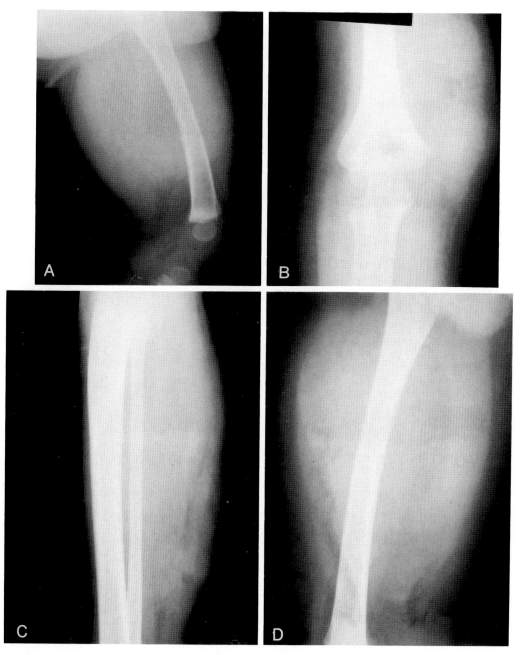

Figure 4.132. Soft tissue masses. A. Large, relatively discrete mass due to rhabdomyosarcoma in infant. **B.** Two inflammatory masses (inflamed nodes) around the elbow. Note indistinct margin of the masses secondary to edema. **C.** Large arteriovenous malformation of calf. Note tortuous and trailing blood vessels. **D.** Note radiolucency of this large lipoma of the thigh in a young child.

or multiple, (b) solid (straight, lumpy, or wavy), (c) spiculated (radiating outward), and (d) markedly elevated or ballooned (Table 4.42). Most often, periosteal new bone is deposited in response to some disease arising from within the bone itself (i.e., osteomyelitis, trauma, subperiosteal bleeding, bone infarction, bone tumor). In such cases, as the disease breaks through the cortex (i.e., pus, blood, edema, tu-

mor), periosteal elevation occurs, and in an attempt to heal, new bone is deposited. Less commonly, the periosteum is irritated by adjacent disease, usually inflammatory, in the soft tissues or joints. As far as the joints are concerned, most often the problem is rheumatoid arthritis (8, 9). In the soft tissues, the problem can be cellulitis, deep abscess, pyomyositis, venous stasis, or vascular tumor. Periosteal new

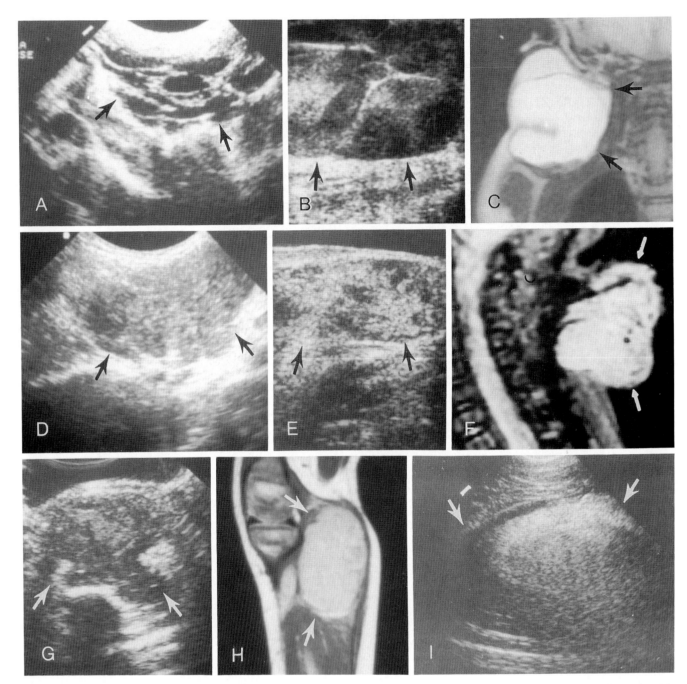

Figure 4.133. Soft tissue masses: ultrasound and MRI findings. A. Typical cystic appearance of lymphangioma *(arrows)*. **B.** Lymphangioma with echogenic debris due to bleeding *(arrows)*. **C.** MR proton density image of lymphangioma *(arrows)*, showing typical high signal in lower compartment and somewhat decreased signal in upper compartment due to bleeding into this compartment. **D.** Hemangioma. Typical course, granular echogenic pattern *(arrows)*. **E.** Another hemangioma *(arrows)* with a similar echogenic pattern but a few anechoic sinusoids. **F.** Magnetic resonance study, T_2-weighted image shows high signal in the hemangioma *(arrows)*. Note the flow void in the feeding and draining vessels. This hemangioma was located on the back. **G.** Rhabdomyosarcoma. Typical echogenic pattern of a solid tumor *(arrows)*. **H.** MR, T_1-weighted image, demonstrates the increased signal in the well-circumscribed rhabdomyosarcoma *(arrows)*. **I.** Typical, finely granular echogenicity of a lipoma *(arrows)*. On MRI, lipomas show high signal on T_1-weighted images and degradation of the signal on T_2-weighted images.

Table 4.42
Periosteal New Bone[a]

Disease	Layered (single or multiple)	Solid (straight, wavy, lumpy)	Markedly Elevated (ballooned)	Spiculated
Infection-inflammation				
Osteomyelitis—neonatal infection (lues, rubella, cmv)	+ +	−	−	−
Bone infarction	+ +	+	−	−
Cellulitis	+ +	+	−	−
Caffey's disease	+ +	+ +	−	−
Rheumatoid arthritis (8,9)	+	−	−	−
Fractures-injury				
Fractures (ordinary)	+ +	+ +	−	−
Fractures (battered child)	+ +	+ +	+ +	−
Fractures (neurogenic)	+ +	+ +	+ +	−
Fractures (pathologic)	+ +	+	−	−
Metabolic disease				
Rickets (healing)	+ +	+	−	−
Scurvy	+ +	−	+	−
Metabolic bone disease in premature	+ +	+	−	−
Hypervitaminosis D	+ +	−	−	−
Hypervitaminosis A	+ +	−	−	−
Thyroid acropachy	+	+ +	−	+
Gangliosidosis (infant)	+ +	−	+ +	−
Mucolipidosis II (infant)	+ +	−	+ +	
Hyperphosphatemia (3,7)	+ +	−	+ +	−
Gaucher disease (12)	+ +	+	−	−
Bone tumors and cysts				
Malignant—primary	+ +	−	−	+ +
Benign with fracture	+ +	+	−	−
Bone metastases	+ +	−	−	+
Leukemia-lymphoma	+ +	−	−	+
Hemangioma (with or without fracture)	+	+	−	−
Infantile fibromatosis (hamartomas)	+ +	−	−	−
Miscellaneous				
Osteoarthropathy	+ +	+ +	−	−
Pachydermoperiostosis (5,6)	+ +	+ +	−	−
Neurofibromatosis	−	−	+	−
Macrodystrophia lipomatosa	+	+	−	−
Normal infants (prematures)	+ +	−	−	−
Vascular soft tissue tumors	+	+	−	−
Mastocytosis (early stages)	+	−	+	−
Prostaglandin E treatment	+ +	−	−	−
Melorheostosis (2).	+ −	+ +	−	−
Venous stasis	+ −	+	−	−

[a] + +, quite common; +, occasional; −, rare or never.

bone deposition also can be seen in rickets, but only in its healing stages.

Another instance when periosteal new bone deposition occurs under somewhat unusual circumstances is when it is deposited in reaction to some distant, non-bony disease process. It then is termed "idiopathic hypertrophic osteoarthropathy" and, as in the adult, the initiating problem can be an intrathoracic tumor, some other distant tumor, pulmonary inflammatory disease, cystic fibrosis, chronic intestinal or liver disease, or cyanotic heart disease (1, 4, 5, 10, 13, 20–22). With the latter, chronic hypoxia is considered the underlying factor, but in the other conditions no specific etiology has been determined. Circulating toxins, hormones, or nonspecific neurologic disturbances often are suggested as possible etiologies.

In other cases the problem is familial (5, 6) and finally, it should be mentioned that when a bone becomes demineralized, the last layer of normal periosteal new bone previously deposited becomes visible as a thin, white line (Fig. 4.134). In such cases, it should be noted that the apparent layer of periosteal new bone does not bulge or deviate away from the

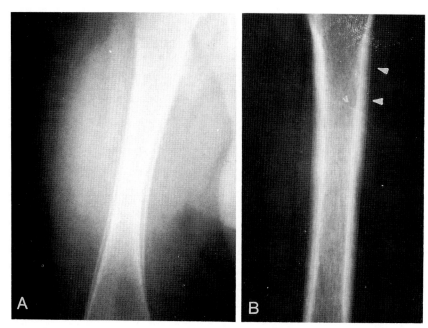

Figure 4.134. True vs. pseudoperiosteal new bone deposition. A. Note typical, outwardly displaced, true periosteal new bone deposition in premature infant. **B.** Pseudoperiosteal new bone deposition *(arrows)* secondary to demineralization revealing last layer of normally deposited cortical bone.

cortex; **rather it remains in complete alignment with the cortex and attests to its normal heritage.** With pathologic deposition, the reverse is true.

In general, when one or another of the foregoing periosteal new bone configurations is seen, some underlying disease should be present, but while this is almost irrevocably true in older children, in the very young infant periosteal new bone deposition can be normal (15). **Indeed, this is the only time when it can be normal, and the phenomenon is actually quite common.** Basically, it occurs between the ages of 2 and 6 months (with peak at 3 months), more often in premature infants, and is believed to represent nothing more than exuberant normal diaphyseal new bone deposition (16, 19). It must be differentiated from pathologic periosteal new bone formation, and for the most part one can do this on the basis of its configuration and favorite locations. In this regard, it is a phenomenon of the long bones and most often is seen in the femora (Fig. 4.134A), tibiae, and humeri. In the tibiae, it tends to occur medially more than laterally, and in all the bones it is primarily diaphyseal. In other words, the layer of periosteal new bone is deposited along the diaphysis and disappears before it gets to the metaphysis. Similar diaphyseal new bone deposition preponderance occurs in Caffey disease (infantile cortical hyperostosis) but, generally, concomitant clinical symptoms establish

the latter diagnosis. With normal periosteal new bone, no symptoms are present and roentgenographic identification often is incidental.

Layered Periosteal New Bone

Thin, layered periosteal new bone can occur in single or multiple layers (Fig. 4.135). Its appearance belies a rather active and/or acute disease process; i.e., acute osteomyelitis, bone infarction (usually with sickle cell disease), malignant bone tumors (both primary and secondary), leukemia and lymphoma, prostaglandin therapy (11, 18), healing fractures (ordinary and pathologic), more aggressive histiocytosis-X, rheumatoid arthritis (8, 9), hypervitaminosis A (14), and indolent, adjacent soft tissue inflammations and infections (16). In those cases where the disease process involves the metaphyses, periosteal new bone deposition extends down to the epiphyseal-metaphyseal junction, and when it is extremely aggressive, cortical breakthrough causes such rapid periosteal elevation that an acute triangle is formed at the point of maximal elevation. This has been termed "Codman's triangle" (Fig. 4.135B), and although it can be seen with any aggressive lesion (Fig. 135C), it is most characteristic of malignant bone tumors. Other causes of layered periosteal new bone deposition are listed in Table 4.42.

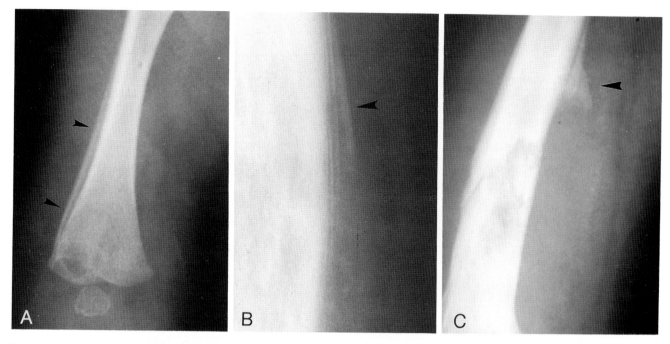

Figure 4.135. Layered periosteal new bone. A. Single layer of periosteal new bone *(arrows)* in infant with osteomyelitis. Note destructive lesion in distal metaphysis. **B.** Multiple layers of periosteal new bone in patient with Ewing sarcoma. Also note Codman triangle *(arrow)*. **C.** Codman triangle in patient with healed, chronic osteomyelitis *(arrow)*.

Solid, Straight, Wavy, or Lumpy Periosteal New Bone

This form of periosteal new bone deposition indicates a slow disease process (Fig. 4.136) and, consequently, is not seen with malignant bone tumors or the usual case of osteomyelitis or bone infarction. However, if bone infection is low grade, or a benign tumor is associated with pathologic fracturing, solid new bone deposition can be seen. Such new bone deposition can be straight or undulating (i.e., lumpy or wavy) and, when undulating, chronic venous stasis, long-standing infection (either bony or soft tissue) (Fig. 4.136B), or chronic stress fractures (Fig. 4.136C) should be considered. Solid, rather straight, periosteal new bone deposition in the fingers occurs with thyroid acropachy, but the problem is rare in children (17), and solid periosteal bone deposition can be seen in histiocytosis-X (Fig. 4.136A). Solid, wavy periosteal bone also is characteristic of melorheostosis (Fig. 4.136D) (2).

Spiculated Periosteal New Bone

In the long bones, spiculated periosteal new bone deposition reflects a very abrupt and rapid elevation of the periosteum. For this reason, it is virtually synonymous with malignant bone tumor, either primary (more common), or secondary (Fig. 4.137). In such cases, periosteal elevation occurs at a rate just slow enough to allow new bone deposition on perpendicularly oriented fibers located between the elevated periosteum and underlying cortex. These fibers, called Sharpey fibers, provide a lattice for calcium deposition which, because of their perpendicular orientation, leads to spiculation. Such spiculation is not seen with osteomyelitis, bone infarction, or trauma. In osteomyelitis, it has been suggested that proteolytic activity of the exudate leads to destruction of the fibers, but this would not explain why spiculated bone is not seen with periosteal elevations secondary to bone infarction or hemorrhage. All of this notwithstanding, when spiculated periosteal new bone is seen one should think of malignant bone tumors such as Ewing sarcoma, osteosarcoma, fibrosarcoma, chondrosarcoma, metastatic disease, leukemia, and occasionally even lymphoma. The only benign tumor that produces some degree of spiculation with any consistency is hemangioma of the bone.

Markedly Elevated (Ballooned) Periosteal New Bone

In these cases, periosteal new bone takes the form of a single, often undulating, layer, widely removed

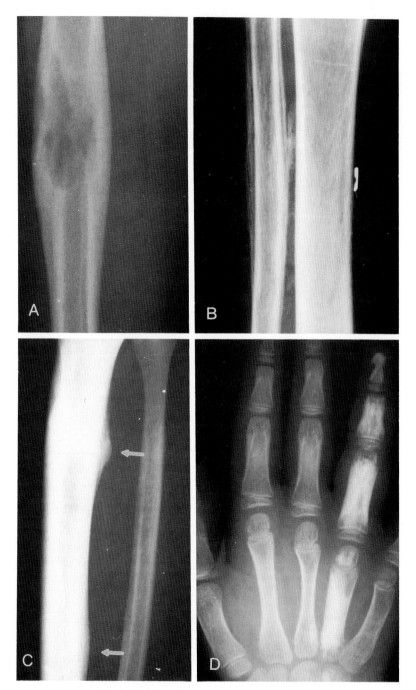

Figure 4.136. Solid, straight, wavy, or lumpy periosteal new bone. A. Solid, dense periosteal new bone in histiocytosis-X. **B.** Solid, thick single layer of periosteal new bone deposition with chronic soft tissue infection. **C.** Lumpy periosteal new bone deposition in healing stress fractures *(arrows)*. **D.** Periosteal thickening (smooth) in melorheostosis.

from the shaft (Fig. 4.138). In some cases, the periosteum is pulled so far away that ballooning occurs. Almost always, the finding is due to extensive subperiosteal bleeding and most often is seen with neurogenic fractures and fractures in the battered child syndrome. In both instances, excessive motion around the fracture site predisposes the patient to marked subperiosteal bleeding and periosteal elevation. Similar bleeding, usually spontaneous or due to minor trauma, also occurs in bleeding disorders, neurofibromatosis (22), and of course, in scurvy. Ballooned periosteal new bone deposition also occasionally is seen in mastocytosis in its early stages and in hyperphosphatemia (3, 7).

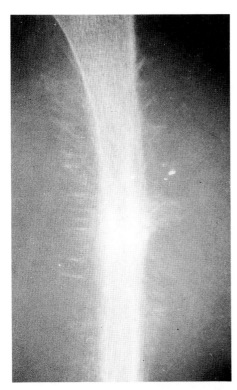

Figure 4.137. Spiculated periosteal new bone. Typical spiculations in malignant bone tumor *(arrow).* Ewing sarcoma.

REFERENCES

1. Athreya BH, Borns P, Rosenlund ML: Cystic fibrosis and hypertrophic osteoarthropathy in children. *Am J Dis Child* 129:634–637, 1975.
2. Beauvais P, Faure C, Montagne JP, Chigot PL, Maroteaux P: Leri's melorheostosis: three pediatric cases and a review of the literature. *Pediatr Radiol* 6:153–159, 1977.
3. Caffey J: Familial hyperphosphatasemia with ateliosis and hypermetabolism of growing bone. *Progr Pediatr Radiol* 4:438–468, 1973.
4. Cavanaugh JJA, Holman GH: Hypertrophic osteoarthropathy in childhood. *J Pediatr* 66:27–40, 1965.
5. Chamberlain DS, Whitaker J, Silverman F: Idiopathic osteoarthropathy and cranial defects in children (familial idiopathic osteoarthropathy). *AJR* 93:408–415, 1965.
6. Currarino G, Tierney RC, Giesel RG, Weihl C: Familial idiopathic osteoarthropathy. *AJR* 85:633–644, 1961.
7. Dunn V, Condon VR, Rallison ML: Familial hyperphosphatasemia: diagnosis in early infancy and response to human thyrocalcitonin therapy. *AJR* 132:541–545, 1979.
8. Goel KM, Rawson SP, Shanks RA: Radiological assessment of fifty patients with juvenile rheumatoid arthritis: correlation with clinical and laboratory abnormalities. *Pediatr Radiol* 2:51–60, 1974.
9. Kapusta MA, Sedlezky I: Periostitis: an early diagnostic sign of juvenile rheumatoid arthritis. *J Can Assoc Radiol* 18:268, 1967.
10. Kay CJ, Rosenberg MA, Burd R: Hypertrophic osteoarthropathy and childhood Hodgkin's disease. *Radiology* 112:177–178, 1974.
11. Matzinger MA, Briggs VA, Dunlap HJ, Udjus K, Martin DJ, McDonald P: Plain film and CT observations in prostaglandin-induced bone changes. *Pediatr Radiol* 22:264–266, 1992.
12. Miller JH, Ortega JA, Heisel MA: Juvenile Gaucher disease simulating osteomyelitis. *AJR* 137:880–882, 1981.
13. Nathanson I, Riddlesberger MM Jr: Pulmonary hypertrophic osteoarthropathy in cystic fibrosis. *Radiology* 135:649–651, 1980.
14. Seibert JJ, Byrne WJ, Golladay ES: Development of hypervitaminosis A in a patient on long-term parenteral hyperalimentation. *Pediatr Radiol* 10:173–174, 1981.
15. Shopfner CE: Periosteal bone growth in normal infants. *AJR* 97:154–163, 1966.
16. Swischuk LE, Jorgenson F, Jorgenson A, Capen D: Wooden splinter-induced "pseudotumors" and "osteomyelitis-like lesions" of bone and soft tissues. *AJR* 122:176–179, 1974.
17. Thomas J, Collipp PJ, Sharma RK: Thyroid acropachy. *Am J Dis Child* 125:745–746, 1973.
18. Ueda K, Saito A, Nakano H, Aoshima M, Yokota M, Muraoka R, Iwaya T: Brief clinical and laboratory observations: cortical hyperostosis following long-term administration of prostaglandin E in infants with cyanotic congenital heart disease. *J Pediatr* 97:834–836, 1980.
19. Volberg FM Jr, Whalen JP, Krook L, Winchester P: Lamellated periosteal reactions: a radiologic and histologic investigation. *AJR* 128:85–87, 1977.

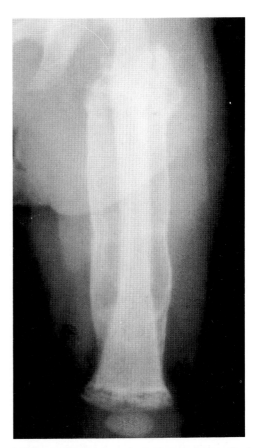

Figure 4.138. Ballooned, periosteal new bone. Typical ballooning in massive subperiosteal bleeding in battered child syndrome *(arrow).*

20. Wadhwa N, Balsam D, Ciminera P: Hypertrophic osteoarthropathy in a young child with adult respiratory distress syndrome (ARDS) secondary to burns. *Pediatr Radiol* 22:539–540, 1992.
21. Wastie ML, Wong HO, Ang AH: Hypertrophic osteoarthropathy in cyanotic congenital heart disease. *Australas Radiol* 17:276–279, 1973.
22. Yaghmai I, Tafazoli M: Massive subperiosteal hemorrhage in neurofibromatosis. *Radiology* 122:439–441, 1977.

BONE TUMORS, CYSTS, AND TUMOR-LIKE LESIONS

In analyzing bone tumors, cysts, and tumor-like lesions, the following roentgenographic features should be considered: (a) whether the lesion is single or multiple; (b) whether it is metaphyseal, diaphyseal, or epiphyseal; (c) whether it occurs in a flat bone, long bone, or both; (d) the type and rate of bone destruction it produces; (e) whether calcification or ossification are associated; (f) whether it is central (medullary) or eccentric (cortical); and (g) whether or not there is an associated soft tissue mass.

Single or Multiple Lesions

For the most part, multiple lesions occur with fibrous dysplasia, multiple enchondromatosis or Ollier disease (unilateral predominance of the enchondromas in this condition is pathognomonic), multiple osteochondromatosis (no unilateral predominance), histiocytosis-X, osteomyelitis, metastatic disease, leukemia, lymphoma, and benign cortical defects. The latter lesions are very common in children and are completely innocuous. Most often, they are seen in the knees and ankles, and their characteristics are discussed in greater detail in the next section.

Location of the Lesion

It is helpful to note whether a lesion occurs in a **long or flat bone** and, if in a long bone, whether it is **diaphyseal, metaphyseal, or epiphyseal.** Thereafter, one should determine whether the lesion is **central (medullary) or eccentric (cortical).** Primarily **diaphyseal** lesions are not that common, but of those that are malignant, Ewing sarcoma should be considered first. On the benign side of the ledger, one should consider histiocytosis-X (2) and possibly fibrous dysplasia. With osteomyelitis, bone infarction, most other bone tumors, metastatic disease, and bone cysts, the **metaphyses** are favored.

As far as **eccentricity of a lesion** is concerned, most lesions are central and located in the medullary cavity of the bone. However, benign cortical defects

and their related lesion, the nonossifying fibroma, characteristically are eccentric (Fig. 4.139*A*). These tumors, probably one and the same (36), are separated primarily by size. When they are large and cystic, they are termed "nonossifying fibromas," and when small and less prominent, they are called "benign cortical defects." Both can exist in the same individual and, many times, especially with benign cortical defects (27), the lesions are multiple. They occur primarily around the knees and ankles, and although benign cortical defects may appear cyst-like en face, on tangent their cortical location is clearly apparent (see Fig. 4.32*D*). Once these roentgenographic criteria are met for a solitary lesion, the diagnosis virtually is assured. When low-grade osteomyelitis produces such a defect, differentiation may be more difficult, but clinical symptoms should separate the two conditions. In addition, in osteomyelitis the defect almost always extends to the epiphyseal line. Indeed, very often the adjacent epiphysis is involved and so is the joint. When nonossifying fibromas are large, they are susceptible to pathologic fracture, but this does not occur with the smaller ones or with benign cortical defects. With time, both lesions tend to disappear spontaneously, and thus, neither lesion requires any specific therapy. The natural course is for the lesions to become obliterated by healing and bony sclerosis (Fig. 4.139*B*).

In contradistinction to benign cortical defects and nonossifying fibromas, benign unicameral bone cysts characteristically are central (26). They expand the cortex and are quite radiolucent (Fig. 4.139*C*), and because they are expansile their cortex becomes quite thin and susceptible to pathologic fracture. Histologically, they are full of serous fluid and, consequently, when such fractures occur, a piece of the cyst wall can fall into the cyst cavity. Roentgenographically, the phenomenon results in the "fallen fragment" (30) sign (Fig. 4.139*C*).

Bone cysts, much as nonossifying fibromas and benign cortical defects, heal by slow, spontaneous obliteration, but often the process is hastened by repeated fracturing or surgical filling with bone chips. Steroid injections also seem to accomplish the same objective (11). Overall, bone cysts have a tendency to recur, at least until the patient passes out of adolescence. Eighty percent occur in the proximal humerus and femur (26), but most of these are seen in the proximal humerus. Of course, they can occur in other long bones and even in flat bones (34).

Lesions located within the **epiphysis** are far less common than those seen in the metaphysis. When they do occur, they usually are accounted for by one

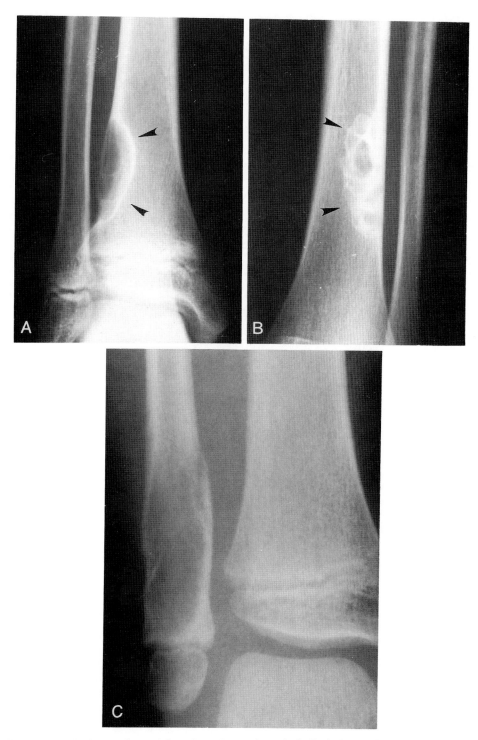

Figure 4.139. Solitary bone lesion: value of location. A. Typical eccentric location of nonossifying fibroma *(arrow)*. **B.** Another typical eccentric nonossifying fibroma in its healing stage *(arrow)*. **C.** Typical central, metaphyseal location of benign bone cyst with a "fallen fragment sign" due to a piece of cortex in the cyst.

of the following conditions: osteomyelitis (14, 31) (Fig. 4.140A), osteochondritis dissecans, histiocytosis-X (rather rare in epiphysis), benign bone cysts (also rare in epiphysis), normal epiphyseal de-

fects (common in knees), monarticular rheumatoid arthritis (Fig. 4.140B), tuberculous arthritis (12), fungal arthritis, traumatic avulsions, and, rarely, intraosseous ganglions (see Table 4.22) (9). Tumors

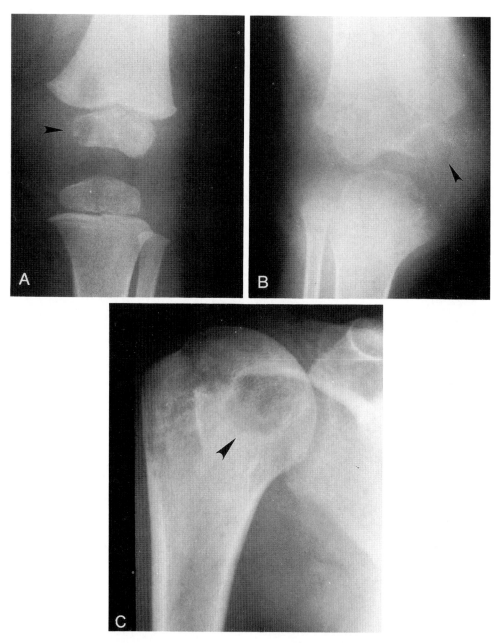

Figure 4.140. Solitary bone lesions: epiphyseal location. A. Note radiolucent defect in the distal femoral epiphysis *(arrow).* Above it is another radiolucent defect in the metaphysis. Both were caused by osteomyelitis. **B.** Large defect in distal femur secondary to erosion in monarticular rheumatoid arthritis *(arrow).* **C.** Classic appearance of chondroblastoma in young adult *(arrow).* Note its epiphyseal-metaphyseal location. For other lesions producing epiphyseal defects, see Figure 4.58.

causing epiphyseal defects are rare, except for chondroblastomas. This tumor, more a problem of older children, characteristically involves the epiphysis (25) and extends across the epiphyseal line into the metaphysis (Fig. 4.140C). The other tumor, notoriously involving the epiphysis, is the giant cell tumor. However, this is not a common tumor in children, and moreover, it does not produce an isolated epiphyseal defect.

Type and Rate of Bone Destruction

Bone destruction can be rapid or slow, and can occur from diseases arising from within the bone, or from those arising in adjacent tissues. The latter, for the most part, occurs with soft tissue bone tumors, chronic tendon avulsions, and periosteal lesions such as the rare periosteal sarcoma and cortical, eccentric giant cell tumor. Soft tissue radiography and MRI

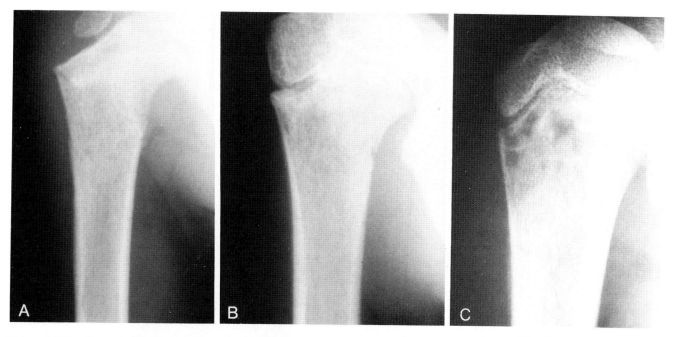

Figure 4.141. Bone destruction: aggressive, moth-eaten appearance. A. Typical moth-eaten, coarsely trabeculated, destruction due to tumor (metastatic neuroblastoma). **B.** Similar appearance due to acute osteomyelitis. **C.** More extensive and coarse appearing destruction in osteomyelitis.

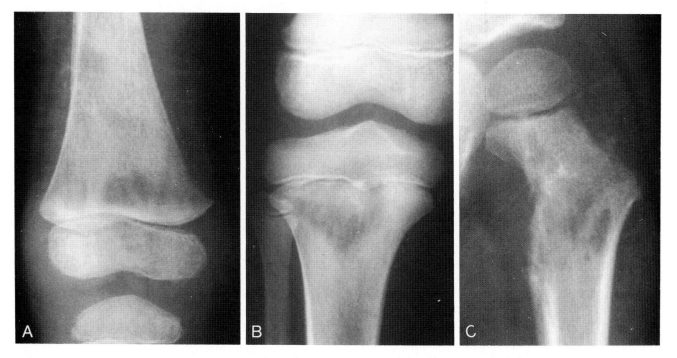

Figure 4.142. Bone destruction: aggressive homogeneous appearance. A. Rather homogeneous bone destruction in metastatic neuroblastoma. Also note permeative pattern in some areas. **B.** Aggressive, rather homogeneous destruction in osteomyelitis. **C.** Homogeneous destruction in histiocytosis-X. In all cases, note lack of any significant peripheral sclerosis.

are quite useful for delineating many of these lesions. Arteriography still can be employed, but is utilized primarily for defining the degree of vascularity in or around a tumor.

As far as destruction from within is concerned, it can be (a) aggressive and moth-eaten, (b) aggressive and homogeneous, or (c) slow, and variably expanding (Figs. 4.141–144). The more active the de-

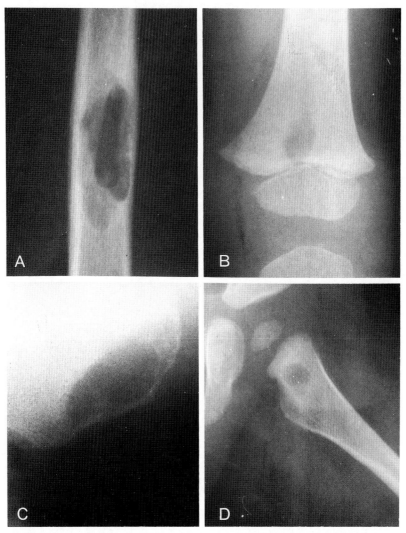

Figure 4.143. Punched out lytic lesions. A. Typical punched out lesion of histiocytosis-X *(arrow).* Often these lesions are more dramatically displayed in the calvarium. **B.** Smaller lesion of histiocytosis-X. **C.** Somewhat similar lesion in the iliac wing of a patient with disseminated coccidiomycosis. **D.** Small focus of osteomyelitis.

structive process, the less distinct and sclerotic is the margin of the lesion and, conversely, the slower the rate of destruction, the more discrete and sclerotic the margin. When rapid destruction results in a moth-eaten appearance of the bone, and the cortex is penetrated, the term "permeative" is applied. Cortical penetration also commonly occurs with aggressive homogeneous destruction, and in either case, when this happens periosteal elevation and new bone deposition is seen. For the most part, diseases producing moth-eaten destruction include acute osteomyelitis, aggressive fibromas (15), metastatic disease, leukemia, lymphoma, malignant bone tumors, and bone infarction (Fig. 4.141).

Aggressive destruction leading to a more homogeneous pattern of destruction (Fig. 4.142) is seen with

osteomyelitis, cat-scratch disease (4), bone infarction, some cases of leukemia (22, 35), lymphoma, or metastatic disease, and the histiocytosis-X-eosinophilic granuloma group of lesions (2) (Fig. 4.142). When these lesions are sharp-edged or "punched out" and their margins nonsclerotic, one should first consider histiocytosis-X (2) and then osteomyelitis, especially fungal (Fig. 4.143). Other conditions to be considered include all of the neonatal infections (i.e., rubella, CMV, syphilis), multiple fibromatosis or hamartomatosis of bone, fibrous dysplasia, malignant fibrous histiocytoma (10), osteitis fibrosa cystica, bone infarcts associated with pancreatitis (6, 13, 16, 17), and intraosseous bleeding with blood dyscrasias such as hemophilia. In these latter cases, cystic expansion of the bone eventually may result. When

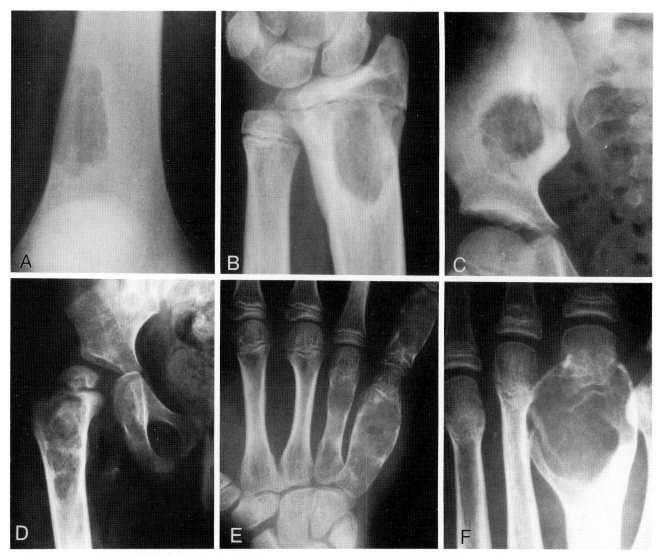

Figure 4.144. Bone destruction: nonaggressive. A. Slow bone destruction with minimal sclerosis in nonossifying fibroma. **B.** Slow destruction with more sclerosis in low grade osteomyelitis (i.e., Brodie abscess). Note extension into epiphysis. **C.** Slow destruction with sclerosis in benign bone cyst of iliac wing. **D.** Slow destruction with considerable sclerosis in chronic, cystic tuberculosis of the bone. Also note epiphyseal involvement. **E.** Slow destruction with expansion of bone in multiple enchondromatosis. **F.** Slow destruction with marked expansion in solitary enchondroma.

homogeneous bone destruction is focal, and associated with considerable sclerosis of its margins, a slower disease process should be inferred, and then one should consider lesions such as bone cysts, low-grade or antibiotic modified (7, 33) osteomyelitis (Brodie abscess), fibrous dysplasia, chondromyxoid fibroma, hemangioma, lymphangioma, and intraosseous ganglion (Fig. 4.144). The densest, thickest margins are seen with osteomyelitis (8, 12), Brodie's abscess (18), some cases of chondromyxoid fibroma, fibrous dysplasia, and intraosseous ganglia (9). The thinnest sclerotic margins are seen with unicameral bone cysts, aneurysmal bone cysts (5, 19, 21,

24, 28), giant cell tumors, some cases of fibrous dysplasia, hemangiomas (3), hemophilic pseudotumors (1, 2), lymphangiomas, and a few enchondromas.

When any of the foregoing, slow-growing lesions are multiloculated, the two best possibilities are unicameral bone cyst (all compartments communicate and thus the cyst is still unicameral) or fibrous dysplasia (Fig. 4.145). Somewhat similar configurations can be seen with multiple enchondromatosis, malignant fibrous histiocytoma, the brown tumor of hyperparathyroidism, giant cell tumors, aneurysmal bone cysts, and hemangiomas (32) or lymphangiomas (29)

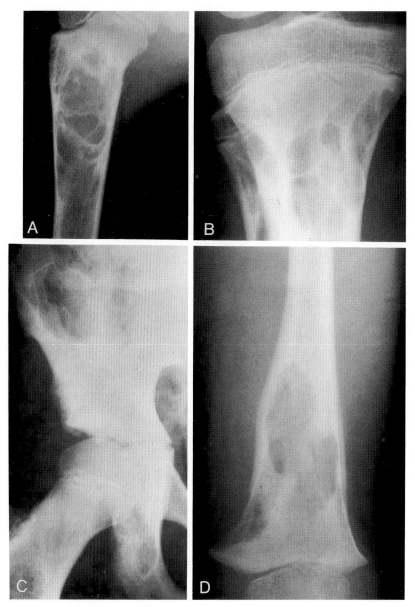

Figure 4.145. Multiloculated cystic lesions. A. Multiloculated unicameral bone cyst. **B.** Multiloculated fibrous dysplasia, with pathologic fracture. **C.** Multiloculated lymphangioma of bone. **D.** Somewhat multiloculated cystic destruction in histiocytosis-X.

of bone (Fig. 4.145C). Less commonly, one might encounter chondromas or chondromyxoid fibromas producing multiloculated lesions. However, the latter tend not to be as multiloculated and their sclerotic margins are broader. Occasionally, histiocytosis-X lesions also can appear somewhat multiloculated (Fig. 4.145D).

Finally, a note may be made regarding certain bone tumors that produce rather elongated lesions. For the most part, these are benign tumors, and include fibrous dysplasia and multiple enchondromas (Ollier disease) (23). In fibrous dysplasia, the lesions are quite variable and may be associated with areas of radiolucency, bone expansion, cystic change, sclerosis, or smudgy, expanded bone (Fig. 4.146). With multiple enchondromatosis, the lesions often consist of broad, radiolucent stripes extending for some distance into the diaphysis of the long bones (Fig. 4.147). Some of these lesions become somewhat bulbous, and occasionally may be difficult to distinguish from an osteochondroma or exostosis. Multiple enchondromatosis, or Ollier disease, tends to be predominantly, if not entirely, unilateral in its distribution, and eventually some of the cartilaginous lesions may calcify in characteristic, popcorn fashion (Fig. 4.148A).

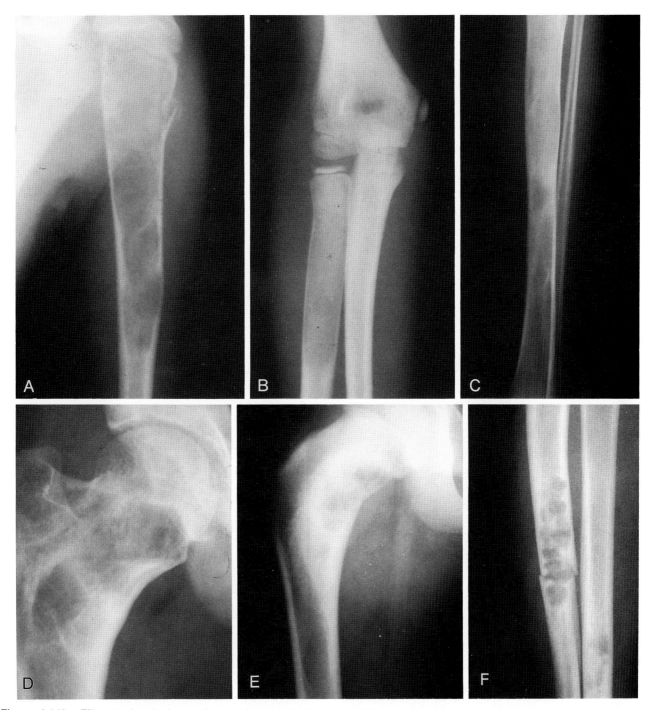

Figure 4.146. Fibrous dysplasia: various lesion types. A. Long multiloculated, expanding lesion of fibrous dysplasia of humerus. Note pathologic fracture. **B.** Long expanding lesion of radius with smudgy, ground glass appearance. **C.** Long, mixed lytic and blastic lesion of tibia in fibrous dysplasia. **D.** Multiloculated, expanding lytic lesion of upper femur. **E.** Sclerosing, slightly loculated lesion in another patient. **F.** Small locules in multiloculated lesion of fibrous dysplasia with pathologic fracture.

Calcification or Ossification

Very few bone lesions calcify or ossify and almost always when calcifications are seen they are irregular, and occur in some type of cartilage tumor (e.g., enchondroma, chondroblastoma [Fig.4.148A]). Ossi-fication, often profound, is characteristic of osteogenic sarcoma and usually is rather amorphous (Fig. 4.148B). Metastatic lesions from osteogenic sarcoma also can ossify, and these are best known in the lung. Punctate calcifications are pathognomonic of hemangiomatous or lymphangiomatous tumors, but these

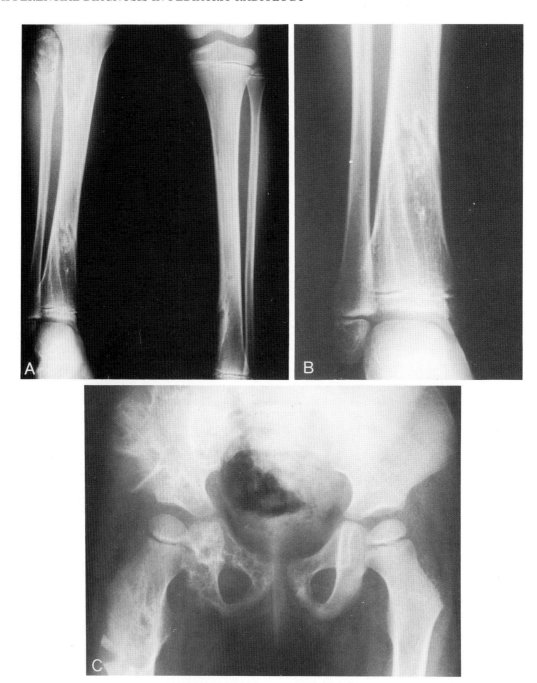

Figure 4.147. Lesions of multiple enchondromatosis. A. Note unilateral predominance of long radiolucent lesions in the tibial metaphyses on the right. **B.** Closeup of lower tibial lesion to show elongated pattern of tumor. **C.** Another patient with less linear enchondromas. Note unilateral distribution.

tumors most often are soft tissue tumors and involve the bones only secondarily. The calcifications, of course, are calcified phleboliths (see Fig. 4.130B).

Soft Tissue Components

Soft tissue components of a bony lesion result only when the disease process within the bone breaks through the cortex and extends into the soft tissues. This occurs, for the most part, with infection and malignant bone tumors. Occasionally, expansile bone cysts or benign bone tumors become so large that they produce associated bulging of the soft tissues, but there is no actual extension of the lesion into the soft tissues if no fracture occurs.

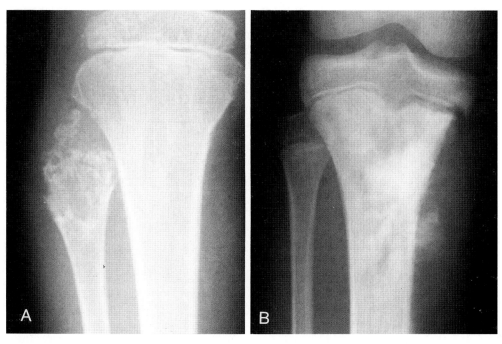

Figure 4.148. Calcification-ossification in bone tumors. A. Typical, irregular calcification of cartilage in enchondroma. Patient with Ollier disease. **B.** Sclerosis due to new bone formation in osteogenic sarcoma of tibia.

REFERENCES

1. Brant EE, Jordan HH: Radiologic aspects of hemophilic pseudotumors in bone. *AJR* 115:525–539, 1972.
2. Bollini G, Jouve JL, Gentet JC, Jacquenier M, Bouyala JM: Bone lesions in histiocytosis X. *J Pediatr Orthop* 11:469–477, 1991.
3. Brower AC, Culver JE Jr, Keats TE: Diffuse cystic angiomatosis of bone: report of two cases. *AJR* 118:456–463, 1973.
4. Carithers HA: Cat-scratch disease associated with an osteolytic lesion. *Am J Dis Child* 137:968–970, 1983.
5. Carlson DH, Wilkinson RH, Bhakkavisiam A: Aneurysmal bone cysts in children. *AJR* 116:644–650, 1972.
6. Cohen H, Haller JO, Friedman AP: Pancreatitis, child abuse, and skeletal lesions. *Pediatr Radiol* 10:175–177, 1981.
7. Davis LA: Antibiotic modified osteomyelitis. *AJR* 103:608–610, 1968.
8. Echeverria J, Kaude JV: Multifocal tuberculous osteomyelitis. *Pediatr Radiol* 7:238–240, 1978.
9. Feldman F, Johnston A: Intraosseous ganglion. *AJR* 118:328–343, 1973.
10. Feldman, F, Lattes R: Primary malignant fibrous histiocytoma (fibrous xanthoma) of bone. *Skeletal Radiol* 1:145–160, 1977.
11. Fernbach SK, Blumenthal DH, Poznanski AK, Dias LS, Tachdjian MO: Radiographic changes in unicameral bone cysts following direct injection of steroids: a report of 14 cases. *Radiology* 140:689–695, 1981.
12. Goldblatt M, Cremin BJ: Osteoarticular tuberculosis: its presentation in colored races. *Clin Radiol* 29:669–677, 1978.
13. Goluboff N, Cram R, Ramgotra B, Singh A, Wilkinson GW: Polyarthritis and bone lesions complicating traumatic pancreatitis in two children. *Can Med Assoc J* 118:924–928, 1978.
14. Green NE, Beauchamp RD, Griffin PO: Primary subacute epiphyseal osteomyelitis. *J Bone Joint Surg* 63A:107–114, 1981.
15. Herring JA, Watts HG, Enneking WF: Aggressive fibromatosis. *J Pediatr Orthop* 7:107–108, 1987.
16. Hollingworth P, Isaacs D, Dydder G: Recurrent osteolytic lesions and subcutaneous fat necrosis in association with a developmental pancreatic cyst. *Arch Dis Child* 54:790–792, 1979.
17. Keating JP, Shackelford GD, Shackelford PG, Ternberg JL: Pancreatitis and osteolytic lesions. *J Pediatr* 81:350–353, 1972.
18. Kozlowski K: Brodie's abscess in the first decade of life. *Pediatr Radiol* 10:33–37, 1980.
19. Kozlowski K, Middleton RWD: Aneurysmal bone cysts-review of 10 cases. *Australas Radiol* 24:170–175, 1970.
20. Krill CE Jr, Mauer AM: Pseudotumor of calcaneus in christmas disease. *Pediatrics* 77:848–855, 1970.
21. Kubicz S: Radiological aspects of aneurysmal bone cysts in children. *Ann Radiol* 13:211–218, 1970.
22. Kushner DC, Weinstein HJ, Kirkpatrick JA: The radiologic diagnosis of leukemia and lymphoma in children. *Semin Roentgenol* 15:316–334, 1980.
23. Mainzer F, Hanagi H, Steinbach HL: The variable manifestations of multiple enchondromatosis. *Radiology* 99:377–388, 1971.
24. Locher GW, Kaiser G: Giant-cell tumors and aneurysmal bone cysts of ribs in childhood. *J Pediatr Surg* 10:103–108, 1975.

25. McLeod RA, Beabout JW: The roentgenographic features of chondroblastoma. *AJR* 118:464–471, 1973.
26. Norman A, Schiffman M: Simple bone cysts: factors of age dependency. *Radiology* 124:779–782, 1977.
27. Prentice AID: Variations on fibrous cortical defect. *Clin Radiol* 25:531–533, 1974.
28. Pullan CR, Alexander JW, Halse PC: Aneurysmal bone cyst: a report of three cases. *Arch Dis Child* 53:899–901, 1979.
29. Reilly BJ, Davidson JW, Bain H: Lymphangiectasis of the skeleton: a case report. *Radiology* 103:385–386, 1972.
30. Reynolds J: The "fallen fragment sign" in the diagnosis of unicameral bone cysts. *Radiology* 92:949–953, 1969.
31. Rosenbaum DM, Blumhagen JD: Acute epiphyseal osteomyelitis in children. *Radiology* 156:89–92, 1985.
32. Schajowicz F, Aiello C, Francone M, Giannini R: Cystic angiomatosis. *J Bone Joint Surg* 60B:100–106, 1978.
33. Season EH, Miller PR: Primary subacute pyogenic osteomyelitis in long bones in children. *J Pediatr Surg* 11:347–353, 1976.
34. Shulman HS, Wilson SR, Harvie JN, Cruickshand B: Unicameral bone cyst in a rib of a child. *AJR* 128:1058–1060, 1977.
35. Simmons CR, Harle TS, Singleton EB: The osseous manifestations of leukemia in children. *Radiol Clin North Am* 6:115–130, 1968.
36. Steiner GC: Fibrous cortical defect and nonossifying fibroma of bone: a study of the ultrastructure. *Arch Pathol* 97:205–210, 1974.

Syndromology

The identification of syndromes, dwarfs, and dysplasias is an important part of pediatric radiology, but there are so many syndromes to remember and so many findings to consider that the problem becomes overwhelming. Of course, if one deals with the problem on a regular basis, identification becomes a little easier, but never is it completely without difficulty. For this reason, one needs to devise a system of analysis and, in this regard, one might begin by noting that the most useful information is derived from examination of the long bones, hands, pelvis, and spine. Additional information is available from examination of the skull, feet, and other flat bones, but almost always, if one cannot make a diagnosis from the bones noted in the first group, difficulty persists. Differential diagnoses and more details for the various skeletal findings to be noted in the ensuing discussion are available throughout this chapter and in a number of currently available syndrome books (1–4). The following is a brief resume only, and only one possible approach to the evaluation of syndromes.

LONG BONE FINDINGS

One of the first long bone observations to be made concerns bone length, and although occasionally the bones are too long, most often the problem is shortening. In this regard, once shortening is noted, one should try to determine whether it is the proximal (humerus, femur), middle (tibia, fibula, radius-ulna), or distal (hands, feet) segment of the extremity that bears the brunt of the shortening. Proximal segment predominance is referred to as rhizomelic, and middle segment as mesomelic shortening. Distal segment shortening as a predominant or isolated phenomenon is rather uncommon, and then generally is referred to as peripheral dysostosis. For a list of conditions with overly long or short bones, see Tables 4.3 and 4.5.

After major segment predominance has been assessed, one should try to decide whether the problem in the individual bone is diaphyseal, metaphyseal, or epiphyseal. Diaphyseal predominance is easiest to assess because in such cases the metaphyses and epiphyses appear normal or near normal. Abnormal **diaphyseal changes** can be grouped as follows: (a) thin or overtubulated bones (see Table 4.5); (b) short, squat, or undertubulated bones (see Table 4.3); and (c) diaphyseal sclerosis caused by periosteal deposition. **Metaphyseal abnormalities** consist of (a) splaying, (b) cupping, (c) widening, and (d) irregularity (see Tables 4.24–4.26). **Abnormalities of the epiphysis** usually consist of (a) smallness, (b) fragmentation or irregularity, and (c) calcification (see Tables 4.15–4.22). In most instances, it is relatively easy to determine whether the epiphysis or metaphysis is bearing the brunt of the abnormality; but, in some cases, epiphyseal maldevelopment is so profound that secondary metaphyseal changes are induced (i.e., it is surmised that, because the epiphysis is underdeveloped, injury to the growth plate causes subsequent metaphyseal growth disturbances). In such cases, it is important to appreciate that the epiphyseal changes are the primary problem because, otherwise, an erroneous diagnosis will result. For the most part, this phenomenon occurs with the pseudoachondroplasia syndromes, and almost always one is dealing with multiple epiphyseal dysplasia or spondyloepiphyseal dysplasia (see Fig. 4.4*B*).

HAND AND FOOT ABNORMALITIES

With these abnormalities, it is the hand that "pays off" more than the foot, because hand changes are easier to assess and usually more striking.

Changes in the hands include the following: spade-shaped hand, shortening of the metacarpals (either selective or generalized), shortening of various phalanges, shortening of the thumb, triphalangeal thumb, incurving of the fifth digit, cone-shaped epiphyses, polydactyly, and syndactyly (see Tables 4.29–4.32). In addition to assessing the small bones of the hands and feet, the carpal and tarsal bones should be assessed for irregularity, smallness, scalloping, and fusion (see Table 4.34).

PELVIC CHANGES

For the most part, pelvic changes are most useful for the diagnosis of the various chondrodystrophies, storage diseases, and certain chromosomal abnormalities. Although, in the past, much was made regarding these pelvic configurations, they are now used less than other abnormalities of the skeletal system. Nonetheless, one still should be familiar with the differential diagnosis for the following: (a) short, squared off iliac wings; (b) iliac wings with a narrow waist; (c) increased and decreased acetabular angles; and (d) absence of portions of the pubic bones (see Table 4.35).

SPINE ABNORMALITIES

Assessment of the spine can be very helpful in establishing diagnoses in confusing syndromes and dwarfs, especially in the neonatal period (see Fig. 5.26). However, as with the rest of the skeleton, one should have some idea as to which findings are most helpful. In this regard, it is worthwhile looking at the following: (a) the C_1–C_2 area for abnormalities of the dens (see Table 6.25); (b) the presence or absence of clefting abnormalities of the vertebral bodies (see Table 6.7); and (c) the shape of the vertebral bodies. Abnormal shapes consist of (a) platyspondyly (for various types see Table 6.10), (b) cuboid vertebrae (see Table 6.11), (c) round or bullet-shaped vertebrae (see Table 6.14), and (d) notched or beaked vertebrae (see Table 6.16). In addition, one should determine whether the vertebral column is narrowed or normal in diameter. This is important in identifying achondroplasia and other examples of chondrodystrophic dwarfism in which the vertebral canal is narrowed (see Table 6.18).

MISCELLANEOUS FINDINGS

In the long bones, miscellaneous findings include congenital dislocations, synostoses, and abnormalities of mineralization (i.e., demineralization and increased sclerosis). All of these features have been covered in earlier sections. Other abnormalities include exostoses, calcification of cartilage, and twisted bones. The latter almost exclusively occur in the Melnick-Needles syndrome, but also can be seen with neurofibromatosis. Exostoses are seen in a variety of conditions (see Table 4.14), but on a diagnostic basis they are used most often in the multiple exostosis syndrome and in the nail patella syndrome where they take the form of iliac wing exostoses (horns) or Fong lesion. Stippled calcification of cartilage occurs in punctate epiphyseal dysplasia, Zellweger cerebrohepatorenal syndrome, and Warfarin embryonopathy (see Fig. 4.46). In these cases, as well as calcification of the epiphyses, calcification of the cartilages in the pelvis and spine also occurs.

REFERENCES

1. Poznanski AK: *The Hand in Radiologic Diagnosis.* Philadelphia: WB Saunders, 1984.
2. Smith DW: *Recognizable Patterns of Human Malformations: Genetic, Embryologic and Clinical Aspects.* Philadelphia: WB Saunders, 1970.
3. Spranger JW, Langer LO Jr, Weidemann HR: *Bone Dysplasias: An Atlas of Constitutional Disorders of Skeletal Development.* Philadelphia: WB Saunders, 1974.
4. Taybi H, Lachman RS: *Radiology of Syndrome.* 3d ed. Chicago: Year Book Medical Publishers, 1990.

Bone Age Determination

Bone age determination is an important part of pediatric radiology and almost everyone uses the Greulich-Pyle tables (2) for its determination. For the most part these suffice, but other methods of bone age determination (1, 3) are available and, of these, probably the most sensitive is the Elgenmark method (1). In this method, all the ossification centers of the epiphyses and carpal and tarsal bones are counted on one side of the body, and then the total is compared to what should be normal. However, only occasionally does one require this much refinement in bone age determination and, actually, if one is doing a lot of bone age work, one can memorize certain key ossification centers to facilitate rapid assessment. With this method, one still can obtain a reasonably accurate estimate of bone age and, for the most part, the centers include: (a) the capitate and hamate of the wrist; (b) the distal radial and ulnar epiphyses; (c) the epiphysis of the proximal phalanx of the thumb; (d) the pisiform bone; (e) the sesamoid

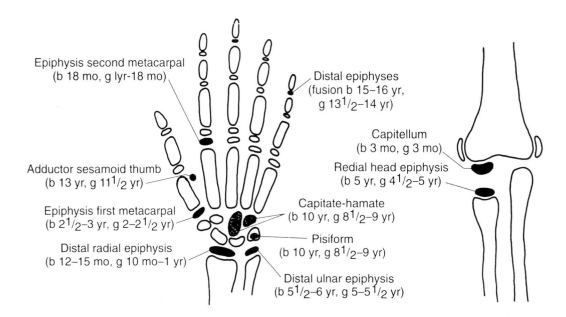

Epiphysis second metacarpal
(b 18 mo, g lyr-18 mo)

Distal epiphyses
(fusion b 15–16 yr,
g 13 1/2–14 yr)

Capitellum
(b 3 mo, g 3 mo)

Adductor sesamoid thumb
(b 13 yr, g 11 1/2 yr)

Redial head epiphysis
(b 5 yr, g 4 1/2–5 yr)

Epiphysis first metacarpal
(b 2 1/2–3 yr, g 2–2 1/2 yr)

Capitate-hamate
(b 10 yr, g 8 1/2–9 yr)

Pisiform
(b 10 yr, g 8 1/2–9 yr)

Distal radial epiphysis
(b 12–15 mo, g 10 mo–1 yr)

Distal ulnar epiphysis
(b 5 1/2–6 yr, g 5–5 1/2 yr)

Figure 4.149. Bone age determination. Utilizing the above data, one can arrive at a reasonably accurate bone age estimate.

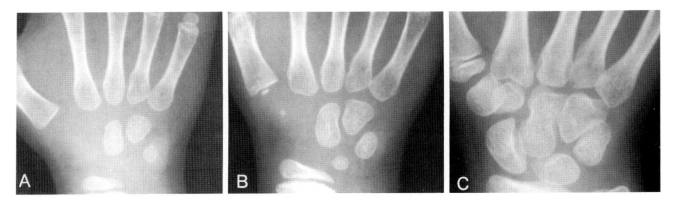

Figure 4.150. Maturation of carpal bones. A. Young infant with rather round carpal bones. **B.** Maturation leads to more angular configuration of these bones. **C.** More maturity leads to larger and much more angular, adult-appearing, bones.

of the thumb; (f) the epiphyses of the terminal phalanges; and, in the elbow: (g) the capitellum; and (h) the radial head epiphysis (Fig. 4.149).

In addition to the foregoing considerations, one or two other practical points about bone age determination might be made. For example, one should appreciate the fact that girls mature earlier than do boys and, as age progresses, the difference becomes greater. Furthermore, rate of bone maturation differs somewhat from one race to another (Blacks mature faster than Whites), and to some extent from one socioeconomic group to another (lower socioeconomic groups mature later). More important, how-

ever, is the fact that, in certain endocrinologic abnormalities, the ossification centers come in less regularly and, in some cases, seemingly haphazardly. In other words, one center might come in unexpectedly and yet another, which should have come in, is delayed. In these cases, it is important to assess as many centers as possible (this is the time to use the Elgenmark method) and, in addition, to appreciate how mature the individual bones appear. This is best accomplished with the carpal bones, which appear more and more angular as they become more mature (Fig. 4.150). In infants they are round and smooth, while in teenagers they are quite angular.

Nonetheless, in some cases, it is still difficult to establish an absolutely accurate bone age, and then it probably is more important to note degree of change from one examination to another.

REFERENCES

1. Elgenmark O: Normal development of the ossific centers during infancy and childhood: clinical, roentgenologic and statistical study. *Acta Paediatr* 33(suppl 1):1–79, 1946.
2. Greulich WW, Pyle JS: *Radiographic Atlas of Skeletal Development of Hand and Wrist.* 2d ed. Stanford, CA: Stanford University Press, 1959.
3. Sontag LW, Snell D, Anderson M: Rate of appearance of ossification centers from birth to the age of five years. *Am J Dis Child* 58:949–956, 1939.

ADVANCED AND DELAYED BONE AGE

Bone age deviations from normal are numerous and can be seen with endocrinologic, metabolic, and dysplastic bone disease. Most of the conditions producing such changes are listed in Table 4.43, and the information has been derived from experience and a number of extensive publications on the subject (1–3).

REFERENCES

1. Kuhns LR, Finnstrom O: New standards of ossification of the newborn. *Radiology* 119:655–660, 1976.
2. Smith DW: *Recognizable Patterns of Human Malformations: Genetic, Embryologic and Clinical Aspects.* Philadelphia: WB Saunders, 1970.
3. Taybi H: *Radiology of Syndromes.* Chicago: Year Book Medical Publishers, 1975.

Rickets: Roentgenographic Differential Diagnosis

Rickets has a number of causes and roentgenographically can be mimicked by conditions such as metaphyseal dysostosis and hypophosphatasia. However, once one decides that rickets is the problem, very often the type can be determined from roentgenographic examination of the knees and wrists

Table 4.43
Altered Bone Age

Retarded bone age
  Achondrogenesis
  Achondroplasia
  Aminopterin-induced syndrome
  Camptomelic syndrome
  Carpenter syndrome (acrocephalopolysyndactyly)
  Cephaloskeletal dysplasia (Taybi-Lindner syndrome)
  Cerebrohepatorenal syndrome (Zellweger syndrome)
  Chondrodysplasia punctata
  Chondroectodermal dysplasia (Ellis-van Creveld syndrome)
  Cleidocranial dysostosis
  Cloverleaf skull syndrome
  Cornelia de Lange syndrome
  Cushing syndrome
  Diastrophic dwarfism
  Epiphyseal dysplasia (multiple and spondylo)
  Failure-to-thrive
  Fanconi anemia
  Generalized gangliosidosis
  Hypothyroidism
  Leprechaunism
  Lesch-Nyhan syndrome
  Lightwood syndrome
  Lorain-Levi syndrome
  Mesomelic dwarfism: Nievergelt type
  Metatropic dwarfism
  Morquio disease
  Mucolipidoses
  Mucopolysaccharidoses
  Noonan syndrome
  Pierre-Robin syndrome
  Prader-Willi syndrome
  Riley-Day syndrome
  Rubella, congenital
  Rubinstein-Taybi syndrome
  Russell-Silver syndrome
  Saldino-Noonan syndrome
  Small for gestational age
  Spondyloepiphyseal dysplasia
  Thanatophoric dwarfism
  Trisomy-18
  Trisomy-21
  Turner syndrome
  Von Gierke syndrome
  Weill-Marchesani syndrome
  Wilson syndrome
  XXXXY syndrome
Accelerated bone age
  Acrodysostosis
  Adrenogenital syndrome
  Asphyxiating thoracic dystrophy
  Beckwith-Wiedemann syndrome
  Chondroectodermal dysplasia
  Cockayne syndrome
  Cushing syndrome
  Diastrophic dwarfism
  Homocystinuria
  Hyperthyroidism
  Lawrence-Seip syndrome
  Marshall syndrome
  McCune-Albright syndrome
  Majewski syndrome
  Peripheral dysostosis
  Saldino-Noonan syndrome
  Sotos syndrome
  Typus edinburgensis

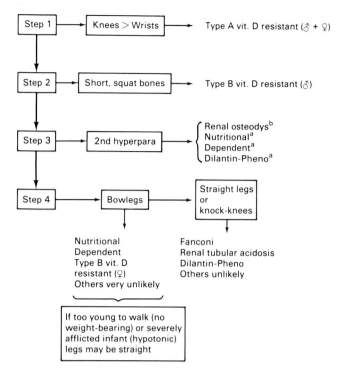

Figure 4.151. Roentgenographic scheme for diagnosis of rickets. Step 1 identifies patients with type A hypophosphatemic vitamin D-resistant rickets. **Step 2** identifies type B hypophosphatemic vitamin D-resistant rickets in males. Females with this form of rickets are not identified in this step, and with all other patients are described in the next step. **Step 3** identifies patients with renal osteodystrophy and the occasional case of severe nutritional, dependent, or Dilantin-phenobarbital rickets. **Step 4** deals with the remaining patients and allows one to offer a practical, short differential diagnosis in each instance. A few severe cases only (a). Accounts for most cases (b).

alone (2). This can be accomplished by the application of the following four steps (Fig. 4.151).

STEP 1: DISTRIBUTION OF EPIPHYSEAL-METAPHYSEAL CHANGE

In this step, one must decide whether the rachitic changes are uniformly distributed throughout the skeleton or most prominent in the lower extremities. This is a very important determination, for it serves to specifically identify a certain group of patients with hypophosphatemic vitamin D-resistant rickets (2). The preponderance of lower extremity changes in these patients has been known for some time, and their characteristically bowed legs with medial widening of the epiphyseal plates of the distal femur and proximal tibia also are well known (Fig. 4.152A). In the more severely afflicted individuals, similar changes are seen in the proximal femur and distal tibia, but in the upper extremity, changes usually

are entirely absent. If they occur, they consist of nothing more than slight broadening or cupping of the ulna (Fig. 4.152B).

Widening of the epiphyseal plates medially is a stress-related phenomenon wherein increased compressive forces occur laterally and diastatic forces result medially (1). Support for this concept exists in the fact that, if these patients are first seen with straight legs, epiphyseal plate widening is uniform from side to side and, if knock-knees occur, widening of the epiphyseal plates occurs laterally. However, most cases of this type of hypophosphatemic rickets, designated type A (2), show bowing and medial epiphyseal plate widening.

Unfortunately, not all patients with hypophosphatemic vitamin D-resistant rickets show the foregoing discrepancy of knee and wrist findings. Indeed, there are some patients who demonstrate equal changes in the upper and lower extremities and a rather severe modeling error of the long bones. This undertubulation error results in very short, squat bones, and this type of rickets is identified by step 2.

STEP 2: PRESENCE OR ABSENCE OF A GENERALIZED MODELING ERROR LEADING TO SHORT, SQUAT BONES

Very severe cases of any type of rickets can result in some bone growth impairment, but when severe shortening of the long bones is seen, one should begin to suspect the second type of hypophosphatemic vitamin D resistance, that is, type B rickets (2). Overall, the bones in these patients have a rather distinctive appearance (Fig. 4.153) because all of the bones appear quite short and squat. Very often the humerus seems to take the brunt of the abnormality and appears clublike, indeed, rather similar to that seen in Hurler disease (Fig. 4.153).

The changes just described for this type of hypophosphatemic rickets are seen in males. In females, the findings are not nearly as striking, and this discrepancy reflects the sex-linked inheritance pattern in hypophosphatemic vitamin D-resistant rickets (i.e., males generally show greater change than do females). However, because the females do not show the same findings they usually are not identified in step 2; rather they are identified in step 4.

STEP 3: PRESENCE OF SECONDARY HYPERPARATHYROIDISM

Roentgenographic evidence of secondary hyperparathyroidism in a patient with rickets usually denotes the presence of renal osteodystrophy. Hyper-

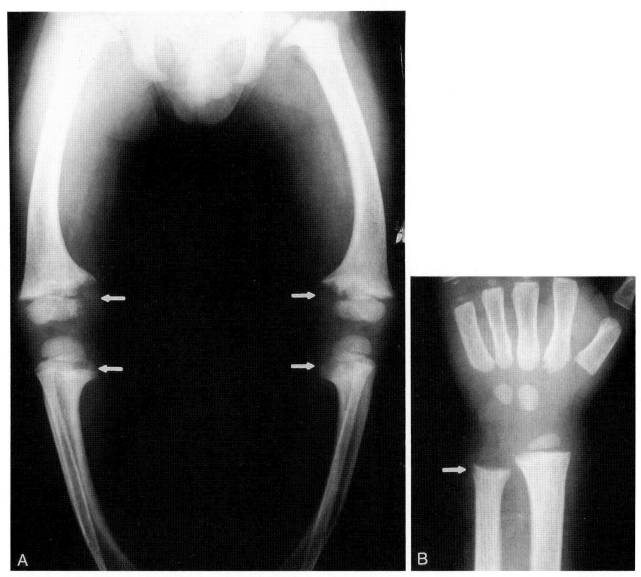

Figure 4.152. Rickets: step 1. Identifies type A hypophosphatemic rickets. Note characteristic bowing of lower extremities and widening of the medial aspects of the epiphyseal plates *(arrows)*. **B.** Wrist is almost normal; only slight cupping of the ulna *(arrow)* is seen. In most cases, not even this finding is present.

parathyroidism in these patients occurs because their renal diseases are such that there is impairment of both tubular and glomerular function. Impairment of glomerular function leads to phosphorous retention, and this causes the parathyroid glands to overreact and secondary hyperparathyroidism to develop. Invariably, secondary hyperparathyroidism becomes the predominant feature in the bones of these patients (Fig. 4.154).

Secondary hyperparathyroidism manifests in subperiosteal bone resorption, endosteal bone resorption, and generalized bony demineralization. Subperiosteal and endosteal resorption of bone most often is

seen in the (a) middle phalanges of the hands; (b) upper, inner proximal tibial metaphyses; (c) femoral neck; (d) distal clavicles; (e) distal radius and ulna; and (f) lamina dura of the teeth. These findings are well known and usually not present in any other type of rickets. However, we have noted that they can occur in infants with nutritional or dependent rickets, and older children with Dilantin-phenobarbital rickets. All of these patients have very severe rickets, and we believe that secondary hyperparathyroidism in them is induced by the prolonged and profound hypocalcemia present when rickets is this severe. This point notwithstanding, however, sec-

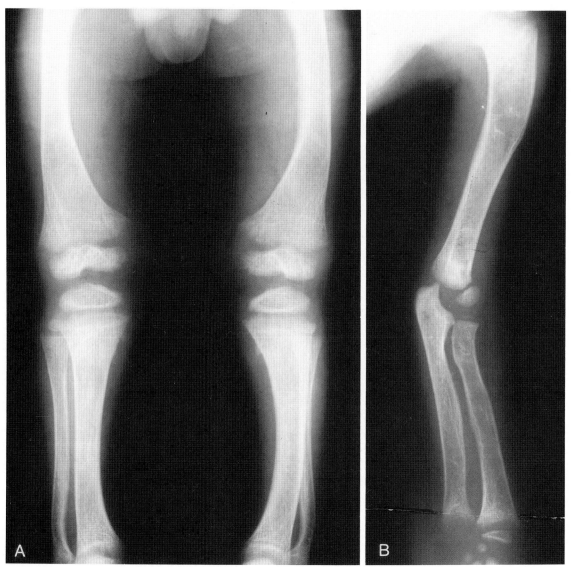

Figure 4.153. Step 2. Identifies type B hypophosphatemic rickets—male. A. Note short, squat undertubulated bones. Also note bowing and uniformity of epiphyseal-metaphyseal change. **B.** Upper extremity showing similar findings. Note that changes in the wrist are equal to those in the knees and the Hurler-like appearance of the humerus.

ondary hyperparathyroidism generally is a feature of patients with renal disease that causes glomerular dysfunction. This leads to renal osteodystrophy, and the identification of this condition is the main function of step 3. All patients remaining at this point are described in step 4.

STEP 4: PRESENCE OR ABSENCE OF BOWLEGS, KNOCK-KNEES, OR STRAIGHT LEGS

Whether bowlegs, knock-knees, or straight legs are determined to be present in rickets is surpris-

ingly valuable in the further differentiation of rickets. Bowlegs generally occur in patients who have normal muscle tone and are ambulant. If they are not ambulant, mild or no bowing at all is seen, and if a patient is nonambulant and has poor muscle tone, straight legs result. If hypotonia and ambulation exist together, knock-knees develop. One can use these observations to further differentiate one form of rickets from another (Fig. 4.155).

Generally speaking, bowlegs occur in patients with both types A and B hypophosphatemic vitamin D-resistant rickets, and the majority of patients with nutritional or dependent rickets. If, however, pa-

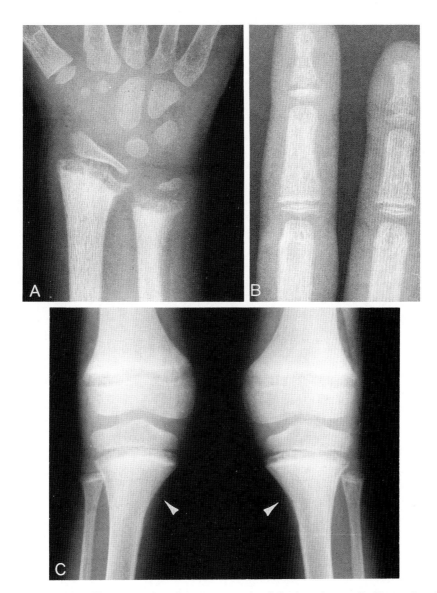

Figure 4.154. Rickets: step 3. Identifies secondary hyperparathyroidism. A. Note typical coarse trabecular pattern, loss of cortical distinction, and subperiosteal resorption in the distal ends of the long bones. **B.** Note subperiosteal bone resorption over the phalanges. **C.** Subperiosteal bone resorption present along the upper medial tibial aspects *(arrow)*.

tients with the latter two forms are too young to walk, or so severely afflicted that they are not ambulant, they show straight legs, or mild bowing only. Other patients showing straight legs, and almost all those showing knock-knees, include patients with Fanconi syndrome (with or without cystinosis), renal tubular acidosis, Dilantin-phenobarbital rickets, and renal osteodystrophy. For the most part, these patients are chronically ill and have decreased muscle tone.

The scheme just outlined deals with untreated rickets diagnosed after the age of 6 months. At less than 6 months of age, only certain forms of rickets

are manifest, and these include congenital (maternal vitamin D deficiency) rickets, rickets secondary to prematurity (metabolic disease of the premature), and rickets secondary to proximal renal tubular acidosis. In terms of our classification, all of these patients demonstrate a uniform distribution of epiphyseal-metaphyseal change, straight legs or mild bowing only (they are nonambulant), no signs of secondary hyperparathyroidism, and no evidence of a modeling error of the long bones. All would be identified in step 4 as would patients with rickets secondary to hormonally active bone tumors or other bone lesions producing distant rachitic changes.

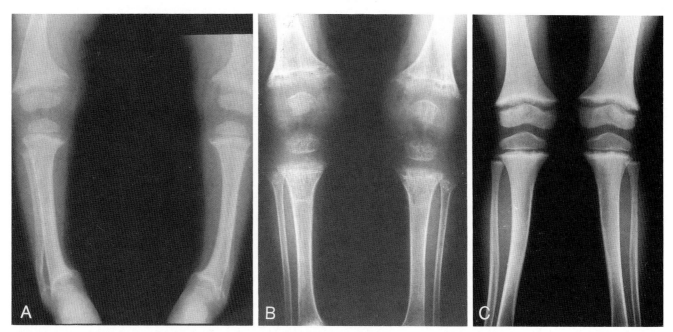

Figure 4.155. Rickets: step 4. Further differentiation based on presence or absence of bowlegs, knock-knees, or straight legs. A. Bowlegs in patient with vitamin D-dependent rickets. This patient was ambulant. **B.** Straight legs in patient with very severe dependent rickets. Patient was virtually nonambulant. **C.** Knock-knees in patient with Fanconi (cystinosis) rickets. This patient was ambulant and hypotonic.

REFERENCES

1. Bateson EM: Non-rachitis bow leg and knock-knee deformities in young Jamaican children. *Br J Radiol* 39:92–101, 1966.

2. Swischuk LE, Hayden CK Jr: Rickets: a roentgenographic scheme for diagnosis. *Pediatr Radiol* 8:203–208, 1979.

Size Abnormalities

When making head size assessments, and the skull is enlarged, it is important to determine whether it is enlarged out of proportion to the face or whether both are enlarged proportionately. The latter is less common and most often is seen in normal but large children and in children with gigantism. When the skull is enlarged relative to the face, the problem can be (a) absolute calvarial enlargement or (b) hypoplasia of the jaw and face. The latter problem is discussed in Chapter 2, and this section deals only with absolute calvarial enlargement.

LARGE HEAD (TABLE 5.1)

The commonest cause of an enlarged head in the pediatric age group is hydrocephalus (Fig. 5.1). For the most part this occurs in infancy while the cranial sutures are still open; when hydrocephalus develops in older children and adolescents, calvarial enlargement is minimal or absent. The etiology of hydrocephalus may be congenital or acquired, and, although calvarial configurations differ in some of the conditions, final diagnosis generally is relegated to CT, MRI, or, in early infancy, ultrasonography. Congenital causes include aqueductal stenosis, stenosis of the foramen of Monroe (unilateral ventricular enlargement), the Arnold Chiari malformation (downward displacement of the medulla and fourth ventricle), and Dandy-Walker cyst (obstruction of the foramina of the fourth ventricle). More commonly, however, hydrocephalus is acquired, and due to meningeal adhesions secondary to meningitis or intracranial hemorrhage. Adhesions can result from trauma-induced subarachnoid bleeding (common in

the battered child syndrome) and, occasionally, with bleeding secondary to blood dyscrasias. In premature neonates, bleeding usually is secondary to prematurity and hypoxia. In all of these cases, adhesions lead to decreased cerebrospinal fluid absorption and subsequent communicating hydrocephalus, and a similar phenomenon can occur when the meninges are infiltrated in the storage diseases.

Hydrocephalus also can result from tumors and cysts compressing and obstructing the normal cerebrospinal fluid pathways. If large enough, a mass can produce calvarial enlargement because of size alone. Finally, hydrocephalus should be differentiated from hydranencephaly, another cause of calvarial enlargement. In this rare condition, there is virtually complete destruction of the brain in utero, probably due to occlusion of the internal carotid arteries. The vertebral arteries remain patent, so the cerebellum, pons, and midbrain are present, but the cerebral hemispheres are replaced by a membranous sac. As the sac becomes filled with fluid, the calvarium enlarges.

Subdural hematoma is another relatively common cause of calvarial enlargement and, when bilateral, produces characteristic biparietal widening of the skull (see Fig. 5.7D). Children with benign subdural effusions generally exhibit similar cranial enlargement. Enlargement of the head also is seen in a number of syndromes, and in most of these conditions it is the brain that is large. Such conditions include cerebral gigantism (Sotos) syndrome, the Russell-Silver (hemiatrophy) syndrome, cleidocranial dysplasia, Bannayan syndrome, Proteus syndrome, Robinow syndrome, Zellweger syndrome, Ruvalcaba-Myhre-Smith syndrome, the craniometaphyseal dysostoses, and most of the chondro-

Table 5.1
Large and Small Head

Large head

Hydrocephalus Subdural hematoma Subdural effusions	Common
Chondrodystrophies Calvarial thickening[a]	Moderately common
Cleidocranial dysplasia Craniometaphyseal dysplasia Pyle disease Beckwith-Wiedemann syndrome Russell-Silver dwarf Storage diseases Neurofibromatosis	Uncommon
Sotos syndrome Bannayan syndrome Proteus syndrome Robinow syndrome Zellweger syndrome Ruvalcaba-Myhre-Smith syndrome Alexander disease Familial megalencephaly Lipomatosis-hemangiomatosis syndrome Large brain tumor or cyst	Rare

Small head

Brain atrophy Poor brain growth[b]	Common
Universal craniosynostosis	Rare

[a] See Table 5.2.
[b] Multiple causes.

dystrophies (e.g., achondroplasia, achondrogenesis, thanatophoric dwarfism, Kniest syndrome, and metatropic dwarfism). Alexander disease is a rare leukoencephalopathy associated with increased intracranial pressure and macrocephaly (4). Enlargement of the head also is seen in neurofibromatosis (5, 8), but the etiology is unknown. A similar phenomenon has been documented with multiple cutaneous hemangiomas (7) and lipomas (9). Unilateral megalencephaly is an anomaly due to abnormal neuronal migration that causes the involved hemisphere to be enlarged with loss of the normal gyral pattern (3, 6).

Familial megalencephaly is a relatively rare cause of calvarial enlargement. The condition is characterized by a large brain and mental retardation (2), but a benign form without retardation also has been documented (1). Calvarial enlargement due to enlargement of the brain also occurs with the storage diseases (i.e., the mucopolysaccharidoses, mucolipidoses, and generalized gangliosidosis). Finally, it should be noted that the head can enlarge anytime the calvarial bones become excessively thickened (see Thickening of the Calvarium).

REFERENCES

1. Asch AJ, Myers GJ: Benign familial macrocephaly: report of a family and review of the literature. *Pediatrics* 57:535–539, 1976.
2. DeMeyer W: Megalencephaly in children. *Neurology* 22:634–643, 1972.
3. Fitz CR, Harwood-Nash DC, Boldt DW: The radiographic

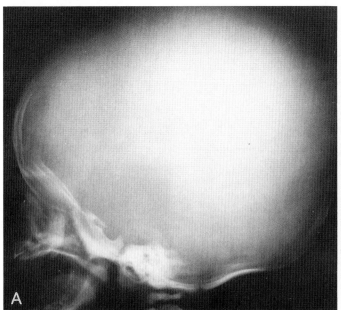
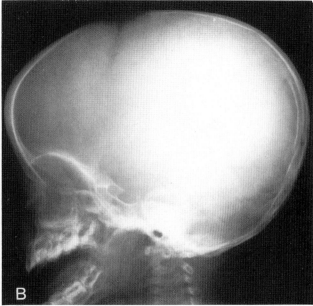

Figure 5.1. Large head. A. Large head in hydrocephalus. In this patient the face appears small because the head is so large. **B.** Large head in patient with achondroplasia. There is a certain degree of maxillary hypoplasia in this condition, but still the head is larger than normal. Also note the elongated sella, a common finding in achondroplasia.

features of unilateral megalencephaly. *Neuroradiology* 15:145–148, 1978.

4. Hess DC, Fischer AO, Yaghmai F, Figueroa R, Akamatsu Y: Comparative neuroimaging with pathologic correlates in Alexander's disease. *J Child Neurol* 5:248–252, 1990.
5. Holt JF, Kuhns LR: Macrocranium and macrocephaly in neurofibromatosis. *Skeletal Radiol* 1:25–28, 1976.
6. Kalifa GL, Chiron C, Sellier N, Demange P, Pongot G, Lalande G, Robain O: Hemimegalencelaphy: MR imaging in five children.
7. Stephan MJ, Hall BD, Smith DW, Cohen MM Jr: Macrocephaly in association with unusual cutaneous angiomatosis. *J Pediatr* 87:353–359, 1975.
8. Weichert KA, Dine MS, Benton C, Silverman FN: Macrocranium and neurofibromatosis. *Radiology* 107:163–166, 1973.
9. Zonana J, Rimoin DL: Macrocephaly with multiple lipomas and hemangiomas. *Pediatrics* 89:600–603, 1976.

SMALL HEAD (TABLE 5.1)

Radiographic assessment of the small head initially is made from the lateral skull film. However, when doing so one should exercise caution, because in some cases the head appears small on lateral view (short from front to back) but is compensatorily wide on frontal view. In some patients this is due simply to lying supine for a prolonged period and the actual head circumference may be normal. On the other hand, when a head is small in both parameters the most common cause is brain atrophy (Fig. 5.2A). The causes of brain atrophy are too numerous to list here but include ischemia or infarction, encephalitis, and

a wide variety of syndromes and degenerative neurologic conditions. In such cases, calvarial smallness is associated with progressive narrowing of the sutures, thickening of the calvarium, and, in more advanced cases, overgrowth of the air-filled paranasal sinuses and mastoid air cells. In addition, one usually sees loss of normal inner table convolutions and, in advanced cases, a small sella. All of these changes are due to decreased intracranial pressure and are distinctly different from those seen when the head is small because of primary craniosynostosis. In universal craniosynostosis, all the sutures fuse prematurely, the head becomes round and small, and the intracranial pressure increases. Indeed, virtually every finding (except for spreading of the sutures) of chronically increased intracranial pressure is present; these include markedly increased inner table convolutions, demineralization of the dorsum of the sella and posterior clinoids, and even enlargement of the sella (Fig. 5.2B).

Abnormal Calvarial Configurations

Generally, abnormal calvarial configurations consist of the following: (a) deformity associated with primary craniosynostosis; (b) postural flattening; (c) unilateral smallness; (d) frontal bossing; (e) biparietal bossing; and (f) localized bulging.

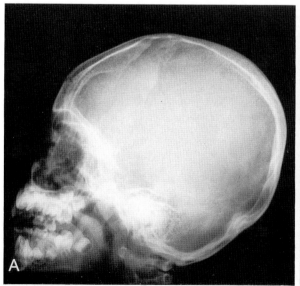 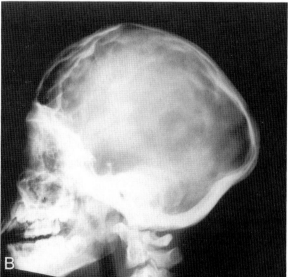

Figure 5.2. Small head. A. Note that the head is small in proportion to the face. Also note the absence of convolutional markings and rather poorly defined cranial sutures. In addition, the calvarium is markedly thickened. These findings are consistent with decreased intracranial pressure, and in this patient the problem was brain atrophy. **B.** Small head in universal craniosynostosis. Note the pronounced inner table convolutions and enlargement of the sella (increased intracranial pressure). All of the sutures are obliterated because they have closed prematurely, but the brain is still growing, leading to the prominent inner table convolutions.

DEFORMITY WITH CRANIOSYNOSTOSIS

A lengthy discussion of primary craniosynostosis is beyond the scope of this book, but it might at least be noted that the type of calvarial deformity is determined by which suture is involved (2, 4). These deformities are summarized in Table 5.2, and in addition in some patients more than one suture can be involved. In such patients, calvarial configurations can be rather bizarre, and one of the most bizarre is the cloverleaf or Kleeblattschädel skull (1, 3, 5). In this condition the skull bulges in cloverleaf fashion over the bregma and both parietal regions (see Fig. 5.7). The deformity can occur in isolated form or in association with other anomalies, and has been recorded with thanatophoric dwarfism (3).

In most patients, primary craniosynostosis can be diagnosed radiographically. When a suture closes prematurely, radiographs usually show one or more of the following findings: (a) the specific calvarial deformity for the suture; (b) narrower than normal sutures with unusually sharp edges; (c) sclerosis along the suture edges; (d) actual bony fusion (usually incomplete bridging) of the suture; (e) bony ridging along the suture; and (f) locally increased convolutional markings (Fig. 5.3). The latter finding is variable and due to pressure from the locally crowded brain. In isolated sagittal synostosis, because such confinement of the brain is minimal, convolutional markings usually are normal. They are more prominent with coronal and lambdoid synostosis (especially if unilateral) and with closure of multiple sutures (Fig. 5.3C). When all sutures are involved, microcephaly also is present, and this leads to severe confinement of the brain. Indeed, in this situation inner table convolutions usually are markedly increased and intracranial pressure is elevated.

In patients with complex forms of craniosynostosis, the exact patterns of suture closure are more difficult to determine with plain radiographs. In such cases, three-dimensional CT reconstruction has been shown to be helpful (6). In the majority of patients, craniosynostosis is an isolated abnormality. However, it can also be associated with a variety of syndromes, the most well-known of which include Crouzon syndrome (craniofacial dysostosis) and the acrocephalosyndactyly syndromes. In addition, the cranial sutures may close prematurely when poor brain growth or brain atrophy is present. In such secondary forms of craniosynostosis, although the sutures are obliterated and the skull remains small, the characteristic skull deformities or abnormal sharp appearance of the sutures seen with primary suture closure is not demonstrated.

REFERENCES

1. Angle CR, McIntire MS, Moore RC: Cloverleaf skull: Kleeblattschädell deformity syndrome. *Am J Dis Child* 114:198–202, 1967.
2. Ebel KD: Craniostenosis-roentgenological and craniometric features. *Pediatr Radiol* 2:1–14, 1974.
3. Iannaccone G, and Gerlini G: The so-called "cloverleaf skull syndrome": a report of 3 cases with a discussion of its relationships with thanatophoric dwarfism and the craniostenoses. *Pediatr Radiol* 2:175–184, 1974.
4. Nathan MH, Collins VP, Collins LC: Premature unilateral synostosis of the coronal suture. *AJR* 85:433–446, 1961.
5. Wollin DG, Binnington VI, Partington MW: Cloverleaf skull. *J Can Assoc Radiol* 19:148–154, 1968.
6. Vannier NW, Hildebolt CF, March JL, Pilgram TK, McAlister WH, Shackelford CD, Offutt CJ, Knapp RH: Craniosynostosis: diagnostic value of three-dimensional CT reconstruction. *Radiology* 173:669–673, 1989.

POSTURAL FLATTENING

Basically, there are two types of postural flattening and both occur over the occiput, i.e., asymmetric flattening and symmetric flattening. The first is more common and results from infants lying on their backs with the head rotated to one side. This occurs in neurologically compromised infants, but also in some perfectly normal infants who just seem to prefer lying that way. Flattening of the entire occiput usually is seen in retarded children who constantly lie on their backs (Fig. 5.4). Although the

Table 5.2
Calvarial Configurations in Primary Craniosynostosis

Suture	Calvarial configuration	Descriptive terms
Sagittal	Long, narrow head	Scaphocephaly or dolichocephaly
Bilateral coronal	Short, wide head, hypertelorism proptosis, small anterior fossa	Brachycephaly or bradycephaly
Metopic	Frontal wedging or keel-shaped head	Trigonocephaly
Bilateral lambdoid	Shallow posterior fossa, prominent bregma	Turricephaly
Unilateral coronal	Unilateral, frontal flattening, uptilting of orbit and tilting of nasal septum	Plagiocephaly
Unilateral lambdoid	Unilateral posterior flattening	Plagiocephaly
All sutures	Small, round head	Microcephaly

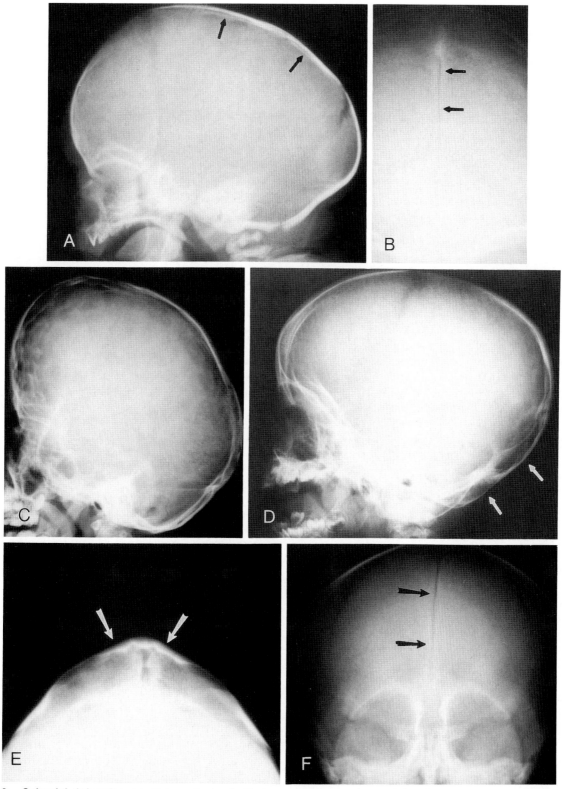

Figure. 5.3. Calvarial deformity: craniosynostosis. A. Typical elongated head in sagittal synostosis. Also note the thickening of the parietal bone *(arrows).* **B.** Frontal view showing very sharp, straight sagittal suture, partially bridged *(arrows).* **C.** Longstanding coronal synostosis in Crouzon syndrome. Note marked brachycephaly, pronounced flattening of the front of the head, and increased convolutional markings over the frontal region. **D.** Occipital flattening. Note flattening of the lower occipital region *(arrows),* characteristic of lambdoid synostosis. **E.** Metopic synostosis. Typical pointed forehead *(arrows)* constituting trigonocephaly. **F.** Frontal view demonstrates hypotelorism and a sharp, straight, closing metopic suture *(arrows).*

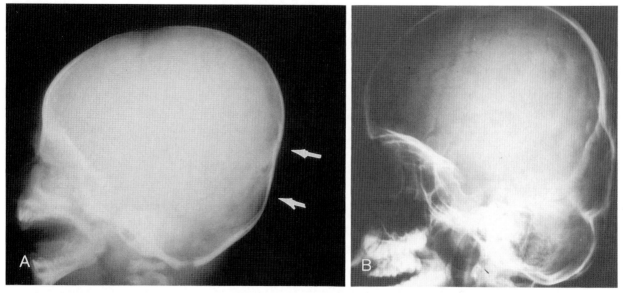

Figure 5.4. Postural flattening. A. Note occipital flattening *(arrows)* in a retarded child. **B.** Exaggerated long-standing flattening in an older retarded child.

finding occasionally can be seen in some normal infants (inherited calvarial shape) and some who are not retarded (i.e., perhaps just chronically immobilized), most often it is seen in the retarded child.

UNILATERAL SMALL HEAD

To a minor degree, unilateral calvarial smallness is present in many if not most normal individuals. This type of asymmetry continues into the face, but usually goes unnoticed by the casual observer. When more severe, it becomes more apparent clinically and radiographically, and then must be differentiated from unilateral smallness due to underlying brain atrophy. In these cases, the brain is atrophic on one side, and in addition to the calvarium being smaller on that side, the ipsilateral bones often are thickened, and the petrous pyramid and sphenoid wing are elevated (Fig. 5.5). There also may be associated upward slanting of the orbit and secondary enlargement of the paranasal sinuses and mastoid air cells on the involved side. The entire complex of findings is known as the Dyke-Davidoff-Masson syndrome (1), and underlying brain atrophy is clearly demonstrable with CT.

Unilateral smallness of the calvarium also occurs with unilateral lambdoid or coronal synostosis (see previous section) and in the Silver syndrome. In this latter condition, also known as congenital hemiatrophy, the more profound changes occur in the lower extremities. However, the upper extremities also may be small and, in some cases, the ipsilateral side

of the skull also is small. Other features of the syndrome include gonadal abnormalities and inguinal hernias (2–4). When the head is enlarged in these patients, with one side still smaller than the other, the condition is referred to as the Russell-Silver syndrome. Both conditions are interrelated and probably are one and the same.

REFERENCES

1. Dyke CG, Davidoff LM, Masson CG: Cerebral hemiatrophy with homolateral hypertrophy of the skull and sinuses. *Surg Gynecol Obstet* 57:588–600, 1933.
2. Marks LJ, Bergeson PS: The Silver-Russell syndrome. *Am J Dis Child* 131:447–451, 1977.
3. Moseley JE, Moloshok RE, Freiberger RH: The Silver syndrome: congenital asymmetry, short stature, and variations in sexual development. *AJR* 97:74–81, 1966.
4. Silver HK: Asymmetry, short stature and variations in sexual development: a syndrome of congenital malformations. *Am J Dis Child* 107:495–515, 1964.

FRONTAL BOSSING

Frontal bossing is a common finding in children and seldom is normal. Most often it occurs with the chondrodystrophies (e.g., achondroplasia, achondrogenesis, thanatophoric dwarfism, metatropic dwarfism, diastrophic dwarfism) and hydrocephalus (Fig. 5.6). However, it also is seen with cleidocranial dysostosis, pyknodysostosis, megalencephaly, diaphyseal dysplasia, the storage diseases, chronic subdural hematoma (biparietal widening is more common), and with conditions associated with thick-

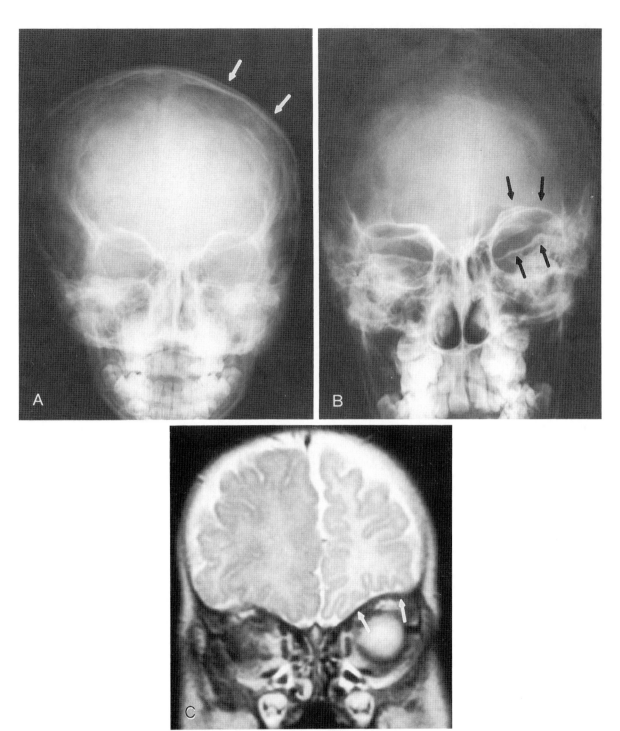

Figure 5.5. Unilateral calvarial smallness: unilateral atrophy. A. Note flattening of the parietal bone *on the left (arrows)*. The ipsilateral sphenoid wing is slightly elevated and the entire hemicranium is smaller than the one *on the right*. **B.** Another patient with classic roundness and elevation of the roof of the involved orbit *(upper arrows)*. Also note accelerated ipsilateral frontal sinus development and elevation of the petrous bone *(lower arrows)* as seen through the orbit. In addition, note that the floor of the middle cranial fossa is elevated as compared to the right cranial fossa. **C.** MRI in another patient shows atrophy of the left cerebral hemisphere, increase in the cerebrospinal fluid space, and slight elevation of the left supraorbital ridge *(arrows)*.

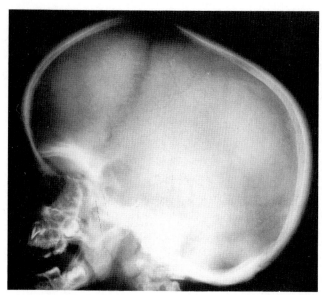

Figure 5.6. Frontal bossing. Characteristic frontal bossing in achondroplasia.

ening of the frontal bone such as chronic anemias, osteopetrosis, healing rickets, or hypophosphatasia (see Thickening of the Calvarium).

BIPARIETAL BOSSING

Biparietal bossing is not as common as frontal bossing and, as far as syndromes are concerned, the one best known to produce such bossing is bilateral coronal synostosis, isolated or associated with Crouzon disease. Gross, biparietal (actually bitemporal) bossing is seen in the rare craniosynostosis syndrome known as cloverleaf skull or Kleeblattschädel (Fig. 5.7A and B). Rather prominent biparietal bossing also is seen in cleidocranial dysostosis (Fig. 5.7C), pyknodysostosis, and chronic bilateral subdural hematomas (Fig. 5.7D).

LOCALIZED BULGES

These can result from lesions causing pressure erosion of the calvarium from within, lesions of the calvarium itself, or scalp abnormalities. Those conditions involving the scalp include a variety of tumors and cysts and localized subgaleal bleeds. Most often the findings are self-evident, and underlying calvarial abnormality may or may not be present. This depends on whether the overlying lesion is causing any destruction or erosion of the bone. As far as calvarial lesions are concerned, the most common problem is a cephalhematoma. When healed, the degree of bulging is minimal and radiographically one sees localized thickening and sclerosis of the calvarium only

(see Fig. 5.10A). In early infancy, before the cephalohematoma has fully healed, the bulge may be more prominent and clinically can be misinterpreted as a depressed skull fracture. The reason for this is that the edge of the calcifying cephalohematoma feels much like the edge of a depressed fracture (Fig. 5.8A).

Other causes of localized calvarial bulging include intradiploic dermoid cysts, histiocytosis-X, fibrous dysplasia, chronic anemias, metastatic lesions (Fig. 5.8D), and, rarely, primary calvarial bone tumors. In chronic anemia, the entire calvarium is thickened in many cases, but in others only a small part is affected, and then a localized calvarial bulge results. This is most likely to occur with iron deficiency and sickle cell anemia.

Intracranial lesions producing localized bulging of the skull also usually produce inner table thinning. The problem must be long standing and conditions leading to the finding include porencephalic cysts (Fig. 5.8B), arachnoid cysts, large intracranial tumors, and, occasionally, unilateral subdural hematomas. With the latter condition, bulging usually is subtle and, if tumors are present, they usually are large and occur in infancy.

A leptomeningeal cyst, although not causing actual bulging of the calvarium, does cause a scalp bulge. In such cases, a skull fracture leads to tearing of the dura, and through this tear the arachnoid membrane herniates. Slowly, as the herniation pulsates, there is erosion of the calvarium along the fracture site. Eventually, an elongated or rounded area of bone destruction results. It has a discreet but minimally sclerotic edge (see Fig. 5.29D) and a fluctuant overlying mass. Often there is some degree of adjacent focal brain atrophy in these patients, a finding readily demonstrable with CT.

Thickening of the Calvarium

Thickening of the calvarium can be generalized, confined to the base, or focal in the vault. Furthermore, in some cases it can be associated with homogeneous sclerosis, while in others sclerosis is spotty. In still others vertical striations of the diploë exist. Conditions producing these combinations of changes are listed in Tables 5.3 and 5.4.

GENERALIZED THICKENING

The commonest cause of generalized calvarial thickening, **associated with homogeneous, in-**

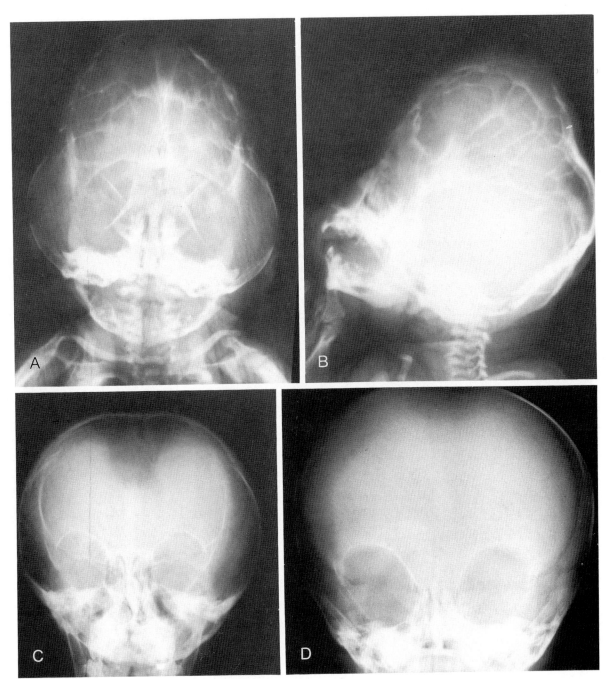

Figure 5.7. Biparietal bossing. A. Pronounced biparietal (actually bitemporal) bulging in cloverleaf skull. **B.** Lateral view shows bulging of the upper portion of the calvarium, the third component of the cloverleaf. Also note prominent convolutions characteristic of this craniosynostosis syndrome. **C.** Biparietal prominence in cleidocranial dysostosis. **D.** Biparietal prominence in chronic bilateral subdural hematoma.

creased density of bone, is normal variation. Thereafter, one should consider one of a number of sclerosing bone dysplasias (Fig. 5.9A) (4) or long-standing decreased intracranial pressure (1, 9, 14). The latter occurs with cerebral atrophy and after successful shunting for hydrocephalus. In either case, it is the prolonged decrease in intracranial pressure that leads to inward growth of the calvarium and thickening of the bones (Fig. 5.9B). In atrophy, the phenomenon also is referred to as hyperostosis cranii ex vacuo. Generalized thickening with increased density of the calvarium also is seen in healing renal osteodystrophy, especially in patients receiving dialysis.

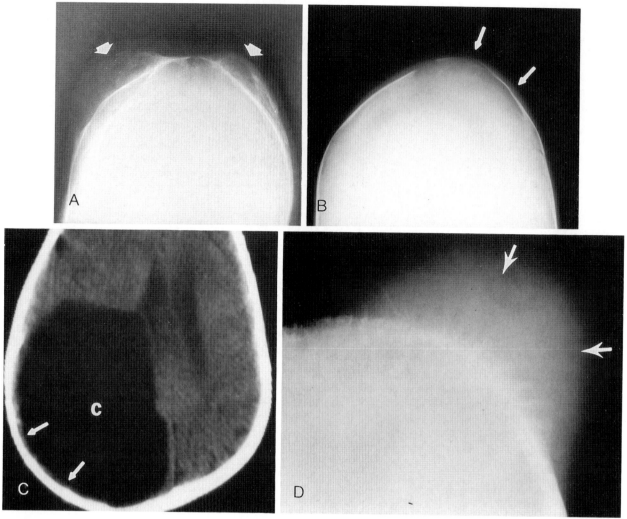

Figure 5.8. Localized bulges. A. Note bilateral, calcifying cephalohematomas *(arrows)*. The rim of the one *on the right* is incompletely calcified and clinically could be misinterpreted for a depressed skull fracture. **B.** Localized bulging of the calvarium *(arrows)* due to a large congenital porencephalic cyst. **C.** Marked bulging of the calvarium *(arrows)* secondary to a large, communicating porencephalic cyst *(C)*. **D.** Localized bulging with spiculation of bone due to metastatic neuroblastoma *(arrows)*.

Generalized calvarial thickening, with **inhomogeneous sclerosis or no sclerosis** at all, is seen in a number of metabolic and hematologic conditions (Table 5.3). In the hematologic conditions, in addition to thickening the diploë of the calvarial bones also shows vertical striation (Fig. 5.9C). This phenomenon most commonly is seen with chronic anemias such as sickle cell disease, iron deficiency anemia, thalassemia, congenital spherocytosis, and polycythemia (3, 6, 13, 17). The changes often are more focal with iron deficiency and sickle cell anemia than with the other anemias. Occasionally, similar focal findings are seen with leukemia, lymphoma, or metastatic disease, and almost always the latter is metastatic neuroblastoma. In some cases of metastatic neuroblastoma, in addition to the vertical stri-

ations in the calvarium, spiculated periosteal new bone is seen, and the sutures usually are spread. Widened sutures indicate increased intracranial pressure, usually caused by metastases to the brain or meninges. In all of these hypertrophied marrow or infiltrative problems, the vertical diploic striations result from pressure atrophy of smaller trabeculae. A similar phenomenon, but with concentric lamellations, has been described with sickle cell disease (19), and we have seen it with neuroblastoma metastases (see Fig. 5.10D).

When metabolic disease produces thickening of the calvarium, no striations are seen but the bones may show patchy sclerosis. For the most part, the following conditions should be considered: hyperparathyroidism, hyperphosphatemia, hypophos-

Table 5.3
Generalized Calvarial Thickening (with or without Sclerosis)

Homogeneous sclerosis

Normal
Decreased intracranial pressure
  Brain atrophy
  Posthydrocephalus shunting
	Common

Dilantin therapy Hypervitaminosis D Hypoparathyroidism Idiopathic hypercalcemia Storage diseases Osteopetrosis Healing rickets[a]	Uncommon
Acrodysostosis Cockayne syndrome Craniometaphyseal dysplasia[b] Jansen metaphyseal dysostosis Lipodystrophy Osteopathia striata Otopalatodigital syndrome Pyknodysostosis Proteus syndrome Van Buchem osteosclerosis Fluorosis Melorheostosis Kenny-Caffey syndrome[c] Myelosclerosis Myotonic dystrophy	Rare

Nonhomogenous sclerosis, or no sclerosis

Chronic anemia[d]
  Thalassemia, sickle cell disease,
  iron deficiency anemia, heredi-
  tary spherocytosis
	Common

Hyperparathyroidism Active and healing rickets	Moderately common
Dilantin therapy Polycythemia Metastatic disease[e]	Uncommon
Hyperphosphatasia Hypophosphatasia Leukemia-lymphoma[e]	Rare

[a]With bossing.
[b]Pyle disease.
[c]Tubular stenosis of long bones.
[d]Often show vertical striations.
[e]May show vertical striations.

phatasia, pseudo-pseudohypoparathyroidism (18), lipodystrophy, and healing rickets. In hyperparathyroidism the skull may appear very mottled, the "salt and pepper skull" (Fig. 5.9D), and with hyperphosphatemia the thick skull may be lamellated. Generalized irregular thickening of the calvarium can be seen in fibrous dysplasia (Fig. 5.9G), and the findings also can be focal (see Fig. 5.11D).

LOCALIZED THICKENING OF THE SKULL

Much as with generalized thickening, thickening of the skull on a localized basis may or may not be associated with sclerosis. When **sclerosis is present,** the most common problem is a healing cephalohematoma (Fig. 5.10A). Most often this is encountered in the postnatal period, but it also can be seen in older infants. Peculiar localized thickening occurs in the frontal bone in chronic head bangers (20), and we have seen a similar problem in a young child who was battered in the form of repeated insults to the temples. Localized sclerosis with thickening also can occur with chronic osteomyelitis, adjacent cellulitis, healing histiocytosis-X, tuberous sclerosis (Fig. 5.10B), the chronic anemias (especially sickle cell disease and iron deficiency anemia), leukemia, and metastatic neuroblastoma. The latter three usually show vertical striations (Fig. 5.10D), but also can show concentric lamellations.

Very large areas of increased sclerosis and thickening of the calvarium almost always are due to the hyperostotic form of fibrous dysplasia. Very often the

Table 5.4
Localized Thickening of the Calvarium

Localized thickening of the calvarium

Cephalohematoma—healed[a] Trauma[a]	Common
Fibrous dysplasia[b] Anemia[c] Chronic infection[a] Cerebral hemiatrophy[a]	Moderately common
Meningioma[b,c] Hemangioma[a–c] Other primary bone tumors[b]	Rare

Base of skull thickening

Bone dysplasias	Common
Fibrous dysplasia	Moderately common
Meningioma[b] Chordoma of clivus Chronic infection of nasopharynx[a]	Rare
Other tumors of clivus	Very rare

[a]Sclerotic.
[b]Sclerotic or lytic.
[c]Vertical striations.

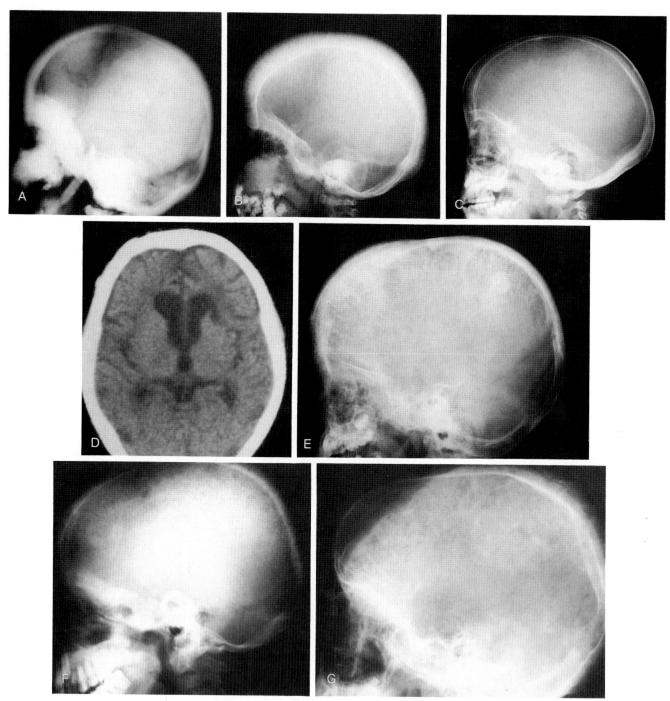

Figure 5.9. Generalized calvarial thickening. A. Typical thickening of the calvarium with increased sclerosis in osteopetrosis. **B.** Thickening due to Cooley anemia. Note vertical striations. **C.** Thickening of the calvarium secondary to decreased intracranial pressure in brain atrophy. **D.** CT study in another patient demonstrating a thick calvarium secondary to atrophy (note large ventri- cles and prominent sulci). **E.** Generalized bony calvarial thickening with marked spiculation secondary to metastatic neuroblastoma. **F.** Thickened salt-and-pepper skull in hyperparathyroidism (secondary hyperparathyroidism in renal osteodystrophy). **G.** Fibrous dysplasia with generalized, irregular lucent and hyperostotic thickening of the calvarium.

base and frontal regions of the skull are involved (see Fig. 5.11D and E). Focal thickening with sclerosis of the skull due to other bone tumors is rather uncommon, but can be seen with some hemangiomas

(Fig. 5.10E), osteomas, and, rarely, with osteogenic sarcoma or rhabdomyosarcoma (2).

Localized thickening **without sclerosis** is not particularly common and most often is seen with fi-

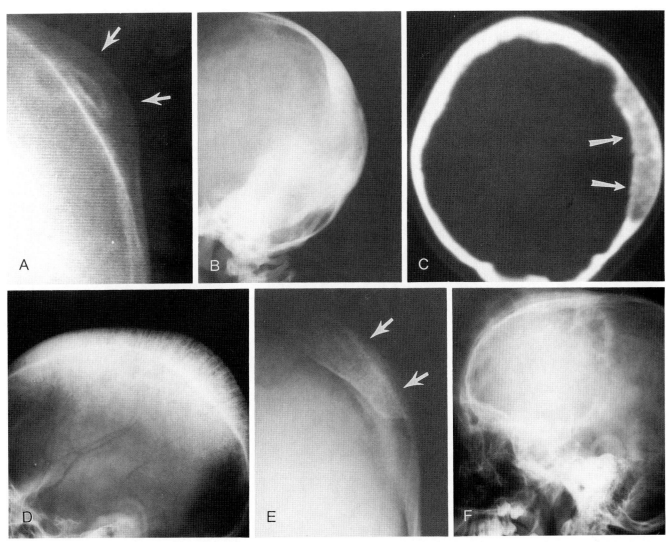

Figure 5.10. Localized thickening of the calvarium. A. Thickening of the calvarium due to partially healed cephalohematoma *(arrows)*. **B.** Occipital thickening *(arrows)* in tuberous sclerosis. **C.** Localized calvarial thickening *(arrows)* due to fibrous dyspla-sia. **D.** Localized thickening, with vertical striations in sickle cell disease. **E.** Localized thickening with some honeycombing and striations in osseous hemangioma *(arrows)*. **F.** Frontal thickening with lysis in meningioma.

brous dysplasia. It also can be seen with the rare meningioma occurring in childhood (Fig. 5.10*F*) and aneurysmal bone cyst of the cranial vault (2). Thickening and sclerosis of most or all of one side of the calvarium in association with ipsilateral smallness of the calvarium reflects underlying cerebral atrophy, as in the Dyke-Davidoff-Masson syndrome.

THICKENING OF THE BASE OF THE SKULL

Predominant thickening of the skull base occurs with bone dysplasias such as osteopetrosis (Fig. 5.11*A*) (7, 8), craniometaphyseal dysplasia (including Pyle disease), Englemann-Camurati diaphyseal dysplasia, Melnick-Needles osteodysplasia, Jansen metaphyseal dysostosis (10), osteopathia striata with cranial sclerosis (16), cleidocranial dysostosis, the otopalatodigital syndrome (Fig. 5.11*B*), and melorheostosis. Tumors or tumor-like conditions leading to thickening of the base of the skull include fibrous dysplasia (most common), meningioma, chordoma of the clivus (11, 12), chondrosarcoma (5), and tumors of the nasopharynx. Thickening of the base of the skull also can occur with chronic nasopharyngeal infections (15), but all of these conditions are rare in children. Chondromas can be identified by the characteristic calcification with which they are associated (Fig. 5.11*C*), and fibrous dysplasia can be lytic or sclerotic (Fig. 5.11*D* and *E*). Meningioma usually is osteolytic.

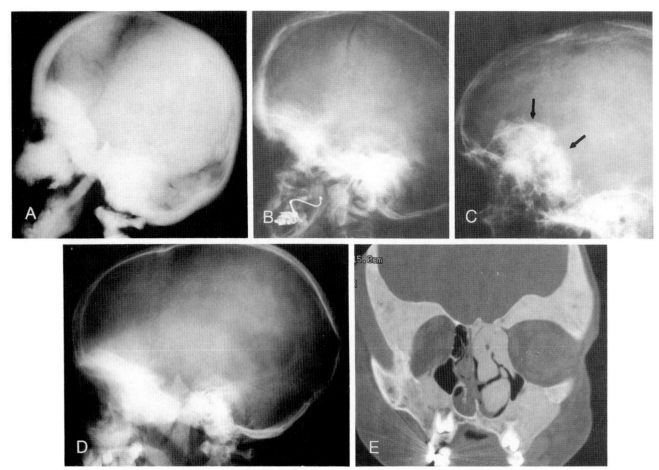

Figure 5.11. Thickening of the base of the skull. A. Thickening and sclerosis of the base of the skull in osteopetrosis. All of the other bones, including the facial bones, also are sclerotic and slightly thickened. **B.** Basal sclerosis and thickening in otopalatodigital syndrome. **C.** Focal calvarial thickening due to enchondroma *(arrows)*. **D.** Marked sclerosis of the base of the skull in fibrous dysplasia. **E.** CT of same patient demonstrates marked thickening of the floor of the anterior fossae which then extends into the lateral skull walls and into the maxillary regions, especially *on the left*. Thickening also extends into the turbinate bones *on the left*.

REFERENCES

1. Anderson R, Kieffer SA, Wolfson JJ, Peterson HO: Thickening of the skull in surgically treated hydrocephalus. *AJR* 110:96–101, 1970.
2. Arthur RJ, Brunelle F: Computerised tomography in the evaluation of expansile lesions arising from the skull vault in childhood: a report of 5 cases. *Pediatr Radiol* 18:294–301, 1988.
3. Burko H, Mellins HZ, Watson J: Skull changes in iron-deficiency anemia simulating congenital hemolytic anemia. *AJR* 86:447–452, 1961.
4. Cook JV, Phelps PD, Chandy J: Van Buchem's disease with classical radiological features and appearances on cranial computed tomography. *Br J Radiol* 62:74–77, 1989.
5. Cook PL, Evans PG: Chondrosarcoma of the skull in Maffucci's syndrome. *Br J Radiol* 50:833–836, 1977.
6. Dykstra OH, Halbertsma T: Polycythemia vera in childhood. *Am J Dis Child* 60:907–916, 1940.
7. Elster AD, Theros EG, Key LL, Chen MYM: Cranial imaging in autosomal recessive osteopetrosis, Part II: skull base and brain. *Radiology* 183:137–144, 1992.
8. Elster AD, Theros EG, Key LL, Chen MYM: Cranial imaging in autosomal recessive osteopetrosis, Part I: facial bones and calvarium. *Radiology* 183:129–135, 1992.
9. Griscom NT, Kook Sang O: The contracting skull; inward growth of the inner table as a physiologic response to diminution of intracranial content in children. *AJR* 110:106–110, 1970.
10. Holthusen W, Holdt JF, Stoeckenius M: The skull in metaphyseal chondrodysplasia type jansen. *Pediatr Radiol* 3:137–144, 1975.
11. Kendall BE, Lee BCP: Cranial chordomas. *Br J Radiol* 50: 687–698, 1977.
12. Lim GHK: Clivus chordoma with unusual bone sclerosis and brainstem invasion. *Australas Radiol* 19:242–250, 1975.
13. Moseley JE: Skull changes in chronic iron deficiency anemia. *AJR* 85:649–652, 1961.
14. Moseley JE, Rabinowitz JG, Dziadiw R: Hyperostosis cranii ex vacuo. *Radiology* 87:1105–1107, 1966.

Table 5.5
Thinning of the Calvarium

Generalized

Long standing hydrocephalus[a] Osteogenesis imperfecta Normal, in premature infants	Common
Advanced rickets Craniolacunia or lacunar skull Trisomies	Moderately common
Cleidocranial dysplasia Hypophosphatasia	Uncommon
Aminopterin embryonopathy Aplasia cutis Melnick-Needles syndrome Progeria	Rare

Localized

Intracranial cysts	Common
Neurofibromatosis Chronic subdural hematoma	Moderately common
Localized or unilateral hydro- cephalus Intracranial tumor Aneurysmal bone cyst	Uncommon

[a] Untreated.

15. Nemir RL, Branom-Genieser N, Balasubramanyam P: Extensive sclerosis of the base of the skull due to primary nasal tuberculosis. *Pediatr Radiol* 8:42–44, 1979.
16. Paling MR, Hyde I, Dennis NR: Osteopathia striata with sclerosis and thickening of the skull. *Br J Radiol* 54:344–348, 1981.
17. Powell JW, Weens HS, Wenger NK: The skull roentgenogram in iron deficiency anemia and in secondary polycythemia. *AJR* 95:143–147, 1965.
18. Steinback HL, Young DA: The roentgen appearance of pseudohypoparathyroidism (PH) and pseudo-pseudo-hypoparathyroidism (PPH), differentiation from other syndromes associated with short metacarpals, metatarsals, and phalanges. *AJR* 97:49–66, 1966.
19. Williams AO, Lagundoye SB, Johnson CL: Lamellation of the diploe in the skulls of patients with sickle cell anemia. *Arch Dis Child* 50:948–952, 1975.
20. Williams JP, Fowler GW, Pribram HF, Delaney CA, Fish CH: Roentgenographic changes in headbangers. *Acta Radiol Diagn* 13:37–42, 1972.

Thinning of the Calvarium

Just like thickening, thinning of the calvarium can be generalized or localized (Table 5.5). **Localized thinning** usually is due to a slowly growing and eroding intracranial lesion such as a porence-phalic cyst (Fig. 5.12*A*), an arachnoid or leptomeningeal cyst, or a tumor. However, similar thinning can be seen with chronic subdural hematomas and unilateral hydrocephalus due to unilateral foramen of Monroe obstruction. The plain film findings in all of these conditions, of course, are nonspecific.

Aneurysmal bone cysts also can produce localized thinning of the calvarium (Fig. 5.12*B*), and isolated thinning of a sphenoid wing or other parts of the calvarium, occurs with neurofibromatosis (Fig. 5.12*C* and *D*). The latter is believed to be secondary to a nonspecific mesenchymal defect of bone development. This type of bone abnormality is common in neurofibromatosis. When the defect in the sphenoid bone is extensive, only a membrane remains and pulsating exophthalmos results.

As far as **generalized thinning** of the calvarium is concerned, it almost always is part of some bone dysplasia or syndrome (Table 5.5). However, the problem also normally occurs in infancy in the premature infant. The most common dysplasia to produce calvarial thinning is osteogenesis imperfecta, but other conditions to be considered include aminopterin embryonopathy, aminopterin-like syndrome, cleidocranial dysplasia, aplasia cutis congenita, hypophosphatasia, Melnick-Needles osteodysplasia, progeria, some of the trisomies, and longstanding hydrocephalus.

Abnormalities of the Sutures

The cranial sutures are visible and open throughout childhood but normally appear wider in infants. Abnormal sutures can appear either too wide or too narrow. Furthermore, either problem can be generalized or may involve one or two sutures only. The following is a discussion of these problems.

SUTURES TOO WIDE (TABLE 5.6)

Generalized widening of the sutures may be real and due to increased intracranial pressure, or only apparent and due to underossification of the calvarial bone edges (Fig. 5.13). When calvarial underossification is the cause, most often one is dealing with a demineralizing metabolic bone disease or a bone dysplasia where membranous bone ossification is impaired. These conditions are listed in Table 5.6. In addition, delayed ossification causing unduly wide-appearing sutures is common in premature infants.

True spreading of the sutures occurs from any cause of increased intracranial pressure, including

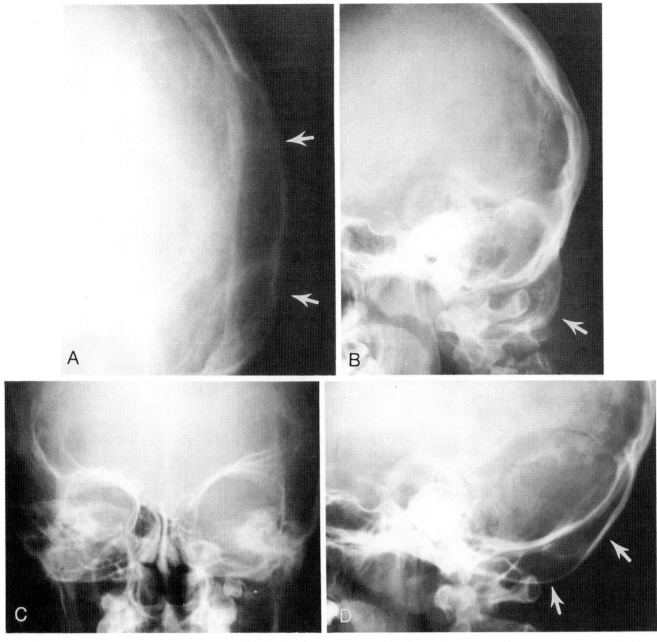

Figure 5.12. Thinning of the calvarium: localized. A. Note localized thinning of the calvarium due to an acquired porencephalic cyst *(arrows)*. Also note calcification just above the area of thinning. **B.** Thinning due to expanding aneurysmal bone cyst *(arrows)*. **C.** Absence of sphenoid wing *on the left,* due to thinning in neurofibromatosis. Also note that the left orbit is large. **D.** Occipital thinning in neurofibromatosis *(arrows)*.

meningitis, cerebritis, abscess, intracranial hemorrhage, cerebral edema, brain tumor, hydrocephalus, hydranencephaly, megalencephaly, expanding cysts, subdural hematoma or hygroma, pseudotumor cerebri (7), lead encephalopathy, hypervitaminosis A encephalopathy (3), and other encephalopathies. In all of these conditions, suture spread appears about the same and, when marked, is easy to assess (Fig. 5.13).

Lesser degrees of spread are more difficult to evaluate, especially in children less than 2 to 3 years of age in whom a certain degree of prominence of the coronal suture is normal (5, 6). Most likely this type of spread is physiologic and attests to the relatively rapid growth of the brain at that age. As an aid to differentiating this type of suture spread from pathologic spread, one should look at the sagittal suture. If the sagittal suture also is wide pathologic spread

Table 5.6
Wide Sutures

Normal 　Neonate 　Infant—coronal Intracranial: 　Bleeding, contusion[a] 　Infection[a] 　Edema Hydrocephalus[a]	Common
Intracranial tumor[a] Rickets[b] Prematurity[b] Intrauterine: 　Growth failure[b] 　Infections[b] Encephalopathy[a] Psychosocial dwarfism[a]	Moderately common
Large intracranial cysts[a] Hypothyroidism[b] Cleidocranial dysplasia[b] Hyperparathyroidism[b] Osteogenesis imperfecta[b]	Uncommon
Megalencephaly[a] Hydranencephaly[a] Aminopterin-induced syndrome[b] Hypophosphatemia[b] Pachydermoperiostosis[b] Progeria[b] Pyknodysostosis[b] Jansen-type metaphyseal dysostosis[b] Treated hypothyroidism[a] Pseudotumor cerebri[a]	Rare

[a] Increased pressure.
[b] Pseudospread due to defective ossification.

usually is present, but if the sagittal suture is normal physiologic spread is more likely. Physiologic spreading of the sagittal suture does not occur as readily as it does with the coronal suture and indeed may never occur. Evaluation of the sutures in the neonate is even more difficult, because the normal sutures can be as wide as 1 cm or more. This appearance can last for as long as 1 month after birth, but usually somewhere during the first month of life the sutures become more "normal" in appearance.

Generalized calvarial suture spread may also occur after head trauma. Of course, if there is significant intracranial injury, a rise in intracranial pressure is expected. However, spreading of the sutures also can occur in the absence of such injury and is due to expanded brain volume secondary to vasodilatin.

Finally, it should be noted that at times rather marked, generalized suture spread occurs with psychosocial dwarfism (1, 2, 4). Although these children

are emotionally deprived, growth of the body and brain is retarded, possibly as a result of temporary impairment of growth hormone production. When these children are removed from their adverse environment, rebound growth of the body and brain occur. So exuberant is this phenomenon that intracranial pressures rise and the sutures spread. It is important not to misinterpret this exaggerated normal phenomenon for a pathologic state. Similar rebound growth can be seen under other circumstances where body and brain growth are impaired for some time (e.g., treated hypothyroidism).

Localized spread of one or more sutures almost invariably is related to calvarial trauma. In such cases, a fracture may extend directly into the suture, or the suture alone can "fracture" or "widen." The term "diastatic sutural fracture" is applied to this type of injury, and then it is important to compare the involved suture with that on the other side (Fig. 5.13D). Of course, if the suture is unpaired interpretation is a little more difficult.

REFERENCES

1. Afshani E, Osman M, Girdany BR: Widening of cranial sutures in children with deprivational dwarfism. *Radiology* 109:141–144, 1973.
2. Capitanio MA, Kirkpatrick JA: Widening of the cranial sutures, a roentgen observation during periods of accelerated growth in patients treated for deprivation dwarfism. *Radiology* 92:53–59, 1969.
3. Lippe B, Hensen L, Mendoza G, Finerman M, Welch M: Chronic vitamin A intoxication. *Am J Dis Child* 135:634–636, 1981.
4. Sondheimer FK, Grossman H, Winchester P: Suture diastasis following rapid weight gain: pseudo-pseudotumor cerebri. *Arch Neurol* 23:314–318, 1970.
5. Swischuk LE: The growing skull. *Semin Roentgenol* 9:115–124, 1974.
6. Swischuk LE: The normal pediatric skull: variations and artifacts. *Radiol Clin North Am* 10:277–290, 1972.
7. Weisberg LA, Chutorian AM: Pseudotumor cerebri of childhood. *Am J Dis Child* 131:1243–1248, 1977.

NARROWED OR OBLITERATED SUTURES

Sutures can become narrowed or frankly obliterated on a primary or secondary basis, but the latter probably is more common (Table 5.7). Primary obliteration or craniosynostosis has been discussed earlier (see Table 5.2), and is common. Its etiology is unknown, but the general belief is that it is related to an abnormality of dural development in the fetus. Any of the sutures in almost any combination can be involved and, radiographically, in addition to calvarial deformity, one can see (a) narrower and sharper than normal sutures, (b) variable sclerosis along the

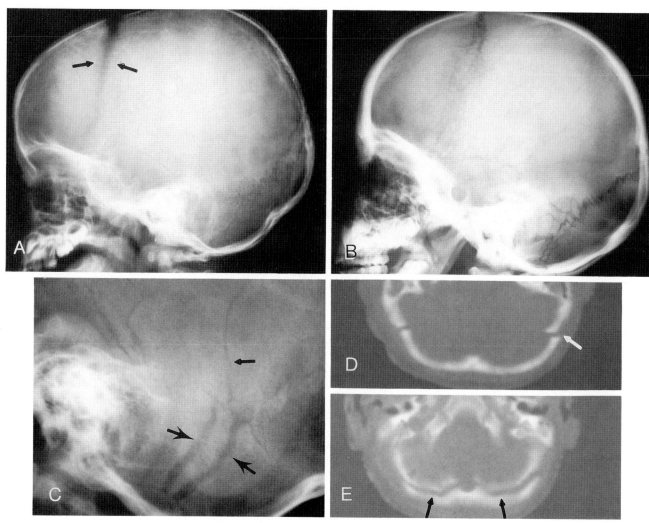

Figure 5.13. Sutures too wide. A. Note typical widening of the coronal suture *(arrows)* due to increased intracranial pressure. **B.** Prominent (more radiolucent than normal) sutures in patient with hypothyroidism. **C. Spread sutures: focal.** Note bilaterally spread occipitomastoid sutures *(large arrows)*. Also note the associated linear fracture *(small arrow)*. The spread sutures repre-sent diastatic sutural fractures in association with the linear fracture. **D.** CT of the same patient shows the sutural widening bilaterally and the bony displacement *on the left (arrow)*. **E.** Lower cut demonstrates the bilateral diastatic sutural fractures *(arrows)*.

suture edges, and, in some cases, (c) actual bony bridging (see Fig. 5.3). Primary craniosynostosis usually is an isolated abnormality (8), but it also can be seen with certain syndromes. For example, the coronal and sagittal sutures frequently are involved in Crouzon syndrome and in the acrocephalosyndactyly syndromes (Apert, Pfeiffer, Carpenter). Presumed primary, but perhaps secondary, synostosis also is seen in Jansen metaphyseal dysostosis, the Rubinstein-Taybi syndrome, punctate epiphyseal dysplasia, aminopterin fetopathy, and the idiopathic hypercalcemia or Williams syndrome.

When suture synostosis occurs on a secondary basis, the cause is (a) decreased intracranial pressure or (b) some bony hypermetabolic state (2). Decreased intracranial pressure can occur with brain atrophy or after successful ventricular shunting for hydrocephalus (1, 3, 4, 6). In either case, because intracranial pressure is decreased on a prolonged basis, the calvarial bones, rather than being kept apart, are allowed to approach each other and narrow the sutures. Eventually, they fuse and become obliterated. In addition, in these patients the calvarium becomes thickened, the sella becomes small, and the paranasal sinuses and mastoid air cells may show compensatory overgrowth. The findings are quite different from those in primary synostosis (compare Fig. 5.14A and B).

Table 5.7
Narrowed or Obliterated Sutures

Primary synostosis[a]
Decreased intracranial pressure[b]
  Atrophy
  Shunted hydrocephalus
	Common

Healing rickets[b]	Moderately common
Storage diseases[b] Chronic anemias[b] Hyperthyroidism[b] Crouzon disease Acrocephalosyndactyly syndromes	Uncommon
Hypervitaminosis D[b] Hyperparathyroidism[b] Hypophosphatasia[b] Idiopathic hypercalcemia[b] Jansen metaphyseal dysostosis Rubinstein-Taybi syndrome Punctate epiphyseal dysplasia Aminopterin-induced syndrome	Rare

[a] See Table 5.2.
[b] Secondary synostosis.

Hypermetabolic conditions leading to premature synostosis of the calvarium include hyperthyroidism (5, 7), healing rickets, hypophosphatasia (in active or healing stage), and hypervitaminosis D. Premature closure of the sutures also occurs in the various storage diseases and chronic anemias (Fig. 5.14C). It is not known why the phenomenon occurs in storage diseases, but it may be that there also is some degree of hypermetabolism present. Decreased intracranial pressure seems unlikely, because most of these patients demonstrate megalencephaly rather than small atrophic brains. In the chronic anemias, local hypermetabolism secondary to bone marrow overgrowth probably is the cause of premature suture closure (see Fig. 5.14C).

REFERENCES

1. Anderson R, Kieffer SA, Wolfson JJ, Long D, Peterson HO: Thickening of the skull in surgically treated hydrocephalus. *AJR* 110:96–101, 1970.
2. Duggan C, Keener E, Brit G: Secondary craniosynostosis. *AJR* 109:277–293, 1970.
3. Griscom NT, Kook Sang O: The contracting skull: inward growth of the inner table as a physiologic response to diminution of intracranial content in children. *AJR* 110:106–110, 1970.
4. Kaufman B, Weiss MH, Young HF, Nulsen FE: Effects of prolonged cerebrospinal fluid shunting on the skull and brain. *J Neurosurg* 38:288–297, 1973.
5. Menking FWM, Schmid WU, Ebel KD, Holthusen WH, Schmidt WWT: Premature craniosynostosis associated with hyperthyroidism. *Ann Radiol* 15:279–284, 1972.
6. Moseley JE, Rabinowitz JG, and Dziadiw R: Hyperostosis cranii ex vacuo. *Radiology* 87:1105–1107, 1966.
7. Riggs W Jr, Wilroy RS Jr, Etteldorf JN: Neonatal hyperthyroidism with accelerated skeletal maturation, craniosynostosis, and brachydactyly. *Radiology* 105:621–625, 1972.
8. Tait MV, Gilday DL, Ash JM, Boldt DJ, Harwood-Nash DCF, Fitz CR, Barry J: Craniosynostosis: correlation of bone scans, radiographs and surgical findings. *Radiology* 133:615–621, 1979.

Convolutional Marking Abnormalities

Inner table convolutions are a normal feature of the childhood skull and result from the gyri of the normally pulsating brain pounding against the inner table. Usually they are not present at birth but become variably prominent after the first year of life. In terms of pathologic change, convolutional markings can become too prominent or may not be prominent enough. Generally, when they are too prominent there is a condition causing increased intracranial pressure, and when they are not prominent enough decreased intracranial pressure is the culprit (Table 5.8).

INCREASED CONVOLUTIONAL MARKINGS

The commonest cause of increased inner table convolutional markings is chronically increased intracranial pressure, but the finding is a late manifestation of the problem. Consequently, it should be seen in association with other signs of chronically increased intracranial pressure—for example, spread sutures, demineralization of the sella, truncation of the posterior clinoids, and, in some cases, actual sellar enlargement (Fig. 5.15A). These additional features are important because they serve to distinguish children with chronically increased intracranial pressure from some who are normal but yet demonstrate alarmingly prominent convolutional markings. In the latter case, the findings are entirely normal and not associated with any signs of chronically increased intracranial pressure (Fig. 5.15B).

In most cases of chronically increased intracranial pressure, the problem is a slowly expanding intracranial lesion (i.e., tumor, cyst, hydrocephalus). In such cases there is time for increased convolutions to develop, but if spread is acute (e.g., intracranial bleed, meningitis, brain abscess, cerebritis), no in-

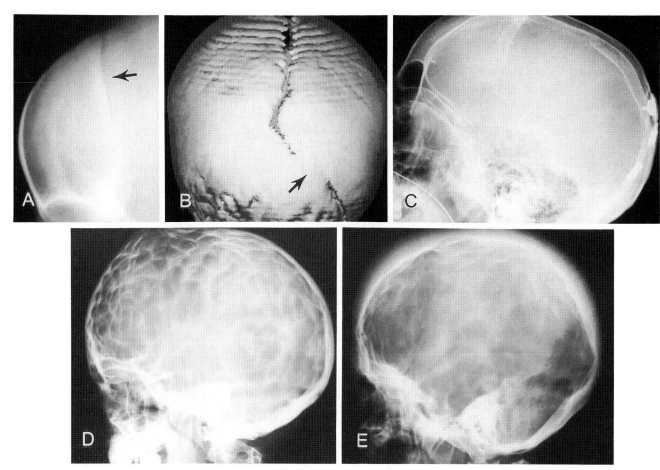

Figure 5.14. Obliterated or prematurely fused sutures. A. Primary coronal synostosis. Note the exceptionally sharp-appearing coronal suture *(arrow)*. This indicates premature closure. **B.** Three-dimensional CT reconstruction demonstrates closure of the right lambdoid suture and partial closure of the left lambdoid suture *(arrow)*. The sagittal suture is normal and open. **C.** Note the absence of sutures in this patient with brain atrophy, a small head, thickened calvarium, and overgrowth of the sinuses and mastoid air cells. **D.** Obliterated sutures in primary craniosynostosis. Note increased convolutional markings due to brain crowding and increased pressure. **E.** Obliterated sutures, increased intracranial pressure, and exaggerated convolutional markings in secondary synostosis in a patient with chronic anemia due to stematocytosis.

crease in convolutional markings occurs. Another situation in which increased convolutional markings are seen is with universal craniosynostosis (Fig. 5.15C). In these patients, premature union of the calvarium causes it to be small and unable to accommodate the normally growing brain. As a result, intracranial pressures rise and inner table convolutions become more prominent. Such a phenomenon can occur with primary or secondary synostosis, and the latter occurs in conditions such as healing rickets, hypophosphatasia, hypercalcemia, and in chronic anemias such as Cooley anemia. In all of these conditions, it is believed that local bone hypermetabolism predisposes to closure of the sutures.

Locally increased convolutional markings are less common and are not as dire a finding. Most commonly, the problem is premature closure of one, or perhaps two, cranial sutures causing localized crowding of the brain.

Lacunar skull, craniolacunia, or Lückenschadel skull represents another condition where inner table markings are increased (1, 2). However, the problem is not increased intracranial pressure but rather faulty inner table bone formation (Fig. 5.16). Lacunar skull is seen almost exclusively in patients with meningoceles, meningomyeloceles, or encephaloceles, and then only in neonates. By the age of 6 to 8 months, virtually no lacunar skull deformity remains, regardless of whether the head becomes larger or smaller. This is an important point, for many patients with lacunar skull have associated hydrocephalus (e.g., Arnold-Chiari malformation, aqueductal stenosis), and it is tempting to assign the increased convolutional pattern to chronically in-

Table 5.8
Convolutional Marking Abnormalities

Increased		
Normal	}	Common
Chronic increased intracranial pressure		
Lacunar skull	}	Moderately common
Primary synostosis[a]		
Primary synostosis[b]		
Secondary synostosis		
Rickets		
Hypophosphatasia		
Hyperthyroidism	}	Uncommon
Chronic anemia		
Cloverleaf skull[c]		
Metaphyseal dysostosis		
Decreased		
Atrophy	}	Common
Shunted hydrocephalus		
Severe failure to thrive	}	Moderately common
Psychosocial dwarfism		
Hypothyroidism	}	Uncommon

[a] Local.
[b] Universal.
[c] Primary synostosis.

creased intracranial pressure. However, the true cause of lacunar skull is dysplastic bone formation associated with focal dural defects.

DECREASED CONVOLUTIONAL MARKINGS

As noted earlier, it is normal for convolutional markings to be sparse or absent in neonates and young infants in their first year of life. Indeed, even up to the age of 3 or 4 years, some children show very little in the way of inner table convolutional markings, but thereafter at least some should be present. When the brain fails to grow normally (e.g., brain atrophy, severe failure to thrive, deprivational dwarfism, hypothyroidism), inner table convolutional markings may not develop. In any of these conditions, if the problem is reversible, once appropriate treatment is instituted convolutional markings usually return (Fig. 5.17), and, indeed, in some cases become quite prominent. This, of course, does not occur with brain atrophy.

Another relatively common cause of decreased inner table convolutional markings is shunted hydrocephalus. In patients with successful ventricular shunting intracranial pressures are decreased and because of this, the calvarium can become thickened,

the sutures prematurely closed, and convolutional markings less prominent or absent.

REFERENCES

1. McRae DL: Observations on craniolacunia. *Acta Radiol Diagn* 5:55–64, 1966.
2. Shopfner CE, Jabbour JT, Vallion RM: Craniolacunia. *AJR* 93:343–349, 1965.

Abnormalities of Calvarial Density

For the most part any conditions causing increased or decreased density of the skeleton cause similar findings in the skull (see Table 4.1 and 4.2). Those cases where abnormalities of calvarial density are accompanied by thickening of the skull are listed in Table 5.3. Multiple or patchy calvarial densities can be seen on a normal basis and are due to variable thickness of the skull. However, scattered areas of increased density also are seen in tuberous sclerosis (1), acromegalic gigantism, and, occasionally, with metastatic disease, leukemia, or lymphoma. In addition, patchy calvarial densities alternating with areas of radiolucency are seen in more florid cases of hyperparathyroidism.

REFERENCE

1. Medley BE, McLeod RA, Houser OW: Tuberous sclerosis. *Semin Roentgenol* 11:35–54, 1976.

Radiolucent Lines in the Calvarium

The commonest radiolucent lines in the calvarium are those caused by vascular grooves, sutures, synchondroses, and fractures (4). A detailed discussion of all possible appearances of these structures is beyond the scope of this book, and is covered in detail elsewhere (6). The following comments are merely a resume.

Normal sutures are the structures that most commonly cause radiolucent lines in the calvarium of children, but they usually pose a diagnostic problem only when rotation of the skull places them in a peculiar projection. As a safeguard, then, it behooves one to know the positions into which these sutures are projected with rotation of the head. In addition, it is important to note that most of the troublesome sutures (squamosal, lambdoid, other posterior fossa sutures) are paired, and such pairing should be sought for constantly. Utilizing this rule, even if a

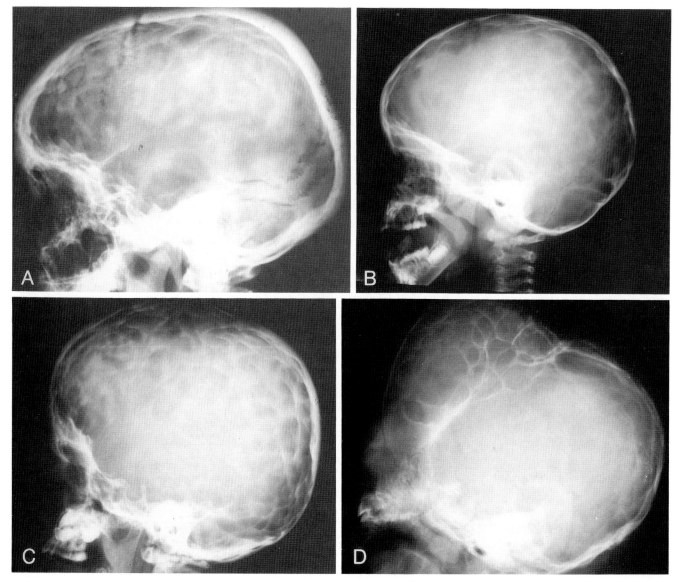

Figure 5.15. Increased convolutional markings. A. Increased convolutional markings due to chronically increased intracranial pressure. Patient with long-standing brain tumor. Note spread sutures and enlarged sella. **B.** Normal patient with prominent convolutional markings. Note normal sutures and normal sella. **C.** Increased convolutional markings in premature synostosis of the sutures. Note absence of suture visualization and slight enlargement of the sella. **D.** Localized increased convolutional markings due to brain crowding in focal synostosis of the metopic and coronal sutures.

suture has the appearance of a fracture, if it is located in the expected position, and if it is one of a pair, then most likely it is a suture. If on the other hand one already has identified both sutures of any given pair and another similar line is seen, even though it is located where one might expect a suture it is probably a fracture.

Knowledge of normal accessory sutures is also important and, for the most part, these include the posterior parietal fissure, intraparietal accessory suture (near horizontal in the parietal bone) (2, 5, 6), the basal synchondroses (3), the metopic suture (7), and

the midline occipital fissure (1). With intraparietal and posterior parietal fissures, the fact that these structures often are paired and indeed quite symmetric is helpful. In addition, the posterior parietal fissure occurs in the lower third of the parietal bone. Consequently, if a similar finding is seen in the upper part of the parietal bone a fracture should be suspected. Intraparietal sutures are quite common and most tend to be relatively horizontal in position. However, occasionally vertical intraparietal sutures are encountered, and in some cases so many of these sutures are present that an eggshell fracture of the calvarium is mimicked. If one cannot decide whether a radiolucent line is a fracture, other factors such as type of injury, location of injury, and overlying soft tissue swelling can be utilized. Ultimately, if none of these potentially helpful considerations produce results, a bone scan may be helpful. Fractures should be positive and sutures negative.

Vascular grooves producing radiolucent lines in the calvarium are not a problem if they are tortuous or branching, but if they are straight they also can

be misinterpreted for fractures. One of the most commonly misinterpreted vascular grooves is that which occurs in the frontal bone. It is produced by the supraorbital artery, and when it is straight or gently curving it can mimic a fracture. Diploic veins over the parietal bone are no particular problem because they have a stellate configuration, but the superficial branch of the temporal artery as it crosses the temporal bone can be mistaken for a fracture. The middle meningeal artery usually is recognized for what it is, and only its posterior branch as it travels horizontally commonly is misinterpreted for a fracture.

Fractures usually occur at or near the site of injury. However, if the injury is sustained by a blow against a broad surface, the fracture may occur at some distance away from the point of impact. Nonetheless, fractures usually are not difficult to identify. With a depressed fracture, a V-shaped configuration of the fracture line, sclerosis along one of the fracture line edges, and increased density of some of the depressed fragments can aid in diagnosis. Increased density in these fractures results from overlapping of the fracture fragments or visualization of the fragments on tangent.

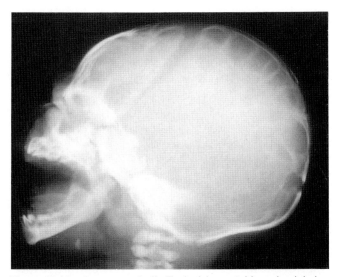

Figure 5.16. Lacunar skull. Typical inner table calvarial defects of lacunar skull. These are not due to increased pressure and are not the same as the increased convolutions seen in Figure 5.15.

REFERENCES

1. Franken EA: The midline occipital fissure: diagnosis of a fracture versus anatomic variants. *Radiology* 93:1043–1046, 1969.
2. Shapiro R: Anomalous parietal sutures and the bipartite parietal bone. *AJR* 115:569–577, 1972.

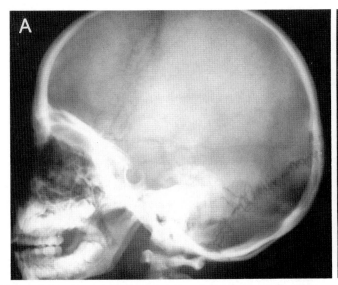
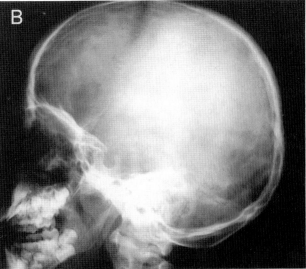

Figure 5.17. Decreased convolutional markings. A. Patient with hypothyroidism and paucity of convolutional markings. Also note prominence of the sutures and roundness of the sella (cherry sella). **B.** After treatment, note the increase in convolutional markings, slight spread of the sutures, and change in sellar configuration. All of these changes are due to maturation and accelerated brain growth.

3. Shopfner CE, Wolfe TW, O'Kell RT: The intersphenoid synchondrosis. *AJR* 104:184–193, 1968.
4. Swischuk LE: The growing skull. *Semin Roentgenol* 9:115–124, 1974.
5. Swischuk LE: The normal pediatric skull variations artifacts. *Radiol Clin N Am* 10:227–290, 1972.
6. Swischuk LE: *Emergency Radiology of the Acutely Ill or Injured Child*. 3rd ed. Baltimore: Williams & Wilkins, pp. 602–624.
7. Torgerson J: A roentgenologic study of the metopic suture. *Acta Radiol* 33:1–11, 1950.

Abnormalities of the Sella

The sella can be larger than normal, smaller than normal, or of abnormal shape. If it is enlarged, pathology is present, but if it is smaller than normal

Table 5.9
Sellar Size Abnormalities and Configurations

Sellar size abnormalities		
Large sella		
Intrasellar tumor		
Chronically increased pressure with tumor or hydrocephalus	}	Common
Nelson syndrome		
Hypothyroidism	}	Uncommon
Empty sella syndrome		
Intrasellar cyst		
Chronic pressure with universal craniosynostosis	}	Rare
Small sella		
Normal	}	Common
Atrophy		
Shunted hydrocephalus		
Hypopituitarism	}	Moderately common
Sellar configurations		
Stretched sella	Normal	
	Enlarging head	} Common
Scooped or omega sella	Optic chiasm tumor	} Most common
	Pituitary fossa tumor	
	Unilateral normal	} Relatively rare
Boat-shaped or J-shaped sella	Normal	} Most common
	Chiasmatic or intrasellar tumor	} Relatively rare
	Intrasella cyst	} Rare
Dysplastic sella	Neurofibromatosis	} Most common

pathology may or may not be present. Indeed, most often a small sella is a normal variant. Abnormal shapes of the sella many times are also just normal variations, but there are a few specific configurations that should strongly suggest a pathologic condition. All of these features of the sella are discussed in ensuing paragraphs and summarized in Table 5.9.

LARGE SELLA

The commonest cause of a large sella in the pediatric age group is an intrasellar tumor. Such a tumor may arise within the sella itself (e.g., adenoma; Fig. 5.18A) (5) or from the para-sellar regions. The best example of the latter is craniopharyngioma. The common occurrence of calcification (irregular or curvilinear) in this tumor aids in its diagnosis (Fig. 5.18B). The sella also can enlarge in the late stages of chronically increased intracranial pressure, but the finding usually takes months to develop (see Fig. 5.15A and C). In such cases, enlargement probably results from bone erosion secondary to intrasellar subarachnoid space distension and dilation.

The sella also enlarges in response to rebound hypertrophy of the pituitary gland secondary to end organ failure. Such rebound hypertrophy of the pituitary gland following bilateral adrenal ablation is known as Nelson syndrome (8, 9). A similar phenomenon occurs with hypothyroidism (6). In either condition, if pituitary hypertrophy is long standing an actual adenoma may develop in the pituitary gland. In most cases of rebound hypertrophy the enlarged sella is quite round, and in hypothyroidism it has been termed the "cherry" sella (see Fig. 5.13B).

The sella rarely can enlarge when a subarachnoid cyst enters the pituitary fossa. Such cysts can be congenital or acquired. The latter occurs after intracranial bleeds, infections, or infiltration with the storage diseases (4). Dilation of the arachnoid space in the pituitary fossa, as occurs in the empty sella syndrome, is relatively rare in children (3). Finally, the sella can enlarge on a nonneoplastic basis in neurofibromatosis. In such cases the finding represents yet another manifestation of the mesenchymal developmental defect that affects many of the bones in patients with this condition (see Fig. 5.21).

SMALL SELLA

The commonest cause by far of a smaller than normal sella is normal variation (Fig. 5.18C). However, in children a small sella also commonly is seen in hypopituitarism and with decreased intracranial

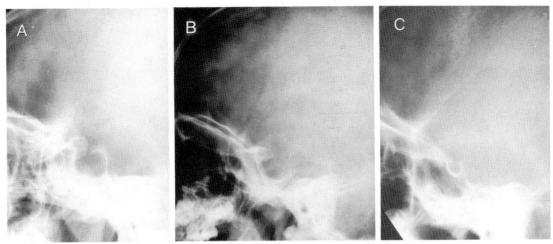

Figure 5.18. Small and large sellas. A. Large sella due to adenoma of pituitary gland. **B.** Craniopharyngioma causing a large sella. Note curvilinear intra- and suprasellar calcification. **C.** Small sella in normal child. A small sella also can be seen in hypopituitarism. For a slightly large, rounded cherry sella of hypothyroidism, see Figure 5.17A.

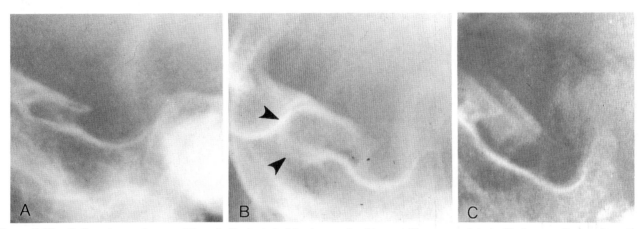

Figure 5.19. Sellar shape abnormalities. A. Typical stretched sella. **B.** Typical scooped or omega sella. **C.** Boat-shaped or J sella. For conditions associated with these sellar configurations see description in text.

pressure (1, 7). The latter can occur with brain atrophy or after successful shunting for hydrocephalus. In either case, the sella becomes small in response to chronically decreased intracranial pressure. The phenomenon is the reverse of that which occurs when the sella enlarges in response to chronically increased intracranial pressure. With decreased intracranial pressure other findings accompany the small sella, and these include (a) inward thickening of the calvarium, (b) absence of convolutional markings, and (c) prominence of the paranasal sinuses and mastoid air cells.

SHAPE ABNORMALITIES

Shape abnormalities of the sella include (a) the stretched sella, (b) the scooped or omega sella, (c) the boat-shaped or J sella (Fig. 5.19), and (d) the dysplastic sella. In addition, one may encounter a number of nonspecific and usually clinically insignificant changes in configuration of the anterior clinoids, the middle clinoids, and the bridged sella (Fig. 5.20). The stretched sella often is misinterpreted for the J-shaped sella, but the two should be separated for they represent changes due to different problems. **The stretched sella** most often occurs in normal children, but it also is seen with any cause of calvarial enlargement. In these latter cases it seems that as the calvarium enlarges there is undue stretching to the base of the skull and subsequent elongation of the chiasmatic sulcus, flattening of the tuberculum sella, and shallowness of the pituitary fossa. The stretched sella is seen in the various storage diseases, chondrodystrophies, hydrocephalus, and megalencephaly.

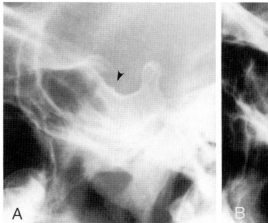

Figure 5.20. Miscellaneous sellar variations. A. Note small middle clinoids *(arrow)*, which often can be larger. **B.** Typical bridged sella due to ossification of diaphragma sella *(arrows)*. Often the sella also is small in these patients. Neither of these findings is of any clinical significance.

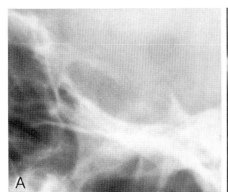
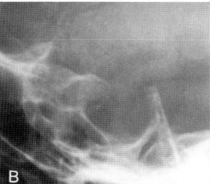
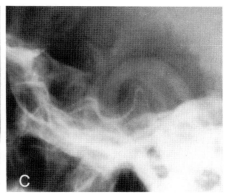

Figure 5.21. Dysplastic sella. A–C. Three cases of sellar and, in some cases, adjacent sphenoid wing dysplasia in neurofibromatosis. None of these patients had intra- or parasellar tumors.

The **scooped or omega sella** is actually a misnomer, because the configuration is formed by an enlarged chiasmatic groove. This sellar abnormality almost always denotes the presence of a tumor of the optic chiasm. Most often the tumor is an optic glioma, but it can be a neurofibroma or any other tumor that might occur in the area. Only occasionally is this configuration seen in a normal individual, and in such cases the groove enlargement is usually unilateral.

The **J or boat-shaped sella** differs from the stretched sella in that the tuberculum sella is completely flattened or eroded and the entire sella is more boat-shaped (2). This type of sellar configuration occasionally is seen in normal children. More often it occurs when an optic glioma extends into the pituitary fossa or an intrasellar tumor extends into the optic chiasm. Occasionally it can be seen with a subarachnoid cyst that extends into the sella.

A **dysplastic sella** is most commonly seen in patients with neurofibromatosis. Indeed, except for a few minor congenital variations in configuration of the sella, neurofibromatosis essentially is the sole culprit. In this condition, sellar configurations are almost endless (Fig. 5.21).

REFERENCES

1. Fisher RL, DiChiro G: The small sella turcica. *Neuroradiology* 91:996–1008, 1964.
2. Kier EL: "J" and "omega" shape of sella turcica. *Acta Radiol* 9:91–94, 1969.
3. Merle P, Georget, AM, Goumy P, Jarlot, D: Primary empty sella turcica in children: report of two familial cases. *Pediatr Radiol* 8:209–212, 1979.
4. Neuhauser EBD, Griscom NT, Gilles FH, Crocker AC: Arachnoid cysts in the Hurler-Hunter syndrome. *Ann Radiol* 11:453–469, 1968.
5. Richmond IL, Wilson CB: Pituitary adenomas in childhood and adolescence. *J Neurosurg* 49:163–168, 1978.

6. Swischuk LE, Sarwar M: The sella in childhood and hypothyroidism. *Pediatr Radiol* 6:1–3, 1977.
7. Swischuk LE, Sarwar M: The sella turcica (some lesser known dynamic features). *CRC Crit Rev Diagn Imaging* 11:37–55, 1978.
8. Weinstein M, Tyrrell B, Newton T: The sella turcica in Nelson's syndrome. *Radiology* 118:363–365, 1976.
9. Young LW, Lim GHK, Forbes GB, Bryson MF: Postadrenalectomy pituitary adenoma (Nelson's syndrome) in childhood: clinical and roentgenologic detection. *AJR* 126:550–559, 1976.

Foramen Magnum Abnormalities

Foramen magnum abnormalities consist primarily of size and configuration disturbances (Table 5.10). These abnormalities usually are visible on plain films but are more clearly demonstrated with CT. The most common abnormality of configuration is asymmetric smallness, which for the most part occurs with fusion (occipitalization) of C_1 to the base of the skull (Fig. 5.22A). In such cases, union of C_1 to the base of the skull is bony, and in some cases the narrowed foramen magnum can produce pressure on the brainstem and upper cervical cord. This is aggravated by the frequently associated finding of upward displacement of the dens (basilar invagination) (see Fig. 5.23).

Enlargement of the foramen magnum is seen with cervical-occipital meningoceles, the Arnold-Chiari malformation, syringobulbia, and posterior fossa cysts extending into the spinal canal. The most common of these cysts is the Dandy-Walker cyst (Fig. 5.22B). Other cysts of the posterior fossa herniating through the foramen magnum are rather uncommon and so are tumors and cysts of the cervical spine rising upward and enlarging the foramen magnum. Overall, the Arnold-Chiari malformation is the most common cause of a large foramen magnum (Fig. 5.22C) due to the downward displacement of the fourth ventricle and medulla. A final cause of enlargement of the foramen magnum is underdevelopment of the upper cervical spine, especially the posterior elements, and concomitant abnormal development of the foramen magnum.

A smaller than normal foramen magnum usually is seen in the chondrodystrophies and, of these, achondroplasia is the most common (Fig. 5.22D). Others include achondrogenesis, thanatophoric dwarfism, metatropic dwarfism, and diastrophic dwarfism. In any of these conditions, failure of adequate growth of the cartilaginous base of the skull leads to constriction of the foramen magnum. In milder cases the abnormality is of no serious consequence, but when the abnormality is severe hydrocephalus can result (2). The foramen magnum also may be smaller than normal with occipitalization of C_1 (Fig. 5.22A) and, finally, it should be noted that the foramen magnum often is normally irregular in the neonate. Ossification of the base of the skull is incomplete and thus many extra ossification centers and irregularities of ossification result (1).

Table 5.10
Foramen Magnum Abnormalities

Enlargement	
Arnold-Chiari malformation Cervical occipital encephaloceles	Common
Dandy-Walker cyst	Moderately common
Other posterior fossa cysts Cervical cord tumor Syringobulbia Posterior fossa tumor	Rare
Small foramen magnum	
Chondrodystrophies	Common
Bilateral or unilateral occipitalization	Uncommon
Irregular foramen magnum	
Normal neonatal ossicles	Common
Unilateral or bilateral occipitalization	Uncommon

REFERENCES

1. Caffey J: The accessory ossicles of the supra-occipital. *AJR* 70:401–412, 1953.
2. Cohen ME, Rosenthal AD, Matson DD: Neurologic abnormalities in achondroplastic children. *J Pediatr* 71:367–376, 1967.

Basilar Invagination

Basilar invagination is an abnormality that consists of upward displacement of the odontoid process into the foramen magnum. The high position of the dens can result in compression of the upper cervical cord or brainstem. This problem can result from congenital malformation of the cranio-cervical junction or acquired softening of the skull base. When congenital it is frequently associated with other craniocervical anomalies, the most common of which is congenital occipitalization of C_1. In this condition, the atlas is fused to the occiput of the skull, and it is the close apposition of the atlas to the base of the skull

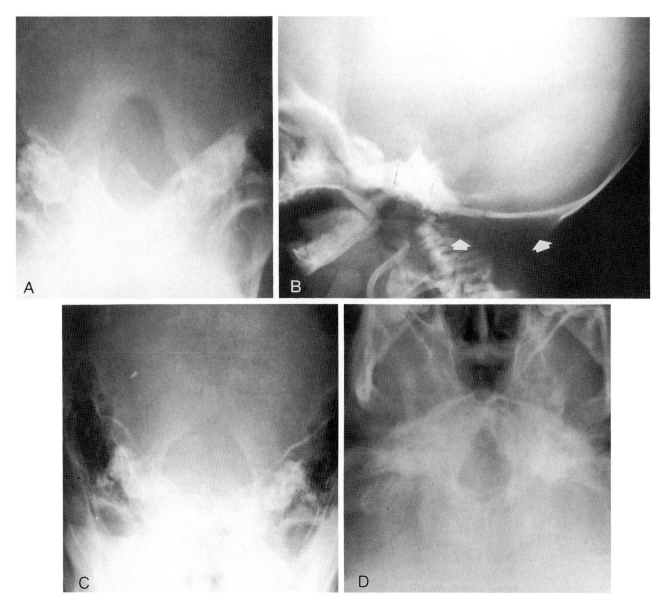

Figure 5.22. Abnormalities of the foramen magnum. A. Asymmetrically deformed, small foramen magnum secondary to unilateral occipitalization of C$_1$. **B.** Large foramen magnum in Dandy-Walker cyst which extends into the cervical canal *(arrows).* **C.** Large foramen magnum in older patients with Arnold-Chiari malformation. **D.** Small foramen magnum in achondroplasia.

that causes the dens to ride high (Fig. 5.23). Basilar invagination due to hypoplasia of C$_1$ is seen in a variety of syndromes (e.g., achondroplasia, Morquio disease, trisomy-21).

A less common cause of basilar invagination in children is softening of the base of the skull. This most commonly occurs with osteogenesis imperfecta, but the problem can also develop in hyperparathyroidism (primary or secondary with renal osteodystrophy), severe rickets, and in some cases of hypophosphatasia.

The diagnosis of basilar invagination is usually made on plain radiographs that show the high position of the odontoid process in relationship to MacGregor's, Chamberlain's, or McRay's line. MRI is useful for identifying cord compression or associated hydrocephalus or syringomyelia (1, 2).

REFERENCES

1. Calvy TM, Segall HD, Gilles FH, Bird CR, Zee CS, Ahmadi J, Biddle R: CT anatomy of the craniovertebral junction in infants and children. *AJNR* 8:489–494, 1987.
2. DiLorenzo N, Fortuna A, Guidetti B: Craniovertebral junction malformations: clinicoradiological findings, long-term

results and surgical implications in 63 cases. *J Neurosurg* 57:603–608, 1982.

Basal Angle Abnormalities

The basal angle is measured as the angle between lines drawn from (a) the base of the clivus to the center of the sella turcica and (b) the center of the sella turcica to the nasion (base of the nose). This angle normally ranges between 123° and 152°. The angle is decreased (more acute) in trisomy-21, Turner syndrome, acromegaly, craniosynostosis (usually coronal) (see Fig. 5.3*C*), and occasionally in hypothyroidism (1). It is increased (flatter) in Klinefelter syndrome, the XXX syndrome, and eunuchoidism (1). It is also increased in platybasia, which is seen in cleidocranial dysplasia, and bone softening conditions such as osteogenesis imperfecta, hyperparathyroidism, severe rickets, and hypophosphatasia.

REFERENCES

1. Rzymski K, Kosowicz J: Abnormal basal angle of the skull in sex chromosome aberrations. *Acta Radiol* 17:669–675, 1976.

Abnormalities of the Anterior Fontanelle

The anterior fontanelle, of course, should be open at birth and remain open for a few months after birth. Eventually, as the infant grows older, the fon-

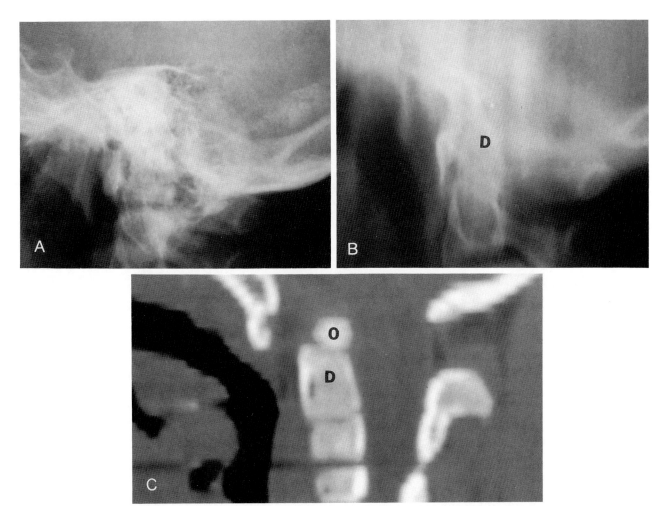

Figure 5.23. High dens position. A. Note difficulty in defining normal anatomy of the base of the skull including C₁ and the dens on plain radiograph. **B.** Tomogram in same patient, demonstrating the slightly high position of the dens *(D)* just protruding into the foramen magnum. This patient had occipitalization of C₁ and minimal basilar invagination. **C.** Another patient whose sagittal CT reconstruction demonstrates a slightly high dens *(D)* with a small os terminale *(O)*. The tip of the dens just enters the foramen magnum.

Table 5.11
Anterior Fontanelle Abnormalities

Large fontanelle	
Premature—normal	
Intrauterine infections	Common
Trisomy-21	
Hypothyroidism	
Severe rickets	
Trisomy-18	Moderately common
Osteogenesis imperfecta	
Cranium bifidum with lacunar skull	
Epiphyseal dysplasia punctata[a]	Uncommon
Cleidocranial dysplasia	
Aminopterin embryonopathy	
Cerebrohepatorenal (Zellweger) syndrome	
Congenital cutis aplasia	
Familial idiopathic osteoarthropathy	
Hypophosphatasia	
Hallerman-Streiff syndrome	Rare
Melnick-Needles syndrome	
Otopalatodigital syndrome	
Pachydermoperiostosis	
Progeria	
Rubinstein-Taybi syndrome	
Small fontanelle	
Craniosynostosis[b]	
Brain atrophy[c]	Common
Shunted hydrocephalus[c]	
Craniosynostosis[d]	
Chronic anemias	
Rickets	Moderately common
Hypophosphatasia	
Normal variation	Rare
Anterior fontanelle bone	
Normal	Common
Large head[e]	Moderately common

[a] Conradi disease.
[b] Primary.
[c] Secondary synostosis.
[d] Secondary.
[e] Hydrocephalus.

tanelle becomes smaller and finally is obliterated. In infancy, two common deviations from this sequence of events can occur—i.e., the anterior fontanelle can be too big or too small. When it is **too large,** there is almost always associated delayed ossification of the membranous bones of the calvarium. This is a common phenomenon in the normal premature infant and occasionally is seen in normal, full-term infants. Pathologically, it occurs with neonatal rubella, almost any cause of intrauterine growth failure (2), hypothyroidism, and bony dysplasias where defective

ossification of the bone is present (Table 5.11). An example of the latter is seen in Figure 5.24A, a case of cleidocranial dysplasia. The anterior fontanelle also is large when the calvarium enlarges, but the fact that it is large in such cases is no surprise. Another relatively common cause of an overly large anterior fontanelle is lacunar skull. In these patients, a temporary cranium bifidum (ossification defect in the midfrontal bone) exists and this defect extends into the anterior fontanelle.

An **overly small** anterior fontanelle occasionally is seen in normal infants, but more often it occurs with primary craniosynostosis or premature closure of the sutures secondary to atrophy of the brain (Fig. 5.24B) or decreased intracranial pressure due to shunting of hydrocephalus. Finally, it might be noted that occasionally one can encounter one or more extra bones in the anterior fontanelle (Fig. 5.24C). These bones can be seen in completely normal patients (1) or in patients with hydrocephalus.

REFERENCES

1. Girdany BR, Blank E: Anterior fontanelle bones. *AJR* 95:148–153, 1965.
2. Philip AGS: Fontanel size and epiphyseal ossification in neonates with intrauterine growth retardation: preliminary communication. *J Pediatr* 84:204–207, 1974.

Wormian Bones

Wormian bones are intrasutural bones that commonly occur in normal infants but also are seen in pathologic conditions (Table 5.12) (1). Most often they are seen along the lambdoid suture (Fig. 5.25), and as far as pathologic conditions are concerned, the ones most commonly encountered are osteogenesis imperfecta and cleidocranial dysplasia. Others include pyknodysostosis, hypophosphatasia, pachydermoperiostosis, some trisomies, idiopathic osteoarthropathy, progeria, hypothyroidism, aminopterin embryopathy, and the Hallermann-Streiff, Zellweger, Hadju-Cheney, kinky hair (Menkes), otopalatodigital, and Prader-Willi syndromes. As a side point, it also has been noted that excess wormian bone formation occurs in some patients with gross central nervous system abnormalities (2). However, it may be that many of these infants have lesser known chromosomal abnormalities.

REFERENCES

1. Cremin B, Goodman H, Spranger J, Beighton P: Wormian bone in osteogenesis imperfecta and other disorders. *Skeletal Radiol* 8:35, 1982.

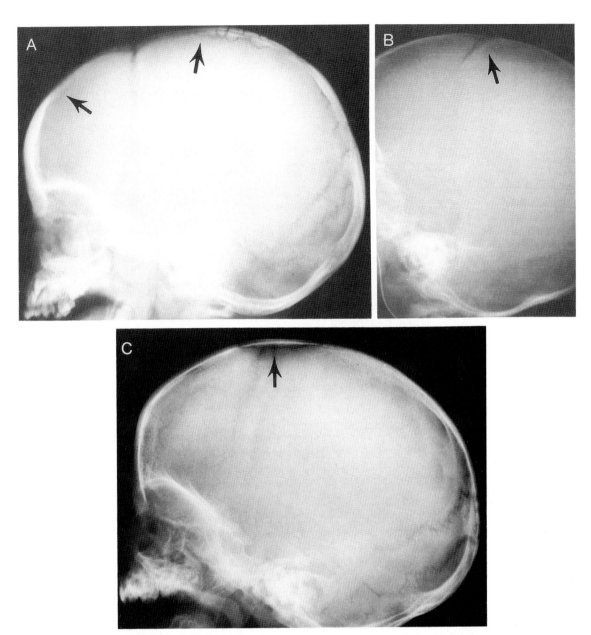

Figure 5.24. Anterior fontanelle abnormalities. A. Large anterior fontanelle *(arrows)* due to underossification in cleidocranial dysostosis. Note the wormian bones along the sagittal and lambdaed sutures. **B.** Small anterior fontanelle *(arrow)* secondary to premature closure of sutures in brain atrophy. **C.** Anterior fontanelle bone *(arrow)*.

2. Pryles CV, Khan AJ: Wormian bones. *Am J Dis Child* 133:380–382, 1979.

Button Sequestrum

A button sequestrum occurs when a round destructive lesion of the calvarium is associated with a small sclerotic piece of sequestered bone in its center. It is not particularly common in children and, although it can occur in a number of conditions, in childhood it most often is seen with osteomyelitis or eosinophilic granuloma (1–3). However, other causes to be considered include dermoid cysts, healing of a burr hole, fibrous dysplasia, hemangioma, epidermoid cysts, and radiation necrosis. In adults it has been noted with Paget disease, multiple myeloma, and meningioma, but only the latter condition might be seen in the child.

REFERENCES

1. Satin R, Usher MS, Goldenberg M: More causes of button sequestrum. *J Can Assoc Radiol* 27:288–289, 1976.

Table 5.12
Wormian Bones

Normal (especially lambdoid) suture }	Common
Osteogenesis imperfecta Cleidocranial dysplasia Cretinism Some trisomies Healing rickets	Moderately common
Pyknodysostosis Hypophosphatasia Pachydermoperiostosis Idiopathic osteoarthropathy Hallermann-Streiff syndrome Aminopterin embryonopathy Kinky hair or Menkes syndrome Cutis aplasia congenita Hadju-Cheney syndrome Zellweger syndrome Otopalatodigital syndrome Prader-Willi syndrome Progeria	Rare

2. Sholkoff SD, Mainzer F: Button sequestrum revisited. *Radiology* 100:649–652, 1971.
3. Wells PO: The button sequestrum of eosinophilic granuloma of the skull. *Radiology* 67:746–747, 1956.

Calvarial Bone Destruction

The causes of bone destruction of the calvarium are essentially the same as those for long bones (see Chapter 4), and in general calvarial destruction may be described as (a) mottled and permeative, or (b) discretely lytic (Table 5.13).

MOTTLED OR PERMEATIVE DESTRUCTION

This type of bone destruction most often is due to infection, metastatic disease, or the leukemia-lymphoma group of diseases. It also occurs with primary bone tumors but in the calvarium these are rare. When multiple areas of mottled destruction are seen, the best possibilities are metastatic disease and the leukemia-lymphoma group of diseases (Fig. 5.26A). In infection such destruction usually is solitary (Fig. 5.26B). An example of focal mottled destruction due to infection is Pott's puffy tumor (Fig. 5.26D), a subperiosteal abscess of the frontal bone that is associated with sinusitis (3). Diffuse, permeative destruction can be mimicked in hyperparathyroidism, where severe demineralization and osteo-

malacia are the causes of the mottled appearance (Fig. 5.26C).

DISCRETELY LYTIC DESTRUCTION

With this type of destruction, the lesion, once again, may be solitary or multiple. Most of these lesions are characterized by areas of rather homogeneous osteolysis rimmed by varying degrees of sclerosis. However, before such lesions of the skull are discussed, it should be mentioned that the commonest radiolucent defects in the calvarium are the normal fontanelles. The anterior and posterior fontanelles are not a diagnostic problem, but the third or accessory parietal fontanelle, the lateral fontanelles, and the metopic fontanelle can present difficulties.

The third or accessory fontanelle occurs in the midline, along the sagittal suture, and above the posterior fontanelle (Fig. 5.27A and B). This is in the same location that normal, persistent parietal foramina occur (Fig. 5.27C) (6). Probably all of these defects are related. They may vary widely in size, but usually they are quite symmetric and bilateral. The metopic fontanelle is rather rare, but occurs in the midline below the anterior fontanelle. The lateral fontanelles occur at the confluence of the posterior fossa sutures, but seldom are they large enough to cause a diagnostic problem. Furthermore, since the posterior fossa sutures join at their site, they readily are identified as normal structures. Other discretely lytic, nonpathologic areas of radiolucency in the skull can be seen with intradiploic venous lakes and pacchionian granulations (Fig. 5.27D). These skull impressions are not as common in children as in adults and clinically no masses are associated with these lesions.

Pathologic entities producing solitary or multiple lytic lesions include conditions such as histiocytosis-X, epidermoid inclusion cysts, dermoids, osteomyelitis, fibrous dysplasia, leptomeningeal cyst, congenital occipital dermal sinus (8), encephalocele, hyperparathyroidism, and metastatic disease (Table 5.13). Examples of a variety of these lytic lesions are demonstrated in Figures 5.28 through 5.31. Encephaloceles tend to occur in the midline, most often in the occipital region and then in the frontal area (see Fig. 5.48A). They can, however, occur along the base of the skull and even laterally. Osteomyelitis and metastatic disease can occur anywhere in the skull and so can fibrous dysplasia. Metastatic lesions usually have little sclerosis around their edges (Fig. 5.29C), while sclerosis is variable with fibrous dysplasia (Fig. 5.29B). Although some degree of sclero-

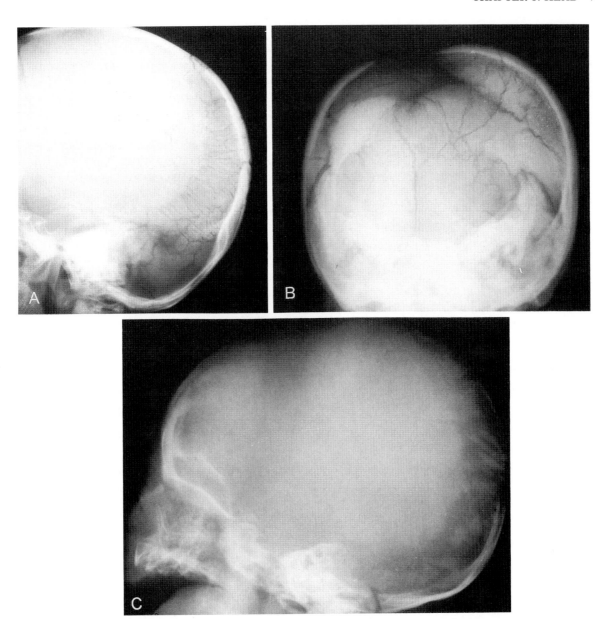

Figure 5.25. Wormian bones. A. Note extensive wormian bone formation along the lambdoid suture and posterior parietal regions. Patient with cleidocranial dysostosis. **B.** Another patient with cleidocranial dysostosis demonstrating more extensive wor-mian and mosaic bone formation. **C.** Wormian bone formation in the posterior parietal region and lambdoid suture areas in osteogenesis imperfecta.

sis usually is present with osteomyelitis, the lesions of eosinophilic granuloma and histiocytosis-X typically are extremely radiolucent, sharp-edged, and not rimmed by sclerosis (Figs. 5.29A and 5.31A).

Epidermoid inclusion cysts of the skull most commonly occur in the frontoparietal region but can be seen almost anywhere. They appear as round or oval lesions with smooth margins usually with a definite, sclerotic border, and can measure anywhere from 1 to 3 cm in diameter (Fig. 5.28). Leptomeningeal cysts occur at the site of old fractures, where associated dural tears allow the arachnoid membranes to herniate through the fracture. With subsequent normal pulsation of the brain, gradual erosion along the margins of the herniation occurs, and chronic widening with scalloping of the fracture line is seen. Eventually, a cyst-like calvarial defect is formed. The defect usually is oval or oblong and peripheral sclerosis is absent or minimal (Fig. 5.29D). Minimal brain herniation through the defect can occur and post-traumatic encephalomalacia of the underlying brain may be seen with CT or MRI.

Table 5.13
Calvarial Destruction

Permeative or mottled	
Metastatic disease[a]	
Infection[b,c]	} Common
Leukemia-lymphoma[a]	} Uncommon
Primary bone tumor	
Hyperparathyroidism	} Rare
Solitary or multiple discretely lytic lesions	
Histiocytosis-X[a]	
Fibrous dysplasia[c]	
Encephaloceles[b]	
Normal and accessory fontanelles	} Common
Osteomyelitis[b]	
Metastatic disease	
Venous lakes[a,b]	
Healing cephalohematoma[b]	
Epidermoid inclusion cyst[d]	} Moderately common
Leukemia-lymphoma[a]	
Leptomeningeal cysts[b]	
Pachyonnian granulations[b]	
Neurofibromatosis[e]	} Uncommon
Scalp tumor or cyst	
Congenital dermal sinus[b]	
Aneurysmal bone cyst[d]	
Intraosseous hematoma	
Hemangioma of calvarium[b]	
Calvarial dermoids[b]	
Congenital syphilis	
Primary bone tumor	} Rare
Radiation necrosis	
Intradiploic ectopic neural tissue[b]	
Caffey disease	
Reparative granuloma	
Cranial fascitis	
Large lytic areas	
Fibrous dysplasia[b]	
Infection[b]	} Common
Histiocytosis-X	
Postoperative bone flap necrosis	} Uncommon
Chordoma of clivus	
Meningioma	
Nasopharyngeal tumors and polyps	} Rare
Neurofibromatosis[f]	
Radiation necrosis	

[a] Frequently multiple.
[b] Variable but not markedly sclerotic edge.
[c] Occasionally multiple.
[d] Markedly sclerotic edge.
[e] Lambdoid defect.
[f] Sphenoid wing.

Rarer causes of solitary lytic lesions of the calvarium include intraosseous hematoma (trauma, head bangers, hemophilia), hemangioma (Fig. 5.29E) (may be a honeycombed radiolucency), congenital syphilis, sarcoidosis, neurofibromatosis (defect along lambdoid suture) (Fig. 5.30A), primary bone tumor (5), scalp tumor or cyst causing erosion of the calvarium, leukemia or lymphoma, congenital dermal sinus (usually midline in the occipital or frontal region) (8), radiation necrosis, intradiploic ectopic neural tissue, giant cell reparative granuloma (2), cranial fascitis (4), Caffey disease (1, 7), and healing cephalohematoma (Fig. 5.30B). Of the foregoing conditions, the most likely to produce multiple discrete lytic lesions are histiocytosis-X, metastatic disease, and leukemia-lymphoma (Fig. 5.31). Rarely, multiple discrete defects occur in hyperparathyroidism (Fig. 5.31D).

REFERENCES

1. Boyd RDH, Shaw DG, Thomas BM: Infantile cortical hyperostosis with lytic lesions in the skull. *Arch Dis Child* 47:471–472, 1972.
2. Cohen D, Granda-Ricart MC: Giant cell reparative granuloma of the base of the skull in a 4-month-old infant—CT findings. *Pediatr Radiol* 23:319–320, 1993.
3. Feder HM Jr, Cates KL, Cementina AM: Pott puffy tumor: a serious occult infection. *Pediatrics* 79:625–629, 1987.
4. Hunter NS, Dulas DI, Chadduck WM, Chandra R: Cranial fascitis of childhood. *Pediatr Radiol* 23:398–399, 1993.
5. Kornreich L, Grunebaum, Ziv N: Osteogenic sarcoma of the calvarium in children: CT manifestations. *Neuroradiology* 30:439, 1988.
6. Murphy J, Gooding CA: Evolution of persistently enlarged parietal foramens. *Radiology* 97:391–392, 1970.
7. Neuhauser EBD: Infantile cortical hyperostosis and skull defects. *Postgrad Med* 48:57–59, 1970.
8. Shackelford GD, Shackelford PG, Schwetschenau PR, McAlister WH: Congenital occipital dermal sinus. *Radiology* 111:161–166, 1974.

Intracranial Calcifications

Intracranial calcifications, like calcifications anywhere in the body, can be irregular, curvilinear, serpentine, or punctate. In some cases more than one type is seen at the same time, but most often one form prevails. Many times, by utilizing the location and configuration of a calcification, one can determine its most likely etiology (Table 5.14). Although many calcifications are visible radiographically, ultrasound and especially CT are more sensitive for the detection of small calcifications (28).

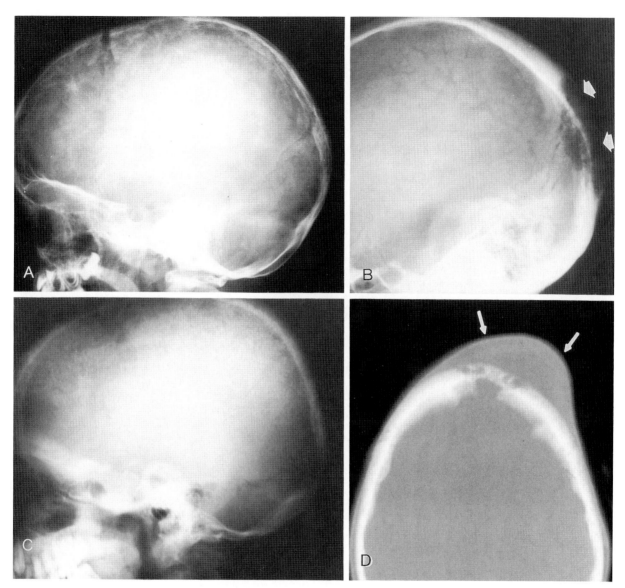

Figure 5.26. Mottled calvarial destruction. A. Note mottled destruction due to neuroblastoma. **B.** Permeative destruction due to osteomyelitis-coccidiomycosis *(arrow).* **C.** Mottled pseudodestruction secondary to hyperparathyroidism. **D.** Mottled calvarial destruction with marked soft tissue swelling over the frontal bone *(arrows)* due to Pott's puffy tumor (osteomyelitis secondary to sinusitis).

IRREGULAR CALCIFICATIONS

When irregular calcifications are small they may appear punctate, but true punctate calcifications are discussed later. Irregular calcifications most commonly are seen after infection, infarction, or intracranial bleeding, and with intracranial tumors. Less commonly they are seen with metabolic hypercalcemic states. If irregular calcifications are seen in and around the sella, the most common cause is tumor and most often the tumor is craniopharyngioma (Fig. 5.32A) (14, 18, 22, 24). Occasionally, it can be an atypical teratoma (38) or other tumor. With craniopharyngioma, in addition to irregular calcification curvilinear calcification in the walls of these frequently cystic tumors is common (see Fig. 5.34A).

Irregular calcifications in the basal ganglia can be idiopathic (23), but also are seen with pseudohypoparathyroidism (Fig. 5.32B), tuberous sclerosis (13, 21), CMV infection (5, 39, 43), toxoplasmosis (26), AIDS encephalopathy (12, 30), nephrogenic diabetes insipidus (41), and following radiation therapy. When irregular calcifications are located around the posterior portion of the third ventricle in the region

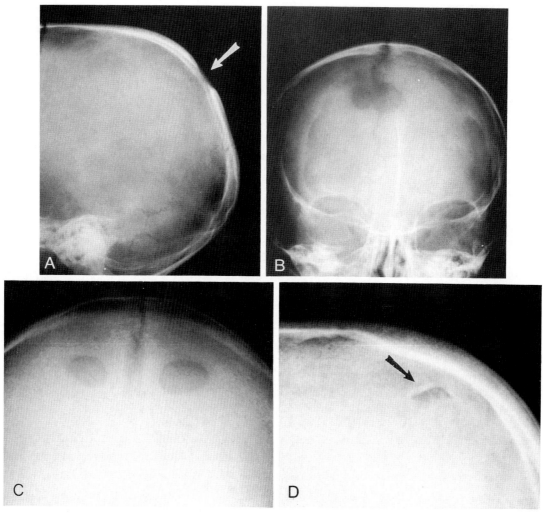

Figure 5.27. Solitary calvarial defects. A. Typical location of the accessory or third fontanelle *(arrows).* **B.** Frontal view showing the same defect. **C.** Typical posterior parietal foramina. **D.** "Lytic" defects in the calvarium due to the pacchionian granulations *(arrows).*

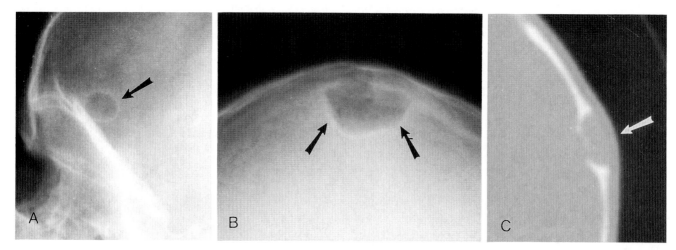

Figure 5.28. Solitary lytic lesions of calvarium. A. Typical epidermoid (congenital cholesteatoma) of frontal bone *(arrow).* Note sclerosis around its edge. **B.** Large external table epider-moid *(arrows).* **C.** CT scan in another patient demonstrates characteristic epidermoid inclusion cyst *(arrow).* Note that it expands both the inner and outer tables.

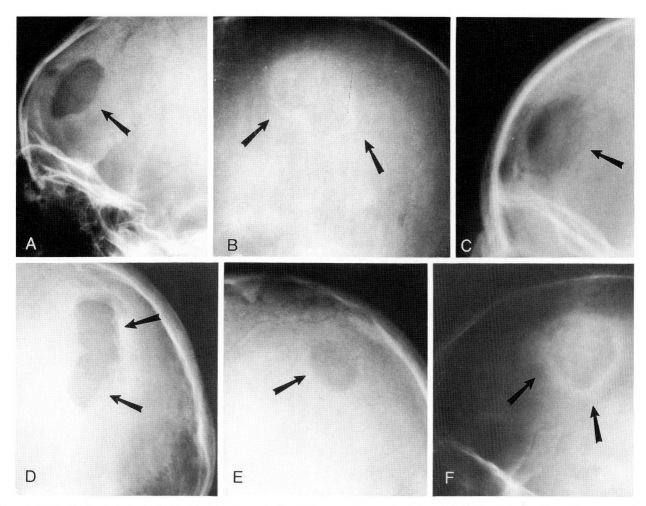

Figure 5.29. Solitary lytic lesions of calvarium. A. Typical eosinophilic granuloma with no sclerosis around its edges *(arrows)*. **B.** Vague, lytic area with minimal sclerosis in fibrous dysplasia *(arrow)*. **C.** Solitary lytic area due to metastatic neuroblastoma *(arrow)*. Note absence of sclerosis. **D.** Typical lepto- meningeal cyst *(arrows)*. Note oblong configuration and minimal sclerosis. **E.** Cranial hemangioma *(arrows)*. In some cases a latticework or honeycombed appearance is seen in these lesions. **F.** Large epidermoid cyst with moderate sclerosis *(arrows)*. This epidermoid cyst was located predominantly in the external table.

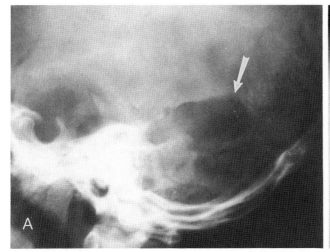
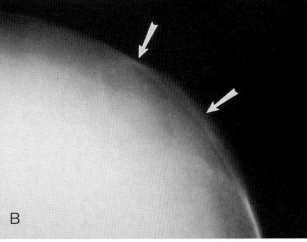

Figure 5.30. Solitary lytic lesions of calvarium. A. Note characteristic lambdoid defect in neurofibromatosis *(arrow)*. **B.** Pseu- docystic lesion of the calvarium due to a healing cephalohematoma in an infant *(arrows)*.

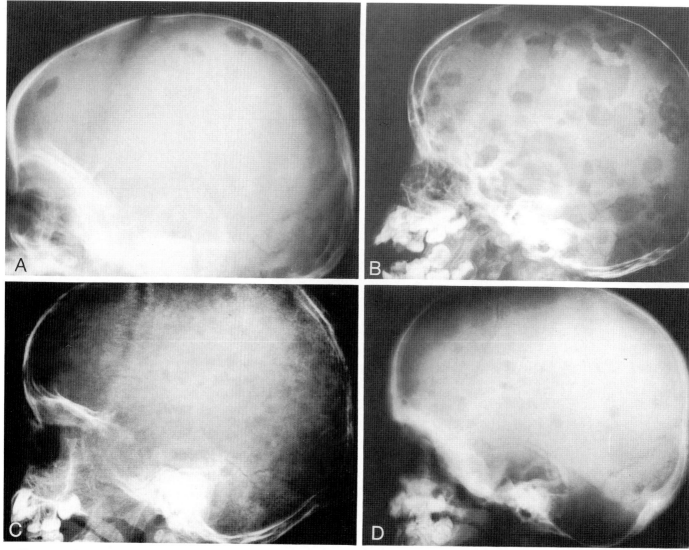

Figure 5.31. Multiple lytic lesions of calvarium. A. Typical nonsclerotic, punched-out lesions of histiocytosis-X. **B.** More extensive lesions producing geographic skull. **C.** Multiple areas of moth-eaten destruction in metastatic neuroblastoma. **D.** Multiple lytic lesions in hyperparathyroidism (renal osteodystrophy). Also note increased density of calvarium. (Courtesy of Derek Harwood-Nash, M.D., Toronto.)

of the pineal gland, almost always they are secondary to atypical teratoma. These tumors can coexist with another similar lesion just anterior and inferior to the third ventricle (38). Physiologic, irregular calcifications of the glomi of the choroid plexus of the lateral ventricles are not as commonly encountered in children as in adults (Fig. 5.32C) and, rarely, irregular calcifications behind the pineal gland can be seen in a thrombosed vein of Galen aneurysm (46).

Irregular calcifications located anywhere in the brain usually are due to old infection, bleeding, infarction, or brain tumor (Fig. 5.32D and E). The most common intracranial tumors that exhibit such calcifications include ependymoma (1, 37), oligodendroglioma (40), and primitive neuroectodermal tumor (20).

Similar calcifications also can be seen in meningioma (fine and sandlike, or irregular), hemangioma, teratoma (39), intracranial neuroblastoma (17), ganglioglioma (8), and along the base of the skull with chordoma or other cartilaginous tumors of the calvarium. Metastatic disease to the brain seldom calcifies in children, except in infants with retinoblastoma (11).

Irregular calcifications distributed around the walls of the ventricles almost always indicate intrauterine infection, and the organism most likely to cause this type of calcification is CMV (Fig. 5.33A and B) (32). Most often, associated brain atrophy and a small skull are present. Although the configuration is not entirely specific for CMV, the virus still

Table 5.14
Intracranial Calcification

Location	Type				
	Punctate	Irregular	Curvilinear	Serpentine	Linear
Pituitary fossa	**25, 40**	**25**			
Para- and suprasellar	25		25		
Basal ganglia	**1, 2, 13, 20, 41, 42**				
Anterior III ventricle	23, 24, 27, 37				
Pineal post. III ventricle	**11, 27, 38**	**11**	**11**		
Convexities	2–6, 8, 9	9	9	18, 19, 22	
Brain substance (anywhere)	**1, 2, 4, 5, 7**	**1, 2, 5, 7, 8**	**12**	**31**	
	24, 43	**10, 20, 26, 28**			
		36			
Periventricular		1, 2	1, 2		
Entire brain		**3**			
Falx-tentorium					14–17, 21
Glomi of choroid plexus,	**39**				

Key: 1. cytomegalovirus; 2. toxoplasmosis; 33 herpes simplex; 4. rubella; 5. tuberculosis; 6. meningitis; 7. brain infection-abscess; 8. intracranial bleeding; 9. subdural hematoma, hygroma; 10. cerebral infarction; 11. vein of Galen aneurysm; 12. other aneurysms; 13. pseudohypoparathyroidism; 14. hypervitaminosis D; 15. hyperparathyroidism; 16. idiopathic hypercalcemia; 17. other hypercalcemic states; 18. folic acid deficiency; 19. methotrexate therapy; 20. tuberous sclerosis; 21. basal cell nevus syndrome; 22. Sturge-Weber disease; 23. Fahr syndrome; 24. lissencephaly; 25. craniopharyngioma; 26. teratoma; 27. atypical teratoma (pinealoma); 28. glioma-astrocytoma; 29. meningioma; 30. ependymoma; 31. hemangioma; 32. oligodendroglioma; 33. hemangioblastoma; 34. metastatic retinoblastoma; 35. metastatic neuroblastoma; 36. neuroblastoma (primary); 37. lipoma corpus callosum; 38. normal pineal; 39. normalglomi choroid plexus; 40. pituitary stone; 41. AIDS encephalopathy; 42. idiopathic; 43. cysticecosis.

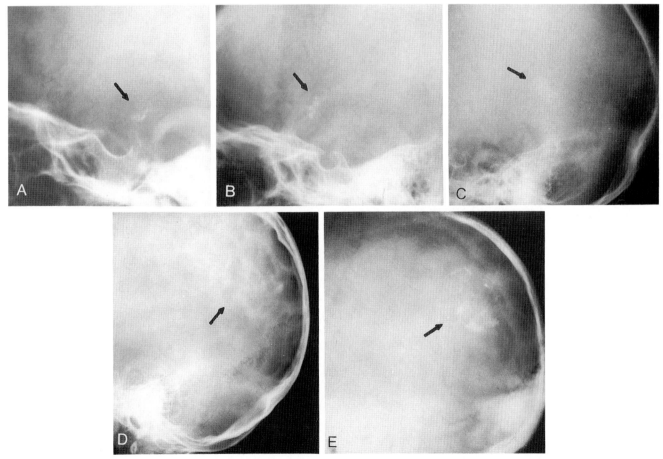

Figure 5.32.   Irregular intracranial calcifications. A. Irregular calcification in craniopharyngioma *(arrow).* **B.** Typical irregular calcifications in the basal ganglia of a patient with pseudohypoparathyroidism *(arrow).* **C.** Typical location of normal irregular calcifications in the glomi of the choroid plexus of the lateral ventricles *(arrows).* These calcifications, on frontal view, are usually bilateral. **D.** Irregular calcification in an old brain infarction *(arrow).* **E.** Irregular calcification in parasagittal meningioma.

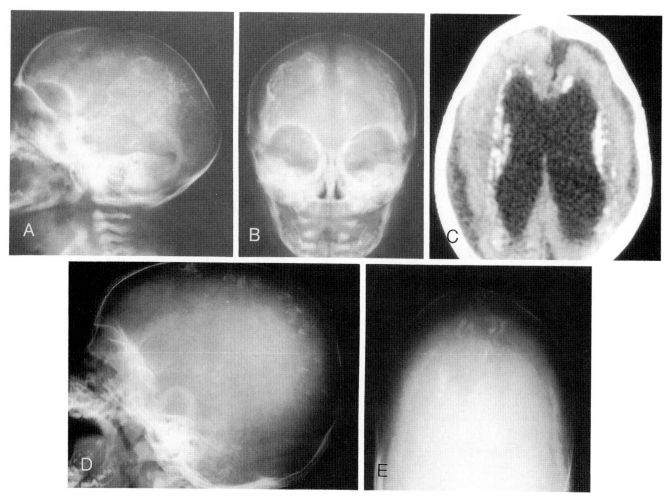

Figure 5.33. Irregular intracranial calcifications. A. Typical periventricular calcifications of cytomegalovirus infection. **B.** Frontal view demonstrating periventricular configuration. Note that the head is small. **C.** CT scan in another patient demon-strates typical periventricular calcifications of CMV infection. **D.** Typical scattered, flaky calcifications of toxoplasmosis. **E.** Frontal view demonstrating parasagittal location of the calcifications.

should be one's first diagnostic choice (42). Similar calcifications produced by other intrauterine infections are far less common. CMV infection also can cause calcifications elsewhere in the brain substance (3, 5, 43), but the periventricular distribution is most common and characteristic (Fig. 5.33C).

In toxoplasmosis, the head may be small due to atrophy or large due to hydrocephalus. Irregular, flaky calcifications can coexist and can be located almost anywhere (e.g., over the meninges, around the ventricles, in the basal ganglia, along the brain base) (Fig. 5.33D) (26). Seldom, however, are they as distinctly periventricular as in CMV infection. When very dense calcifications virtually outline the external surface of a small, atrophic brain, herpes simplex should be considered as the cause (27, 35). Rubella produces diffuse or focal calcifications (29, 31).

Irregular calcifications over the convexities of the brain or along the undersurface of the superior sagittal sinus most commonly are due to old, subdural hematomas. However, they also can be seen with subdural hygroma, healed meningitis, subdural abscess, and in leukemia and lymphoma after methotrexate treatment (36). More often, however, the latter calcifications are more serpentine and mimic those of Sturge-Weber disease (7, 25). Ill-defined, irregular calcifications located in the midline around the anterior third ventricle have been seen in ferrocalcinosis, or Fahr disease (2, 9).

CURVILINEAR AND LINEAR CALCIFICATIONS

Curvilinear calcifications almost always occur in a cyst, cystic tumor, or vascular lesion (Fig. 5.34).

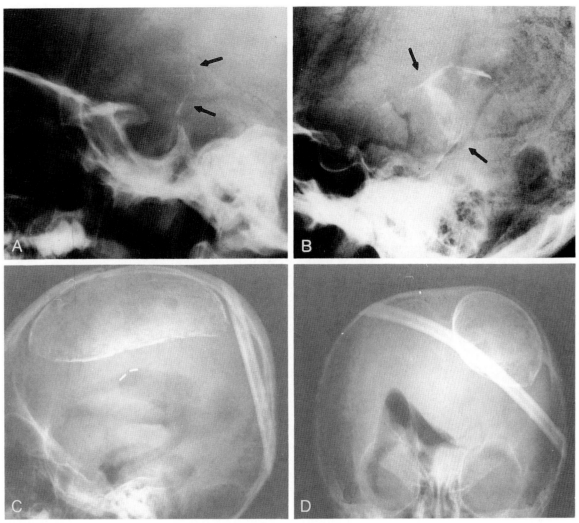

Figure 5.34. Curvilinear and linear calcifications. A. Typical curvilinear calcification of cystic craniopharyngioma *(arrows).* **B.** Calcified congenital aneurysm in young adult *(arrows).* **C.** Curvi- linear, sheath-like calcification in old subdural hematoma. **D.** Frontal view of the same patient.

They are not particularly common in children, except when they occur in cystic craniopharyngioma (Fig. 5.34*A*). Curvilinear calcifications in aneurysms, either congenital or mycotic, are rare in children (Fig. 5.34*B*). Similar calcifications over the convexities can be seen with old subdural hematomas, hygromas, or abscesses (Fig. 5.34*C* and *D*).

Purely linear calcifications usually are located in the falx, tentorium, or petroclinoid ligaments, but none are common in children. Although idiopathic calcification of these structures occasionally occurs, when seen in children it is more likely to be due to the basal cell nevus syndrome or a hypercalcemic state such as hypervitaminosis D (Fig. 5.35), hyperparathyroidism, or idiopathic hypercalcemia.

SERPENTINE CALCIFICATIONS

These calcifications usually occur within large blood vessels or over the gyri of the brain. Blood vessel calcifications are rare, even in arteriovenous malformations and hemangiomas, and actually when one sees a serpentine calcification in a child, most often the problem is the Sturge-Weber syndrome. In this condition, a diffuse leptomeningeal angiomatosis leads to gyral calcifications that most commonly arise in the second and third cortical layers. Radiographically, these calcifications produce double tract serpentine configurations, which are virtually pathognomonic (Fig. 5.36). Most often they occur in the temperoparietal or occipital regions (6). Similar calcifications have been seen in leukemia and lymphoma, viral encephalitis (19), tuberous sclerosis (34, 45), after methotrexate therapy (7, 25, 36), and with folic acid deficiency (15). Somewhat serpentine calcifications occasionally are seen in the rare oligodendroglioma.

PUNCTATE CALCIFICATIONS

The commonest punctate calcification in an adult is the normally calcified pineal gland, but normal pineal gland calcification usually is not encountered in children until after 6 years of age (33). Even then, it is uncommon until adolescence (Fig. 5.37A).

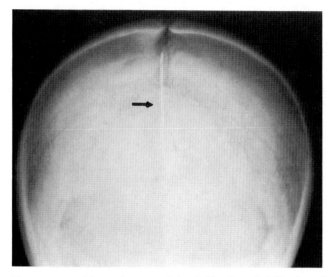

Figure 5.35. Linear intracranial calcification. Calcification of falx in hypervitaminosis D.

Larger, similar calcifications in the pineal gland can be seen with atypical teratoma (Fig. 5.37B) (10), and a small punctate calcification just anterior to and above the pineal gland occasionally is seen in the calcified splenium of the normal corpus callosum (Fig. 5.37C). Nonspecific punctate calcifications due to inflammatory disease of the brain, hemorrhage, or infection are not particularly common (Fig. 5.37D). A small punctate calcification just anterior to the third ventricle has been documented in congenital lissencephaly (44), a condition characterized by severe mental retardation and lack of normal cerebral gyri. Calcification in the same location occurs with lipoma of the corpus callosum, where the presence of an area of fat density surrounding the calcification usually secures the diagnosis. Both of these findings can be seen on plain films and with CT and MRI.

Small punctate- or comma-shaped calcifications can be seen with cysticercosis, but the condition is common only in the southern regions of this country. A normal reverse, small, comma-shaped calcification, seen in the habenular commissure just behind the pineal gland, is not commonly encountered in children. Finally, a small punctate calcification occasionally can be encountered in the pituitary fossa, the so-called "pituitary stone" (Fig. 5.37E). The finding is of no particular clinical consequence (4, 16).

REFERENCES

1. Armington WG, Osborn AG, Cubberley DA, Harnsberger HR, Boyer R, Naidich TP, Sherry RG: Supratentorial ependymoma: CT appearance. *Radiol* 157:367–372, 1985.

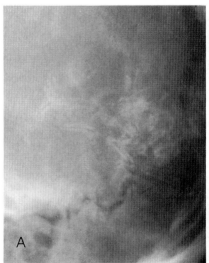
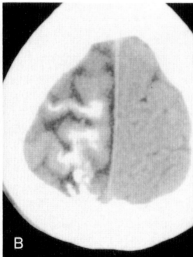
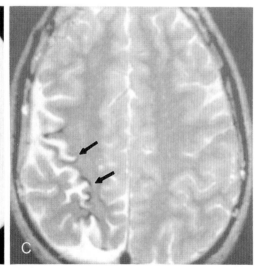

Figure 5.36. Serpentine calcifications. A. Typical serpentine calcifications of Sturge-Weber syndrome. **B.** CT study in another patient demonstrates similar calcifications over the convexity *on the right.* **C.** MR study in the same patient demonstrates the typical low signal layers of calcification *(arrows).* Note associated atrophy with increase of cerebrospinal fluid in the sulci.

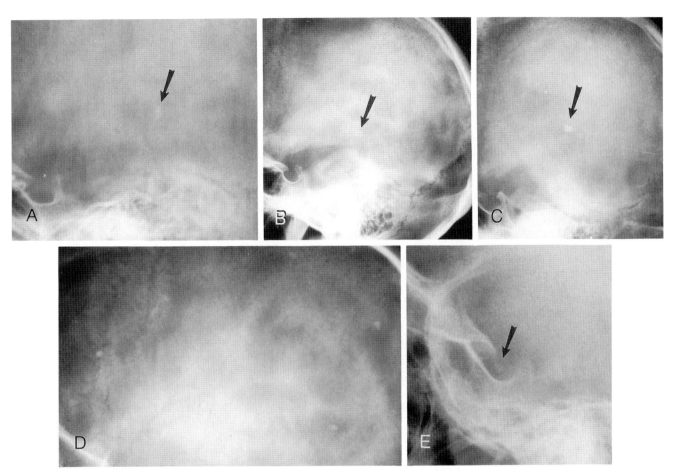

Figure 5.37. Punctate intracranial calcifications. A. Typical normal pineal calcification in a 10-year-old child *(arrow).* **B.** Large pineal calcification in atypical teratoma (ectopic pinealoma). **C.** Calcification in splenium of normal corpus callosum. **D.** Punctate calcifications *(arrows)* secondary to healed intracranial tuberculosis. **E.** Punctate calcification due to a pituitary stone *(arrow).*

2. Babbitt DP, Tang T, Dobbs J, Berk E: Idiopathic familial cerebrovascular ferrocalcinosis (Fahr's disease) and review of differential diagnosis of intracranial calcification in children. *AJR* 105:352–358, 1969.

3. Bale JF, Bray PF, Bell WE: Neuroradiologic abnormalities in congenital cytomegalovirus infection. *Pediatr Neurol* 1:42, 1985.

4. Barson AJ, Symonds J: Calcified pituitary concretions in the newborn. *Arch Dis Child* 52:642–645, 1977.

5. Boesch CL, Issakainen J, Kewitz G, Kikinis R, Martin E, Boltshauser E: Magnetic resonance imaging of the brain in congenital cystomegalovirus infection. *Pediatr Radiol* 19:91–93, 1989.

6. Boltshauser E, Wilson J, Hoare RD: Sturge-Weber syndrome with bilateral intracranial calcification. *Radiology* 121:767–768, 1976.

7. Borns PF, Rancier LF: Cerebral calcification in childhood leukemia mimicking Sturge-Weber syndrome: report of two cases. *AJR* 122:52–55, 1974.

8. Castillo M, Davis PC, Takei Y, Hoffman JC Jr: Intracranial ganglioglioma: MR, CT, and clinical findings in 18 patients. *AJR* 154:607–612, 1990.

9. Chalkias SM, Magnaldi S, Cova MA, et al: Fahr disease: significance and predictive value of CT and MR findings. *Eur Radiol* 2–6:570, 1992.

10. Chang T, Teng MM, Gno W, Sheng WC: CT of pineal tumors and intracranial germ cell tumors. *AJNR* 10:1039, 1989.

11. Davis LA, Diamond I: Metastatic retinoblastoma as a cause of diffuse intracranial calcification. *AJR* 78:437–439, 1957.

12. Epstein LG, Berman CZ, Sharer LR, Khademi M, Deposito F: Unilateral calcification and contrast enhancement of the basal ganglia in a child with AIDS encephalopathy. *AJNR* 8:163–165, 1987.

13. Fitz CR, Harwood-Nash DCF, Thompson JR: Neuroradiology of tuberous sclerosis in children. *Radiology* 110:635–642, 1974.

14. Freeman MP, Kessler RM, Allen JH, Price AC: Craniopharyngioma: CT and MR imaging in nine cases. *J Comput Assist Tomogr* 11:810–814, 1987.

15. Garwicz S, Mortensson W: Intracranial calcification mimicking the Sturge-Weber syndrome: a consequence of cerebral folic acid deficiency. *Pediatr Radiol* 5:5–9, 1976.

16. Glasser SP, Earll JM: Pituitary "stone": an unusual calcification. *JAMA* 203:367–369, 1968.

17. Horten BC, Rubinstein LJ: Primary cerebral neuroblastoma: a clinicopathological study of 35 cases. *Brain* 99:735–756, 1976.

18. Hurst RW, McIlhenhy J, Park TS, Thomas WO: Neonatal craniopharyngioma: CT and ultrasonographic features. *J Comput Assist Tomogr* 12:858, 1988.

19. Ketonen L, Koskiniemi JL: Gyriform calcification after herpes simplex virus encephalitis. *J Comput Assist Tomogr* 7:1070, 1983.

20. Kingsley DP, Hardwood-Nash DC: Radiological features of the neuroectodermal tumors of childhood. *Neuroradiology* 26:463–467, 1984.

21. Lagos JD, Holman CB, Gomez MR: Tuberous sclerosis: neuroroentgenologic observations. *AJR* 104:171–176, 1968.

22. Londen CN, Martinez CR, Gonzalvo AA, Cahill DW: Intrinsic third ventricle craniopharyngioma: CT and MR findings. *J Comput Assist Tomogr* 13:362, 1989.

23. Macpherson RI, Hoogstraten J, Tjaden R: Calcification of the basal ganglia in infancy. *J Can Assoc Radiol* 20:159–163, 1969.

24. Majd M, Farkas J, LoPresti JM, Chandra R, Hung W, Lussenhop AJ: A large calcified craniopharyngioma in the newborn. *Radiology* 99:399–400, 1971.

25. Mueller S, Bell W, Seibert J: Cerebral calcifications associated with intrathecal methotrexate therapy in acute lymphocytic leukemia. *J Pediatr* 88:650–653, 1976.

26. Mussbichler H: Radiologic study of intracranial calcifications in congenital toxoplasmosis. *Acta Radiol Diagn* 7:369–379, 1968.

27. Noorbehesht B, Enzmann DR, Sullender W, Bradley JS, Arvin AM: Neonatal herpes simplex encephalitis: correlation of clinical and CT findings. *Radiology* 162:813–19, 1987.

28. Norman D, Diamond C, Boyd D: Relative detectability of intracranial calcifications on computed tomography and skull radiography. *J Comput Assist Tomogr* 2:61–64, 1978.

29. Parisot S, Droulle P, Feldman M, Pineaud P, Marchal C: Unusual encephaloclastic lesions with paraventricular calcification in congenital rubella. *Pediatr Radiol* 21:229–230, 1991.

30. Price DB, Inglese CM, Jacobs J, Haller JO, Kramer J, Hotson GC, Loh JP, Schlusselberg D, Menez-Bautista R, Rose AL, Fikrig S: Pediatric AIDS neuroradiologic and neurodevelopmental findings. *Pediatr Radiol* 18:445–448, 1988.

31. Rowen M, Singer MI, Moran ET: Intracranial calcifications in the congenital rubella syndrome. *AJR* 115:86–91, 1972.

32. Sackett GL, Ford MM: Cytomegalic inclusion disease with calcification outlining the cerebral ventricles. *AJR* 76:512–515, 1956.

33. Schey WL: Intracranial calcifications in childhood, frequency of occurrence and significance. *AJR* 122:495–502, 1975.

34. Sener RN, Meral A, Farmaka H, Kalender N: CT of gyriform calcification in tuberous sclerosis. *Pediatr Radiol* 22:525–26, 1992.

35. South MA, Tompkins W, Morris R, Rawls WE: Congenital malformation of the central nervous system associated with genital type (type II) herpes virus. *Am J Pediatr* 75:13–18, 1969.

36. Spehl M, Flament J, Maurus R, Delalieux G, Brihaye J, Cremer N: Diffuse intracranial calcification appearing during the follow-up of acute lymphoblastic leukemia. *Ann Radiol* 17:417–422, 1974.

37. Swartz JD, Zimmerman RA, Bilanium LT: Computed tomography of intracranial ependymomas. *Radiology* 143:97–101, 1982.

38. Swischuk LE, Bryan RN: Double midline intracranial atypical teratomas (a recognizable neuroendocrinologic syndrome). *AJR* 122:517–524, 1974.

39. Takaku A, Mita R, Suzuki J: Intracranial teratoma in early infancy. *J Neurosurg* 38:265–268, 1973.

40. Tice H, Barnes PD, Goumnerova L, Scott RM, Tarbell NJ: Pediatric and adolescent oligodendrogliomas. *AJNR* 14:1293–1300, 1993.

41. Tohyama J, Inagaki M, Koeda T, Ohno K, Takeshita K: Intracranial calcification in siblings with nephrogenic diabetes insipidus: CT and MRI. *Neuroradiology* 35:553–55, 1993.

42. Tucker AS: Intracranial calcifications in infants. *AJR* 86:458–461, 1961.

43. Voigt K, Sauer M, Luthardt T: Unusual roentgenological findings in cytomegalic inclusion body disease: large and circumscribed calcareous deposits of the basal ganglia and scattered calcifications of the parieto occipital cortex. *Pediatr Radiol* 3:47–49, 1975.

44. Wesenberg RL, Juhl JH, Daube JR: Radiological findings in lissencephaly (congenital agyria). *Radiology* 87:436–444, 1966.

45. Wilms G, Van Wijck E, Demaerel P, Smet MH, Plets C, Brucher JM: Gyriform calcifications in tuberous sclerosis simulating the appearance of Sturge-Weber disease. *AJNR* 13:295–97, 1992.

46. Wilson CB, Roy M: Calcification within congenital aneurysms of the vein of Galen. *AJR* 91:1319–1326, 1964.

Intracranial Radiolucencies (Air and Fat)

Abnormal intracranial radiolucency is due to either abnormal accumulations of fat or the presence of intracranial gas. As far as fat is concerned, almost always when the finding is seen on plain films the problem is lipoma of the corpus callosum (1, 3, 4). Characteristically, there is an area of fatty density in the midline anteriorly (Fig. 5.38), and the lesion is exceptionally well delineated with CT or MRI. These lipomas can occur as isolated lesions or in association with other intracranial anomalies. Fat also can be present in dermoids, and previously undetected intracranial epidermoid cysts are being documented more frequently with CT and MRI. Indeed, in some cases fat-fluid levels have been demonstrated in these lesions (2, 5, 6). Other common locations for intracranial lipomas are the hypothalamus and the quadrigeminal plate region.

As far as intracranial air is concerned, almost always it is secondary to trauma, either penetrating or with fractures involving the paranasal sinuses or mastoid air cells. The finding is very important to note, especially in trauma cases, and once again is demonstrable both with plain films and CT (Fig.

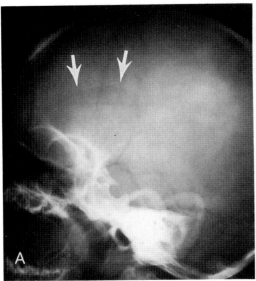

Figure 5.38. Intracranial radiolucencies. A. Typical location of fatty density in a midline lipoma *(arrows)*. **B.** CT scan in an-other patient demonstrates the midline lipoma *(arrow)* with an associated punctate calcification.

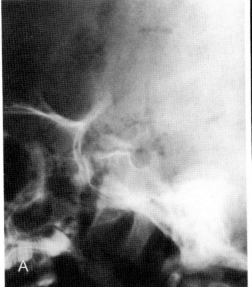
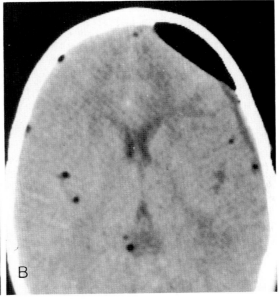

Figure 5.39. Intracranial radiolucencies. A. Scattered radiolucencies due to intracranial air after trauma. **B.** CT scan in an-other patient demonstrating scattered bubbles of air and a large collection of air over the left frontal lobe.

5.39*A* and *B*). Seldom is intracranial gas due to a gas-forming infection. Iatrogenic intracranial gas now is most often postsurgical. Massive air embolus is rare, but can lead to air being seen in the various vessels of the brain.

REFERENCES

1. Beltinger C, Saule: Imaging of lipoma of the corpus callosum and intracranial dermoids in the Goldenhar syndrome. *Pediatr Radiol* 18:72–73, 1988.
2. Cornell SH, Graf CJ, Dolan KD: Fat-fluid level in intracranial epidermoid cyst. *AJR* 128:502–503, 1977.
3. Fisher RM, Cremin BJ: Lipoma of the corpus callosum: diagnosis by ultrasound and magnetic resonance. *Pediatr Radiol* 18:409–410, 1988.
4. Kushnet MW, Goldman RL: Lipoma of the corpus callosum associated with a frontal bone defect. *AJR* 131:517–518, 1978.
5. Laster DW, Moody DM, Ball MR: Epidermoid tumors with intraventricular and subarachnoid fat: report of two cases. *AJR* 128:504–507, 1977.
6. Maravilla KR: Intraventricular fat-fluid level secondary to

rupture of an intracranial dermoid cyst. *AJR* 128:500–501, 1977.

Abnormalities of the Mastoid Air Cells and Petrous Bone

MASTOID SCLEROSIS AND LYSIS

The commonest cause of **sclerosis** of the mastoid bone around the mastoid air cells is chronic middle ear infection. In such cases, with time the mastoid air cells can disappear entirely and the bone becomes very dense (Fig. 5.40*A*). Next most common among the causes of mastoid sclerosis are the various bone dysplasias producing skull base thickening (see Table 5.4). Occasionally, one may encounter a sclerotic, primary bone tumor (Fig. 5.40*B*) and, in addition, sclerosis of the mastoid region can occur after radiation therapy for tumors and histiocytosis-X.

The most common causes of **lysis** or **destruction** of the petrous bone are mastoid abscess (Fig. 5.41*A*) and histiocytosis-X (Fig. 5.41*B*). Destruction secondary to cholesteatoma accompanying chronic middle ear inflammatory disease is uncommon in children (Fig. 5.41*C*). If the cholesteatoma is large enough the destruction can be seen on plain films, but usually CT or MRI is required to demonstrate the earliest changes (i.e., destruction of the scutum) (1).

Occasionally, a tumor can cause destruction of the petrous bone and, of the primary tumors, the most common in childhood is rhabdomyosarcoma (Fig. 5.41*D*). Meningioma causing destruction of the petrous bone is rare in childhood and the next most common cause of such destruction is leukemia or lymphoma. Metastatic disease always is a possibil-

ity, but it is unusual for it to selectively go to the petrous bone.

REFERENCES

1. Ishii K, Takahashi S, Matsumoto K, Kobayashi T, Ishibashi T, Sakamoto K, Soda T: Middle ear cholesteatoma extending into the petrous apex: evaluation by CT and MR imaging. *AJNR* 12:719–24, 1991.

DECREASED AERATION OF MASTOID AIR CELLS

The commonest cause of decreased aeration of the mastoid air cells is middle ear infection. With chronic infection there is inhibition of air cell development and in long-standing cases air cells virtually are absent. In such cases the petrous bone also is sclerotic (Fig. 5.42*A*). However, when the air cells are normally developed but aeration is decreased, the cause of opacification is edema or exudate secondary to acute infection (Fig. 5.42*B*), or blood associated with a basal skull fracture (Fig. 5.42*C*). In addition to these causes, any of the conditions producing frank bone destruction mentioned in the preceding section can produce associated mastoid air cell underaeration.

Internal Auditory Canal Abnormalities

Basically, abnormalities of the internal auditory canals consist of size and contour changes. Smallness of the canals can occur on a congenital basis and with any condition leading to hyperostosis or thickening of the base of the skull (see Table 5.4). Contour

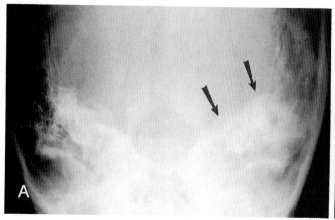

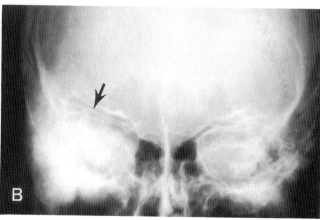

Figure 5.40. Mastoid sclerosis. A. Note dense, sclerotic, virtually airless mastoid bone secondary to chronic infection *(arrows).*

B. Marked sclerosis of mastoid bone secondary to primary osteogenic sarcoma *(arrows).*

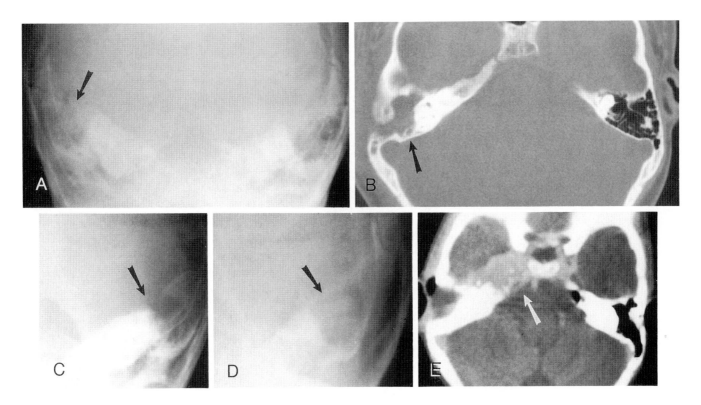

Figure 5.41. Mastoid destruction. A. Haziness with early destruction of the right mastoid bone *(arrow)* due to abscess. **B.** CT study in another patient more clearly demonstrates the destructive process *(arrow)*. **C.** Mastoid destruction secondary to histio- cytosis-X *(arrow)*. **D.** Large cholesteatoma *(arrow)* producing mastoid destruction. **E.** Mastoid destruction secondary to rhabdomyosarcoma, seen on CT *(arrow)*.

changes usually consist of canal enlargement and are seen with intracanalicular tumors or neurofibromatosis. In adults, acoustic neuromas account for most cases of internal auditory canal enlargement, but this tumor is not common in children. Meningiomas also are uncommon in children and, actually, in children, if the canals appear wider than normal, one should first consider normal variation. An unusual cause of enlargement is dural ectasia, as seen in neurofibromatosis type I (1, 2). In such cases no tumor is present, but rather dural ectasia, as part of the generalized mesenchymal abnormality in neurofibromatosis, leads to widening of the canals (Fig. 5.43). The abnormality is similar to that seen with posterior scalloping and spinal canal widening in neurofibromatosis (see Fig. 6.12*B*).

REFERENCES

1. Hill MD, Oh KS, Hodges FH: Internal auditory canal enlargement in neurofibromatosis without acoustic neuroma. *Radiology* 122:730, 1977.
2. Sarwar M, Swischuk LE: Bilateral internal auditory canal enlargement due to dural estasia in neurofibromatosis. *AJR* 129:935–936, 1977.

Abnormalities of the Orbit

ORBITAL CALCIFICATIONS

The commonest intraorbital calcification is that seen with retinoblastoma. Such calcifications are not always easy to detect radiographically, but are more readily demonstrable with CT (1) (Fig. 5.44*A*). Calcification is said to occur in as many as 90% of cases of retinoblastoma (3), usually with a granular and irregular pattern. Following enucleation for the treatment of retinoblastoma, it has been reported that calcification of a scleral-wrapped implant can occur, representing dystrophic calcifications rather than tumor recurrence (4). Irregular intraorbital calcifications also occur in ocular dermoids, retrolental fibroplasia (usually in and around the limbus of the lens), infection, trauma, with foreign bodies, and in hypercalcemic states such as hypervitaminosis D, hyperparathyroidism, and idiopathic hypercalcemia (2, 5). In retrolental fibroplasia, the lens itself can be outlined with calcification (Fig. 5.44*B*).

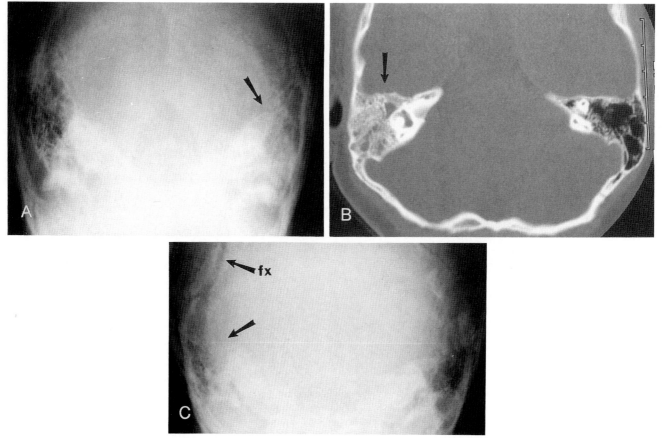

Figure 5.42. Decreased mastoid air cell aeration. A. Decreased aeration and development of mastoid air cells in chronic middle-ear inflammation *(arrow)*. **B.** CT scan in another patient demonstrates haziness (due to fluid) of mastoid air cells *on the* right *(arrow)* secondary to mastoiditis. **C.** Markedly decreased aeration of mastoid antrum and air cells *(arrow)* secondary to bleeding after fracture. Note diastatic lambdoid suture fracture *(fx)*.

Finally, it might be noted that in some patients with certain degrees of steepness on the Waters view, the lenses appear denser than the soft tissues. In such cases one should not mistake this normal finding for calcification (Fig. 5.44C).

REFERENCES

1. Danziger A, Price HI: CT findings in retinoblastoma. *AJR* 133:695–697, 1979.
2. Fleischner FG, Shalek SR: Conjunctival and corneal calcification in hypercalcemia: roentgenologic findings. *N Engl J Med* 241:863–865, 1949.
3. Mafee MF, Goldberg MF, Greenwald MJ, Schulman J, Malmed A, Flanders AE: Retinoblastoma and simulating lesions: role of CT and MR imaging. *Radiol Clin North Am* 25:667–682, 1987.
4. Summers CG: Calcification of scleral-wrapped orbital implant in patients with retinoblastoma. *Pediatr Radiol* 23:34–36, 1993.
5. Taybi H: Ocular calcification and retrolental fibroplasia. *AJR* 76:583–593, 1956.

ORBITAL SIZE ABNORMALITIES

The orbit can be too large or too small, but seldom are both orbits enlarged. In terms of unilateral enlargement, the commonest cause is a growing orbital tumor in a young infant (Fig. 5.45A and B). Thereafter, one should consider orbital enlargement as part of the skeletal dysplasia of neurofibromatosis (Fig. 5.45C–E). Occasionally, destructive lesions of the orbit can cause slight orbital enlargement, and this can occur with histiocytosis-X (Fig. 5.45F).

A unilateral small orbit most commonly is the result of congenital underdevelopment of the globe (Fig. 5.46A), and the face usually also is underdeveloped on the same side. A small orbit also can be seen after enucleation of the eye (Fig. 5.46C) and in cases where hyperostosis of the calvarium encroaches on the orbit and causes it to be small. This can occur with conditions such as fibrous dysplasia (Fig.

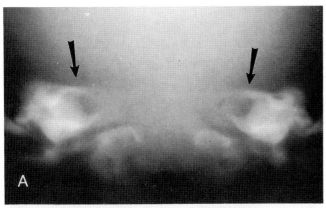

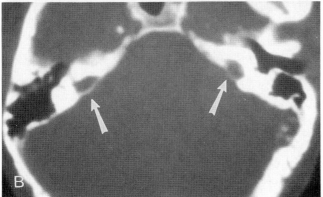

Figure 5.43. Enlarged internal auditory canals. A. Bilateral internal auditory canal enlargement due to dural ectasia in neurofibromatosis. **B.** Bilateral internal auditory canal enlargement *(arrows)* secondary to acoustic neuromas in neurofibromatosis.

5.46*B*), osteopetrosis, and Cooley anemia. Bilaterally small orbits are seen with many of the forebrain hypoplasia syndromes, causing hypotelorism (Fig. 5.47).

HYPOTELORISM

Hypotelorism in its severest form is seen with arrhinencephaly (1), cebocephaly, and the cyclops deformity (Fig. 5.47*A* and *B*). In all of the these conditions the forebrain is poorly developed, and, in addition, the orbits usually are small and round. Hypotelorism also occurs with simple trigonoencephaly secondary to premature closure of the metopic suture. In such cases, the close-set orbits also have a medially slanted, "puzzled" appearance (Fig. 5.47*C*). Mild degrees of hypotelorism are seen with sagittal craniosynostosis and in syndromes such as trisomy-13 and trisomy-21.

HYPERTELORISM

Hypertelorism occurs as a normal familial variant in some infants. In such cases, the deformity usually is mild and probably is not true hypertelorism. The eyes may appear to be set apart more than usual, but when the bony margins of the orbit are measured, intraorbital distance still is normal. It is the clinical appearance of some of these patients that suggests

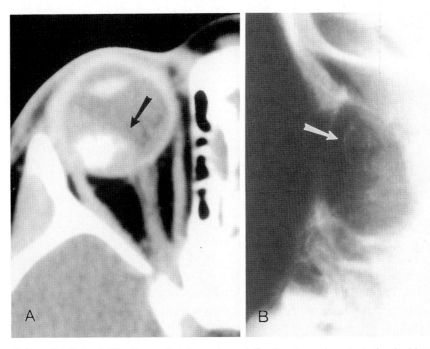

Figure 5.44. Orbital calcifications. A. Intraocular calcification *(arrow)*, typical of retinoblastoma. **B.** Peripheral calcification of the lens *(arrow)* in retrolental fibroplasia.

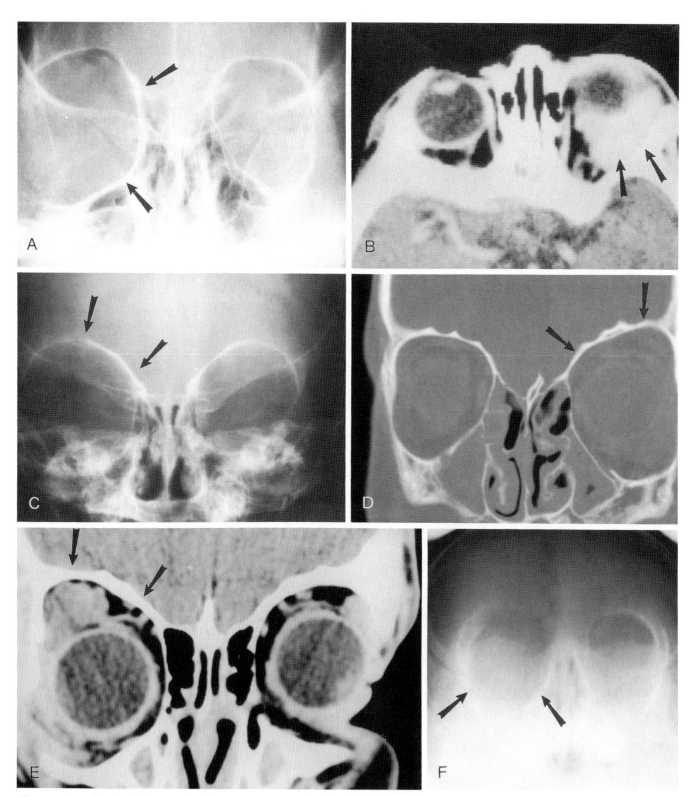

Figure 5.45. Large orbits and orbital masses. A. Large orbit on the right *(arrows)* due to hemangioma. **B.** Another patient with a contrast-enhanced CT scan demonstrating an intraorbital hemangioma *(arrows)* that is also enlarging the orbit. **C.** Large orbit in neurofibromatosis *(arrows)*. Also note associated sphenoid wing thinning. **D.** Another patient with neurofibromatosis demonstra-ting a large dysplastic orbit on the left *(arrows)*. **E.** Large orbit *(arrows)* in a patient with plexiform neurofibromatosis involving the orbit. The tumor is located above the globe which itself is downwardly displaced. **F.** Large orbit *(arrows)* due to bony de-struction with subsequent healing in histiocytosis-X.

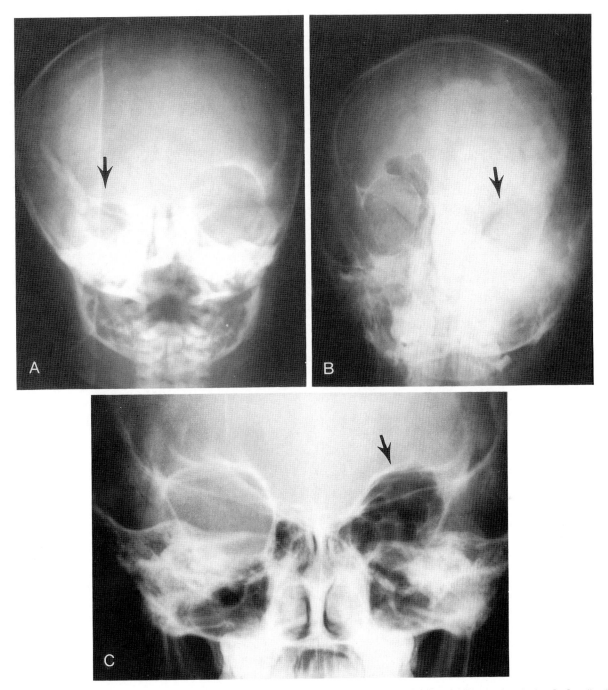

Figure 5.46. Small orbits. A. Congenital underdevelopment of the face and orbit *(arrow)* on the right. **B.** Small orbit *(arrow)* due to hyperostosis secondary to fibrous dysplasia. **C.** Small orbit on the left *(arrow)* after enucleation of the eye.

hypertelorism. True hypertelorism probably is confined to conditions such as frontal encephalocele (Fig. 5.48A), the median cleft face or Greig syndrome (Fig. 5.48B) (3, 4), and bone dysplasias such as cleidocranial dysostosis, Crouzon craniofacial dysplasia, and bilateral craniosynostosis of the coronal sutures. Indeed, mild hypertelorism occurs in so many syndromes that it is of questionable diagnostic value. In the median cleft face syndrome, some patients demonstrate a peculiar bony spicule in the frontal portion of the skull (Fig. 5.48B). Final causes of hypertelorism are nasal tumors such as fibromas and gliomas and chronic nasal polyps such as are seen in cystic fibrosis.

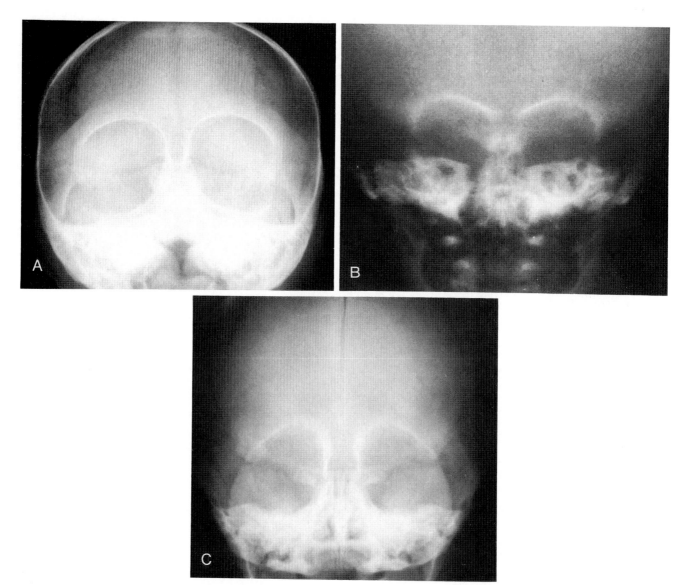

Figure 5.47. Hypotelorism. A. Severe hypotelorism in arrhinencephaly syndrome. **B.** More severe hypotelorism, almost a cyclops deformity in another patient with arrhinencephaly. **C.** Hypotelorism in metopic suture synostosis. Note characteristic "puzzled" appearance of the orbits. In addition, note the characteristic straight, sharp metopic suture indicating impending closure.

ORBITAL MASSES

Orbital masses may be classified as intraocular or extraocular, and the most common intraocular mass is retinoblastoma (Table 5.15). This malignant neoplasm arises from neuroectodermal cells within the retina and usually is unilateral. Bilateral retinoblastoma also can occur and usually is familial. CT typically shows a calcified mass along the posterior aspect of the globe (see Fig. 5.44) (6). A rare congenital intraocular tumor is medulloepithelioma. This tumor arises from the epithelium of the ciliary body and is therefore usually located in the anterior portion of the globe.

The most common primary malignant neoplasm of the orbit outside of the globe is rhabdomyosarcoma. However, it is much less common than retinoblastoma and accounts for only a small percentage of pediatric orbital masses in general. Optic gliomas occur in children, especially in patients with neurofibromatosis type I. Metastatic disease of the orbit is unusual, but it most commonly occurs in children with neuroblastoma or Ewing sarcoma (1, 2). Benign masses are seen more frequently, and dermoid tumor is the most common pediatric orbital neoplasm. Dermoids are usually anterior extraconal masses that characteristically arise in the upper temporal or upper nasal quadrants of the orbit. Most orbital der-

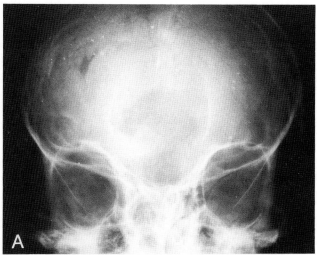

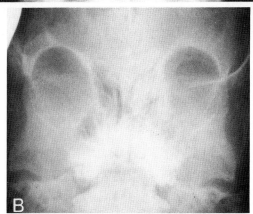

Figure 5.48. Hypertelorism. A. Hypertelorism in frontal encephalocele. Note bony defect. **B.** Grieg syndrome with hypertelorism.

Table 5.15
Orbital Masses

Intraocular		
Retinoblastoma	}	Moderately common
Medulloepithelioma	}	Rare
Extraocular		
Dermoid	}	Moderately common
Hemangioma		
Teratoma		
Lymphangioma		
Rhabdomyosarcoma		
Optic glioma		
Neuroblastoma		
Neurofibroma/schwannoma	}	Rare
Histiocytosis-X		
Metastases		
Orbital varix or arteriovenous malformation		
Granolocytic sarcoma		

moids are of the cystic variety and exhibit slow growth that can result in erosion of the adjacent bone. Hemangiomas, usually the capillary variety, also are a relatively common cause of intraorbital mass in young children (Fig. 4.45B). Other neoplasms are rare and include teratoma, lymphangioma, histiocytosis-X, and neurofibroma or schwannoma (4) (Fig. 4.45E). Vascular malformations are uncommon in the pediatric orbit and include the primary orbital varix and arteriovenous malformations, and, rarely, a meningoencephalocele can extend into the orbit (1).

REFERENCES

1. Albert DM, Rubinstein RA, Scheie HG: Tumor metastases to the eye, Part II: clinical study in infants and children. *Am J Ophthalmol* 3:727–32, 1967.
2. Gallet BL, Egelhoff JC: Unusual CNS and orbital metastases of neuroblastoma. *Pediatr Radiol* 19:287–289, 1989.
3. Hopper KK, Sherman JL, Boal DKB: Abnormalities of the orbit and its contents in children: CT and MR imaging findings. *AJR* 156:1219, 1991.
4. Lallemand DP, Brasch RC, Char DH, Normal D: Orbital tumors in children: Characterization by computed tomography. *Radiol* 151:85-88, 1984.
5. Levy RA, Wald SL, Aitken PA, et al: Bilateral intraorbital meningoencephaloceles and associated midline craniofacial anomalies: MR and three dimensional CT imaging. *AJNR* 10:1272–1274, 1989.
6. Mafee MF, Goldberg MF, Greenwald MJ, Schulman J, Malmed A, Flanders AE: Retinoblastoma and simulating lesions: role of CT and MR imaging. *Radiol Clin North Am* 25:667–682, 1987.

ORBITAL DEFORMITY

Deformity of the orbit is commonly associated with dysmorphism of the skull, and such deformities are most commonly due to premature closure of the cranial sutures. Primary craniosynostosis of the coronal suture causes the ipsilateral orbit to elongate, particularly along its supraorbital margin (harlequin eye deformity), and it is especially easy to detect when the problem is unilateral (Fig. 5.49A). With metopic craniosynostosis, in addition to hypotelorism the superior and medially slanted orbits give the face a puzzled appearance (Fig. 5.47C) (1). Orbital deformity occurs with hypo- and hypertelorism (see Figs. 5.47 and 5.48) (2) and also is seen when the orbit is small for any reason, including thickening of the bone around it (Fig. 5.46).

The orbit also can be deformed when an intraorbital tumor causes enlargement or when bony dysplasia is seen in association with neurofibromatosis (see Fig. 5.45). The bony abnormality in neurofibromatosis type I is believed to be due to mesodermal

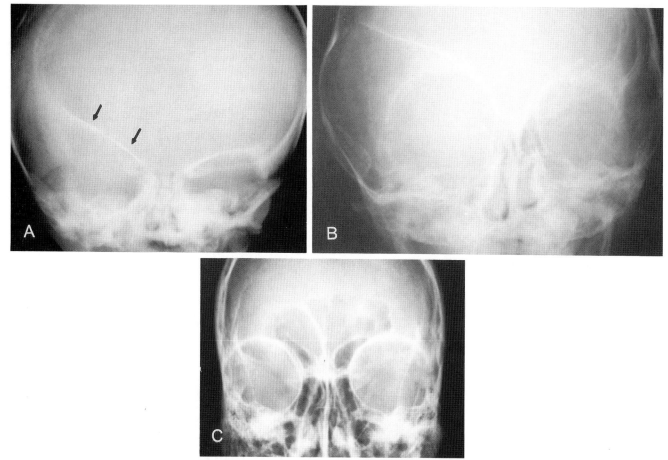

Figure 5.49. Miscellaneous orbital deformities. A. Typical harlequin eye appearance with elevated sphenoid wing on the right *(arrows)* and distorted orbital shape in unilateral coronal synostosis. **B.** Large orbit with dysplastic appearance, including elevated and thinned sphenoid wing with bulging parietal region in neurofibromatosis. **C.** Overly round orbits in a patient with severe brain atrophy. Also note overly large frontal and other sinus cavities.

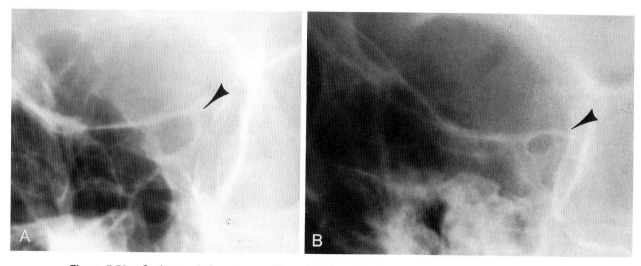

Figure 5.50. Optic canal size abnormalities. A. Enlarged optic canal *(arrow)* in patient with optic glioma. **B.** Small optic canal *(arrow)* secondary to optic nerve atrophy.

dysplasia rather than to erosion by adjacent tumors. The findings consist of enlargement of the orbit, sphenoid wing hypoplasia (empty orbit sign), and an overall dysplastic appearance of the orbit (Fig. 5.49*B*). Finally, frontal encephaloceles can extend inferiorly into the ethmoid air cells to produce flattening or erosive deformities of the medial walls of the orbits, and may be associated with hypertelorism.

Exceptionally round orbits are seen with brain atrophy and may be associated with overgrowth of the frontal or other sinus cavities (Fig. 5.49*C*). This is a common phenomenon of advanced brain atrophy, in which absence of the brain allows the superior orbital margins to become more rounded than usual.

OPTIC CANAL SIZE ABNORMALITIES

Enlargement of the optic canal is almost always secondary to an intracanalicular tumor such as an optic glioma, neurofibroma, or meningioma. In children, optic glioma is most common (Fig. 5.50*A*), and the finding is most easily demonstrated with CT. A small optic canal can be seen with optic nerve atrophy (Fig. 5.50*B*) that is either congenital or postenucleation of the eye. As with the orbit, lesions leading to hyperostosis of the calvarium also cause smallness of the optic canal (e.g., Cooley anemia, hypercalcemia, fibrous dysplasia, osteopetrosis).

PROPTOSIS

Proptosis can occur with intraorbital tumors, intraorbital inflammation secondary to sinusitis, nonspecific intraorbital soft tissue inflammation, Caffey disease (inflammatory hyperostosis of the bone), hyperthyroidism, neoplasm of the retro-orbital bones, fibrous dysplasia involving the bony orbit, and with hyperostosis in conditions such as osteopetrosis and Cooley anemia. Proptosis also can occur with ret-

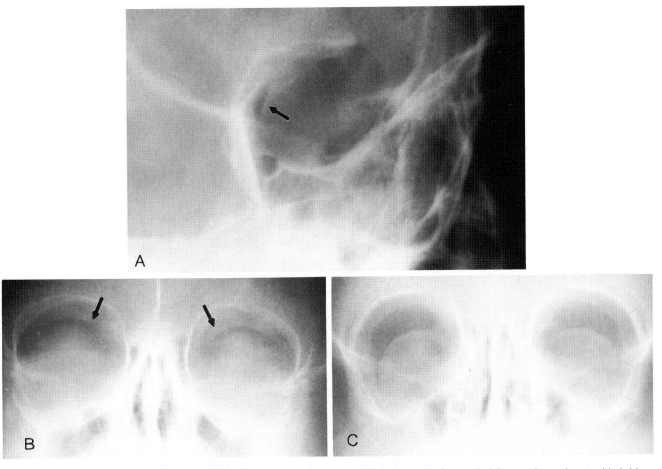

Figure 5.51. Intraorbital air. A. Intraorbital air secondary to fracture through the ethmoid sinuses *(arrow).* **B.** Pseudointraorbital air due to air outlining palpebral fissure *(arrow).* **C.** Pseudoin- traorbital air due to deep-set globes and prominent orbital ridges *(arrows)* in a patient with Cockayne syndrome.

robulbar, intraorbital infarcts in sickle cell disease. A peculiar form of proptosis is that which occurs with thinning of the sphenoid bone due to the skeletal dysplasia of neurofibromatosis. Because the bone is absent, exophthalmos often is pulsatile in these patients.

INTRAORBITAL AIR

Intraorbital air almost always is secondary to penetrating trauma (Fig. 5.51A). However, occasionally such air can be mimicked by air outlining the normal palpebral fissures (Fig. 5.51B) or in patients with sunken eyes and prominent supraorbital ridges (Fig. 5.51C).

REFERENCES

1. Currarino G, Silverman FN: Orbital hypotelorism arhinencephaly and trigonencephaly. *Radiology* 74:206–217, 1960.
2. Keats TE: Ocular hypertelorism (Grieg's syndrome) associated with Springel's deformity. *AJR* 110:119–122, 1970.

CHAPTER

6

THE SPINE

Abnormalities of Mineralization

GENERALIZED ABNORMALITIES

Abnormalities of mineralization consist of (a) demineralization (osteomalacia and osteoporosis), (b) increased density or osteosclerosis, and (c) the **bone-in-bone vertebra.** As far as causes of generalized demineralization and osteosclerosis are concerned, they are the same as those encountered for other parts of the skeleton. For a list of these conditions, see Tables 4.1 and 4.2. The **bone-in-bone** appearance of the vertebral bodies most commonly is seen as a physiologic phenomenon in newborn (often premature) infants (Table 6.1). In such cases, with the stresses of the perinatal period, enchondral bone formation is temporarily impaired and a ring of radiolucency develops. However, the ring is not appreciated until normal growth resumes and a white line of healthy bone is deposited around it (Fig. 6.1A). The finding is comparable to that which occurs with trophic (growth arrest) lines in the long bones and is entirely nonspecific. Occasionally, these growth arrest lines can be seen in older children (Fig. 6.1B).

Table 6.1
Bone-in-Bone and Sandwich Vertebra

Physiologic in premature infant	}	Common
Healing renal osteodystrophy[a]	}	Moderately common
Osteopetrosis[a] Chronic lead poisoning[a] Hypercalcemia Chronic illness-trophic lines[a]	}	Relatively rare

[a] Usually sandwich vertebra.

Otherwise, when a bone-in-bone appearance is encountered, one should consider conditions such as osteopetrosis (Fig. 6.1C), chronic lead poisoning, healing renal osteodystrophy, and, occasionally, hypercalcemia. In these conditions, rather than a ring encircling the entire vertebral body, one usually sees two horizontal white lines at the top and bottom of the body. For this reason, the terms **"sandwich vertebra"** and **"rugger jersey spine"** are utilized.

FOCAL SCLEROSIS

Focal sclerosis of a vertebral body or its posterior elements is not common in children (Table 6.2). Bone islands and osteoblastic metastases are virtually unheard of, and about the only primary malignant bone tumors producing focal sclerosis in the spine are osteogenic sarcoma, lymphoma (3), and Ewing sarcoma (5) (Fig. 6.2). The so-called "solitary sclerotic pedicle" is discussed later with abnormalities of the pedicles. Osteoid osteoma, although rare, probably is the commonest cause of focal sclerosis in the pediatric spine, but, once again, more often tends to involve the pedicles (see Fig. 6.4B). Osteoid osteoma often is a cause of occult pain or undiagnosed scoliosis (1, 2) and, until sclerosis around the aberrant nidus of osteoid tissue becomes apparent, the lesion may elude even the most experienced observer. For this reason, nuclear scintigraphy may be performed as a screening test for the cause of pain. Large osteoid osteomas are termed "giant osteoblastomas" (4) and are more lytic than blastic.

Focal sclerosis of the apophyseal joints, extending into the pedicles, can be seen with congenital abnormalities of joint alignment and articulation. Most

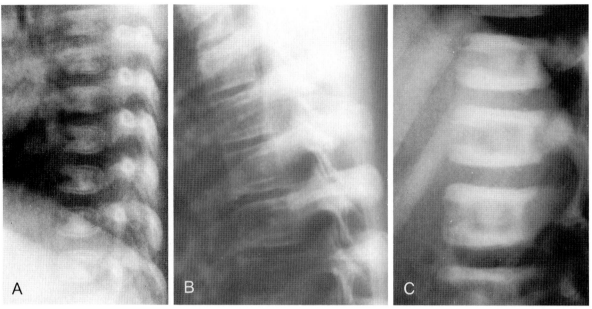

Figure 6.1. Bone-in-bone vertebra. A. Typical bone-in-bone vertebra in newborn infant. **B.** Bone-in-bone vertebra due to growth arrest lines in patient with asthma. **C.** Bone-in-bone appearance in osteopetrosis.

Table 6.2
Focal Sclerosis of Vertebra

Osteoid osteoma Sclerosis with apophyseal joint mal- alignment	Common
Bone islands Osteoblastic metastases Ewing sarcoma Osteogenic sarcoma Lymphoma Tuberous sclerosis Healed trauma, infection	Rare

often this occurs in the lumbosacral region. Other causes of focal sclerosis include healed osteomyelitis, healed histiocytosis-X, healed trauma, and tuberous sclerosis.

REFERENCES

1. Caldicott WJH: Diagnosis of spinal osteoid osteoma. *Radiology* 92:1192–1195, 1969.
2. Keim H, Reina E: Osteoid osteoma as a cause of scoliosis. *J Bone Joint Surg* 57A:159–163, 1975.
3. Mandell GA: Resolution of Hodgkin's induced ivory vertebrae. *Pediatr Radiol* 7:178–179, 1978.
4. Myles ST, MacRae ME: Benign osteoblastoma of the spine in childhood. *J Neurosurg* 68:884–888, 1988.
5. Whitehouse GH, Griffiths GJ: Roentgenologic aspects of spinal involvement by primary and metastatic Ewing's tumor. *J Can Assoc Radiol* 27:290–297, 1976.

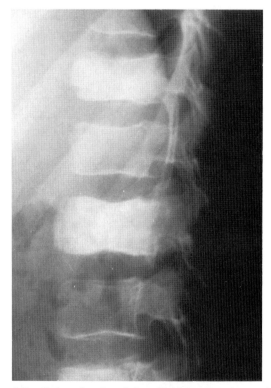

Figure 6.2. Sclerosis of vertebra. Multiple sclerotic vertebra in healed metastatic Ewing sarcoma.

Abnormalities of the Pedicles

Abnormalities of the pedicles consist of (a) abnormal sizes and shapes, (b) absence or destruction, and (c) sclerosis.

ABNORMAL SHAPES

Abnormal shapes of the pedicle include flattened and dysplastic pedicles (Table 6.3), and dysplastic pedicles occur with congenital anomalies such as meningomyelocele, diastematomyelia, Klippel-Feil

Table 6.3
Abnormal Pedicle Shapes

Flattened pedicles		
Normal[a]	}	Common
Intraspinal expanding tumor or cyst	}	Relatively rare
Dysplastic pedicle		
Part of other spinal anomaly	}	Common
Neurofibromatosis	}	Moderately common

[a]Lumbar region.

syndrome, and neurofibromatosis (7). Flattened pedicles occur with intraspinal expanding lesions (i.e., tumor, cyst), and in advanced cases the flattened pedicles are somewhat concave along their inner aspects (Fig. 6.3A). The deformity may be more pronounced on one side than the other and should be differentiated from normal flattening of the pedicles, which most commonly occurs in the upper lumbar region (Fig. 6.3B). Normal pedicles, although flattened, are not eroded or concave along their inner aspects (2) and, overall, comprise the commonest cause of flattened or oval pedicles in childhood.

ABNORMAL SIZE

Pedicles can be too small or too large (Table 6.4), but neither deformity is particularly common in children. Small pedicles most often are congenital in origin (1, 8) (see Fig. 6.28B), but also can result from hypoplasia secondary to previous radiation therapy of lesions such as Wilms tumor. Enlarged pedicles can occur on an isolated basis with contralateral arch deficiency, and are believed to result from compensatory hypertrophy (6). Enlargement of a number of pedicles on one side in the absence of arch deficiency also has been described (4), but the adjacent ribs also appeared expanded and dysplastic, and the problem may have been a disease such as fibrous

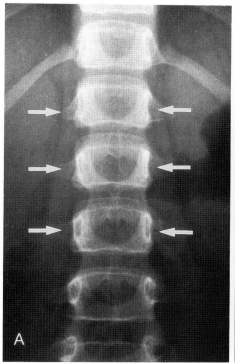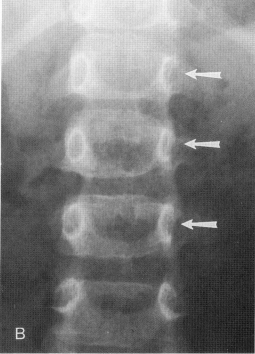

Figure 6.3. Flattened pedicles. A. Flat pedicles due to intraspinal tumor *(arrows)*. **B.** Normal flat pedicles in upper lumbar spine. Note that they do not have a concave inner aspect *(arrows)*. Very often these normal flat pedicles are bilateral.

Table 6.4
Abnormal Pedicle Size

Enlarged pedicle	
Osteoblastoma	
Hemangioma	
Lymphangioma	Relatively rare
Other tumor	
Contralateral arch deficiency	

Small pedicle	
Congenital with other anomaly	Common
Postradiation therapy	Moderately common
Congenital absence or hypoplasia	Relatively rare

Table 6.5
Destroyed, Absent and Sclerotic Pedicles

Destroyed or absent pedicles	
Metastatic disease	Moderately common
Leukemia, lymphoma	
Primary bone tumor	
Histiocytosis-X	Relatively rare
Congenitally absent pedicle	

Sclerotic pedicle	
Osteoid osteoma	Common
Stress with abnormal apophyseal joint alignment	Moderately common
Ewing sarcoma	
Hodgkin lymphoma	Rare
Osteogenic sarcoma	

dysplasia or neurofibromatosis. Pedicles also can enlarge when they are involved by bony tumors such as osteoid osteoma, giant osteoblastoma, hemangioma, lymphangioma, or osteochondroma.

DESTRUCTION OR ABSENCE OF A PEDICLE

Isolated destruction of a pedicle can occur with metastatic disease, leukemia, lymphoma, or a primary bone tumor (Table 6.5). Congenital absence is rare in children (3, 5, 9–11), and the cervical and lumbar spine seem to be the most common locations for this abnormality (Fig. 6.4A). Although the disorder is usually asymptomatic, in some cases pain may be associated (9–11). Presumably, in these cases, unilateral associated neural arch hypoplasia and apophyseal joint instability lead to abnormal mechanical stresses and symptoms.

SCLEROTIC PEDICLE

A sclerotic pedicle is not particularly common in the pediatric age group (12), but it does occur (Table 6.5). The commonest cause is osteoid osteoma (Fig. 6.4B), and the next most common is stress-induced sclerosis secondary to abnormal alignment of apophyseal joints or frank spondylolisthesis. Rarely, one can see a sclerotic pedicle with Ewing sarcoma, Hodgkin lymphoma, or osteogenic sarcoma, and, of course, as a presumed normal variation (Fig. 6.4C).

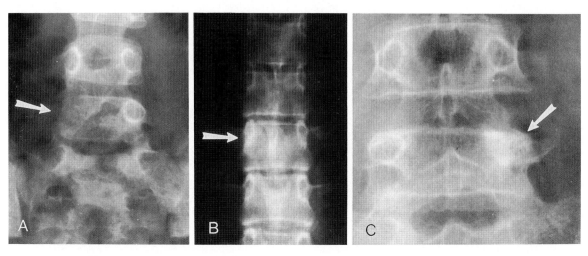

Figure 6.4. Abnormalities of the pedicles. A. Absent pedicle *(arrow)* in patient with trisomy-21. **B.** Slightly sclerotic pedicle *(arrow)* due to osteoid osteoma. **C.** Idiopathic normal sclerotic pedicle *(arrow)*.

REFERENCES

1. Bardsley JL, Hanelin LG: The unilateral hypoplastic lumbar pedicle. *Radiology* 101:315–317, 1971.
2. Benzian SR, Mainzer F, Gooding CA: Pediculate thinning: a normal variant at the thoracolumbar junction. *Br J Radiol* 44:936–939, 1971.
3. Danziger J, Jackson H, Block S: Congenital absence of a pedicle in a cervical vertebra. *Clin Radiol* 26:53–56, 1975.
4. Hart KZ, Brower AC: Unilateral hypertrophy of multiple pedicles. *AJR* 129:739–740, 1977.
5. Kaufman RA, Poznanski AK, Hensinger RN: Congenitally absent thoracic pedicle in a child with rhabdomyosarcoma. *Pediatr Radiol* 9:173–174, 1980.
6. Maldaque BE, Malghem JJ: Unilateral arch hypertrophy with spinous process tilt: a sign of arch deficiency. *Radiology* 121:567–574, 1976.
7. Mandell GA: The pedicle in neurofibromatosis. *AJR* 130:675–678, 1978.
8. Morin ME, Palacios E: The aplastic hypoplastic lumbar pedicle. *AJR* 122:639–642, 1974.
9. Oestreich AE, Young LW: The absent cervical pedicle syndrome: a case in childhood. *Am J Roentgenol Radium Ther Nucl Med* 107:505–510, 1969.
10. Polly DW Jr, Mason DE: Congenital absence of a lumbar pedicle presenting as back pain in children. *J Pediatr Orthop* 11:214–219, 1991.
11. Wiener MD, Martinez S, Forsberg DA: Congenital absence of a cervical spine pedicle: clinical and radiographic findings. *AJR* 155:1037–1041, 1990.
12. Wilkinson RA, Hall JE: The sclerotic pedicle: tumor or pseudotumor? *Radiology* 111:683–688, 1974.

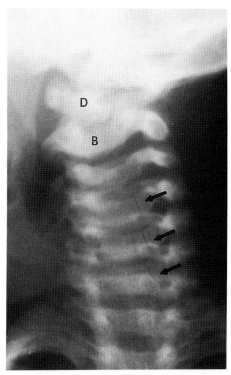

Figure 6.5. Normal posterior arch synchondroses. Note the normal synchondroses in the posterior arches of the cervical vertebra *(arrows)*. Also note the synchondrosis between the dens *(D)* and body *(B)* of C$_2$.

Defects, Hypoplasia, and Absence of the Posterior Arches

Posterior arch abnormalities run the gamut of simple defects (spondylolysis) through varying degrees of hypoplasia and then total absence of the bony elements. The commonest defects of the posterior vertebral arches consist of the normal synchondroses, which are visualized only on oblique views of the cervical spine (Fig. 6.5). The one occurring between the dens and arch of C$_2$ must be differentiated from the defect caused by a "hangman" fracture (11). Other defects are relatively uncommon but can be congenital or acquired (Table 6.6). Congenital defects occurring in association with anomalies such as meningocele, meningomyelocele, sacral dimple, diastematomyelia, and the like are straightforward. When isolated, however, they always are a problem in differentiation from fractures. The most common such defect is that which occurs in the posterior arch of C$_1$ (6, 10), and the resulting configurations are endless and bizarre (Fig. 6.6A and B). However, the smooth pointed or triangular appearance of the fragments or wide gap between them should

Table 6.6
Posterior Arch Defects or Underdevelopment

Congenital defects C$_1$ Spondylolysis-spondylolisthesis[a] Normal synchondroses between body and arches	Common
Fractures with hyperextension injury[b] Congenital defects with myelomeningocele, etc. Neurofibromatosis[c] Spondyloepiphyseal dysplasia[c] Spondylometaphyseal dysplasia[c] Storage diseases[c]	Moderately common
Congenital defects other than C$_1$ Defects acquired after infection, tumor, etc. Chondrodystrophies[c]	Rare

[a]Lower lumbar spine.
[b]Hangman fracture of C$_2$ and other levels.
[c]Underdevelopment.

suggest a congenital etiology. When the defects are more vertical and narrow, they may mimic fractures such as those seen with hyperextension injuries (see Fig. 6.7A). Congenital defects can be recognized at any level because of their smooth, sclerotic margins and lack of motion on flexion (Fig. 6.6C). With fractures the defect produced usually is narrow and does

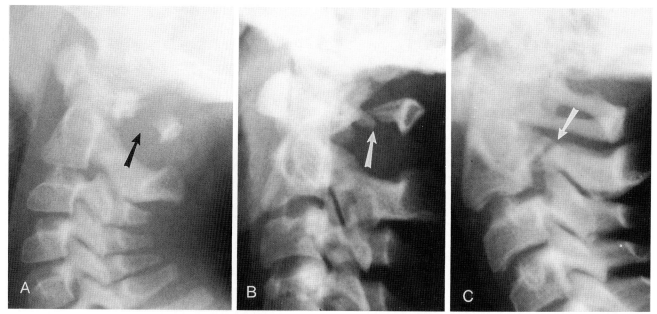

Figure 6.6. Posterior arch defects of C$_1$ and C$_2$. A. Large congenital defect of C$_1$ *(arrow)*. **B.** Smaller defect *(arrow),* associated with peculiarly shaped bony remnants. **C.** Congenital defect of posterior arch of C$_2$ *(arrow)*. Note smooth, somewhat sclerotic edges. With flexion, the configuration did not change. (Part **C** courtesy of John Dorst, M.D.)

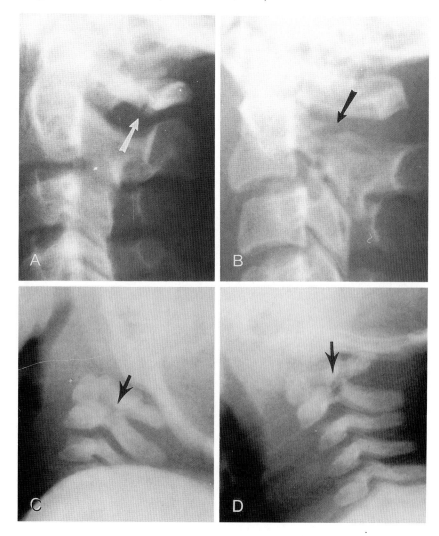

Figure 6.7. Fractures of C$_1$ and C$_2$. A. Thin, discrete defect with sharp edges due to fracture *(arrow)* secondary to hyperextension injury of C^1. **B.** Typical hangman fracture *(arrow)*. Note irregular and indistinct margins of defect. **C.** Hangman fracture in infant *(arrow)*. **D.** With flexion, the fracture line widens *(arrow)*. (Parts **C** and **D** courtesy of Richard Heller, M.D.)

not demonstrate sclerotic edges. Furthermore, once initial spasm (splinting) dissipates, motion through the fracture site occurs (Fig. 6.7C and D). At the level of C_2 these fractures are referred to as "hangman" fractures (4).

The defect of spondylolysis (Fig. 6.8A), and subsequent spondylolisthesis, usually is seen in the lower lumbar spine. The problem is believed to be a chronic stress fracture (2, 8), but it is possible that such fractures might have a greater tendency to occur in neural arches that are to some degree congenitally hypoplastic.

Spondylolysis at other levels is much less common (1, 3, 5, 9). Overt fractures resulting in the same problem in this area are also less common than they are at the C_2 level (i.e., hangman fracture). Arch defects secondary to infections, histiocytosis-X, tumors, or other conditions are rare. Extensive congenital defects of the neural arches (dysplastic arches) can be associated with considerable instability of the spine and are most likely to occur in the cervical region. These widespread defects can occur on an isolated basis (Fig. 6.8B), but also can be seen with neurofibromatosis. Hypoplasia of the neural arch, with or without associated dysplasia or defect, is most commonly seen at the C_1 level. Most often this occurs on an isolated basis, but it is also seen in association with trisomy-21 (7) and syndromes such as spondyloepiphyseal dysplasia, spondylometaphyseal dyspla-

sia, the storage diseases, and chondrodystrophies in general. These patients may or may not demonstrate associated atlantoaxial instability.

REFERENCES

1. Azouz EM, Chan JD, Wee R: Spondylolysis of the cervical vertebrae: report of three cases, with a review of the English and French literature. *Radiology* 111:315–318, 1974.
2. Beeler JW: Further evidence on the acquired nature of spondylolysis and spondylolisthesis. *AJR* 108:796–798, 1970.
3. Charlton OP, Gehweiler JA Jr, Morgan CL, Martinez S, Daffner RH: Spondylolysis and spondylolisthesis of the cervical spine. *Skeletal Radiol* 3:79–84, 1978.
4. Elliott JM Jr, Rogers LF, Wissinger JP, Lee JF: The hangman's fracture: fractures of the neural arch of the axis. *Radiology* 104:303–307, 1972.
5. Gehweiler JA Jr, Martinez S, Clark WM, Miller MD, Stewart GC Jr: Spondylolisthesis of the axis vertebra. *AJR* 128:682–684, 1977.
6. Logan WW, Stuart ID: Absert posterior arch of the atlas. *AJR* 118:431–434, 1973.
7. Martich V, Ben-Ami T, Yousefzadeh DK, Roizen NJ: Hypoplastic posterior arch of C1 in children with Down syndrome: a double jeopardy. *Radiology* 183:125–128, 1992.
8. McKee BW, Alexander WJ, Dunbar JS: Spondylosis and spondylolisthesis in children. *J Can Assoc Radiol* 22:100–109, 1971.
9. Moseley I: Neural arch dysplasia of the sixth cervical vertebra "congenital cervical spondylolisthesis." Case report. *Br J Radiol* 49:81–83, 1976.

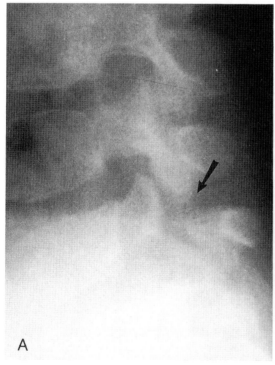
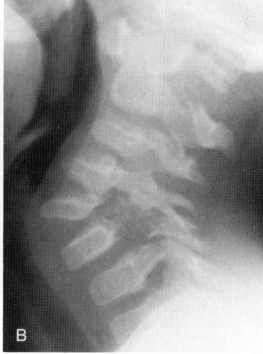

Figure 6.8. Posterior arch defects. A. Spondylolysis *(arrow)* of L_5. **B.** Extensive congenital defects of neural arches in cervical spine, leading to marked instability and, eventually, cord compression.

10. Sauvegrain J, Mareschal JL: Cranio-cervical malformations in childhood: about 35 cases. *Ann Radiol* 15:263–277, 1972.
11. Swischuk LE, Hayden CK Jr, Sarwar M: The dens-arch synchondrosis versus the hangman's fracture. *Pediatr Radiol* 8:100–112, 1979.

Vertical Defects of Vertebral Bodies

The commonest vertical defect of the vertebral bodies is that due to a congenital sagittal cleft (Table 6.7). On frontal view these defects occur in the midsagittal plane and result in a variety of clefting abnormalities ranging from a simple cleft to a typical butterfly vertebra (Fig. 6.9A). Most often seen on an isolated, sporadic basis, they also are common in many syndromes and, in some rare ones, may involve all the vertebral bodies. Congenital coronal defects are less common, and of these the commonest are those seen in neonates in the lower thoracic and upper lumbar regions (Fig. 6.9B). These clefts tend to occur more frequently in boys than in girls, and are a common feature of trisomy-13 (1, 2, 4) and the rhizomelic form of punctate epiphyseal dysplasia. They are believed by some to result from persistent notochordal remnants (5), but more likely they are congenital ossification defects.

Acquired vertical defects of the vertebral bodies for the most part occur with compression fractures resulting from anterior flexion or combined anterior flexion-axial compression injuries (3). In such cases, a vertical fracture of the vertebral body in the sagittal plane occurs and is clearly demonstrable with ordinary or computed tomography (Fig. 6.9C). In infants, a pseudofracture or defect is produced when the normal, posterior, midsagittal neural arch synchondroses are superimposed over the vertebral bodies.

Table 6.7
Vertical Defects of Vertebral Bodies

Pseudodefect—posterior arch synchondrosis	Common
Sagittal cleft vertebra	
Compression fractures	Moderately common
Coronal cleft vertebra	Relatively rare

REFERENCES

1. Cohen J, Currarino G, Neuhauser EBD: Significant variant in the ossification centers of the vertebral bodies. *AJR* 76:469–475, 1956.
2. Fielden P, Russell JGB: Coronally cleft vertebra. *Clin Radiol* 21:327–328, 1970.
3. Richman S, Friedman RL: Vertical fracture of cervical vertebral bodies. *Radiology* 62:536, 1954.
4. Rowley KA: Coronal cleft vertebra. *J Fac Radiol* 6:267–274, 1955.
5. Wollin DG, Elliott GB: Coronal cleft vertebrae and persistent notochordal derivatives of infancy. *J Can Assoc Radiol* 12:781–80, 1961.

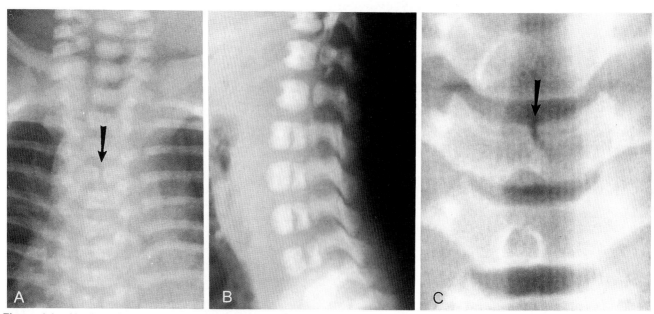

Figure 6.9. Vertical defects of vertebral bodies. A. Typical defect of sagittal cleft (butterfly) vertebra *(arrow)*. **B.** Coronal cleft vertebrae in lumbar region *(arrow)*. **C.** Vertical cleft *(arrow)* due to fracture associated with anterior compression fracture of vertebral body.

Prominent Central Vein Grooves (Table 6.8)

Normally, in infants the anterior central vein groove is readily visible, and in some infants the posterior groove also is seen (3). This is an entirely normal finding (Fig.6.10A), and can be seen even in some young children. The groove does, however, become more prominent and persists longer in the immature spine of hypothyroidism (see Fig. 6.18D). It also is more prominent in osteopetrosis (Fig. 6.10B), and has been noted to be more prominent in marrow packing disorders such as thalassemia major, sickle cell anemia (2), Gaucher disease, leukemia, lymphoma, and metastatic neuroblastoma (1).

REFERENCES

1. Mandell GA, Kricun ME: Exaggerated anterior vertebral notching. *Radiology* 131:367–369, 1979.
2. Riggs W Jr, Rockett JF: Roentgen chest findings in childhood sickle cell anemia: a new vertebral body finding. *AJR* 104:838–845, 1968.
3. Wagoner G, Pendergrass EP: The anterior and posterior "notch" shadows seen in lateral roentgenograms of the vertebrae of infants. *AJR* 42:663–670, 1939.

Vertebral Destruction

Destruction of the vertebra occurs for the same reasons as bone destruction in general. With vertebral body destruction, however, it is important to note whether associated disk destruction is present. Disk destruction is manifest primarily by disk space narrowing and is the hallmark of infection (Fig. 6.11A). With destruction secondary to tumor, pri-

Table 6.8
Prominent Central Vein Grooves

Normal—infants	} Common
Hypothyroidism Osteopetrosis	} Moderately common
Thalassemia major Sickle cell disease Gaucher disease Leukemia Lymphoma Metastatic neuroblastoma	} Relatively rare

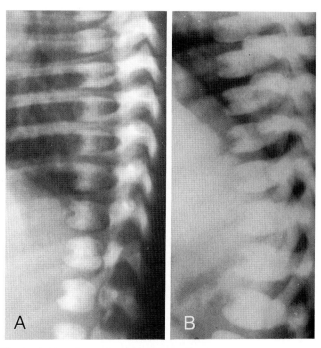

Figure 6.10. Central vein grooves. A. Note prominent, normal anterior central vein grooves in vertebrae of an infant. The posterior grooves are less visible in the thoracic region. **B.** Prominent central vein grooves in a young child with osteopetrosis.

mary or secondary, or histiocytosis-X, the disk usually is preserved (Fig. 6.11B and C). It is only with fungal infections such as coccidiomycosis, aspergillosis, and actinomycosis that destruction of a vertebral body secondary to infection often is associated with preservation of the disk space (Fig. 6.11D).

The commonest cause of vertebral destruction is infection, but destruction secondary to metastatic tumor and histiocytosis-X also is common. With histiocytosis-X, especially marked degrees of vertebral compression and flattening often are seen, and the end result is a plate-like, classic **vertebra plana** (see Fig. 6.14B). Vertebral destruction secondary to primary bone tumors and aneurysmal bone cysts is uncommon. With the latter, often there is preceding bubbly expansion of the compressed vertebral body (see Fig. 6.19A).

Vertebral Scalloping

The commonest cause of vertebral scalloping is that due to normal variation (Table 6.9), and most often this occurs along the posterior aspect of the vertebral bodies in the lumbar region (Fig. 6.12A). Less commonly, but certainly not rarely, normal anterior scalloping is seen in approximately the same

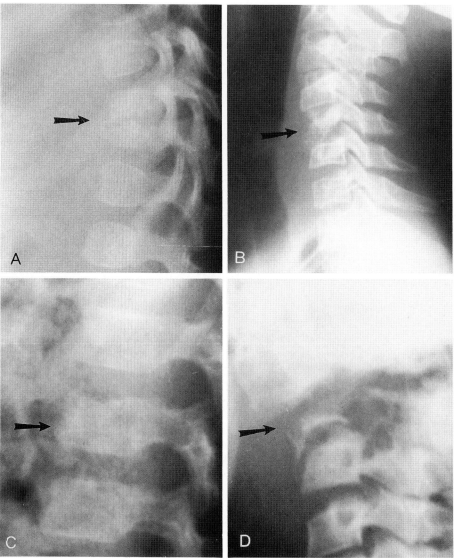

Figure 6.11. Vertebral destruction. A. Note destruction of two vertebral bodies and intervening disk space *(arrow)* due to bacterial osteomyelitis. **B.** Histiocytosis-X. Nearly complete destruction of a cervical vertebra *(arrow)* with relative if not absolute preservation of the disk spaces above and below. **C.** Slightly compressed, destroyed vertebral body secondary to metastatic disease *(arrow)*. Note that the disk spaces are preserved. **D.** Complete destruction of C$_2$ by actinomycosis *(arrow)*. Note preservation of disk space below.

area (Fig. 6.12B). However, as opposed to posterior scalloping, which rarely if ever extends into the thoracic region, normal anterior scalloping commonly extends into the lower thoracic spine. It does not involve the upper thoracic or cervical spine to any degree. Normal scalloping also can be seen along the lateral aspects of the vertebral bodies, especially in the lower thoracic and upper lumbar region.

As far as pathologic scalloping is concerned, most often it is seen posteriorly and is due to an expanding intraspinal lesion. The lesion may be neoplasm, cyst, syringomyelia, hydromyelia, or uncontrolled communicating hydrocephalus (2). Posterior scalloping also can be seen with dural ectasia, and the most common condition to be associated with this phenomenon is neurofibromatosis (Fig. 6.12C). In these patients, it is not an intraspinal tumor which produces the scalloping, but rather a defect in mesenchymal development that leads to a combination of defective bone formation and dural space ectasia with resultant expansion of the spinal canal. In addition to neurofibromatosis, the problem is seen in

Table 6.9
Vertebral Scalloping

Posterior		
Normal—lumbar	}	Common
Intraspinal tumor, cyst	⎫	
Neurofibromatosis[a]		
Achondroplasia, other chondrodys-trophies[b]	}	Moderately common
Storage diseases	⎭	
Ehler-Danlos syndrome[a]	⎫	
Marfan syndrome[a]		
Hydromyelia, syringomyelia	}	Rare
Uncontrolled communicating hydro-cephalus	⎭	
Anterior		
Normal—lower thoracic and upper lumbar	}	Common
Neurofibromatosis[c]	⎫	
Leukemia, lymphoma[d]	}	Moderately common
Metastatic disease[d]	⎭	
Adjacent intraabdominal tumors, cysts[e]	}	Rare

[a] Dural ectasia.
[b] Small canal.
[c] Dysplastic vertebra.
[d] Destruction.
[e] Erosion.

Marfan syndrome, Ehlers-Danlos syndrome, and idiopathically (1).

Increased posterior scalloping also occurs with chondrodystrophies such as achondroplasia (Fig. 6.12D), diastrophic dwarfism, and thanatophoric dwarfism (see Table 6.9). In most of these conditions, the spinal canal also is narrower than normal, and it is the crowding of the normally growing spinal cord that causes pressure scalloping of the vertebral bodies. In later life these patients often suffer from early and severe compression of the spinal cord and nerve roots.

As far as pathologic anterior scalloping is concerned, the causes are relatively few. However, this scalloping can be seen with adjacent eroding tumors, destruction of the vertebra by lymphoma or metastatic disease, and most often, as an inherent mesenchymal dysplasia in neurofibromatosis (Fig. 6.13E). Erosions secondary to adjacent aortic aneurysms are uncommon in children.

When both exaggerated posterior and anterior scalloping occur together, a spindle- or spool-shaped vertebra results. To a mild degree, this can be seen in the chondrodystrophies and storage diseases and even in normal children. In more pronounced form, however, it is seen in trisomy-21, some of the other trisomies, Melnick-Needles osteodysplasia, and neurofibromatosis (see Fig. 6.24).

REFERENCES

1. Katz SG, Grunebaum M, Strand RD: Thoracic and lumbar dural ectasia in a two year old boy. *Pediatr Radiol* 6:238–240, 1978.
2. Mitchell GE, Lourie H, Berne AS: The various causes of scalloped vertebrae with notes on their pathogenesis. *Radiology* 89:67–74, 1967.

Vertebral Body Shape Abnormalities

Vertebral shape abnormalities include (a) flat vertebrae (platyspondyly), (b) cuboid vertebrae, (c) biconcave vertebrae, (d) tall vertebrae, (e) round or oval vertebrae, (f) expanded vertebrae, (g) wedged vertebrae, (h) hooked or beaked vertebrae, and (i) spool-shaped vertebrae.

FLAT VERTEBRAE

Flat vertebrae usually result from compression fractures or developmental abnormalities (Table 6.10). Occasionally, especially in the thoracic spine, a little flattening of the vertebrae can be seen in normal children and, indeed, some children may appear to have slight anterior wedging. Often anterior wedging also occurs with pathologic vertebral flattening, but in all cases it is important to note whether the flattening phenomenon is isolated to one or two vertebral bodies or generalized throughout the spine. If all of the vertebral bodies are flattened, a bony dysplasia (Fig. 6.13A and B) or severe osteoporosis or osteomalacia (Fig. 6.13C) should be considered (1, 2). If only one or two vertebral bodies are flattened, one should consider either an ordinary or pathologic fracture.

Conditions leading to universal platyspondyly include spondyloepiphyseal dysplasia, Morquio disease (storage disease that resembles spondyloepiphyseal dysplasia), achondrogenesis, thanatophoric dwarfism, metatropic dwarfism, Kniest syndrome, and Dyggve-Melchior-Clausen syndrome (findings resemble Morquio disease or spondyloepiphyseal dysplasia). In spondyloepiphyseal dysplasia, Morquio's

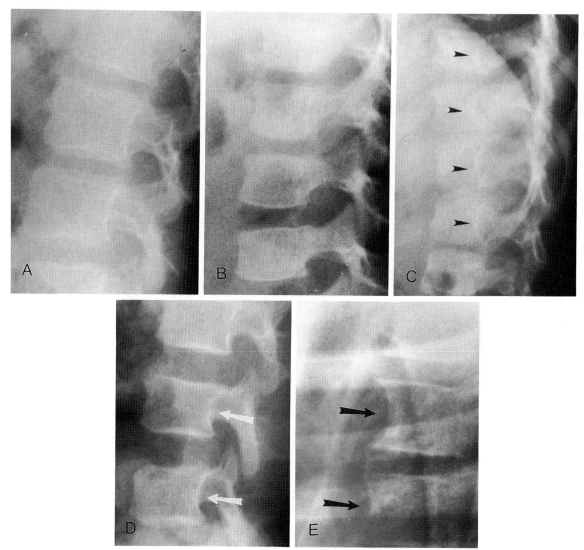

Figure 6.12. Vertebral scalloping. A. Normal posterior lumbar vertebral scalloping. **B.** Normal anterior lumbar and lower thoracic vertebral scalloping. **C.** Pathologic scalloping due to dural ectasia in neurofibromatosis *(arrows)*. **D.** Pathologic posterior scalloping *(arrows)* in achondroplasia. **E.** Pathologic anterior scalloping of thoracic vertebra in neurofibromatosis *(arrows)*.

disease, and Dyggve-Melchior-Clausen syndrome, the vertebral bodies often also are **pear-shaped** (Fig. 6.13D). When universal platyspondyly is seen in osteogenesis imperfecta, the problem is multiple compression fractures, and a mixture of flat and biconcave vertebrae can result.

As noted earlier, when only one or two vertebral bodies are flattened, and especially if they are **anteriorly wedged,** one should consider compression fracture. Such fractures, regular or pathologic, commonly occur with hyperflexion or axial compression injuries (Fig. 6.14A). When a vertebra is flattened entirely, the term **"vertebra plana"** is utilized, and most often is seen in histiocytosis-X. Indeed, in some cases the vertebral body becomes wafer thin (Fig. 6.14B). Other conditions leading to single or multiple, but not universal, vertebral body compression include metastases, leukemia, osteogenesis imperfecta, and any cause of osteomalacia or osteoporosis.

REFERENCES

1. Kozlowski K: Platyspondyly in childhood. *Pediatr Radiol* 81–88, 1974.
2. Schorr S, Legum C: Radiological aspects of the vertebral components of osteochondrocysplasias. *Br J Radiol* 50:302–311, 1977.

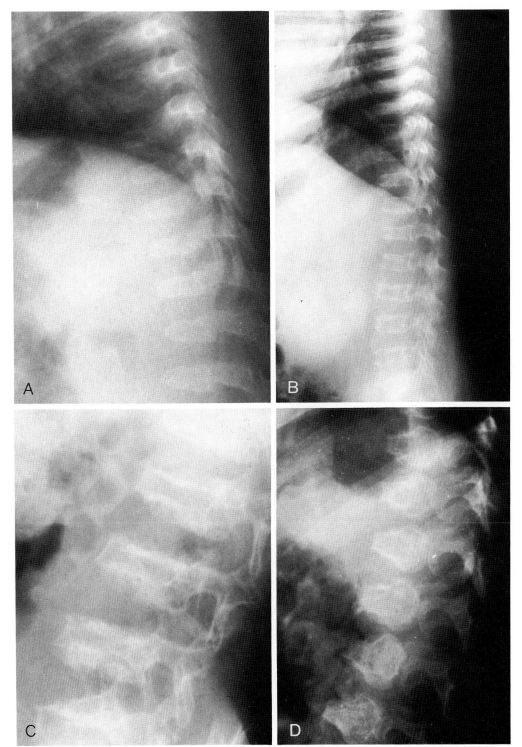

Figure 6.13. Flat vertebra. A. Flat vertebra in Morquio disease. **B.** Flat vertebra in spondyloepiphyseal dysplasia. **C.** Flat vertebra due to severe osteoporosis in Cushing syndrome. **D.** Flat, pear-shaped vertebra in spondyloepiphyseal dysplasia.

Table 6.10
Flat Vertebrae

Single or multiple but not all vertebral bodies	
Fracture Eosinophilic granuloma Histiocytosis-X	Common
Metastatic disease Congenital variation Osteogenesis imperfecta Osteomalacia-osteoporosis Leukemia-lymphoma	Moderately common
All vertebral bodies	
Severe osteoporosis-osteomalacia[a,c] Sickle-cell disease[c]	Common
Severe osteogenesis imperfecta[a,c] Other anemias[a,c] Leukemia, lymphoma[a,c] Spondyloepiphyseal dysplasia[a,b]	Moderately common
Thanatophoric dwarfism[a] Metatropic dwarfism[a] Morquio disease[b]	Relatively rare
Achondrogenesis Kniest syndrome[a] Dyggve-Melchior-Clausen syndrome[b]	Rare

[a] Uniformly flat.
[b] Pear-shaped.
[c] Biconcave.

Table 6.11
Cuboid Vertebrae

Normal[a] Achondroplasia	Common
Hypochondroplasia Other chondrodystrophies Storage diseases	Moderately common
Short rib-polydactyly syndrome	Rare

[a] Cervical and thoracolumbar spine.

CUBOID VERTEBRAE (TABLE 6.11)

Cuboid vertebrae can be encountered in the cervical spine or lower thoracolumbar region on a normal basis. When abnormal, these vertebrae are seen throughout the spine and for the most part occur in chondrodystrophies such as achondroplasia (Fig. 6.15A), thanatophoric dwarfism, diastrophic dwarfism, hypochondroplasia, and the short rib-polydactyly syndromes of Saldino-Noonan and Majewski. In these latter conditions, the vertebrae also are quite hypoplastic and in severe cases more rounded. Somewhat cuboid-shaped vertebrae also occur in the storage diseases (Fig. 6.15B).

BICONCAVE VERTEBRAE (TABLE 6.12)

The best known and one of the most common biconcave or fish vertebra configurations occurs with

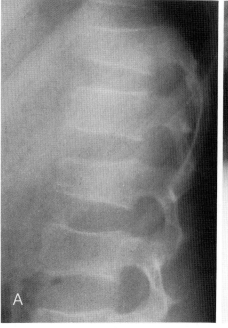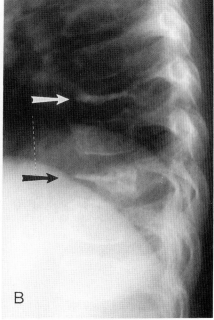

Figure 6.14. Flat vertebral bodies. A. Anteriorly wedged, flat body due to compression fracture in patient with lymphoma. **B.** Typical vertebra plana, wafer-thin, compressed vertebra in histiocytosis-X *(arrows).*

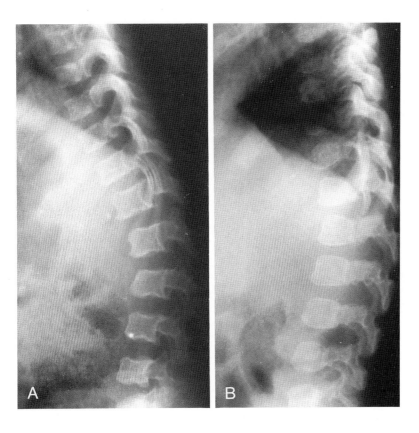

Figure 6.15. Cuboid vertebrae. A. Cuboid vertebrae in achondroplasia. **B.** Mucopolysaccharidosis with cuboid vertebrae.

Table 6.12
Biconcave Vertebrae

Sickle cell disease[a] Osteoporosis-osteomalacia	Common
Osteogenesis imperfecta Renal osteodystrophy Normal Schmorl's nodes	Moderately common
Thalassemia[b] Gaucher disease[b] Homocystinuria[b]	Relatively rare

[a]Often step-like depression.
[b]Occasionally step-like depression.

sickle cell disease (1, 2). In these patients it is believed that endplate infarction causes bone necrosis and subsequent expansion of the normally turgid disks into the vertebrae. Because of the infarction, the depression has a typical square-cornered, step-like appearance (Fig. 6.16A). However, the step-like configuration does not occur in all cases. Furthermore, similar step-like deformities have been noted with renal osteodystrophy, thalassemia, homocystinuria, and Gaucher disease (3–7).

Biconcave vertebrae without step-like compression usually occur when there is extreme softening of the vertebral bodies. In such cases, the turgid

disks once again expand and bulge into the vertebral bodies (Fig. 6.16B). Some of the more common conditions in which this occurs are listed in Table 6.10. Basically, however, they include the more severe forms of osteomalacia and osteoporosis as seen with conditions such as osteogenesis imperfecta, rickets, hypophosphatasia, steroid therapy, hyperparathyroidism, Cushing syndrome, severe malnutrition, and marrow packing disorders such as sickle cell disease, Cooley anemia, lymphoma, and metastases. A complete list of conditions leading to osteomalacia or osteoporosis is presented in Tables 4.1 and 4.2. A mild degree of concavity of the vertebral endplates is seen in some normal individuals and is due to the normally prominent nucleus pulposus of the intervertebral disks (Fig. 6.16C).

REFERENCES

1. Hansen GC, Gold RH: Central depression of multiple vertebral end-plates: a "pathognomonic" sign of sickle hemoglobinopathy in Gaucher's disease. *AJR* 129:343–344, 1977.
2. Riggs W, Rockett JF: Roentgen chest findings in childhood sickle cell anemia: a new vertebral body finding. *Am J Roentgenol Radium Ther Nucl Med* 104:838–845, 1968.
3. Rohlfing BM: Vertebral end-plate depression: report of two patients without hemoglobinopathy. *AJR* 128:599–600, 1977.

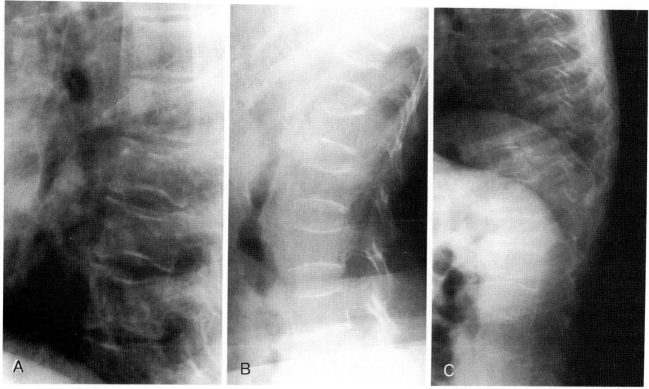

Figure 6.16. Biconcave vertebrae. A. Biconcave vertebrae with step-like central depressions in sickle cell disease. **B.** Biconcave vertebrae, associated with grossly expanded disks in pa-

tient with leukemic and steroid induced osteoporosis. **C.** Mild biconcave vertebrae due to normally prominent nucleus pulposus.

Table 6.13
Tall Vertebrae

Trisomy-21	Common
Other causes of hypotonia	

4. Schwartz AM, Homer MJ, McCauley RGK: Step-off vertebral body: Gaucher's disease versus sickle cell hemoglobinopathy. *AJR* 132:81–85, 1979.
5. Cassady JR, Berdon WE, Baker DH: The "typical" spine changes of sickle-cell anemia in a patient with thalassemia major (Cooley's anemia). *Radiology* 89:1065–1068, 1967.
6. Westerman MP, Greenfield GB, Wong PWK: "Fish vertebrae," homocystinuria, and sickle cell anemia. *JAMA* 230:261–262, 1974.
7. Ziter FMH Jr: Central vertebral end-plate depression in chronic renal disease: report of two cases. *AJR* 132:809–811, 1979.

TALL VERTEBRAE (TABLE 6.13)

Tall vertebrae, for the most part, are seen in hypotonic infants and children. Absence of vertical stresses cause the vertebrae to become tall (1) and canine in shape. The configuration can be seen in a variety of syndromes where hypotonia exists and,

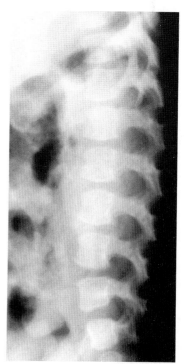

Figure 6.17. Tall vertebrae. Typically tall vertebrae in retarded patient. Note slight spool-shaped appearance of the vertebrae, not an uncommon associated finding.

thus, with many underlying neurologic or neuromuscular disorders (Fig. 6.17).

REFERENCE

1. Gooding CA, Neuhauser EBD: Growth and development of the vertebral bodies in the presence and absence of normal stress. *AJR* 93:388–393, 1965.

ROUND VERTEBRAE (TABLE 6.14)

Normal round vertebral bodies commonly are seen in the neonatal period in the thoracolumbar junction (Fig. 6.18A). As the infant grows older, the vertebrae become more rectangular in shape and eventually, as the ring epiphyses develop, their corners become quite square. In some children, under normal circumstances, the ringed epiphyses may be late in appearing, and then a rounded-to-oval vertebral body configuration temporarily persists (Fig. 6.18B). The same problem occurs with certain pathologic conditions. Basically, these include (a) vertebral body underdevelopment in association with anomalies such as meningomyelocele (Fig. 6.18C) (1), and (b) retarded bone maturation as seen in untreated hypothyroidism (Fig. 6.18D). Round (actually more oval) vertebrae due to underdevelopment are seen in the pear-shaped flattened vertebrae occurring in certain bone dysplasias (see Fig. 6.13D).

REFERENCE

1. Kramer PPG, Scheers IM: Round anterior margin of lumbar vertebral bodies in children with a meningocele. *Pediatr Radiol* 17:263, 1987.

EXPANDED VERTEBRAE (TABLE 6.14)

Isolated, expanded vertebrae are seen with bone cysts and tumors, and the most common bone cyst in the spine is the usually bubbly-appearing aneurysmal bone cyst (Fig. 6.19A). These lesions also can extend into the posterior elements, and a similar configuration can be seen with giant cell tumors. The latter, however, are uncommon in children. Cystic, somewhat honeycombed expansion also occurs with hemangiomas (Fig. 6.19B) and lymphangiomas, and sclerotic, expanded vertebrae can be seen with treated Ewing sarcoma (see Fig. 6.2A). Expanded vertebrae also occur with giant osteoid osteoma (osteoblastoma), and the vertebrae can expand in all directions with severe flexion or axial compression fractures.

Table 6.14
Round and Expanded Vertebrae

Round vertebrae1	
Normal neonate[a]	} Common
Meningocele	
Hypothyroidism	} Moderately common
Short rib-polydactyly syndromes	} Rare
Bone dysplasias[b]	
Expanded vertebrae	
Compression fracture with expansion	} Common
Aneurysmal bone cyst	} Relatively rare
Hemangioma-lymphangioma	
Osteoblastoma	} Rare
Ewing sarcoma[c]	

[a] Especially thoracolumbar junction.
[b] With pear-shaped vertebrae (see Table 6.10).
[c] Sclerotic-treated.

WEDGED VERTEBRAE (TABLE 6.15)

Wedging of the vertebrae can occur anteriorly or laterally, but anterior wedging is more common and is usually due to a fracture (Fig. 6.20A). Occasionally, mild anterior wedging, especially in the thoracic region, can be seen in normal individuals. This configuration may be difficult to differentiate from minor compression fractures. In the upper cervical spine, wedging of C_3 is a common phenomenon in infants and young children, and probably is due to normal hypermobility and flexibility of the upper cervical spine in this age group (1). Such physiologic wedging most commonly occurs at the level of C_3 but occasionally also can be seen at C_4 (Fig. 6.20B). As the child grows older this configuration disappears and, in addition, in any age group it should be remembered that anterior compression fractures of C_3 are very rare.

Other than the foregoing circumstances, wedging abnormalities of the vertebra usually are pathologic and due to acute (Fig. 6.20A) or chronic (Fig. 6.20C) compression. On a chronic basis, such wedging can be seen with Scheuermann disease and hypotonia resulting from any number of causes (Fig. 6.20C). Wedging of the vertebral bodies also occurs with scoliosis or kyphosis, and with scoliosis, usually is more lateral. Compression fractures can occur in normal bone or in bone weakened by problems such as tumor or infection.

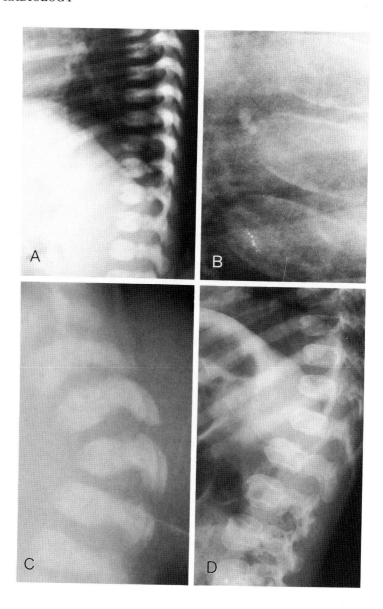

Figure 6.18. Round vertebrae. A. Normal, round vertebrae in neonate. **B.** Oval to round vertebrae in normal child with delayed appearance of ringed epiphyses. **C.** Meningomyelocele. Note acute kyphosis and many, rounded hypoplastic vertebral bodies. **D.** Round-to-oval vertebrae in a child with untreated hypothyroidism. Also note persistent prominence of the anterior and posterior central vein grooves.

REFERENCE

1. Swischuk LE, Swischuk PN, John SD: Wedging of C₃ in infants and children: usually a normal finding and not a fracture. *Radiology* 188:523–526, 1993.

HOOKED OR BEAKED VERTEBRAE (TABLE 6.16)

The hooked or beaked vertebra can show a smooth or irregular hook, but in either case, results from acute or chronic hyperflexion (4). There may or may not be associated disk material extrusion (1, 3), but when extrusion occurs **the notch is irregular and there is associated narrowing of the disk space.** For the most part, irregular beaking is seen with overt hyperflexion, either acute or chronic compression fractures (Fig. 6.20A). Chronic hyperflexion occurs with Scheuermann disease (Fig. 6.21B), and whenever chronic hypotonia is present. Acute trauma, causing notching, most often is accidental, but the finding also can be seen in the battered child syndrome (5).

When nuclear material is extruded anteriorly at an angle, it can keep the free, triangular bony fragments separate and result in the so-called "limbus" vertebra (Fig. 6.21B). This abnormality now is readily demonstrable with MRI (Fig. 6.21C).

When a **smooth, hooked, or beaked vertebra is seen,** the problem still is hyperflexion, but in these cases hyperflexion is prolonged, and irregular fragmentation of the vertebral corners does not occur. Rather, there is a smooth notching deformity (Fig.

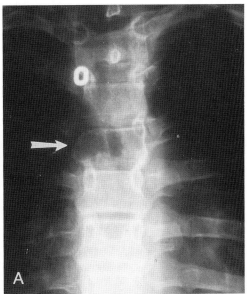

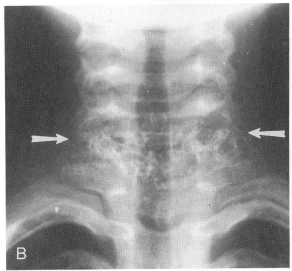
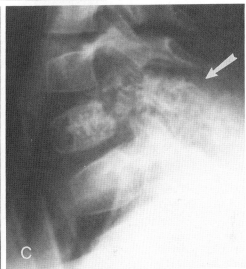

Figure 6.19. Expanded vertebrae. A. Slightly expanded, radiolucent, bubbly-appearing aneurysmal bone cyst *(arrow).* **B.** Markedly expanded, bubbly-appearing vertebra secondary to hemangioma *(arrows).* **C.** Lateral view showing extension into posterior elements *(arrow).*

Table 6.15
Wedged Vertebrae

Anterior compression fracture Scoliosis[a]	Common
Kyphosis[b] Scheuermann disease Normal[c] Hemivertebrae-sagittal[a]	Moderately common
Hemivertebrae-coronal[d] Gibbus[e]	Relatively rare

[a] Lateral wedging.
[b] Various causes.
[c] Thoracic spine minimal.
[d] Gibbus.
[e] Other causes (see text).

6.22). Smooth notching most commonly is seen in normal infants, at the thoracolumbar junction (Fig. 6.22A). The deformity usually is rather mild and entirely reversible. It results because of exaggerated thoracolumbar kyphosis secondary to hypotonia, which is normal in infancy. The problem is exaggerated when the infant is placed in a sitting position. On a pathologic basis, hypotonia also is the basic underlying problem, but there may be abnormality of bone maturation in addition. Most commonly this form of notched vertebra is seen in the various storage diseases (Fig. 6.22B) and hypothyroidism (Fig. 6.22C) (2). Occasionally, it also is seen in some cases of achondroplasia, the hypotonic trisomies (4), and, indeed, in any condition where

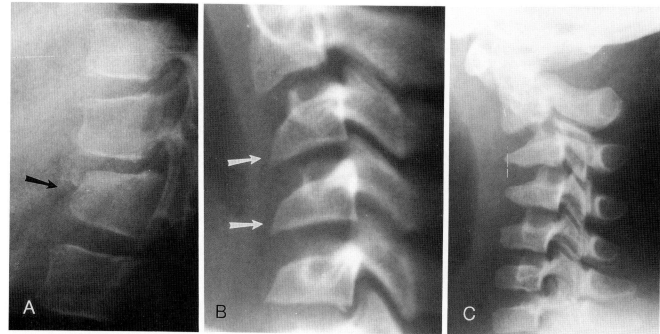

Figure 6.20. Wedged vertebrae. A. Typical wedged vertebra due to flexion-type fracture *(arrow).* The vertebra above also is slightly flattened and a small corner fracture is present. **B.** Nor-mal, anterior wedging of C_3 and C_4 *(arrows).* **C.** Severe anterior wedging due to chronic hyperflexion of cervical spine in patient with pseudohypoparathyroidism and hypotonia.

Table 6.16
Hooked or Beaked Vertebrae

Normal in infants[a]	} Common
Storage diseases Hypothyroidism Acute and chronic trauma Scheuermann disease Neurogenic or neuromuscular dis-ease with hypotonia	} Moderately common
Achondroplasia Bone dysplasia in neurofibromatosis	} Relatively rare

[a]Thoracolumbar junction.

neuromuscular hypotonia exists. In any of these cases, regression of the deformity occurs if hypotonia is reversed (Fig. 6.23).

REFERENCES

1. Begg AC: Nuclear herniation of the intervertebral disc; their radiological manifestations and significance. *J Bone Joint Surg* 36B:180–193, 1954.
2. Evans PR: Deformity of vertebral bodies in cretinism. *J Pediatr* 41:706–712, 1952.
3. Rabinowitz JG, Sacher M: Gangliosidosis (GM₁): a reevalu-ation of the vertebral deformity. *AJR* 121:155–158, 1974.
4. Swischuk LE: The beaked, notched, or hooked vertebra: its significance in infants and young children. *Radiology* 95:661–664, 1970.
5. Swischuk LE: Spine and spinal cord trauma in the battered child syndrome. *Radiology* 92:733–738, 1969.

SPOOL-SHAPED VERTEBRAE

Spool-shaped vertebrae are not particularly com-mon. In the normal lumbar spine, where mild de-grees of anterior and posterior scalloping are com-mon, a mild spool-shaped deformity can be seen. In exaggerated form, however, spool-shaped vertebrae are seen with the tall vertebrae of hypotonia (see Fig. 6.17) and with bony dysplasias such as the Mel-nick-Needles osteodysplasia syndrome, neurofibro-matosis (Fig. 6.24), trisomy-21, some other trisomies, and some chondrodystrophies and storage diseases.

ABSENT VERTEBRAL BODIES

Occasionally, on a congenital basis an entire ver-tebral body is absent and spondylolisthesis results. However, most often only a part of the vertebral body is absent (see Fig. 6.32B), and then either a sa-gittal or coronal cleft hemivertebra is seen. An ab-sent vertebral body also is seen when it is destroyed by a disease process such as metastatic disease, the

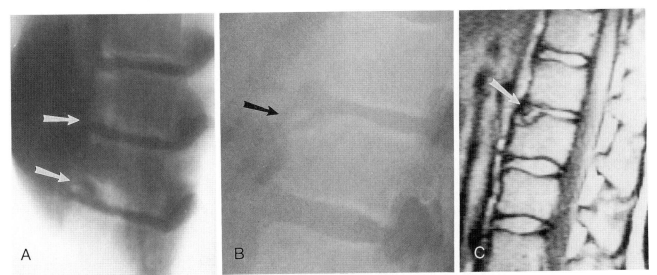

Figure 6.21. Hooked or beaked vertebrae: irregular hooking or beaking. A. Irregular notching on a chronic basis in Scheuermann disease *(arrows)*. **B.** Limbus vertebra. Note irregular notching *(arrow)* due to extrusion of nuclear material into the vertebral body. **C.** MRI clearly demonstrates the extruded nuclear material *(arrow)* under the triangular bony fragment.

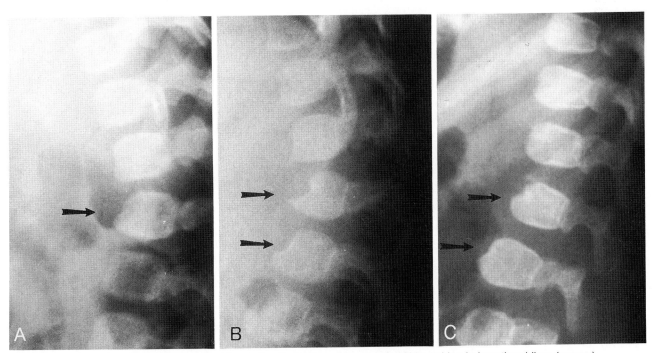

Figure 6.22. Smooth notching or beaking. A. Normal notching in infant *(arrow)*. **B.** Severe notching in Hurler disease *(arrows)*. **C.** Mild notching in hypothyroidism *(arrows)*.

leukemia-lymphoma group of diseases, osteomyelitis, and histiocytosis-X (see Fig. 6.11*B*).

BLOCK VERTEBRAE (TABLE 6.17)

Block vertebrae are associated with an extremely narrow or totally obliterated disk. Most often, such blocking or fusion is congenital and very often is seen in the C$_2$–C$_3$ area (Fig. 6.25*A*). Such blocking can be seen in isolated form or in association with the Klippel-Feil syndrome (1–7). In this latter condition, numerous, bizarre fusion-segmentation anomalies of the cervical spine exist (Fig. 6.25*B*). The result is a short neck and varying degrees of torticollis.

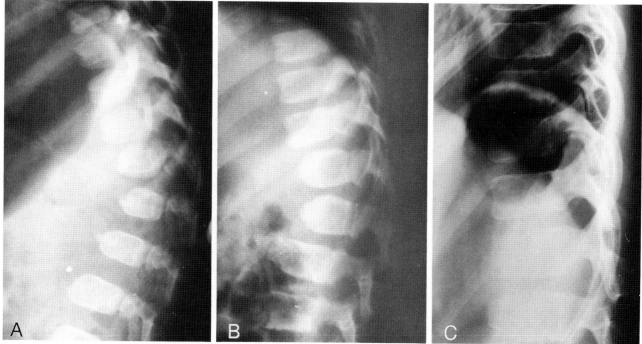

Figure 6.23. Smooth notching with regression. A. Severe notching in hypothyroidism. **B.** Somewhat later, after therapy was initiated, changes were less pronounced. **C.** Patient is now an adolescent and only minimal deformity remains.

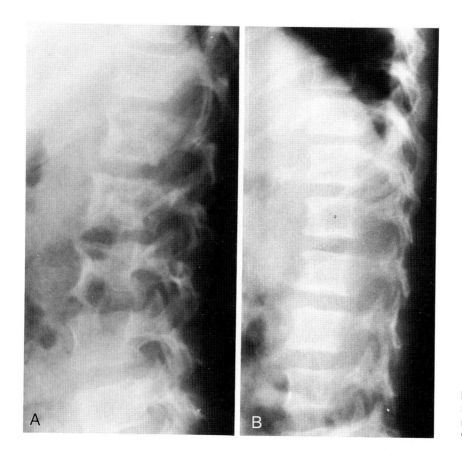

Figure 6.24. Spool-shaped vertebrae. A. Spool-shaped vertebrae in neurofibromatosis. **B.** Melnick-Needles osteodysplasia with spool-shaped vertebrae.

Table 6.17
Block Vertebrae

Congenital—with spinal dysraphism }	Common

Congenital
  Isolated
  Klippel-Feil syndrome
Acquired; after infection }
	Moderately common

Acquired—after trauma Scheuermann disease }	Relatively rare

In spite of the severe bony abnormality, neurologic deficit is uncommon. Sprengel deformity of the scapula (elevated, rotated scapula) is commonly associated (8), and some of these patients may have renal agenesis and/or congenital deafness. Block vertebrae are less common elsewhere and, in fact when seen, usually are not totally blocked but associated with a very narrow disk (see Fig. 6.36A).

Acquired block vertebrae result when intervening disks are destroyed and subsequent healing occurs. Very often, a kyphotic or frank gibbus deformity results (see Fig. 6.43A). Most often, the cause is infection, but occasionally it is severe discovertebral

trauma. On a chronic basis, this latter phenomenon occurs in Scheuermann disease. Ankylosing spondylitis also can lead to acquired block vertebrae, but the condition is rare in children.

REFERENCES

1. Hensinger R, Lang J, MacEwen G: Klippel-Feil syndrome: constellation of associated anomalies. *J Bone Joint Surg* 56A:1246–1253, 1974.
2. Moore W, Matthews TJ, Rabinowitz R: Genitourinary anomalies associated with the Klippel-Feil syndrome. *J Bone Joint Surg* 57A:355–357, 1975.
3. Palant DI, Carter BL: Klippel-Feil syndrome and deafness: a study with polytomography. *Am J Dis Child* 123:218–221, 1972.
4. Ramsey J, Bliznak J: Klippel-Feil syndrome with renal agenesis and other anomalies. *AJR* 113:460–463, 1971.
5. Sherk HH, Shut L, Chung S: Iniencephalic deformity of the cervical spine with Klippel-Feil anomalies and congenital elevation of the scapula: report of three cases. *J Bone Joint Surg* 56:1254–1259, 1974.
6. Shoul ML, Ritvo M: Clinical and roentgenographic manifestations of the Klippel-Feil syndrome. *AJR* 68:369–385, 1952.
7. Stark EW, Borton TE: Hearing loss and the Klippel-Feil syndrome. *Am J Dis Child* 123:233–235, 1972.
8. Wilson MG, Mikity VG, Shinno NW: Dominant inheritance of Sprengel's deformity. *J Pediatr* 79:818–821, 1971.

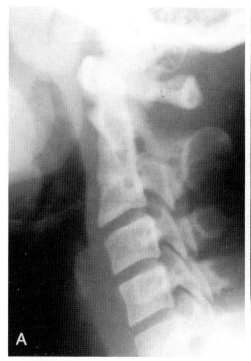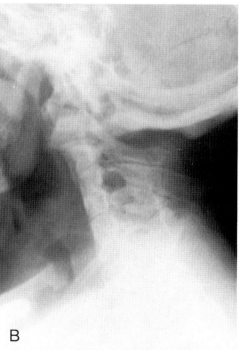

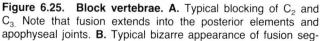

Figure 6.25. Block vertebrae. A. Typical blocking of C$_2$ and C$_3$. Note that fusion extends into the posterior elements and apophyseal joints. **B.** Typical bizarre appearance of fusion segmentation anomalies, including blocking, in the Klippel-Feil syndrome.

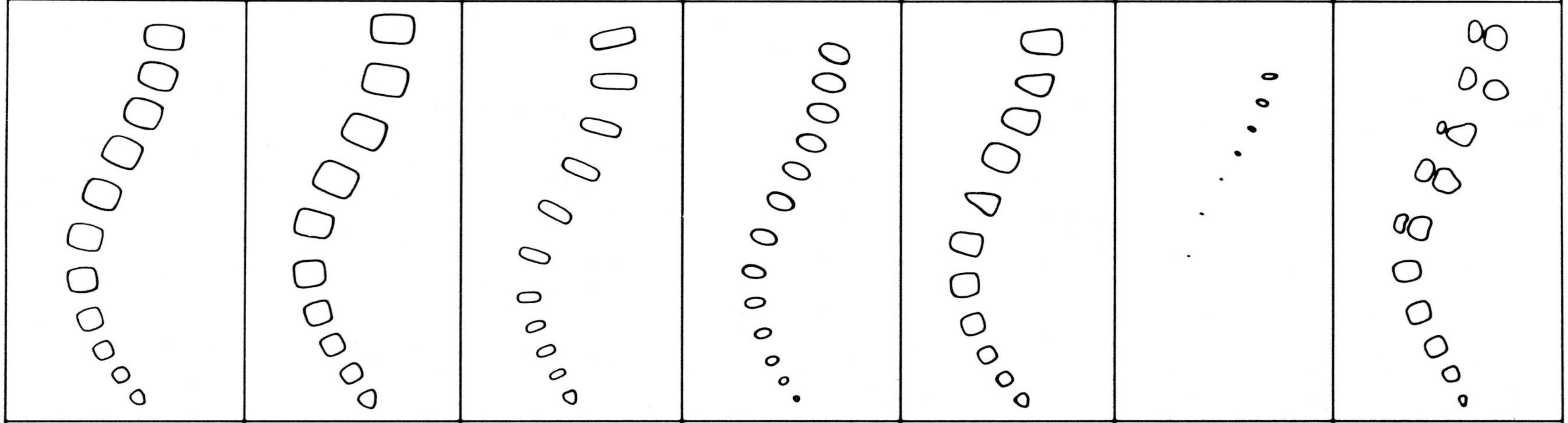

NORMAL	CUBOID-RECTANGULAR	FLAT	FLAT (OVAL)	FLAT (COMPRESSED)	ABSENT HYPOPLASTIC	SEGMENTED
Asphyxiating thoracic dystrophy	Achondroplasia	Thanatophoric dwarfism	Spondyloepiphyseal dysplasia	Osteogenesis imperfecta	Achondrogenesis	Spondylothoracic dysplasia
Ellis-van Creveld	Hypochondroplasia	Metatropic dwarfism	Hypochondrogenesis		Hypophosphatasia	Dyssegmental dwarfism
Camptomelic dwarfism	Short-ribbed polydactyly syndromes	Kneist syndrome			Osteogenesis imperfecta (Type II) congenita	Chondrodystrophia calcificans congenita (dominant)
Diastrophic dwarfism	Rhizomelic	Kneist-like syndromes				
Mesomelic dwarfism	Chondrodystrophia calcificans congenita (recessive)					

Figure 6.26. Vertebral configurations in neonatal dwarfism. Note the various vertebral body configurations and the list of entities most commonly encountered with each of these configurations.

Vertebral Bodies in Neonatal Dwarfism

In cases of neonatal dwarfism, often it is of value to begin the assessment of the underlying bony abnormalities by evaluating the spine, especially on lateral view (1). The method is not foolproof, but it has been a good starting point for us. Depending on whether the vertebral bodies are normal, cuboid-rectangular, flat, oval, compressed, absent, hypoplastic, or segmented, one can provide a practical differential diagnosis for each configuration as a starting point in one's analysis (Fig. 6.26).

REFERENCE

1. Swischuk LE, John SD, O'Keeffe F: Short-limbed neonatal dwarfism: a classification based on the appearance of the spine. Presented at the 76th annual meeting of the Radiological Society of North America, Chicago, IL, 1990.

Spinal Canal Diameter Abnormalities

The abnormal spinal canal can be too wide or too narrow (Table 6.18), but before you consider canal diameter abnormalities, remember that the normal spinal canal, on frontal view, usually appears wide in the cervicothoracic (Fig. 6.27A) and lumbosacral regions of infants. As far as pathologic widening is concerned, the commonest cause is a congenital anomaly such as a meningocele or meningomyelocele. Less commonly, other dysraphic problems such as diastematomyelia (Fig. 6.27E), congenital dermal sinus, and a variety of intraspinal tumors or cysts

Table 6.18
Spinal Canal Diameter Abnormalities

Enlarged	
Normal, cervical and lumbosacral Meningocele-meningomyelocele	} Common
Diastematomyelia Intraspinal tumor, cyst Syringomyelia, hydromyelia	} Relatively rare
Narrowed	
Chondrodystrophies[a]	} Commonest
Congenital narrowing	} Rare

[a]Achondroplasia, etc.

can be encountered (Fig. 6.27B). Another rare cause of spinal canal enlargement often seen in the cervical region is syringomyelia (Fig. 6.27C and D). Syringomyelia in children is usually congenital, and frequently accompanies Arnold-Chiari malformations; however, acquired lesions due to trauma, infection, or tumor also occur. Meningomyeloceles most often are seen in the lumbosacral region and the cervicothoracic junction. Diastematomyelia (1, 2) most commonly occurs at the thoracolumbar junction and, if the transfixing bony spicule is visualized, the diagnosis is assured (Fig. 6.27E). However, many times the spicule is fibrous or cartilaginous and the split cord must be imaged in some other way (Fig. 6.27F). Clinically, as the spicule transfixes the spinal cord, it prevents its normal ascent, causes it to stretch, and induces neurologic symptoms. In all of these conditions, the underlying cord problems are most readily demonstrated with MRI.

Narrowing of the spinal canal most often is generalized and almost always is the result of impaired enchondral bone formation seen with an underlying bony dysplasia. Of these, the chondrodystrophies are most common, and the best example is achondroplasia (Fig. 6.28). Similar narrowing, however, is seen with achondrogenesis, thanatophoric dwarfism, metatropic dwarfism, diastrophic dwarfism, the Kniest syndrome, and some of the storage diseases. A congenitally small spinal canal, under other circumstances, is uncommon in childhood.

REFERENCES

1. Hilal S, Marton D, Pollack E: Diastematomyelia in children: radiographic study of 34 cases. *Radiology* 112:609–621, 1974.
2. Neuhauser EBD, Wittenborg MH, Dehlinger K: Diastematomyelia. *Radiology* 54:659–664, 1950.

Intervertebral Foramen Abnormalities

The intervertebral foramina can be larger or smaller than normal (Table 6.19). The latter is quite uncommon and almost always is secondary to congenital maldevelopment of the vertebra, as seen with congenital abnormalities such as the Klippel-Feil syndrome, fused vertebra, unilateral bar leading to scoliosis, diastematomyelia, and meningomyelocele (Fig. 6.29A). Small intervertebral foramina secondary to posttraumatic and/or degenerative arthritis are rare in children.

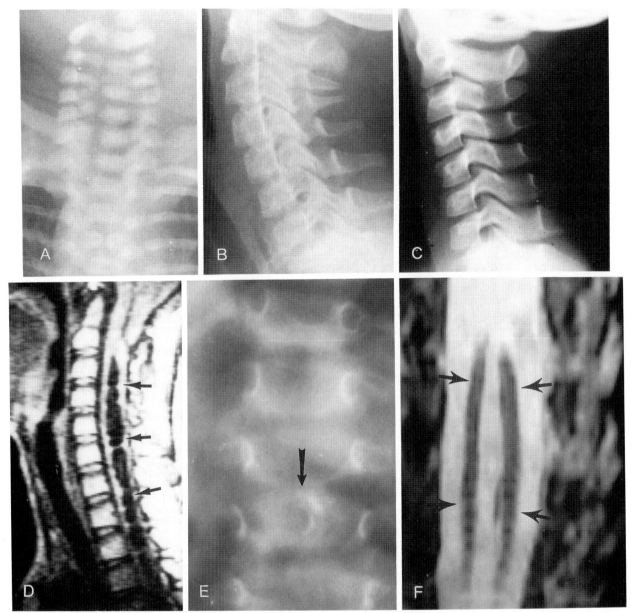

Figure 6.27. Enlarged spinal canal. A. Normal, pseudowidened, cervical spinal canal in infant. **B.** Widening of the canal in the cervical region due to an intraspinal tumor. **C.** Spinal canal widening due to syringomyelia. **D.** MRI demonstrating marked dilation of the central canal *(arrows)* in syringomyelia. **E.** Tomogram showing widening of the canal with flattening of the pedicles in diastematomyelia. Note the bony spicule *(arrow).* **F.** MRI in another patient demonstrates the split cord *(arrows)* of diastematomyelia.

Large intervertebral foramina are more common and can be seen with absence or hypoplasia of a neural arch or an expanding intracanalicular tumor. With regard to the latter, one should think first of a dumbbell-type lesion with intraspinal and extraspinal components (Fig. 6.29B). In children, tumors of the nerve roots (e.g., neurofibroma) are uncommon and, actually, in younger children a dumbbell tumor is more apt to be a neuroblastoma or ganglioneuroma (2, 4). Rarely, a paraspinal sarcoma can produce such a dumbbell configuration.

Other causes of large intervertebral foramina include the bony dysplasia and associated dural ectasia seen in neurofibromatosis, lateral meningoceles, posttraumatic nerve root avulsion diverticula, and hypertrophic interstitial polyneuritis (5). None are

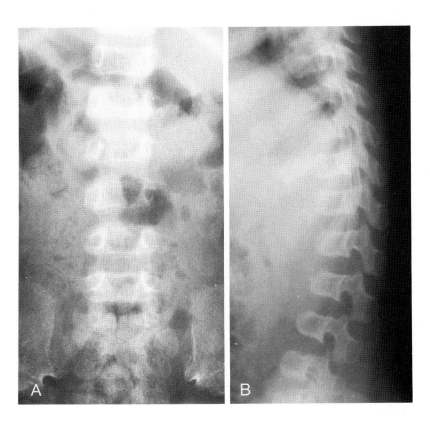

Figure 6.28. Narrow spinal canal. A. Note generalized narrowing of spinal canal, manifested by rather uniform interpedicular distance. Normally, the canal should be wider in the thoracolumbar junction and lower cervical regions. This patient was an achondroplast. **B.** Lateral view showing generalized narrowing of the spinal canal and some exaggerated posterior scalloping.

Table 6.19
Intervertebral Foramen Size Abnormalities

Small

Congenital with other anomalies	}	Common
Posttraumatic	}	Relatively rare

Enlarged

Congenital with dysraphism anomalies	}	Commonest
Dumbbell tumor[a] Neurofibromatosis[b]	}	Moderately common
Intraspinal tumor[c] Posttraumatic nerve root diverticulum Congenital absence or hypoplastic pedicle Lateral meningocele Interstitial polyneuritis Dural ectasia, idiopathic	}	Rare

[a] Usually neuroblastoma-ganglioneuroma.
[b] Bony dysplasia-dural ectasia.
[c] Other.

particularly common in children. Occasionally, dural ectasia also can be seen with the Marfan and Ehler-Danlos syndromes, and on an idiopathic basis (1, 3).

REFERENCES

1. Binet EF, Lustgarten MD: Enlarged neural foramen in a child. *NY State J Med* 7:449–452, 1971.
2. Fagan CJ, Swischuk LE: Dumbbell neuroblastoma or ganglioneuroma of the spinal canal. *AJR* 120:453–640, 1974.
3. Katz SG, Grunebaum M, Strand RD: Thoracic and lumbar dural ectasia in a two-year old boy. *Pediatr Radiol* 6:238–240, 1978.
4. King, D, Goodman J, Hawk T, Boles ET, Sayers MP: Dumbbell neuroblastomas in children. *Arch Surg* 110:888–891, 1975.
5. Patel DV, Ferguson L, Schey WL: Enlargement of the intervertebral foramina: an unusual cause. *AJR* 131:911–913, 1978.

Dislocated Vertebral Bodies (Table 6.20)

Vertebral body dislocation usually results from trauma but also can be seen with disk or vertebral body infection and destruction, and with severe congenital defects of the vertebral bodies and neural arches. However, physiologic anterior displacement in the upper cervical spine is the commonest cause of vertebral body displacement in childhood. Almost always such displacement occurs anteriorly on flexion (Fig. 6.30A), but it also can occur posteriorly

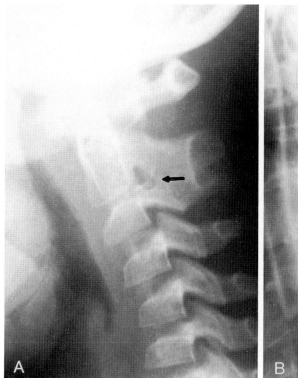
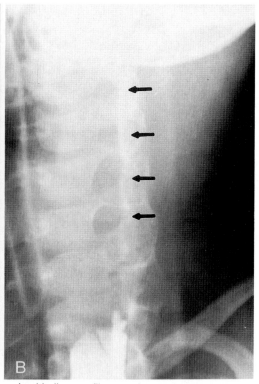

Figure 6.29. Intervertebral foramen size abnormalities. A. Small intervertebral foramen secondary to fusion of posterior elements of C₂-C₃ *(arrow).* **B.** Large intervertebral foramina due to dumbbell neurofibroma *(arrows).* Note complete block on this myelogram.

Table 6.20
Vertebral Body Dislocation

Physiologic—cervical spine	}	Common
Traumatic dislocation Lumbar spondylolysis-spondylo- listhesis	}	Moderately common

Dislocation
  With infection
  With congenital anomalies
	}	Relatively rare

on extension (Fig. 6.30B). When such dislocations occur at multiple levels, as shown in Figure 6.30A and B, accepting them as physiologic is not difficult, but when the phenomenon is isolated to one level, solving the problem can be more difficult. Most often, such isolated dislocation occurs anteriorly at the C₂–C₃ level of the cervical spine (Fig. 6.31A). Indeed, so disturbing is the finding that one's first consideration usually is that of pathologic dislocation. Pathologic dislocation does occur at this level with a hangman's fracture (Fig. 6.31C), and to facilitate differentiating of the two conditions, one can utilize the posterior cervical line (1). This line, applied from the anterior cortex of the spinous process of C₁ to the anterior cortex of the spinous process of C₃, should not pass more than 1 to 1.5 mm anterior to the cortex of the spinous process of C₂ (1). If it does, a fracture should be suspected (Fig. 6.31C), and, contrarily, if it falls within normal range, no matter how serious the problem appears, physiologic dislocation only is present (Fig. 6.31B). **This line, however, does not totally exclude ligamentous injury with no bony displacement.** Indeed, the line will be normal under such circumstances. One must then exercise caution. Only later, when the pain subsides, does the ligament injury come to the forefront, because the patient's neck becomes more mobile and displacement is seen. Therefore, the posterior cervical line is to be used only when C₂ is displaced forward on C₃ (1), because it was designed to differentiate physiologic from pathologic displacement of these two vertebrae and not to exclude every possible injury.

As far as true, traumatic dislocations of the vertebral bodies are concerned, most often these occur anteriorly, in the cervical spine, and are the result of flexion-rotation or whiplash injuries (Fig. 6.32A). In

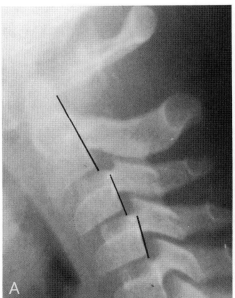 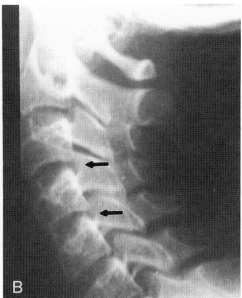

Figure 6.30.   Displaced vertebral bodies. A. Physiologic anterior displacement of cervical vertebral bodies at multiple levels.

B. Physiologic posterior displacement of the cervical vertebrae at two levels *(arrows).*

any of these cases, disruption of the disk space and its surrounding ligaments is the cause of dislocation. Lateral dislocation also occurs with trauma, but is less common and usually is due to severe, combined rotation-flexion or extension injuries. Dislocations associated with disk (Fig. 6.32C) or apophyseal joint infection are relatively uncommon and so are congenital dislocations due to absence, or large defects, of the vertebral bodies and neural arches (Fig. 6.32B).

REFERENCE

1. Swischuk LE: Anterior displacement of C_2 in children: physiologic or pathologic? A helpful differentiation. *Radiology* 122:759–763, 1977.

Spinous Tip Malalignment

Midline malalignment of the spinous tips occurs with rotatory injuries resulting in unilateral locked or perched facets. In such cases, the spinous tips above and below the level of rotation are offset. In other words, they do not follow a straight line down the midsagittal plane (Fig. 6.33A). A note of caution is offered here: one should be aware that congenital anomalies of the spinous tips may make the tips appear displaced.

Increased vertical intraspinous distance is seen with hyperflexion injuries causing rupture of the posterior ligaments (Fig. 6.33B), and also with Chance fractures (1–3) of the thoracolumbar spine. This type of spinous malalignment also can be mimicked by anomalous maldevelopment of the posterior elements. In addition, in infants and young children the distance between the spinous tips of C_1 and C_2 on flexion normally is quite wide (Fig. 6.33C).

REFERENCES

1. Chance GQ: Note on type of flexion fracture of spine. *Br J Radiol* 21:452–453, 1948.
2. Smith WE, Kaufer H: Patterns and mechanisms of lumbar injuries associated with lap-seat belts. *J Bone Joint Surg* 51A:239, 1969.
3. Steckler RM, Epstein JA, Epstein BS: Seat belt trauma to lumbar spine: unusual manifestation of seat belt syndrome. *J Trauma* 9:508–513, 1969.

Abnormalities of the Apophyseal Joints

Deformities of the apophyseal joints associated with congenital anomalies of the spine are straightforward. Apart from this, apophyseal joint abnormalities are rather uncommon in children, but basically consist of joints being too wide, too narrow, or dislocated. Joints that are too wide result from injuries associated with ligamentous tears, and widening often is accentuated with traction (Fig. 6.34A). Many

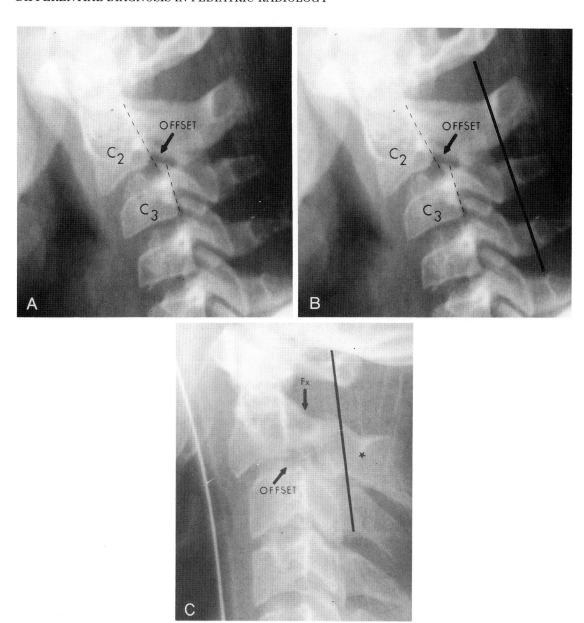

Figure 6.31. Physiologic vs. pathologic dislocation C_2-C_3. **A.** Note dislocation or offsetting of C_2 on C_3. Spine is flexed. **B.** Posterior cervical line touches the cortex of C_2 because the posterior elements of C_2 have moved forward with the body. No true dislocation is present. **C.** Hangman fracture *(Fx)* with anterior dis-placement of C_2. Because of the fracture, the posterior elements of C_2 remain posterior, while C_1 and the body and dens of C_2 move forward. Because of this the distance between the posterior cervical line and spinous process of C_2 now is increased well beyond 1.5 mm. This signifies pathologic dislocation.

times these injuries are the result of flexion-rotation forces. The apophyseal joints then may become dislocated in the "locked," or "perched," facet position (6.34*B*). In other cases, usually with flexion injuries, the joints are wide and V-shaped (Fig. 6.34*C*).

Congenital narrowing of the apophyseal joints does occur and actually most often takes the form of fusion (Fig. 6.34*D*). However, narrowing of the apophyseal joints also occurs with rheumatoid ar-

thritis (Fig. 6.35). Many times these changes lag behind clinical symptoms, and most often joint involvement first is noted at the C_2–C_3 area or in the lower cervical spine. In the most severe form of rheumatoid arthritis, that is, Still disease, one occasionally can have obliteration of all of the apophyseal joints and ankylosis to the point of bamboo spine formation (Fig. 6.35). Narrowing of the apophyseal joints also can occur with traumatic dislocation and with pyogenic infection causing destruction.

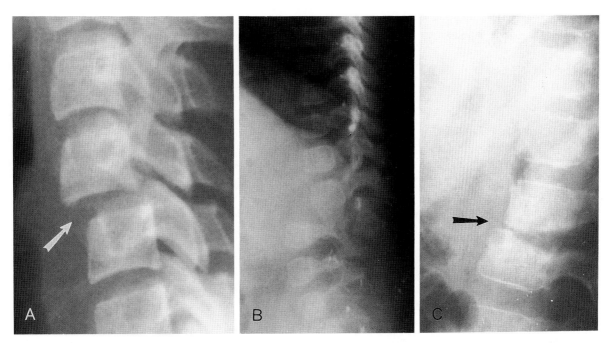

Figure 6.32. Vertebral body dislocation. A. Anterior dislocation of C_6 on C_7 *(arrow)*, due to unilateral locked facet. Also note that the disk space is narrow, which occurs with this type of injury. **B.** Gross dislocation due to congenital absence of vertebral body and partial absence of posterior elements. **C.** Dislocation secondary to diskitis *(arrow)*.

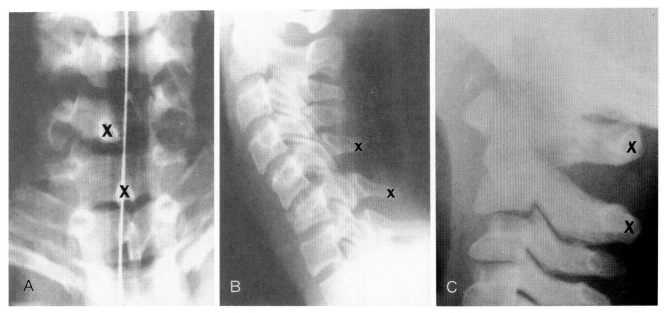

Figure 6.33. Spinous process tip malalignments. A. Note lateral displacement of the lower spinous process as compared with the upper spinous process *(x's)* due to rotatory subluxation. **B.** Widening of the interspinous distance *(x's)* due to ligamentous injury secondary to flexion injury of the cervical spine. **C.** Normal increased distance between the spinous process of C_1 and C_2 *(x's)* in infancy.

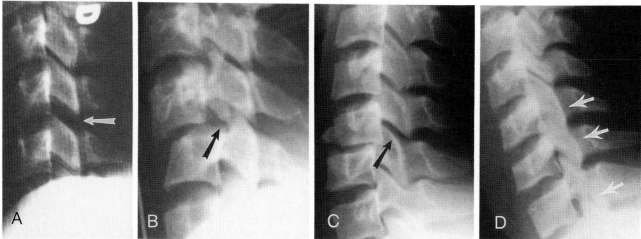

Figure 6.34. Apophyseal joint abnormalities. A. Widening of the apophyseal joint after traumatic dislocation *(arrow).* Patient is in traction. The initial injury was a locked facet. **B.** Dislocated, locked, or jumped facet *(arrow).* **C.** V-shaped, widened apophys-eal joint *(arrow)* due to flexion injury. **D.** Congenital narrowing of the lower cervical and upper thoracic apophyseal joints *(arrows).* Also note associated rudimentary disk at the C$_7$-T$_1$ level.

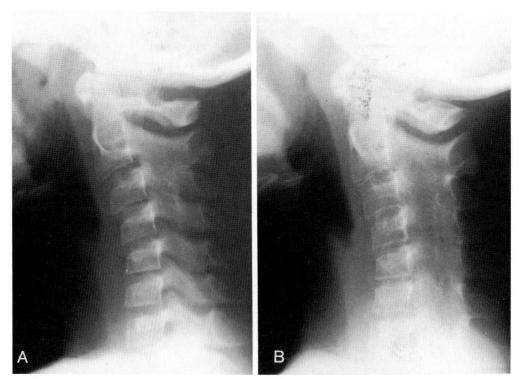

Figure 6.35. Apophyseal joint fusion in rheumatoid arthritis. A. Note early fusion of apophyseal joints. **B.** Later, complete fusion and a bamboo spine result. This usually occurs in Still disease.

Disk Abnormalities

The intervertebral disks can be (a) narrower than normal, (b) thicker than normal, or (c) calcified (Table 6.21). When narrow, the disks may be smooth or irregular, but when thick they usually are smooth and biconvex.

DISK NARROWING

Disk narrowing can be due to congenital underde-velopment of a disk (i.e., block vertebra), disk and

Table 6.21
Disk Abnormalities

Narrowed disks		
Infection[a]	}	Common
Scheuermann disease		
Congenital narrowing[b]	}	Moderately common
Acute trauma[c]		
Spondyloepiphyseal dysplasia	}	Relatively rare
Morquio disease		
Cockayne syndrome		
Ruvalcaba syndrome	}	Rare
Ankylosing spondylitis		
Kneist syndrome		
Widened disks		
Osteoporosis, osteomalacia	}	Common
Endplate infarction[d]		
Trauma[e]	}	Moderately common
Disk calcification		
Idiopathic[f]	}	Common
Ochronosis		
Hemochromatosis		
Hyperparathyroidism	}	Rare
Hypervitaminosis D		
Pseudogout		
Ankylosing spondylitis		

[a] Diskitis, spondyloarthritis, osteomyelitis.
[b] Blocked vertebra.
[c] Flexion-rotation.
[d] Sickle cell, Gaucher.
[e] Hyperextension.
[f] Cervical, thoracic.

adjacent vertebral infection or inflammation, and discovertebral trauma. Congenitally narrowed disks can occur anywhere and may be single (Fig. 6.36A) or multiple. Usually there is some underdevelopment of the adjacent vertebral bodies, but the vertebral bodies themselves are rather smooth and otherwise intact. With disk infection or inflammation, disk space narrowing eventually is associated with adjacent vertebral body destruction, but this may not be overtly apparent in the early stages (Fig. 6.36B and C). Such infection can occur anywhere in the spine, but most often it is seen in the upper lumbar region (1, 2, 5, 9, 14). When seen in the thoracic spine, tuberculosis should be considered first, but in other areas, nontuberculous pyogenic infection is more likely.

When disk narrowing associated with adjacent vertebral body destruction occurs in the lumbar spine, often it is referred to as childhood nonspecific diskitis or spondyloarthritis. Opinions differ as to whether the condition is secondary to trauma or in-

fection. However, most favor the latter, even though organisms cannot be cultured from all patients. Most often, symptoms consist of back pain and an inability to bend over. In addition, there may be a limp or actual refusal to walk. The degree and rate of vertebral destruction in the adjacent vertebral bodies is variable, and some cases apparently are self-limiting even without antibiotic therapy. This is one of the reasons why those who favor a traumatic etiology (i.e., subclinical trauma) support the trauma concept. Whatever the cause, the roentgenographic findings are rather characteristic. In the early stages when plain films are inconclusive, nuclear scintigraphy is in order, and currently MRI (3, 13) is very effective in demonstrating the bony and soft tissue changes (Fig. 6.36E).

Disk destruction secondary to infection also can be seen after spinal puncture (7), and has been reported in sarcoidosis (12). It might be noted at this point that with fungal infections such as coccidioidomycosis and aspergillosis (10), even though vertebral body destruction may be extensive, the intervening disks usually remain intact. Disk space narrowing, as it occurs in ankylosing spondylitis in adults (2, 4, 8), is not common in children, primarily because the disease is not common in children (6).

Spine trauma leading to disk disruption almost always is due to flexion or flexion-rotation forces (Fig. 6.37A). Contrarily, with extension injuries there is a tendency for the disk space to become wider than normal (Fig. 6.37A). In Scheuermann disease the cause also probably is trauma, but trauma is subclinical. In these patients, kyphosis of the thoracic spine, in many instances pain, and irregular disk space narrowing constitute the findings (Fig. 6.37B).

Herniation of disk material into the endplates is common, and if it occurs anteriorly, notched or beaked vertebrae result. Disk irregularities similar to those seen in Scheuermann disease have been noted in the Ruvalcaba syndrome (11), Cockayne syndrome, spondyloepiphyseal dysplasia, Morquio disease, and Kneist syndrome. Acute disk herniation leading to narrowed disk spaces is uncommon in children.

REFERENCES

1. Alexander CJ: The aetiology of juvenile spondylarthritis (discitis). *Clin Radiol* 21:178–187, 1970.
2. Dihlmann W, Delling G: Disco-vertebral destructive lesions (so-called Andersson lesions) associated with ankylosing spondylitis. *Skeletal Radiol* 3:10–16, 1978.
3. Forster A, Pothmann R, Winter K, Bauman-Rath CA: Magnetic resonance imaging in non-specific discitis. *Pediatr Radiol* 17:162–163, 1987.

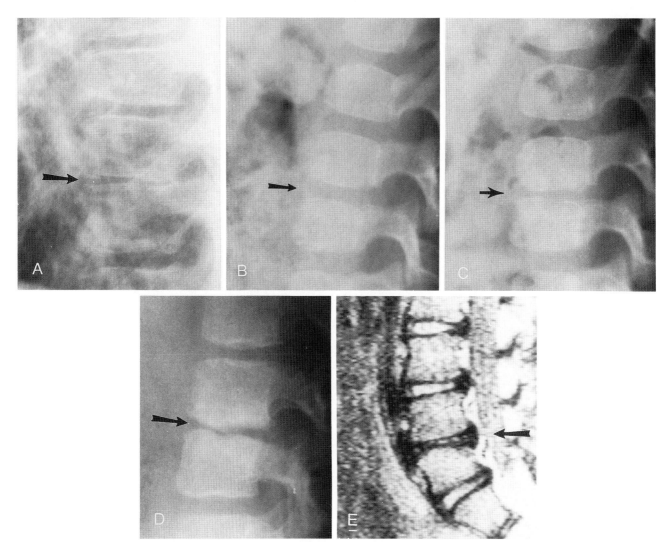

Figure 6.36. Disk narrowing. A. Congenitally narrowed intervertebral disk *(arrows)*. **B.** Early disk narrowing in diskitis *(arrow)*. **C.** Two weeks later, disk narrowing is more pronounced *(arrow)*. Early vertebral destruction also is seen. **D.** Another patient at a later stage, showing pronounced narrowing *(arrow)* along with indistinctness, irregularity, and sclerosis of the end plates. **E.** MRI (T$_1$-weighted) demonstrates loss of signal in the involved disk *(arrow)*.

4. Frank P, Gleeson J: Destructive vertebral lesions in ankylosing spondylitis. *Br J Radiol* 48:755–758, 1975.
5. Jamison RC, Heimlich EM, Miethke JC, O'Loughlin, BJ: Nonspecific spondylitis of infants and children. *Radiology* 77:355–367, 1961.
6. Kleinman P, Rivelis M, Schneider R, Kaye JJ: Juvenile ankylosing spondylitis. *Radiology* 125:775–780, 1977.
7. Lintermans JP, Seyhnaeve V: Spondylitic deformity of the lumbar spine and previous lumbar punctures. *Pediatr Radiol* 5:181–182, 1977.
8. Martel W: Pathogenesis of cervical discovertebral destruction in rheumatoid arthritis. *Arthritis Rheum* 20:1217–1225, 1977.
9. Moes CAF: Spondylarthritis in children. *AJR* 91:578–587, 1964.
10. Rassa M: Vertebral aspergillosis with preservation of the disc. *Br J Radiol* 50:918–920, 1977.
11. Ruvalcaba RHA, Reichert A, Smith DW: A new familial syndrome with osseous dysplasia and mental deficiency. *J Pediatr* 79:450–455, 1971.
12. Stump D, Spock A, Grossman H: Vertebral sarcoidosis in adolescents. *Radiology* 121:153–155, 1976.
13. Szalay EA, Green NE, Heller RM, Horvey G, Kirchner SG: Magnetic resonance imaging in the childhood diagnosis of discitis. *J Pediatr Orthop* 7:164–167, 1987.
14. Wenger DR, Bobechko WP, Gilday DL: The spectrum of intervertebral disc-space infection in children. *J Bone Joint Surg* 60A:100–108, 1978.

THICKENED DISKS

Disks do not thicken per se, but rather they become thick because (a) they expand into softened vertebral bodies or (b) ligament injury allows adjacent vertebral bodies to be separated, causing the disk to expand. The latter occurs, for the most part, with extension injuries of the spine (Fig. 6.37A). Universally thickened disks usually are associated

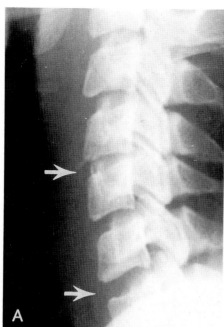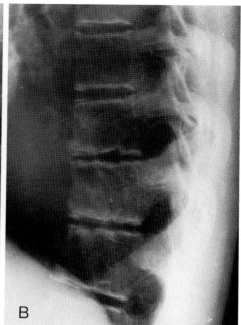

Figure 6.37. Disk narrowing and widening. A. Note disk narrowing due to flexion injury (upper arrow). Note the associated avulsion fracture. Disk widening *(lower arrow)* also is present and is due to an extension injury. This patient had both extension and flexion injuries. **B.** Uniformly thin, irregular disks in Scheuermann disease.

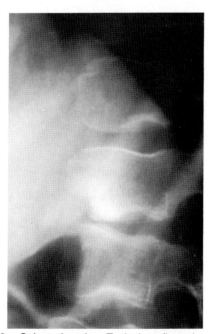

Figure 6.38. Schmorl nodes. Typical configuration of Schmorl nodes with central bulging into the vertebral bodies *(arrows)*. The middle node is smaller because some material has extruded anteriorly and produced a notched vertebra with sclerosis. For the MR appearance of this latter phenomenon see Figure 6.21.

with biconcave vertebral bodies, and very often the problem is extensive osteoporosis or osteomalacia of the spine (see Fig. 6.16B). The disks also become a little widened with endplate infarction, as seen in sickle cell disease (see Fig. 6.16A), and Gaucher

disease. Indeed the disk spaces appear wider than normal with any cause of biconcave vertebral bodies. The disks also are widened with "calcific diskitis," probably due to edema (see Fig. 6.39C and D).

SCHMORL'S NODES

Schmorl's nodes are herniations of the nucleus pulposus into the adjacent vertebral bodies. When they occur in the center, they produce characteristic central bulges into the vertebral bodies (Fig. 6.38) and are most often seen in asymptomatic individuals. If they occur around the periphery of the vertebral body, vertebral notching results (see Fig. 6.21). As indicated earlier, Schmorl's nodes are for the most part asymptomatic, but occasionally they have been known to produce back pain (1).

REFERENCE

1. Walters G, Coumas JM, Akins CM, Ragland RL: Magnetic resonance imaging of acute symptomatic Schmorl's node formation. *Pediatr Emerg Care* 7:294–296, 1991.

DISK CALCIFICATION

Disk calcification is uncommon in children, except as it occurs on an idiopathic basis in the cervical spine (1, 2–4, 7, 10). The etiology of such calcification is unknown, but subclinical trauma or viral infection

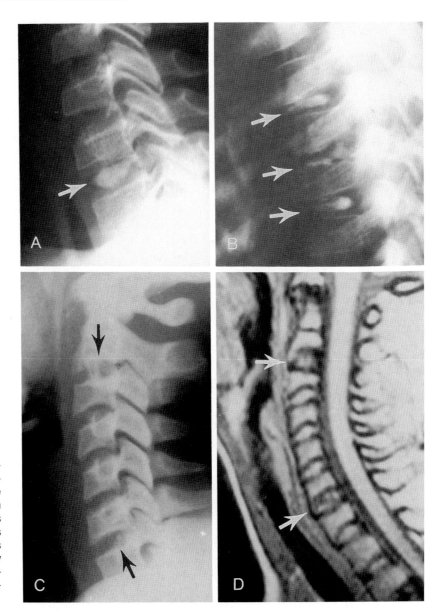

Figure 6.39. Disk calcification. A. Note typical cervical disk calcification *(arrow)*. **B.** Another patient with similar calcifications in the thoracic spine *(arrows)*. **C.** Another patient with slightly widened disk spaces at two levels *(arrows)*. **D.** T$_1$-weighted image demonstrates loss of signal in the disks at these two levels *(arrows)*. (From Swischuk LE and Stansberry SD: Calcific discitis: MRI changes in discs without visible calcification. *Pediatr Radiol* 21:365–366, 1991.)

has been suggested. Most often, these patients have neck pain, a wry neck deformity, and considerable spasm of the paraspinal muscles. The calcified disks, often slightly expanded, are characteristic (Fig. 6.39). The condition is self-limiting and the calcifications tend to disappear with time. In the interval, however, there may be anterior or posterior herniation of the calcifications, but this does not seem to lead to neurologic sequelae (2, 5, 8). Less frequently, these calcifications can be seen in the thoracic or even upper lumbar spine (Fig. 6.39B).

These disks, both calcified and in their edematous precalcification phase, are readily demonstrable with MRI (6, 9). The altered signal in the disks implies an inflammatory or traumatic etiology, probably the former. Indeed, in most of these children a history of significant trauma is not present and certainly not the type of trauma that might result in injury to the disks at multiple levels.

Other causes of disk calcification such as ochronosis, ankylosing spondylitis, gout, hemochromatosis, hyperparathyroidism, hypervitaminosis D, degenerative disease, and pseudogout are very rare in children.

REFERENCES

1. Girodias J-B, Azouz EM, Marton D: Intervertebral disk space calcification: a report of 51 children with a review of the literature. *Pediatr Radiol* 21:541–546, 1991.

2. Heinrich SD, Zembo MM, King AG, Zerkle AJ, MacEwen GD: Calcific cervical intervertebral disc herniation in children. *Spine* 16:228–231, 1991.
3. Henry MJ, Grimes HA, Lane JW: Intervertebral disk calcification in childhood. *Radiology* 89:81–84, 1967.
4. Herring JA, Hensinger RN: Cervical disc calcification. *J Pediatr Orthop* 8:613–616, 1988.
5. Mainzer F: Herniation of the nucleus pulposus. A rare complication of intervertebral disk calcification in children. *Radiology* 107:167–170, 1973.
6. McGregor JC, Butler P: Disc calcification in childhood: computed tomographic and magnetic resonance imaging appearances. *Br J Radiol* 59:180, 1986.
7. Mikity VG, Isenbarger J: Intervertebral disk calcification in children. *AJR* 95:200–202, 1965.
8. Sutton TJ, Turcotte B: Posterior herniation of calcified intervertebral disks in children. *J Can Assoc Radiol* 24:131–136, 1973.
9. Swischuk LE, Stansberry SD: Calcific discitis: MRI changes in disks without visible calcification. *Pediatr Radiol* 21:365–366, 1991.
10. Swick H: Calcification of intervertebral disks in childhood. *J Pediatr* 86:364–369, 1975.

Abnormal Spinal Curvatures

Abnormal curvatures of the spine consists of scoliosis, kyphosis, and lordosis (Tables 6.22 and 6.23). In some patients, kyphosis and scoliosis are combined, but lordosis usually is an isolated problem.

SCOLIOSIS

The commonest cause of scoliosis is paraspinal muscle spasm secondary to some spinal, paraspinal, intraabdominal, or intrathoracic inflammatory or traumatic lesion. After muscle spasm, scoliosis usually is idiopathic in nature. This form of scoliosis is most common in girls and suspected to be due to inherent muscle imbalance (4, 8, 10, 16). Scoliosis of

Table 6.22
Scoliosis

Paraspinal muscle spasm Idiopathic rotoscoliosis	Common
Rotoscoliosis with muscle hypotonia Scoliosis with vertebral anomalies Congenital heart disease	Moderately common

Radiation therapy
Scoliosis
  With intraspinal and spinal tumors,
  cysts
  With neurofibromatosis
  With unilateral bar
	Relatively rare

Table 6.23
Kyphosis

Normal-thoracolumbar in infants Cervical spine angulation, C_2-C_3- normal	Common
Compression fractures[a] Infection with vertebral destruction Congenital spine anomalies Storage diseases Chondrodystrophies and Scheuermann disease	Moderately common
Absent vertebral body Spine and spinal cord tumors Radiation therapy Underlying spinal cord disease[b]	Relatively rare

[a] Regular-pathologic.
[b] Other than tumor.

this type is termed "rotoscoliosis" because, together with a compensatory upper curve, a rotatory arrangement of the vertebral bodies is present. The rotatory component is best assessed by noticing the position of the spinous processes and pedicles (Fig. 6.40A). In mild cases, the rotatory component is barely perceptible, whereas in advanced cases associated kyphosis may be seen. This type of scoliosis also is seen in cases of cerebral palsy and other neuromuscular conditions with muscular imbalance or hypotonia. This type of scoliosis also is commonly seen with congenital heart disease (2, 5, 6, 12, 15).

When scoliosis is due to an underlying spine or spinal cord problem (e.g., tumor, infection, neurofibromatosis), or to an anomaly such as a sagittal hemivertebra or a unilateral bar (7), often it is more angular than rotatory (Fig. 6.40B and C). It is important to appreciate this configuration, for slight degrees of angular scoliosis may provide the first clue to the presence of a significant abnormality of the spine or spinal cord (13). Congenital anomalies of the spine leading to such scolioses are rather straightforward, except for the "unilateral bar," which may require tomography for adequate delineation. In this condition there is fusion in a bar-like fashion of the vertebra on one side, and this inhibits growth to the point of causing scoliosis (Fig. 6.40C). There are numerous methods of measuring scoliosis (4, 9), but the two used most often are the methods of Lippman and Cobb and that of Ferguson (9). Both methods are shown in Figure 6.41.

MRI (11) now is commonly used for the detection of occult spinal pathology in cases of suspicious scoliosis. This is especially true in those cases where excessive pain is present, the curve is angular, and the

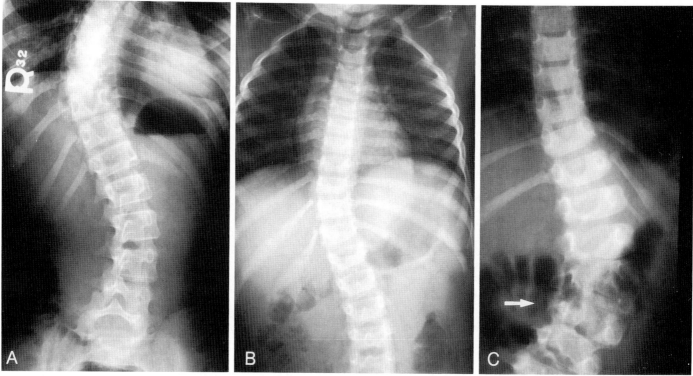

Figure 6.40. Scoliosis. A. Typical rotatory scoliosis. **B.** Angular scoliosis in neurofibromatosis. **C.** Angular scoliosis due to unilateral bar *(arrow)* on the right.

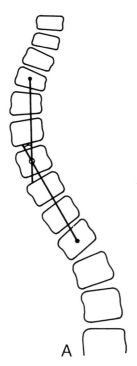

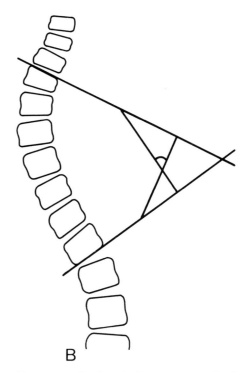

Figure 6.41. Scoliosis measurement. A. Ferguson method of scoliosis measurement. **B.** Lippman-Cobb method of scoliosis measurement. (Redrawn after McAlister WH, Schackelford GD: Measurement of spinal curvatures. *Radiol Clin North Am* 13:113–121, 1975.)

apex of the curve is directed to the left rather than to the right. All of these factors should make one more suspicious of an underlying spinal cord problem, and MRI is excellent for detecting such abnormalities.

KYPHOSIS

The commonest cause of nonpathologic kyphosis is normal physiologic bending of the thoracolumbar spine in infants (Table 6.23). Because of natural hypotonia, especially in the sitting position, kyphosis of the thoracolumbar junction occurs, and can be associated with vertebral notching (see Fig. 6.22A). As these normal infants grow older, muscle tone increases and the kyphosis and notching disappear (14). If, however, hypotonia is pathologic due to any number of causes, kyphosis and notching persist (14). For the most part this occurs in many of the storage diseases, achondroplasia and other chondrodystrophies, some trisomies, hypothyroidism, and any neurologic or neuromuscular condition leading to hypotonia.

Another instance in which kyphosis may appear dramatic and yet be normal is when it occurs at the C_2–C_3 level. Because of muscle spasm or voluntary flexion, a child's head becomes cocked forward. The resulting angulation of C_2 on C_3 may at first erroneously suggest pathologic dislocation (Fig. 6.42). However, when it is noted that C_2 is not anteriorly displaced in C_3 but merely angulated, one can discount thoughts of dislocation. When actual displacement of C_2 on C_3 occurs, differentiation from a hangman's fracture becomes important (see Fig. 6.31).

Localized kyphosis, at any level, is seen with anterior compression fractures of the vertebral bodies (see Fig. 6.20), and with discovertebral infections. In addition, localized kyphosis can be seen secondary to congenital defects of the vertebral bodies, hypoplasia of the vertebral bodies due to radiation therapy, deformity in neurofibromatosis, and with spine and spinal cord tumors. In long-standing infection with healing, especially in cases of tuberculosis, the spine may fuse in a typical **gibbus deformity** (Fig. 6.43A). In some of the other conditions producing focal kyphosis, chronic anterior flexion produces underdevelopment of the vertebral bodies, and a similar gibbus deformity, without vertebral body fusion, can be seen (Fig. 6.43B and C).

Generalized kyphosis also occurs in Scheuermann disease (1, 3), an affliction of teenagers often associated with back pain. The precise cause is not known, but it is believed to represent a problem of subclinical trauma to the vertebral end plates. In essence, it is a traumatic osteochondritis (1), but, in addition, some believe that there may be a genetic predisposition to the problem. The roentgenographic findings are rather typical, with irregular disk space narrowing, anterior wedging of the involved vertebral bodies, and varying degrees of kyphosis (see Fig. 6.37B). In more advanced cases, fusion of the vertebral bodies with a gibbus deformity can result (Fig. 6.43D).

LORDOSIS

The commonest cause of lordosis is normal development of the spine in the lumbar region. However, exaggerated lordosis in the thoracolumbar region occurs with many chondrodystrophies, especially achondroplasia. Lordosis also occurs with lumbar spondylolisthesis. Such defects currently are considered to occur secondary to overt or subclinical trauma. Severe degrees of lordosis also can be seen with extensive contiguous posterior element defects.

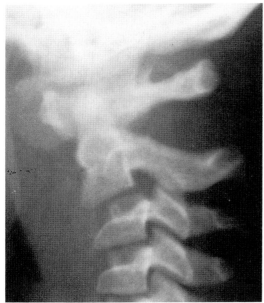

Figure 6.42. Kyphosis. Normal angulation of C_2 on C_3, causing kyphosis, often erroneously suggesting pathologic dislocation.

REFERENCES

1. Alexander CJ: Scheuermann's disease: a traumatic spondylodystrophy? *Skeletal Radiol* 1:209–221, 1977.
2. Fellows KE Jr, Rosenthal A: Extracardiac roentgenographic abnormalities in cyanotic congenital heart disease. *Am J Roentgenol Radium Ther Nucl Med* 114:371–379, 1972.

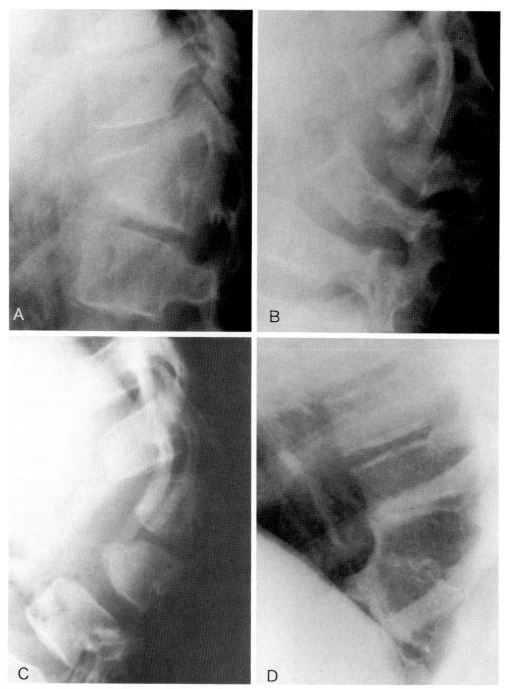

Figure 6.43. Kyphosis-gibbus deformity. A. Typical gibbus deformity due to destroyed, fused vertebra in tuberculosis. **B.** Gibbus deformity in neurofibromatosis. **C.** Gibbus deformity in achondroplasia. **D.** Gibbus deformity secondary to kyphosis and fusion in Scheuermann disease.

3. Halal F, Gledhill RB, Fraser FC: Dominant inheritance of Scheuermann's Juvenile kyphosis. *Am J Dis Child* 132:1105–1107, 1978.

4. Jeffries BF, Tarlton M, De Smet AA, Dwyer SF II, Brower AC: Computerized measurement and analysis of scoliosis: a more accurate representation of the shape of the curve. *Radiology* 134:381–385, 1980.

5. Jordan CE, White RI Jr, Fischer KC, Neill C, Dorst JP: The scoliosis of congenital heart disease. *Am Heart J* 84:463–469, 1972.

6. Luke MJ, McDonnel EJ: Congenital heart disease and scoliosis. *J Pediatr* 73:725–733, 1968.

7. MacEwen GD, Conway JJ, Miller WT: Congenital scoliosis with a unilateral bar. *Radiology* 90:711–715, 1968.

8. McAlister WH, Schackelford GD: Classification of spinal curvatures. *Radiol Clin N Am* 13:93, 1975.

9. McAlister WH, Schackelford GD: Measurement of spinal curvatures. *Radiol Clin N Am* 13:113–121, 1975.
10. Nachemson AJ, Sahlstrandt T: Etiologic factors in adolescent idiopathic scoliosis, spine. *J Bone Joint Surg* 59A:176–184, 1977.
11. Nokes SR, Murtach FR, Jones JD III, Downing M, Arrington JA, Turetsky D, Silbiger ML: Childhood scoliosis: MR imaging. *Radiology* 164:791–797, 1987.
12. Rickles LN, Peterson HA, Bianco AJ, Weidman WH: The association of scoliosis and congenital heart defects. *J Bone Joint Surg* 57A:449–455, 1975.
13. Rothner AD, Keim H, Chutorian AM: Occult neuromuscular disease in 100 consecutive patients with scoliosis. *J Pediatr* 86:748–750, 1975.
14. Swischuk LE: The beaked, notched, or hooked vertebra: its significance in infants and young children. *Radiology* 95:661–664, 1970.
15. Wright WD, Niebauer JJ: Congenital heart disease and scoliosis. *J Bone Joint Surg* 38A:1131–1136, 1956.
16. Young LW, Oestreich AE, Goldstein LA: Roentgenology in scoliosis: contribution to evaluation and management. *AJR* 108:778–795, 1970.

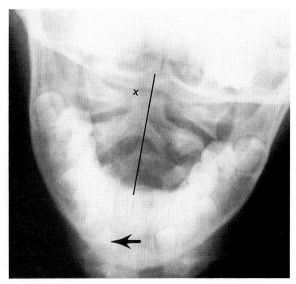

Figure 6.44. Torticollis. Note that the spinous tip of C_2 *(X)* lies on the same side of a line drawn through the dens as does the tip of the mandible *(arrow)*.

Wry Neck or Torticollis

The commonest cause of wry neck or torticollis is muscle spasm, either idiopathic or secondary to inflammation or trauma (Table 6.24) (2, 4). Congenital torticollis can be seen with a shortened, fibrotic sternocleidomastoid muscle. The etiology of idiopathic torticollis is unknown, but it probably represents a mild rotatory subluxation of C_1 on C_2. With true rotatory dislocation of C_1 on C_2, the C_1-dens distance is increased; with idiopathic torticollis it is not.

Wry neck, or torticollis, also can be an initial symptom of upper cervical spine or posterior fossa tumors, and it is also seen in Sandifer syndrome (1, 3). In Sandifer syndrome, gastroesophageal reflux leads to peculiar posturing of the neck and apparent torticollis. Why this occurs is not known, but when the reflux is corrected, the abnormal posture disappears.

On frontal view, with torticollis, the spinous tip of C_2 lies on the same side of a line drawn through the dens as does the tip of the mandible (Fig. 6.44). This does not occur with simple rotation of the spine because with simple rotation the spinous tip of C_2 lies on the other side of the line. On lateral view, the upper cervical spine may appear very disorganized, but it is still important to note the distance between the anterior arch of C_1 and the dens. The reason for this is that idiopathic torticollis is associated with a normal distance while with rotatory dislocation it is increased (see Fig. 6.45C). These rotational abnormalities of C_1–C_2 are best demonstrated with CT, with coronal and saggital reconstruction.

Table 6.24
Torticollis or Wry Neck

Idiopathic Trauma-spasm	Common
Congenital short muscle Upper cervical or posterior fossa tumor	Moderately common
Sandifer syndrome—gastroesophageal reflux	Rare

REFERENCES

1. Bray PF, Herbst JJ, Johnson DG, Book LS, Ziter FA, Condon VR: Childhood gastroesophageal reflux: neurological and psychiatric syndromes mimicked. *JAMA* 237:1342–1345, 1977.
2. Donaldson JS: Acquired torticollis in children and young adults. *JAMA* 160:458–461, 1956.
3. Murphy WJ Jr, Gellis SS: Torticollis with hiatus hernia in infancy. *Am J Dis Child* 131:564–565, 1977.
4. Shapiro R, Youngberg AS, Rothman SLG: The differential diagnosis of traumatic lesions of the occipito-atlanto-axial segment. *Radiol Clin N Am* 11:505–526, 1973.

Upper Cervical Spine Abnormalities
HYPOPLASTIC OR ABSENT DENS

The commonest cause of hypoplasia or absence of the dens is congenital anomaly (Table 6.25) (1, 2, 5,

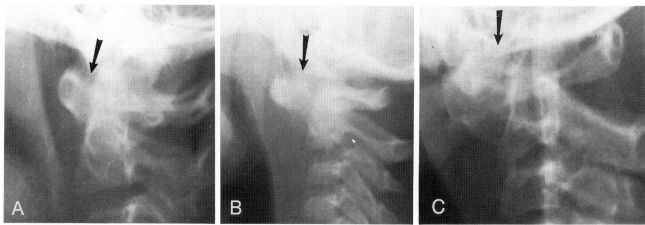

Figure 6.45. Increased C₁-dens distance. A. Normal, generous C₁-dens distance in a child. **B.** Hypoplastic dens and anterior dislocation of C₁ on C₂. C₁-dens distance is markedly increased.

C. Increased C₁-dens distance secondary to rotatory dislocation of C₁ and C₂.

Table 6.25
Hypoplastic or Absent Dens

Congenital anomaly[a]	}	Common
Congenital anomaly[b]	}	Moderately common
Resorption after trauma	}	Relatively rare

[a] With certain syndromes (see text).
[b] Isolated.

6). In such patients there often is an associated problem of C₁–C₂ instability because, along with underdevelopment of the dens, there is generalized underdevelopment of C₁ and C₂ and the stabilizing ligaments (see Fig. 6.45B). In addition, the os terminale, the normal ossification center at the tip of the dens, becomes larger and more bizarre in shape in many cases of dens hypoplasia. When this occurs, it is termed the "os odontoideum" (see Fig. 6.46C). Hypoplasia of the dens also can be acquired and usually is secondary to cervical spine injury in infancy (3, 4). In these cases, blood supply is disrupted and resorption of the dens occurs. Problems with instability also can occur in these patients. Congenital hypoplasia of the dens can occur in normal individuals but has an increased incidence in achondroplasia, trisomy-21, Morquio disease, storage diseases, punctate epiphyseal dysplasia, and spondyloepiphyseal dysplasia.

REFERENCES

1. Garber JN: Abnormalities of the atlas and axis vertebrae-congenital and traumatic. *J Bone Joint Surg* 46A:1782, 1964.
2. Gwinn John L, Smith JL: Acquired and congenital absence of the odontoid process. *AJR* 88:424–431, 1962.
3. Hawkins RJ, Fielding JW, Thompson WJ: Osodontoideum-congenital or acquired: a case report. *J Bone Joint Surg* 58A:413–414, 1976.
4. Ricciardi JE, Kaufer H, Louis DS: Acquired Os odontoideum following acute ligament injury: report of a case. *J Bone Joint Surg* 58A:410–412, 1976.
5. Shapiro R, Youngberg AS, Rothman SLG: The differential diagnosis of traumatic lesions of the occipitoatlanto-axial segment. *Radiol Clin N Am* 11:505–526, 1973.
6. Von Torklus D, Gehle W: *The Upper Cervical Spine.* New York, Grune and Stratton, 1972.

INCREASED C₁-DENS DISTANCE

The C₁-dens distance normally is wider in children than in adults and indeed this is the commonest cause of widening in children (Table 6.26). A distance of 2 to 3 mm is very common and actually measurements of as great as 4 to 5 mm can be seen in 2 to 3% of normal children (4, 8). Nonetheless, pathologic widening still occurs and just because a normal measurement can be in the realm of 4 to 5 mm should not be taken to infer that all such measurements are normal. On the other hand, this does indicate the need for a certain degree of caution in interpreting C₁-dens distance in children (Fig. 6.45A). In addition, it should be noted that the C₁-dens distance can widen by 2 mm with flexion and still be normal.

With pathologic widening of the C₁-dens distance, one should first consider congenital laxity of the ligaments and associated hypoplasia of the dens and C₁ (Fig. 6.45B). This can occur on an isolated basis, but more often is seen in syndromes such as trisomy-21 (6, 9), Morquio disease, the storage diseases (3, 5), and spondylo- and punctate epiphyseal dysplasia (1). In some of these cases, the degree of dislocation is rather profound and neurologic sequelae result.

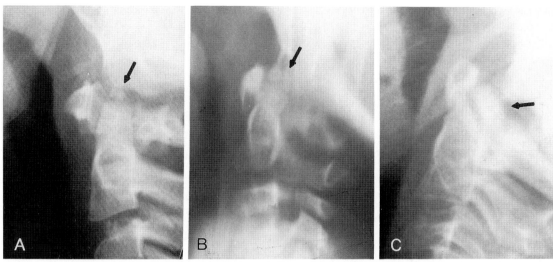

Figure 6.46. Os terminale. A. Normal os terminale *(arrow).* **B.** Slightly larger os terminale with multiple fragments *(arrow).* **C.** Hypoplastic dens and overgrown os terminale, resulting in os odontoideum *(arrow).*

The next most common cause of C_1-dens distance increase is trauma and, for the most part, the injury consists of simple anterior dislocation of C_1 on C_2 or rotatory dislocation of C_1 on C_2 (Fig. 6.45C). After trauma, one might consider laxity of the ligaments predisposing to C_1–C_2 dislocation, as is seen in the collagen vascular diseases (2, 7) and purportedly in retropharyngeal abscess. With the collagen vascular diseases, laxity of the ligaments leads to the dislocation, but whether retropharyngeal abscess causes enough ligament laxity to lead to pathological widening is debatable.

REFERENCES

1. Afshani E, Girdany BR: Atlanto-axial dislocation in chondrocysplasia punctata: report of the findings in 2 brothers. *Radiology* 102:399–401, 1972.
2. Babini SM, Maldonado-Cocco JA, Babini JC, de la Sota M, Arturi A, Marcos JC: Atlantoaxial subluxation in systemic lupus erythematosus: further evidence of tendinous alterations. *J Rheumatol* 17:173–177, 1990.
3. Brill CB, Rose JS, Godmilow L, Sklower S, Hirschhorn K: Spastic quadriparesis due to C_1-C_2 subluxation in Hurler syndrome. *J Pediatr* 92:441–443, 1978.
4. Locke GR, Gardner JI, Van Epps EF: Atlas-dens interval (ADI) in children: a survey based on 200 normal cervical spines. *AJR* 97:135–140, 1966.
5. Pizzutillo PD, Osterkamp JA, Scott CI Jr, Lee MS: Atlantoaxial instability in mucopolysaccharidosis. *J Pediatr Orthop* 9:76–78, 1989.
6. Pueschel SM, Scola FH, Tupper TB, Pezzullo JD: Skeletal anomalies of the upper cervical spine in children with Down syndrome. *J Pediatr Orthop* 10:607–611, 1990.
7. Reid GD, Hill RH: Atlantoaxial subluxation in juvenile ankylosing spondylitis. *J Pediatr* 93:531–532, 1978.
8. Swischuk LE: *Emergency Radiology of the Acutely Ill or Injured Child.* 3d ed. Baltimore, Williams & Wilkins, 1993, p 659.
9. Tredwell SJ, Newman DE, Lockitch G: Instability of the upper cervical spine in Down Syndrome. *J Pediatr Orthop* 10:602– 1990.

Table 6.26
Increased C_1-Dens Distance

Normal	} Common
Congenital hypoplasia of the dens and C_1[a]	} Moderately common

Dislocation of C1–C_2
  Rotatory
  Anterior
	} Relatively rare

Rheumatoid arthritis Morquio disease Other storage diseases	} Rare

[a] Isolated or with syndromes—(see text).

CERVICAL-OCCIPITAL OSSICLES

Because of the complexity of embryologic development of this area, a number of ossicles normally occur at the cervical-occipital junction. Basically, however, ossicles are identified around the lip of the foramen magnum, around the anterior arch of C_1, and over the tip of the dens. The latter is completely normal and is the ossification center for the tip of the dens, the os terminale (Fig. 6.46A and B). The os terminale can overgrow and become quite large with congenital or acquired hypoplasia of the dens. It is then termed the "os odontoideum" (Fig. 6.46C). The most important point about all the remaining ossicles around the cervical occipital junction is not to

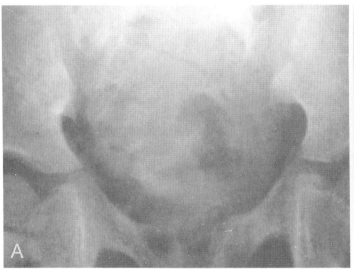
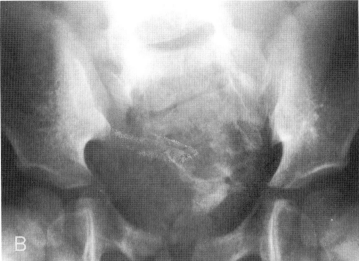
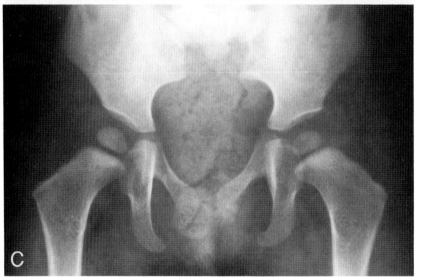

Figure 6.47. Sacral abnormalities. A. Curved or sickle-shaped sacrum in patient with lateral meningocele. **B.** Curved, deformed sacrum with tethered cord. **C.** Absent sacrum. Note close positioning of the iliac wings.

misinterpret them for avulsion fractures. Usually, they are quite smooth and often totally incidental findings. Seldom are they seen in infants and young children, and it is only in adults and teenagers that one encounters them with any regularity. In the adult, however, they are quite common.

Sacral Abnormalities

The sacrum can be destroyed, much as the spine in general, but destructive lesions such as metastatic tumor, histiocytosis-X, or infection occur much less commonly in the sacrum than in the remainder of the spine. In the sacrum, erosion or even frank destruction can be seen with presacral tumors (12), in-

cluding teratoma, sarcoma, and the rare sacral chordoma. Some of these tumors and a variety of presacral cysts can in some cases merely deviate the sacrum.

A curved, or sickle, deformity of the sacrum (Fig. 6.47A) usually signifies some associated sacral anomaly. This can take the form of an anterior, lateral, or intrasacral meningocele or the condition known as "tethered cord" (Fig. 6.47B). In the latter condition, the cord is bound to the abnormal area of sacral development and, with growth, is unable to rise to its normal position. Consequently, there is stretching of the cord and neurologic symptoms develop. Very frequently, an intra- and/or extraspinal lipoma is present. Similar curving deformities and other anomalies also are seen with imperforate anus.

Finally, somewhat similar sacral deformities can be seen in association with presacral teratoma and imperforate anus (1, 2, 6, 7, 14).

Absence of the sacrum (4, 8, 10) results in significant neurologic deficit and a characteristic appearance of the sacrum and pelvis (Fig. 6.44C). In extreme form, the condition is referred to as the caudal regression or mermaid deformity syndrome (3, 5, 9, 13). Sacral hypoplasia or agenesis is believed to result from a vascular insult to the lower spine in fetal life and is more common in infants of diabetic mothers (3, 13). Sacral agenesis also has been noted in association with presacral teratoma (1, 2, 7, 11).

REFERENCES

1. Ashcraft KW, Holder TM: Congenital anal stenosis with presacral teratoma. *Ann Surg* 162:1091–1095, 1956.
2. Ashcraft KW, Holder TM: Hereditary presacral teratoma. *J Pediatr Surg* 9:691–697, 1974.
3. Assemany SR, Muzzo S, Gardner LI: Syndrome of phocomelic diabetic embryopathy (caudal dysplasia). *Am J Dis Child* 123:489–491, 1972.
4. Banta JV, Nichols O: Sacral agenesis. *J Bone Joint Surg* 51:693–703, 1969.
5. Becker MH, Szatkowski JA, Brant EE: Case report 75, diagnosis: caudal regression syndrome. *Skeletal Radiol* 3:191–192, 1978.
6. Cohn J, Bay-Nielsen E: Hereditary defect of sacrum- and coccyx with anterior sacral meningocele. *Acta Paediatr Scand* 58:268–272, 1969.
7. Currarino G, Coin D, Votteler T: Triad of anorectal, sacral, and presacral anomalies. *AJR* 137:395–398, 1981.
8. Dassel PM: Agenesis of the sacrum and coccyx. *AJR* 85:697–700, 1961.
9. Duhamel B: From mermaid to anal imperforation syndrome of caudal regression. *Arch Dis Child* 36:152–155, 1961.
10. Grand M, Eichenfeld S, Jacobson HG: Sacral aplasia (agenesis). *Radiology* 74:611–617, 1960.
11. Kenefick JS: Hereditary sacral agenesis associated with presacral tumors. *Br J Surg* 60:271–274, 1973.
12. Macpherson RI, Young F: Sacrococcygeal tumors. *J Can Assoc Radiol* 21:132–142, 1970.
13. Passarge E, Lenz W: Syndrome of caudal regression in infants of diabetic mothers: observations of further cases. *Pediatrics* 37:672–675, 1966.
14. Tsuchida Y, Watanasupt W, Nakajo T: Anorectal malformations associated with a presacral tumor and sacral defect. *Pediatr Surg Int* 4:398–402, 1989.

Sacroiliac Joint Abnormalities

Widening of the sacroiliac joints can occur with traumatic separation, infection, or inflammation. For discussion of all of these problems, see Chapter 4.

INDEX

Page numbers followed by "*f*" denote figures; those followed by a "*t*" denote tables.

1